DENTAL PRACTICE TOOL KIT

PATIENT HANDOUTS, FORMS, AND LETTERS

DENTAL PRACTICE TOOL KIT

PATIENT HANDOUTS, FORMS, AND LETTERS

with **152** illustrations

ELSEVIER
MOSBY

ELSEVIER
MOSBY

11830 Westline Industrial Drive
St. Louis, Missouri 63146

NOTICE

Dentistry is an ever-changing field. Standard safety precautions must be followed, but as new research and clinical experience broaden our knowledge, changes in treatment and drug therapy may become necessary or appropriate. Readers are advised to check the most current product information provided by the manufacturer of each drug to be administered to verify the recommended dose, the method and duration of administration, and contraindications. It is the responsibility of the licensed prescriber, relying on experience and knowledge of the patient, to determine dosages and the best treatment for each individual patient. Neither the publisher nor the author assumes any liability for any injury and/or damage to persons or property arising from this publication.

The Publishers

International Standard Book Number 0-323-02509-9

Publishing Director: Linda L. Duncan
Executive Editor: Penny Rudolph
Senior Developmental Editor: Kimberly Alvis
Publishing Services Manager: Linda McKinley
Senior Project Manager: Julie Eddy
Book Design Manager: Gail Morey Hudson

Printed in the United States of America

Last digit is the print number: 9   8   7   6   5   4   3   2   1

Consultants and Reviewers

Consultants

David P. Harfst, JD
OHA Media
Ridgeland, Mississippi

Stephen J. Candio, DDS
Private Practice
Preventive, Cosmetic and Family Dentistry
Sparta and Lyndhurst, New Jersey

This project was conceived by Dr. Stephen Candio and developed by David Harfst. We are excited to bring their ideas to fruition.

Reviewers

Darrell Drissell, DDS
Private Practice
Ballwin, Missouri

John H. Francis, DDS
Private Practice (retired)
Suitland, Maryland

Lawrence M. Hoffman, DMD
Private Practice
St. Louis, Missouri

Joe Hwang, DMD
Private Practice
Santa Barbara, California

Ray A. Morse, DMD
Private Practice
Panama City, Florida

How to Use this Book/CD-ROM Package

Congratulations on your selection of *Dental Practice Tool Kit: Patient Handouts, Forms, and Letters* to enhance your patient communications, practice administration, and marketing in your practice. Developed by dental professionals who share your daily concerns and experiences in dental practice, *Dental Practice Tool Kit: Patient Handouts, Forms, and Letters* offers you a vehicle to help ensure patient satisfaction and increase your profitability.

Dental school prepared us to be competent practitioners but never prepared us to practice dentistry in a marketplace with increased competition and complex insurance systems. When you use *Dental Practice Tool Kit: Patient Handouts, Forms, and Letters* to its optimal potential, you can enhance your dental practice, which can lead to an increased revenue from your present patient base and increased referrals.

Today's patients exercise their right to know all options available to them in terms of dental treatment and they seek out dental professionals in whom they can have faith and confidence. The dentist is thus judged by the patient both for quality of service provided and for the ability to communicate clearly.

Incorporating *Dental Practice Tool Kit: Patient Handouts, Forms, and Letters* into the daily practice of dentistry will assist in communicating in a clear, consistent manner that will enhance patient satisfaction. Let's face it: the bottom line is directly related to how well we educate our patients on treatment needs as well as how well the patient accepts our recommendations.

Where to Begin

One of the easiest ways to incorporate the documents included in *Dental Practice Tool Kit: Patient Handouts, Forms, and Letters* into your practice is to browse the Detailed Contents in the book. One quick overview will show you how well the documents are organized. You may want to take note of those documents that you think will be used most often in your practice.

You may also note that the book is organized in two distinct parts: Part One, Business/Front Office Communication, contains the four chapters devoted to documents primarily used by office staff to expedite intraoffice communication, insurance claim processing, patient information, letters to insurance carriers, and referral letters. Part Two, Patient Education, includes 166 patient education and instruction documents and illustrations that are related to eight topic areas:

1. Cosmetic Dentistry
2. Endodontics
3. General Dentistry
4. Orthodontics
5. Pediatric Dentistry
6. Periodontics
7. Prosthodontics
8. Restorative Dentistry

These handouts cover all dental procedures and/or problems and can be given to your patients when they leave your office. Ideally, patients will have no additional questions once they read your informative handout.

Communicate with your Spanish Speaking Patients

Every document in both Parts One and Two of the book/CD-ROM is available in English and Spanish. Never has there been a more convenient way to communicate with your Spanish-speaking patients. Simply "click on" the CD-ROM's Español selection when you want to prepare a handout, form, or letter in Spanish.

CD-ROM Accessibility

The CD-ROM that is included with this book will become absolutely indispensable to you and your front office staff. Every document that you see in the book is available on the CD-ROM. All of the documents are easy to find, and an excellent search feature can take you exactly where you want to go!

After installing *Dental Practice Tool Kit: Patient Handouts, Forms, and Letters* on your computer, it will run seamlessly in Microsoft Word—no need to learn a new program! However, to familiarize yourself with the contents more quickly, it might be best to begin with reviewing this book.

Customized Patient Education Made Easy

Patient education documents or handouts are easy to prepare and use. Each one can be customized to reflect the identity and philosophy of your individual practice. What's more, each document can be personalized for the individual patient. Your patients will feel confident that you have attended to their individual needs, and you will have an excellent record of the instructions you have provided for your patients. Simply select the patient handout that is appropriate for your patient. Choose whether you want to provide the document in Spanish or English. With a few simple keystrokes in Microsoft Word, you can add your patient's name and information and you can insert your own name and practice information.

This is just the beginning of the customization feature! Any wording that is provided for you on the CD-ROM can be edited, expanded upon, or altered in any way. If you have a better way to say something, feel free to change it! The final document will be whatever you want it to be. We have provided you with a firm foundation, and you can do the rest. The final patient education handout that your patient walks away with will be the best possible reflection of your practice.

How to Get Started

We suggest that you have a staff meeting to acquaint your entire team with the documents contained in *Dental Practice Tool Kit: Patient Handouts, Forms, and Letters*. Take this opportunity to determine the best documents and illustrations to use and how to customize them. Show each team member how simple it is to access any handout, form, or letter and begin suggesting ways that all documents can be customized to be a more accurate reflection of your individual practice.

Remember: *Any document can be altered to more accurately reflect the philosophy and environment of your practice. ALL documents have been designed to be altered in whatever way suits YOUR needs.*

Preface

Dental Practice Tool Kit: Patient Handouts, Forms, and Letters was created with today's busy practitioner in mind. We look at it as the perfect practice communication tool. It was created by two dentists who felt a need to communicate effectively with patients and who had experienced a general dissatisfaction with all of the pre-printed patient education pamphlets that were then available. No matter how well the patient handouts were written, they were not suitable because they:

- Did not fit their individual practice philosophy
- Were not well written
- Had to be purchased in expensive bulk lots creating cost and inventory issues
- Did not allow the text to be modified easily as materials and techniques changed
- Used lay terminology and "spoke down" to the patient
- Did not cover enough topics

The dentists determined that because they knew the technical material they could use word processing technology to write their own patient information handouts. They began with the usual post-operative instructions for simple extractions and endodontic therapy.

Dentists who purchase something or seek medical care want to know all about the item or topic. They want to be educated to be able to make informed decisions. They believe that the perfect practice philosophy is to educate patients so that they can make informed decisions about required and elective dental treatment.

Many dentists are excellent communicators, but most often they communicate verbally and they like to communicate *once*. If there is a need to explain something more than once, productivity is lost. Because of the nature of dental explanations and the unease patients feel in the dental environment, many patients tend to remember only two things a dentist tells them: Hello and Goodbye. That is exactly why this product was created.

There was an obvious need to put into writing all the things relating specific dental treatment for that patient, so that no one would have to spend additional time repeating things to the patient. In a written form, the patient information would be available for the patient to review later, to show a spouse, and to begin to become comfortable with the anticipated procedure. Using excellent patient education handouts means that the dentist will receive fewer notes from the staff asking him or her to call the patient to explain again something that had been discussed in the office.

Patient handouts are included for all dental procedures. They were created over time, with changes made along the way, in an attempt to "cover all the bases." Ideally, a patient will read the patient handout and will have no additional questions. Letters to insurance carriers, referral letters, and front office organizational forms are also included. Everything has been streamlined as much as possible in an effort to make the forms useful for multiple-related situations.

The creators of these patient handouts and in-office forms and letters have used every one of the forms at one time or another. They are big fans of having the ability to change, update, and edit any and all forms. Anything included can be easily and neatly rewritten when and where needed.

As far as use of the forms, letters, and handouts go, you won't use every one every day but you will use some every day. Many topics lend themselves to use of more than one related patient education form, to be placed together in a patient information package. For instance, Periodontics, Pediatric Dentistry, Crown and Bridge, and Operative Dentistry procedures can be better explained to the patient when multiple patient information pages are combined and given to the patient. The patient may feel for the first time that he or she truly understands how everything you do works together to produce a final excellent result.

We are confident that as soon as you begin incorporating this customizable CD-ROM into your daily practice, you won't want to work without it again. We hope that your practice will thrive with this excellent new practice management tool.

Contents

Detailed Contents

part one

Business/Front Office Communication

Practice Administration

Content at a Glance: Practice Administration

Patient Contact

New Patient Intake Form
Use to assist the receptionist in obtaining information needed when scheduling new patients.

New Patient Registration
Information needed from patient to process insurance claims.

Initial Patient Visit Record
Track the aspects consistent with Endodontic Therapy: Estimated Lengths under Patient Chart Forms of an initial visit: patient needs, referrals, and discussion topics.

Patient Discussion Checklist
Use to keep track of written information given to patients to reinforce discussions.

Patient Education Documents
Checklist makes sure patients get the information they need and duplicates.

Patient Preferences
Survey of patients' expectations and dental concerns.

Patient Preferences: Child
Survey of parent's expectations and dental concerns for his or her child.

Patient Preferences: Young Adult
Survey of young adult patient's expectations and dental concerns.

Treatment Plan
Use to track a concise history of planned treatment and completion dates. Useful for phased treatments.

Patient Chart Forms

Endodontic Therapy: Estimated Lengths
Keeps track of individual patient's canal lengths throughout all endodontic treatment sessions.

Endodontic Therapy: Informed Consent
Patient's signature indicates an understanding of the endodontic therapy, fees involved, and that questions have been answered to his or her satisfaction.

Extraction: Informed Consent
Patient's signature indicates understanding of reason for dental extraction, possible complications, and that questions have been answered to his or her satisfaction.

Communications

Interoffice Communications

Daily Chart Completion
Use to track the scheduling and treatment needs of patients for front office and as a checklist for completion of all related paperwork.

Dental Hygiene Treatment Directives
Checklist to ensure efficient communication between the dentist and hygienist.

Dental Procedure Codes
A list of CDT-4 codes to use at chairside to communicate treatment rendered on the routing slip.

Content at a Glance: Practice Administration—cont'd

Routing Slips

Use to communicate the treatment provided and needed to the patient to business staff.

Laboratory Communications

Laboratory Cases in Progress

For organizing, scheduling, and tracking lab cases.

Laboratory Work Order

Checklist to provide laboratory with complete instructions for case construction.

Marketing Your Practice

Marketing Tips

Ideas to help plan your marketing strategy.

Press Release Guide

This press release can be used as is or as a base for other press releases. Offers several choices of announcements.

Telephone Lists and Forms

Miscellaneous Calls to be Completed

Use to provide the business staff a list of information needs from other sources.

Patients Who Need to be Rescheduled

List to keep track of appointments that were canceled by patients or were no shows.

Priority Rescheduling

Use to fill openings in the schedule and keep track of patients who would like an earlier or more convenient appointment time when an opening occurs, even on short notice.

Professionals Requesting Patient Information

Track dentist, specialist, or physician calls in relation to a patient's treatment.

HIPAA

Health Insurance Portability and Accountability Act (HIPAA) of 1996

Health Insurance Portability and Accountability Act (HIPAA) of 1996: what it is and what it covers.

HIPAA–Business Associates Contract

List of responsibilities of business associates with respect to protected health information.

HIPAA–Staff Training Registry

List to keep track of employees that have received the office policy regarding the Health Insurance Portability and Accountability Act Privacy Rule.

New Patient Intake Form

Date:_____   **Health Alert:**_____

Patient:_____   **Referred by:**_____

Phone(s): Home:_____   **Work:**_____   **Other:**_____

E-mail:_____

Reason for call:
❏ Toothache or pain, how long?_____
❏ New patient exam
❏ Swelling, where?_____
❏ Lost filling
❏ Denture problems
❏ Broken tooth
❏ Consultation

Remarks (chief complaint). Please state as patient worded it: _____

_____

_____

Last dental or dental hygiene appointment: _____
Attitude: ❏ Pleasant   ❏ Frightened   ❏ Other

Has patient ever been told he or she needed **premedication** before dental appointment?
❏ No   ❏ Yes   Why and what medication?_____
                Name and phone number of physician:_____

Dental insurance?   ❏ Yes   ❏ No
If yes, tell the patient: "In order for you to receive the maximum and quickest reimbursement from your dental insurance, you should bring in your dental benefits booklet and at least one claim form with your section completely filled out and signed. Please be prepared to pay for all diagnostic and emergency treatment when you come in. If further treatment will be needed, you will be informed by the doctor. In this event, a treatment estimate will be made for you and you can make the appropriate financial arrangements. Do you have any questions?"

Tell the patient the anticipated fee for initial oral exam, emergency exam, or radiographs if needed. Tell the patient that the examination fee includes initial examination, diagnosis, treatment plan, and consultation.

Tell the patient: Radiographs (x-rays) may be required for an accurate diagnosis. The doctor will determine what radiographs are necessary when he or she examines you.

Tell the patient: Come in about 15 minutes before the appointment to fill out the health history form. Tell the patient that if an appointment must be canceled, at least a 24-hour advance notice must be given, as a courtesy to the office and other patients.

Call taken by:_____   **Date:**_____

New Patient Registration

Please complete this form. If you have dental insurance, we cannot file a claim for you unless the requested information is accurate. If you have dual dental insurance coverage, complete the information for the secondary carrier. Thank you for your attention to detail.

Patient Name:_____   Date of Birth:_____

Patient SS#:_____
Address:_____
City:_____   State:_____ Zip Code:_____
Home Telephone: (   )_____   Work Telephone: (   )_____
E-mail:_____
Patient's Employer:_____

Insured's Information:

Name:_____   Date of Birth:_____
SS#:_____   Employer:_____
Address:_____
City:_____   State:_____ Zip Code:_____
Home Telephone: (   )_____   Work Telephone: (   )_____

Insurance Information:

Please select the dental insurance carrier: ❑ Traditional   ❑ Delta
❑ AETNA/Prudential PDO   ❑ CIGNA PPO   ❑ MetLife PPO   ❑ BC/BS PPO
Group ID #:_____   Claims Phone #:_____
Claims Submission Address:
Street:_____
City:_____   State:_____ Zip Code:_____

Secondary Insurance Information:

Name:_____   Date of Birth:_____
SS#:_____   Employer:_____
Street:_____
City:_____   State:_____ Zip Code:_____
Home Telephone: (   )_____   Work Telephone: (   )_____

Please select the dental insurance carrier:

❑ Traditional   ❑ Delta
❑ AETNA/Prudential PDO   ❑ CIGNA PPO   ❑ MetLife PPO   ❑ BC/BS PPO
Group ID #:_____   Claims Phone #:_____

Claims Submission Address:

Street:_____
City:_____   State:_____ Zip Code:_____

Initial Patient Visit Record

Patient:_____   **Date:**_____

❑ Time spent with patient:_____

Patient Needs *(date and initial when completed)*
❑ _____ _____ Patient needs   ❑ BW   ❑ FMS   ❑ Treatment plan   ❑ Other_____
❑ _____ _____ Patient needs to receive handouts on topics:_____
❑ _____ _____ Patient needs to view subject visuals:_____
❑ _____ _____ Patient needs our office to call previous dentist for ❑ X-rays   ❑ Charting
                      Dentist's Name:_____   Phone #:_____
                      Date called:_____   Spoke to:_____
❑ Patient informed of periodontal disease:
            Case type: ❑ 1   ❑ 2   ❑ 3   ❑ 4   ❑ 5   ❑ 6   ❑ 7   ❑ 8
            ❑ Generalized   ❑ Localized—specific areas:_____
❑ Patient advised to have the following treatment:
                ❑ Root plane/scale: ❑ Whole mouth   ❑ quadrant _____   ❑ tooth #_____
                ❑ Subgingival irrigation   ❑ Whole mouth   ❑ quadrant _____   ❑ tooth #_____
                ❑ OHI
                ❑ Reevaluation/probing on _____(Date)_____.
                ❑ Adult prophylaxis
❑ Patient advised to be on _____ recare interval.
❑ Comprehensive exam for treatment planning

Patient referred to:
Endodontist
❑ For evaluation of tooth #_____
❑ For treatment of tooth #_____
❑ Endodontist:_____

Oral Surgeon
❑ For extraction of tooth #_____
❑ For evaluation of:_____   Area/tooth_____
❑ Oral surgeon:_____

Orthodontist
❑ For evaluation:_____
❑ For treatment:_____
❑ Orthodontist:_____

Periodontist
❑ For evaluation:_____   Area/tooth_____
❑ For treatment:_____   Area/tooth_____
❑ Periodontist:_____

Discussions with Patient
❑ Patient informed of risks, options, advantages, disadvantages of treatment.
❑ Patient told periodontal treatment must be completed before restorative treatment is begun.
❑ Patient told treatment may change if oral conditions change or are not as expected from exam.
❑ Estimated treatment time and fees discussed with patient.
❑ Patient needs/requests phased treatment.
❑ Patient has objections to treatment: ❑ financial   ❑ time   ❑ emotional
❑ Patient has no further questions.

Patient Discussion Checklist

Patient:_____   **Date:**_____

Dental Information to be Given to Patient

❏ **Office overview**   ❏ Verbal   ❏ Written
                                                           ❏ Welcome to Our Practice

❏ **General dental information**   ❏ Verbal   ❏ Written
                                                           ❏ For a Lifetime of Great Oral Health
                                                           ❏ Initial Oral Examination

❏ **Periodontal disease**   ❏ Verbal   ❏ Written
                                                           ❏ Periodontal Disease
                                                           ❏ Periodontal Disease and Systemic Health

❏ **Hygiene maintenance recare**   ❏ Verbal   ❏ Written
                                                           ❏ Prophylaxis

❏ **Cosmetic dentistry**   ❏ Verbal   ❏ Written
                                                           ❏ Cosmetic Dentistry
                                                           ❏ At-Home Whitening Options
                                                           ❏ Tooth Whitening: Overview and Options
                                                           ❏ Replacing Unesthetic Restorations

❏ **Restorations**   ❏ Verbal   ❏ Written
                                                           ❏ Amalgam Restorations
                                                           ❏ Bonded Resin Restorations
                                                           ❏ Crowns: An Overview
                                                           ❏ Bridges: An Overview
                                                           ❏ Implants: An Overview

❏ **Prevention**   ❏ Verbal   ❏ Written
                                                           ❏ Prevention of Dental Disease in Infants and Children
                                                           ❏ Prevention of Decay
                                                           ❏ Sealants
                                                           ❏ Sealants and Fluoride: Benefits to Adult Patients
                                                           ❏ Supplemental Fluoride
                                                           ❏ Topical Fluoride

❏ **Need for necessary radiographs**   ❏ Verbal   ❏ Written
                                                           ❏ Radiographs

Business Information to be Given to Patient

❏ **Pretreatment information**   ❏ Verbal   ❏ Written
                                                           ❏ Cancellation and No Show Policy
                                                           ❏ Estimate of Fees
                                                           ❏ Next Appointment Procedure
                                                           ❏ Treatment Goals

❏ **Insurance coordination**   ❏ Verbal   ❏ Written
   Financial arrangements   ❏ Dental Insurance Coverage
                                                           ❏ Dental Insurance—Points to Consider
                                                           ❏ Estimate of Fees
                                                           ❏ Financial Arrangements
                                                           ❏ Schedule for Payment

Patient Education Documents

Checked box indicates information to be given to patient. Please date and initial as information is given to patient.

Continued

Patient Education Documents—cont'd

Periodontics
Evaluation and Diseases

Date Initial

Treatment Options

Chemotherapeutics

Prosthodontics

Date Initial

Fixed Restorations
Crowns

Materials Options

Bridges

Implants

Procedures and Applications

Removable Prosthodontics

Restorative Dentistry
Restorations

Date Initial

Corrective Procedures

Continued

Patient Education Documents—cont'd

Patient Preferences

Patient:_____   **Date:**_____

Briefly tell us how you feel about your teeth, your smile, and your dental expectations.

1. What are your expectations from this office?_____
_____
_____

2. Would you like to learn how you can have all of your teeth for the rest of your life?   ❑ yes   ❑ no

3. If you are already missing some teeth, would you like to learn how you can avoid having full dentures?   ❑ yes   ❑ no

4. Do you like your smile?   ❑ yes   ❑ no

5. If the answer is NO, what don't you like and what changes would you like to see?_____
_____
_____

6. If you feel that your teeth have yellowed, or are not white enough, would you like to learn about tooth whitening?   ❑ yes   ❑ no

7. Are you interested in an overall cosmetic dental evaluation?   ❑ yes   ❑ no

8. If you are contemplating a dental cosmetic change, what is most important to you?_____
_____
_____

9. Are you aware of anything that might prevent you from having either basic or cosmetic dental treatment?   ❑ yes   ❑ no

10. Have all your past dental office experiences been positive?   ❑ yes   ❑ no
If NO, please explain:_____
_____

11. Is there anything in particular that you would like us to always do for you?   ❑ yes   ❑ no
If YES, please explain:_____
_____

12. Is there anything in particular that you would like us never to do?   ❑ yes   ❑ no
If YES, please explain:_____
_____

13. Do you have any dental concerns not listed here that you would like to bring to our attention?   ❑ yes   ❑ no
If YES, please explain:_____
_____

Thank you for taking the time to complete this form!

Patient Preferences: Child

Patient: _____   **Date:** _____

Briefly tell us how you feel about your child's teeth and your dental expectations.

1. What are your expectations of this office for your child? _____
_____
_____

2. Would you like to learn how your child can have all of his/her teeth for the rest of his/her life?   ❏ yes   ❏ no

3. Would you prefer to stay in the dental treatment room during your child's visit?   ❏ yes   ❏ no

4. Have your child's past dental office experiences all been positive?   ❏ yes   ❏ no
If NO, please explain: _____
_____

5. Is there anything in particular that you would like us to always do for your child?   ❏ yes   ❏ no
If YES, please explain: _____
_____

6. Is there anything in particular that you would like us never to do for your child?   ❏ yes   ❏ no
If YES, please explain: _____
_____

7. Do you have any dental concerns about your child not listed here that you would like to bring to our attention?   ❏ yes   ❏ no
If YES, please explain: _____
_____

Thank you for taking the time to complete this form!

Patient Preferences: Young Adult

Patient:_____   **Date:**_____

Briefly tell us how you feel about your teeth, your smile, and your dental expectations.

1. What are your expectations of this office?_____
_____
_____

2. Is preventing decay and gum disease and having fresh breath important to you?   ❏ yes   ❏ no

3. Have your past dental office experiences all been positive?   ❏ yes   ❏ no
    If NO, please explain:_____
_____

4. Is there anything in particular that you would like us to always do for you?   ❏ yes   ❏ no
    If YES, please explain:_____
_____

5. Is there anything in particular that you would like us never to do for you?   ❏ yes   ❏ no
    If YES, please explain:_____
_____

6. Do you have any dental concerns not listed here that you would like to bring
    to our attention?   ❏ yes   ❏ no
    If YES, please explain:_____
_____

7. Do you think your teeth are straight enough?   ❏ yes   ❏ no

8. Have you ever seen an orthodontist?   ❏ yes   ❏ no

9. Is there anything about your smile that you don't particularly like?   ❏ yes   ❏ no
    Tell us about it:_____
_____

10. What is your favorite sport and team, what type of music do you like, what is your favorite musical group, and what is the best
    movie you ever saw?

    Sport _____
    Sports team _____
    Music _____
    Musical group _____
    Movie _____

Thank you for taking the time to complete this form!

Treatment Plan

Patient:_____

Procedure	Comment	Treatment Provider	Date of Diagnosis	Date Completed	✓

Endodontic Therapy: Estimated Lengths

Patient:_____   **Date:**_____

Tooth #

	Estimated Length
Canal:	MB is ____ mm to ____ B ____ to ____ P ____ to ____
Date:	DB is ____ mm to ____ L ____ to ____ ML ____ to ____

Working/Apex Locator Length

Canal:	MB is ____ mm to ____ B ____ to ____ P ____ to ____
Date:	DB is ____ mm to ____ L ____ to ____ ML ____ to ____

X-Ray Length

Canal:	MB is ____ mm to ____ B ____ to ____ P ____ to ____
Date:	DB is ____ mm to ____ L ____ to ____ ML ____ to ____

Final Length—Adjusted

Canal:	MB is ____ mm to ____ B ____ to ____ P ____ to ____
Date:	DB is ____ mm to ____ L ____ to ____ ML ____ to ____

Patient:_____   **Date:**_____

Tooth #

	Estimated Length
Canal:	MB is ____ mm to ____ ____ to ____ P ____ to ____
Date:	DB is ____ mm to ____ L ____ to ____ ML ____ to ____

Working/Apex Locator Length

Canal:	MB is ____ mm to ____ B ____ to ____ P ____ to ____
Date:	DB is ____ mm to ____ L ____ to ____ ML ____ to ____

X-Ray Length

Canal:	MB is ____ mm to ____ B ____ to ____ P ____ to ____
Date:	DB is ____ mm to ____ L ____ to ____ ML ____ to ____

Final Length—Adjusted

Canal:	MB is ____ mm to ____ B ____ to ____ P ____ to ____
Date:	DB is ____ mm to ____ L ____ to ____ ML ____ to ____

Endodontic Therapy: Informed Consent

Patient Name:_____   **Date:**_____

I understand that the **endodontic therapy** (root canal therapy) planned for tooth #_____ is attempted when the nerve tissue in the tooth has treatment and is being done on a vital tooth as part of a comprehensive treatment plan. The reason for the nerve death may be decay, infection, trauma, or as part of restorative procedures that require the dentist to prepare the tooth for a large restoration or crown. This procedure has been explained to my satisfaction. I have also been informed that occasionally there are complications that arise during or subsequent to the root canal procedure.

I am aware of possible complications which include: pain, swelling, sensitivity to pressure or normal biting forces. I may have an allergic reaction to medications or anesthetics used. I understand that several radiographs must be taken to help ensure the proper instrumentation of the canal(s) and fit of the root canal filling material.

I understand that treatment may be complicated, have to be modified or even discontinued due to unforeseen difficulties including, but not limited to: calcified canals, perforation of the root or crown, inaccessible or severely twisted canals, internal or external resorption of the tooth, separated or broken files/instruments, or fracture of the root or crown structure. Some of these complications may require that I be referred to an endodontic specialist (endodontist) for further evaluation or treatment. I may have to have this procedure done entirely by an endodontist.

Root canal surgical procedures may be required in the future due to continuing problems with the tooth. The surgery may be needed to remove any cyst(s) or other related infections that either form or do not heal properly.

The visible portion of the tooth and/or root may darken eventually. This could cause a cosmetic problem with the tooth. The tooth could become brittle and be prone to fracture. I understand that it is recommended that this tooth have a full coverage cast restoration (crown or onlay) as soon as the tooth is comfortable. Silver amalgam restorations are not usually indicated for endodontically treated teeth as a final restoration.

The root canal treatment has been explained to me (or a guardian, if the patient is a minor). At this time I have no further questions. I understand that if questions do arise during the course of the root canal treatment, I can ask the treating dentist for further explanations. I understand that there is no warranty or guarantee for this endodontic treatment. I recognize that the only other alternative treatment to the endodontic therapy is to have the tooth extracted. In this event, even more expensive dental treatment may be required.

I consent to this root canal treatment for tooth #_____ to be performed by Dr._____ and any radiographs, medications, or local anesthetics that may have to be used during this therapy. I also understand that the endodontic treatment may require multiple office visits to complete, depending on the number of canals to be treated, degree of difficulty, progress of healing, and resistance of the root infection.

I have been told the estimated costs are:
Endodontic treatment for tooth #_____ $ _____
Final restoration recommended: $ _____
   ❏ Custom cast post
   ❏ Tooth-colored, titanium, or stainless steel post with core buildup
   ❏ Core buildup only
   ❏ Full crown   ❏ Gold onlay   ❏ Porcelain onlay
   ❏ Other:_____

_____   _____
Patient's or Guardian's Signature   Date

Extraction: Informed Consent

Reasons for recommending extraction of a tooth:

- Severe periodontal disease
- Irreversible damage to the nerve tissue inside the tooth
- Failed endodontic therapy
- Extreme fracture or decay of the tooth surface
- Improper positioning of the tooth or for orthodontic purposes

I have been informed of the reason for extraction of tooth #_____ and have been explained what to expect during this procedure. I understand that dental radiographs will be required prior to this extraction, and possibly during the procedure. I understand that I will require an anesthetic and that sutures may be necessary.

I have been given and understand the postoperative instructions. I also understand that if I have been given an antibiotic medication that I am to take them until the entire prescription is *completely* finished. If I have been prescribed a pain medication I will *take it only if necessary*. If the pain medication contains a narcotic such as codeine, operating machinery or driving a motor vehicle will be dangerous and could cause harm to myself or others.

I expect bleeding from the extraction site for the first 24 hours.

If I prefer, I can request that the extraction be done by an oral surgeon.

Some complications of routine extractions include (but are not limited to):

- Fracture of adjacent teeth or restorations
- Postoperative pain—slight, moderate, or severe and lasting from hours to days
- Swelling at and around the extraction site
- Separated root tips or fragments, separated bone fragments
- Temporary or permanent nerve damage to the area resulting in numbness
- Incomplete healing resulting in severe pain (dry socket)
- Fracture of the surrounding bone

If you have any questions about the reason for this extraction, please feel free to ask.

I have read and understand the above information. I have no further questions about the extraction of tooth #_____.

I give my permission to have the tooth extracted.

_____   _____
Patient's or Guardian's Signature   Date

Daily Chart Completion

Treatment Provider: _____

Date: _____

Patient Name	Needs Appointment	Chart Completed	Treatment Plan Needed	Hygiene Needed	New Patient Letter	Check Account Balance	Pre-D Needed	Insurance Completed	Insurance Mailed	Handouts Mailed

Dental Hygiene Treatment Directives

Patient:_____   **Date:**_____

Please perform the following services for the patient. As they are completed, please check off services for review. Numbers adjacent to treatment are appointment sequence and services to be accomplished at that visit.

Service Needed	Sequence	Completed	
___	___	___	Radiographs: BW
___	___	___	Radiographs: FM Series
___	___	___	Radiographs: Other _____
___	___	___	Oral self-care instructions
___	___	___	Disclose
___	___	___	Disclose, review brush and floss each therapy appointment. Have patient demonstrate these techniques. Please date and note on patient's chart as it is accomplished.
___	___	___	Patient advised to purchase an oral irrigator. Please instruct in its use with the periodontal attachment.
___	___	___	OHI instruction includes: ❑ toothbrushing ❑ flossing ❑ proxibrushes ❑ floss threaders ❑ gross debridement ❑ oral irrigator/periodontal attachment
___	___	___	Review periodontal disease process
___	___	___	Periodontal charting
___	___	___	Adult prophylaxis
___	___	___	Full mouth root plane/scale (1 visit)
___	___	___	Quadrant root plane/scale _____ visits ❑ UR ❑ UL ❑ LR ❑ LL ❑ with local anesthesia
___	___	___	Root plane/scale tooth #'s _____
___	___	___	Subgingival irrigation, all pockets 5 mm and over. Specific sites.
___	___	___	Reprobe, reevaluate for localized antimicrobial therapy tooth #'s _____
___	___	___	Place local antimicrobial therapy: tooth #'s _____
___	___	___	Place patient on a _____ month recare interval.
___	___	___	Reprobe appointment after _____ weeks. Evaluate for further periodontal therapy.
___	___	___	Report to Dr. _____ the results of the therapy.
___	___	___	After periodontal treatment, have the patient make a _____ minute appointment with Dr._____ to evaluate and begin other dentistry.
___	___	___	Other: _____

Hygienist's comments, recommendations, or areas needing dentist's evaluation:

_____

_____

_____

Dental Procedure Codes (complete CDT-4)

Diagnostic/Preventives

0120 ___ Periodic exam
0140 ___ Limited oral exam
0150 ___ Comp. oral exam
0160 ___ Extensive oral exam
0170 ___ Limited re-eval
0180 ___ Comp perio eval
0210 ___ FMS
0220 ___ PA 1st film
0230 ___ PA Ea. add. film
0270 ___ BW 1 film
0272 ___ BW 2 films
0274 ___ BW 4 films
0277 ___ Vert BW 4 films
0330 ___ Panoramic
0460 ___ Pulp test
0470 ___ Diag casts
0471 ___ Diag photos
1110 ___ Adult prophy
1120 ___ Prophy - child
1203 ___ Fluoride - child
1204 ___ Fluoride - adult
1330 ___ OHI
1351 ___ Sealant per tooth
1510 ___ Space maint. uni-
1515 ___ Space maint. bi-
1550 ___ Recement space maint.

Restorative
Amalgam

2140 ___ Amalgam-1 surf
2150 ___ Amalgam-2 surf
2160 ___ Amalgam-3 surf
2161 ___ Amalgam-4+ surf

Resin

2330 ___ Resin-1 surf, ant
2331 ___ Resin-2 surf, ant
2332 ___ Resin-3 surf, ant
2335 ___ Resin-4+ inc angle
2390 ___ Comp res crown, ant
2391 ___ Resin-1 surf, post-
2392 ___ Resin-2 surf, post-
2393 ___ Resin-3+ surf, post
2394 ___ Resin-4+ surf, post

Inlay

2510 ___ Inlay-metal 1 surf
2520 ___ Inlay-metal 2 surf
2530 ___ Inlay-metal 3+ surf
2610 ___ Inlay-por/cer 1 surf
2620 ___ Inlay-por/cer 2 surf
2630 ___ Inlay-por/cer 3+ surf
2650 ___ Inlay-comp/res
     1 surf (lab proc)
2651 ___ Inlay-comp/res
     2 surf (lab proc)
2652 ___ Inlay-comp/res 3+ surf
     (lab proc)

Onlay

2543 ___ Onlay-metal 3 surf
2544 ___ Onlay-metal 4+ surf
2642 ___ Onlay-por/cer 2 surf
2643 ___ Onlay-por/cer 3 surf
2644 ___ Onlay-por/4+ surf
2662 ___ Onlay-comp/res
     2 surf (lab proc)
2663 ___ Onlay-comp/res
     3 surf (lab proc)
2664 ___ Onlay-comp/res
     4+ surf (lab proc)

Crowns—Singles

2710 ___ Lab Resin
2740 ___ Porcelain
2750 ___ Porc high noble
2752 ___ Porc to noble
2790 ___ Full cast high noble
2792 ___ Full cast noble
2799 ___ Provisional

Other Restorative

2910 ___ Recement inlay
2920 ___ Recement crown
2930 ___ SS crown-prim
2931 ___ SS crown-perm
2932 ___ Prefab resin crown
2933 ___ SS crown w/resin
2940 ___ Sedative filling
2950 ___ Buildup w/pins
2951 ___ Pin/tooth
2952 ___ Cast post & core
2954 ___ Prefab post & core
2955 ___ Post removal
2960 ___ Labial veneer resin/
     chairside
2961 ___ Labial veneer resin/lab
2962 ___ Labial veneer porcelain/lab
2970 ___ Preformed prov
2980 ___ Crown repair
2999 ___ Unspecified restorative

Endodontics

3110 ___ Pulp cap direct
3220 ___ Pulpotomy
3221 ___ Pulpal debridement
3230 ___ Primary ant therapy
3240 ___ Primary post therapy
3310 ___ Ant RC treatment
3320 ___ Prem RC treatment
3330 ___ Molar RC treatment
3346 ___ Re-treat ant RC
3347 ___ Re-treat pre RC
3348 ___ Re-treat mol RC
3999 ___ Unspecified endo

Periodontics

4210 ___ GV/GP–quad
4211 ___ GV/GP 1-3 teeth
4249 ___ Crown lengthening
4260 ___ Osseous surg–quad
4261 ___ Oss surg 1-3 teeth
4320 ___ Splint intracoron
4321 ___ Splint extracoron
4341 ___ SC/RP per quad
4342 ___ SC/RP 1-3 teeth
4355 ___ Full mouth debride
4381 ___ Site-specific agent
4910 ___ Perio maintenance
4920 ___ Unsched. dressing change
4999 ___ Unspecified perio

Removable Prosthetics

5110 ___ Full denture max
5120 ___ Full denture mand
5130 ___ Immed. full max
5140 ___ Immed. full mand
5211 ___ RPD max resin
     w/clasps
5212 ___ RPD mand resin w/clasps
5213 ___ RPD max cast frame
5214 ___ RPD mand cast frame
5410 ___ Adj. full max
5411 ___ Adj. full mand
5421 ___ Adj. RPD max
5422 ___ Adj. RPD mand
5510 ___ Repair denture base
5520 ___ Repair tooth each
5610 ___ Repair RPD base
5620 ___ Repair RPD frame
5630 ___ Repair/replace clasp
5640 ___ Replace tooth each
5650 ___ Add tooth RPD
5660 ___ Add clasp RPD
5750 ___ Reline full max
5751 ___ Reline full mand
5760 ___ Reline max RPD
5761 ___ Reline mand. RPD
5810 ___ Interim full max
5811 ___ Interim full mand
5820 ___ Interim RPD max
5821 ___ Interim RPD mand
5850 ___ Tissue conditioning max
5851 ___ Tissue conditioning mand

Fixed Prosthetics
Pontic

6210 ___ Cast high noble
6212 ___ Cast noble
6240 ___ Porc. to high noble
6242 ___ Porc to noble
6253 ___ Provisional

Abutments

6545 ___ Cast met/res bond
6720 ___ Resin to high noble
6740 ___ Porc/ceram
6750 ___ Porc to high noble
6752 ___ Porc to noble
6790 ___ Cast high noble
6792 ___ Cast noble
6793 ___ Provisional

Other Fixed Prosthetics

6930 ___ Recement bridge
6970 ___ Cast post and core
6972 ___ Prefab post/core
6973 ___ Core buildup
6975 ___ Coping each tooth
6999 ___ Unspecified fixed prosth

Oral Surgery

7111 ___ Ext. prim remnants
7140 ___ Extraction routine
7210 ___ Extraction surgical
7220 ___ Ext. soft impaction
7230 ___ Ext. partial impact
7240 ___ Ext. full impaction
7250 ___ Ext. surgical root
7285 ___ Biopsy-hard tissue
7286 ___ Biopsy-soft tissue
7287 ___ Brush cytology
7510 ___ Inc & drain abscess

Adjunctive Services

9110 ___ Palliative treatment
9310 ___ Consult 2nd opinion
9430 ___ Office visit-observe
9440 ___ Office visit-aftr hrs
9450 ___ Case presentation
9910 ___ Desensitizing meds
9940 ___ Occlusal guard
9950 ___ Occ. analy mount
9951 ___ Occ. adj. limited
9952 ___ Occ. adj. complete
9970 ___ Enamel microabrasion
9999 ___ Unspecified adjunctive

Routing Slips

Routing Slip

Patient: _____ Provider: _____

Treatment Completed
    Tooth # ____ Procedure Code:_____
    Tooth # ____ Procedure Code:_____
    Tooth # ____ Procedure Code:_____

Hygiene Services
    ❏ Prophylaxis 01110
    ❏ Fluoride 00120
    ❏ Sealants Tooth #_____
    ❏ Root Planing 04341 UL LL UR LR

Predetermination
    Tooth # ____ Procedure Code: _____
    Root Planing/Scaling 04341
    Other _____

Comments: _____

_____

Routing Slip

Patient: _____ Provider: _____

Treatment Completed
    Tooth # ____ Procedure Code:_____
    Tooth # ____ Procedure Code:_____
    Tooth # ____ Procedure Code:_____

Hygiene Services
    ❏ Prophylaxis 01110
    ❏ Fluoride 00120
    ❏ Sealants Tooth #_____
    ❏ Root Planing 04341 UL LL UR LR

Predetermination
    Tooth # ____ Procedure Code: _____
    Root Planing/Scaling 04341
    Other _____

Comments: _____

_____

Routing Slip

Patient: _____ Provider: _____

Treatment Completed
    Tooth # ____ Procedure Code:_____
    Tooth # ____ Procedure Code:_____
    Tooth # ____ Procedure Code:_____

Hygiene Services
    ❏ Prophylaxis 01110
    ❏ Fluoride 00120
    ❏ Sealants Tooth #_____
    ❏ Root Planing 04341 UL LL UR LR

Predetermination
    Tooth # ____ Procedure Code: _____
    Root Planing/Scaling 04341
    Other _____

Comments: _____

_____

Routing Slip

Patient: _____ Provider: _____

Treatment Completed
    Tooth # ____ Procedure Code:_____
    Tooth # ____ Procedure Code:_____
    Tooth # ____ Procedure Code:_____

Hygiene Services
    ❏ Prophylaxis 01110
    ❏ Fluoride 00120
    ❏ Sealants Tooth #_____
    ❏ Root Planing 04341 UL LL UR LR

Predetermination
    Tooth # ____ Procedure Code: _____
    Root Planing/Scaling 04341
    Other _____

Comments: _____

_____

Laboratory Cases in Progress

Tracking Sheet

Patient	Lab	Case	For	Date Sent	Return Date	Back

Laboratory Work Order

Date: _____   Return Date: _____

Patient: _____   Age: _____ Sex: _____

Please Call about Case   yes   no   **Disinfected**   yes   no

Type of Restoration:
- ❑ Single Unit
- ❑ Bridge
- ❑ Full Cast
- ❑ Porcelain
- ❑ Procera
- ❑ Empress I

- ❑ Empress II
- ❑ Targis/Vectris
- ❑ Cristobal Plus
- ❑ LAVA All Ceramic
- ❑ Porcelain/Noble
- ❑ Porcelain/High Noble

- ❑ Inlay
- ❑ Onlay
- ❑ Implant
- ❑ Implant Supported
- ❑ Lab Processed
  Temporary

- ❑ Progressive Loading Temporary
- ❑ Splinted
- ❑ Diagnostic Wax Up
- ❑ Other

Teeth #'s: _____

Finish Line: 360 bevel   270 bevel   Buccal Chamfer   Full Chamfer

Crown Design: Full Minimal Metal Collar (.4 mm maximum)   Buccal Porcelain Butt Joint
              Full Porcelain Margin   Modified Ridge Lap

Enclosed:
- ❑ Full Arch Final Impression
- ❑ Quadrant Impression
- ❑ Occ Registration
- ❑ Withdrawal Impression
- ❑ Full Arch Counter

- ❑ Study Models U L
- ❑ Castings
- ❑ Triple Tray Bite, Counter and Final Impression
- ❑ Face Bow Transfer Table
- ❑ Triple Tray Bite and Counter

Photographs enclosed: yes   no

Shade: _____

- ❑ Please pour impressions   ❑ Return for ditching   ❑ Ditch die(s)   ❑ Mount
- ❑ Return finished, ready for luting or bonding
- ❑ Return for casting try-in and withdrawal impression
- ❑ Apply porcelain return bisque bake   ❑ Apply porcelain and return finished

Special Instructions:

_____

_____

_____

Dr. _____   License # _____

Marketing Tips

This collection is not designed to be a complete marketing package but will provide you with many useful documents to help with your marketing strategy.

Press Releases

The press can be your friend; start by establishing a friendship with someone in the press. Get a contact person on the newspaper that services the area where your patients live. Whenever you add new staff, equipment, techniques, etc., send your contact a press release. Review the **Press Release Guide (p. 27)** in this chapter to help you with these. Many newspapers have column space available for human interest stories of success and opportunities in their community.

Place a simple newspaper advertisement announcing a special event such as an open house or a "Meet the Specialists" day.

Consider sponsoring community events that highlight area businesses; your name and/or advertisement will appear in the pre-event publicity or program. When you are a participant in an event, be sure to have available handouts on "hot" topics such as **Cosmetic Dentistry (p. 119), Tooth Whitening Overview and Options (p. 126), Early Signs of Periodontal Disease (p. 215),** and **For a Lifetime of Great Oral Health (p. 158).**

Continuing Education Bulletin Board

Maintain a bulletin board at your office that lets your patients know about the conferences, training, and other continuing education in which you and your staff participate. Display diplomas, certificates, and letters of commendation as well. Patients are eager to reap the benefits of leading edge research and technology.

New Patients

The **Welcome to the Neighborhood (p. 42)** letter should be sent to all newcomers along with a magnet with your name on it. Contact your community Welcome Wagon, Chamber of Commerce, or Merchants Association; if they don't provide newcomers services, they can probably refer you to someone who does. Offer free, no obligation health information, and invite prospective patients to just visit the practice to show that you care about your community and about patients' needs.

Also, there are several excellent letters in **Patient Letters & Forms (Section 3)** that will be very useful for those who accept your offer and would like more information about your practice. See **Patient Education Documents (pp. 10-11)** for a list of other documents prospective patients may be interested in reading.

The Well-Informed Patient

The main thrust of this publication is patient education. There is no better marketing tool than happy patients who tell all their friends and acquaintances about their dentist who takes the time to explain everything they need to know to make an informed decision. The greater the patients' knowledge, the greater their acceptance of treatment will be. Include the written word to help them keep things straight.

Keeping Track

Much of **Practice Administration (Section 1)** is devoted to forms that help track patient appointments and treatment. These forms are invaluable for a smooth transition from treatment room to the front office. Consider **Laboratory Cases in Progress (p. 23), Patient Education Documents (pp. 10-12), Treatment Plan (p. 16),** and the forms under **Telephone Lists and Forms (pp. 28-31).**

Thank You for Your Referral

Encourage patient referrals by rewarding patients who refer others to you. **Thanks for Your Referral (p. 41)** letters should contain a gift certificate. For a first referral, consider a pizza coupon. The second referral could earn a dinner at a nice restaurant. The third might feature flowers. Use your imagination.

Finances

Properly handled, your financial practices can make you a hero to your patients. Patients can clearly see the need for treatment and want to have the best, but it must be affordable. To help your patient through the financial considerations of dentistry:

1. Always be as up-front as possible in disclosing all of the costs of each treatment option in writing. **Treatment Plan (p. 16) Estimate of Fees (pp. 53-54.)** are good forms to use.
2. Always see that patients know what their means of payment options are in writing. Use **Financial Arrangements (p. 55)** for this.
3. Provide a Truth in Lending form, regardless of whether you intend to charge interest.
4. Be sure your patients have a signed copy of the financial arrangements they have made with you. See **Financial Arrangements (p. 55), Preauthorization of Payment (p. 56),** and **Schedule of Payment (p. 57).**
5. Be sure your patients understand how dental insurers arrive at the reimbursement amount. **Dental Insurance Coverage (p. 48), Dental Insurance: Points to Consider (p. 49),** and **Determination of Insurance Benefits (p. 50)** are useful here.
6. When sending out a letter from the **Insurance Narratives (Section 2),** send the patient a copy as well. This informs the patient of your attempt to obtain proper reimbursement for him or her.
7. Make certain that financial arrangement and consent forms comply with your local and state regulations.

Press Release Guide

Dr. (your name) is pleased to announce (choose one from below)

- the addition of (name) to our staff. (Name) is a (name their profession), who will be (write general duties). (Give a few sentence biography and mention one or two advantages this appointment offers patients.)
- the integration of (name new equipment or technique) into our practice. This new (equipment or technique) will enable us to offer you (name several advantages that this new addition provides for patients).
- that (name), (name their profession) has recently completed (training, certification, etc.) in (name of subject). (Name several advantages that this training offers the patient: may include a new service, more opportunities for an existing popular service, or a more advanced service.)
- the integration of Mosby's *Complete Dental Communication for Patients and Professionals* into his or her practice. This comprehensive software gives Dr._____ enhanced ability to inform all patients, in detail and in writing for their home review, about dental treatment needs and advantages and disadvantages of available options prior to treatment. It also will educate the patient about the many different dental services Dr._____ can provide.

Miscellaneous Calls to be Completed

Person to Call	Phone	Information Needed	Calling for Dr.	Done

Patients Who Need to be Rescheduled

Patient	Phone # (label: home, work, etc.)	Treatment	With Whom	Desired Time	Call Result	Date	Initials

- Keep this form handy; near the phone.
- Place patient name and information on list, one patient per row.
- Contact when the desired opening occurs in the schedule.
- Record results of contact (coming in, etc.), call date, and initials of person placing the call.
- Bring list to doctor's attention weekly, for review.

Priority Rescheduling

Patient	Treatment	Phone # (label: home, work, etc.)	Desired Time	Result	Date	Initials

- Keep this form handy; near the phone.
- Place patient name and information on list, one patient per row.
- Contact when the desired opening occurs in the schedule.
- Record results of contact (coming in, etc.), call date, and initials of person placing the call.
- Bring list to doctor's attention weekly, for review.
- After three attempts to contact, if no appointment scheduled, bring to attention of doctor.

Professionals Requesting Patient Information

Date/Time	Patient	Referring Dentist, Physician	Dentist, Physician Phone #	Subject

■ When patients, other dentists, or physicians call in relation to a patient's treatment, please record the patient's name and information called for in this log.

■ **Be sure to note the call details in the patient's chart as well.** Initial both this log and patient's chart.

■ If the message is long, the appropriate portion of this log may be duplicated for the patient's chart.

■ The treating dentist will review this log **daily.**

Health Insurance Portability and Accountability Act (HIPAA) of 1996

What Is HIPAA?

The Health Insurance Portability and Accountability Act (HIPAA) of 1996 was signed into law by former President Bill Clinton on August 21, 1996. Conclusive regulations were issued on August 17, 2000, to be instated by October 16, 2002. HIPAA requires that the transactions of all patient healthcare information be formatted in a standardized electronic style. In addition to protecting the privacy and security of patient information, HIPAA includes legislation on the formation of medical savings accounts, the authorization of a fraud and abuse control program, the easy transport of health insurance coverage, and the simplification of administrative terms and conditions.

What does HIPAA Cover?

HIPAA encompasses three primary areas, and its privacy requirements can be broken down into three types: privacy standards, patients' rights, and administrative requirements.

1. **Privacy Standards.** A central concern of HIPAA is the careful use and disclosure of protected health information (PHI), which generally is electronically controlled health information that is able to be distinguished individually. PHI also refers to verbal communication, although the HIPAA Privacy Rule is not intended to hinder necessary verbal communication. The U.S. Department of Health and Human Services (USDHHS) does not require restructuring, such as soundproofing, architectural changes, and so forth, but some caution is necessary when exchanging health information by conversation.

   An Acknowledgment of Receipt Notice of Privacy Practices, which allows patient information to be used or divulged for treatment, payment, or healthcare operations (TPO), should be procured from each patient. A detailed and time-sensitive authorization can also be issued, which allows the dentist to release information in special circumstances other than TPOs. A *written consent* is also an option. Dentists can disclose PHI *without* acknowledgment, consent, or authorization in very special situations, for example, perceived child abuse, public health supervision, fraud investigation, or law enforcement with valid permission (i.e., a warrant). When divulging PHI, a dentist must try to disclose only the *minimum necessary* information, to help safeguard the patient's information as much as possible.

   It is important that dental professionals adhere to HIPAA standards because healthcare providers (as well as healthcare clearinghouses and healthcare plans) who convey *electronically* formatted health information via an outside billing service or merchant are considered *covered entities*. Covered entities may be dealt serious civil and criminal penalties for violation of HIPAA legislation. Failure to comply with HIPAA privacy requirements may result in civil penalties of up to $100 per offense with an annual maximum of $25,000 for repeated failure to comply with the same requirement. Criminal penalties resulting from the illegal mishandling of private health information can range from $50,000 and/or 1 year in prison to $250,000 and/or 10 years in prison.

2. **Patients' Rights.** HIPAA allows patients, authorized representatives, and parents of minors, as well as minors, to become more aware of the health information privacy to which they are entitled. These rights include, but are not limited to, the right to view and copy their health information, the right to dispute alleged breaches of policies and regulations, and the right to request alternative forms of communicating with their dentist. If any health information is released for any reason other than TPO, the patient is entitled to an account of the transaction. Therefore, it is important for dentists to keep accurate records of such information and to provide them when necessary.

   The HIPAA Privacy Rule determines that the parents of a minor have access to their child's health information. This privilege may be overruled, for example, in cases where there is suspected child abuse or the parent consents to a term of confidentiality between the dentist and the minor. The parents' rights to access their child's PHI also may be restricted in situations when a legal entity, such as a court, intervenes and when a law does not require a parent's consent. For a full list of patient rights provided by HIPAA, be sure to acquire a copy of the law and to understand it well.

3. **Administrative Requirements.** Complying with HIPAA legislation may seem like a chore, but it does not need to be so. It is recommended that you become appropriately familiar with the law, organize the requirements into simpler tasks, begin compliance early, and document your progress in compliance. An important first step is to evaluate the current information and practices of your office.

   Dentists will need to write a **privacy policy** for their office, a document for their patients detailing the office's practices concerning PHI. The ADA's **HIPAA Privacy Kit** includes forms that you (the dentist) can use to customize your privacy policy. It is useful to try to understand the role of healthcare information for your patients and the ways in which they deal with the information while they are visiting your office. Train your staff; make sure they are familiar with the terms of HIPAA and your office's privacy policy and related forms. HIPAA requires that you designate a privacy officer, a person in your office who will be responsible for applying the new policies in your office, fielding complaints, and making choices involving the minimum necessary requirements. Another person with the role of contact person will process complaints.

A *Notice of Privacy Practices*—a document detailing the patient's rights and the dental office's obligations concerning PHI—also must be drawn up. Further, any role of a third party with access to PHI must be clearly documented. This third party is known as a *business associate* (BA) and is defined as any entity who, on behalf of the dentist, takes part in any activity that involves exposure of PHI. The *HIPAA Privacy Kit* provides a copy of the USDHHS "Business Associate Contract Terms," which provides a concrete format for detailing BA interactions.

The main HIPAA privacy compliance date, including all staff training, was April 14, 2003, although many covered entities who submitted a request and a compliance plan by October 15, 2002, were granted one-year extensions. It is recommended that dentists prepare their offices ahead of time for all deadlines, which include preparing privacy polices and forms, business associate contracts, and employee training sessions.

For More Information on HIPAA
For a comprehensive discussion of all of these terms and requirements, a complete list of HIPAA policies and procedures, and a full collection of HIPAA privacy forms, contact the American Dental Association for a *HIPAA Privacy Kit*. The relevant ADA Web site is www.ada.org/goto/hipaa. Other Web sites that may contain useful information about HIPAA are:
- USDHHS Office of Civil Rights: www.hhs.gov/ocr/hipaa
- Work Group on Electronic Data Interchange: www.wedi.org/SNIP
- Phoenix Health: www.hipaadvisory.com
- USDHHS Office of the Assistant Secretary for Planning and Evaluation: http://aspe.os.dhhs.gov/admnsimp/

Bibliography
1. HIPAA Privacy Kit
2. http://www.ada.org/prof/prac/issues/topics/hipaa/index.html

HIPAA–Business Associates Contract

The Health Insurance Portability and Accountability Act (HIPAA) requires a signed contact between the individual employee designated as the Privacy Officer and the dentist.

   This contract between the office of Dr. _____ (the *entity*) and _____ (the *business associate*) discloses the conditions to satisfactorily ensure compliance with the Privacy Rule of the HIPAA.

During this contract period the business associates must observe the following responsibilities with respect to protected health information:

   A business associate must limit requests for protected health information on behalf of the covered entity to that which is reasonably necessary to accomplish the intended purpose; a covered entity is permitted to reasonably rely on such requests from business associate of another covered entity as the minimum necessary.

   Make information available, including information held by a business associate, as necessary to determine compliance by the covered entity.

   Fulfill an individual's rights to access and amend his or her protected health information contained in a designated record set, including information held by a business associate, if appropriate, and receive an accounting of disclosures by a business associate.

   Mitigate, to the extent practicable, any harmful effect that is known to the covered entity of an impermissible use or disclosure of protected health information by its business associates.

   Business associates cannot use protected health information for their own purposes. This includes, but is not limited to, selling protected health information to third parties for the third parties' own marketing activities, without authorization.

   The covered entity is required to ensure, in whatever reasonable manner deemed effective by the covered entity, the appropriate cooperation by their business associates in meeting these requirements.

   If the covered entity discovers a material breach of violation of the contract by the business associate, it will take reasonable steps to cure the breach or end the contract with the business associate. If termination is not feasible, the covered entity will report the problem to the Department of Health and Human Services Office for Civil Rights.

HIPAA–Staff Training Registry

The Health Insurance Portability and Accountability Act (HIPAA) requires that all employees be inserviced on the dental office's HIPAA policy.

I hereby certify that the following employees of the below named dental office have received the office policy regarding the Health Insurance Portability and Accountability Act Privacy Rule.

Privacy Officer_____   Date_____

Dental Office of   Name_____

                                Address_____

                                City _____ State_____

I understand the office Privacy Policy and procedures needed to protect the private health information of patients and will access only information that is reasonably needed to carry out my duties.

Name   Date

chapter 2

Patient Letters and Forms

Content at a Glance: Patient Letters and Forms

Welcome/Thank You
Evaluation of Our Services
Let patients know you care what they think and prevent misunderstandings on everyone's part. Great for maintaining high-quality care and making that all-important first impression. Solid feedback for treatment improvement.

Pleasure Meeting You
Cement good patient relations with this follow-up letter to a patient whom you have just met for the first time. This must be handwritten to be effective.

Thanks for Your Referral
Thank you note for patient referring a new patient to your practice. Includes sentence indicating you have enclosed a token of your appreciation. This is most effective when handwritten.

Welcome to the Neighborhood
Introduce yourself to new move-ins and give them a positive impression and incentive to drop by for a visit.

Welcome to Our Practice
Introduce yourself to new patients and help them understand your office policies on appointments, financial arrangements, and insurance forms. Ensure them of the thorough explanations and high quality of care they can always expect. Can also be mailed to new patients who have made an appointment.

Office Policy
Cancellation and No-Show Policy
Diplomatic way to inform patients of your and their responsibilities with regard to appointments. Includes information on emergencies, as well as cancellation and no-show charges.

Dental Emergencies
Prevent additional harm or pain by preparing your patients to handle dental emergencies.

How the Health Insurance Portability and Accountability Act (HIPAA) Will Affect Your Next Dental Visit
Reviews the types of health data disclosure allowed under HIPAA.

Insurance
Dental Insurance Coverage
Explain to patients how dental insurance works, their financial responsibility, and how to get a claim submitted.

Dental Insurance: Points to Consider
All insurance coverage is not created equal! A point often missed by many patients. This gives a plain-language overview of many dental benefit concepts.

Determination of Insurance Benefits
Informs patient that the predetermination has been received, payment arrangements can now be made, and treatment begun. Warns of possible time limitations.

Information Request
Expedite insurance claim form problems with this letter to the patient, asking him or her to fill in missing information or contact the office concerning his or her insurance claim form.

Financial
Consent to Payment
An authorization form with selection criteria for actual payment methods to which the patient has agreed.

Estimate of Fees
Informative overview to promote patient understanding of treatment recommendations and the fees involved. Divided into treatment specialties, with separate spaces for insurance and patient financial responsibilities. Gives patients the information they need to make financial arrangements.

Continued

Content at a Glance: Patient Letters and Forms—cont'd

Estimate of Fees (brief form)
A form designed for use in patient communication regarding planned treatment.

Financial Arrangements
Explanation of insurance, possible payment options, fee guarantees, and nonpayment procedures. Gives patients the needed information to choose appropriate financial arrangements.

Preauthorization of Payment
Credit card preauthorization for office to take payment directly from card account on a one-time, weekly, or monthly payment plan. Can be used with "Financial Arrangements" form.

Schedule of Payment
Provides an actual dated schedule of payments. Space for procedure that this schedule covers, total fee, and patient signature.

Treatment
Declination of Treatment
Statement for patients to sign, declining particular treatment that you have recommended.

Dental Cosmetic Evaluation
A form designed to capture all patient-specific cosmetic dental information prior to determining appropriate treatment.

Dental Hygiene Services
This check-off form lets the patient know what has been done at the prophylaxis visit.

Examination/Consultation Overview
General checklist of conditions found and proposed treatment and referrals.

Medical History Update
Allows patient an easy opportunity to update his or her medical history at each appointment. Ensures that you have the latest information, as well as a history of updates.

Next Appointment Procedure
Outlines the next procedure for the patient, the services that will be completed, and the approximate length of time required.

Patient Education Request
For prospective patients, this form is designed as an attachment for "Welcome to the Neighborhood" in this section.

Treatment Goals
Outlines treatment philosophy and engages the patient in the process of treatment determination.

Evaluation of Our Services

Thank you for choosing us as your dental team! We strive to provide you with the best oral care possible by offering you the cutting edge of dental technology and philosophy and we value your feedback. We would appreciate your time in evaluating our services. The information you provide will be used to identify our strengths, as well as areas in which we can make your experience even better. Feel free to comment in the space provided below.

Please circle 1 for Excellent, 2 for Good, 3 for Average, 4 for Fair, and 5 for Poor.

- Was the examination comprehensive?   1   2   3   4   5
- Was this the most thorough examination you have had?   1   2   3   4   5
- How could the examination have been improved? _____

_____

- Were the explanations you were given clear?   1   2   3   4   5
- Did the doctor explain the difference between required and elective dental treatment?   1   2   3   4   5
- Did you understand what dental treatment you need?   1   2   3   4   5
- Did the doctor use adequate visual aids to help explain the dental problems and treatment?   1   2   3   4   5
- Did the doctor give you adequate written information for each dental problem and solution?   1   2   3   4   5
- Did the doctor explain to you the risks, options for treatment, advantages and disadvantages of treatment, consequences of treatment and no treatment for your dental problems?   1   2   3   4   5
- Did the doctor or receptionist clearly explain office financial policy? (Payment is due when treatment is provided, unless prior arrangements have been made.)   1   2   3   4   5
- Would you feel comfortable referring a relative or friend here for his or her dental needs?   1   2   3   4   5

Answer the following questions if you have extensive dental needs.
- If you were referred to a dental specialist, did you understand why?   1   2   3   4   5
- If referred to a specialist, did you understand when you were to see the specialist?   1   2   3   4   5
- If referred to a specialist, did you understand when you would have treatment by our office?   1   2   3   4   5
- Did the doctor explain that your dental treatment can be phased over a period of time?   1   2   3   4   5

We appreciate anyone you refer here and will treat him or her with the same respect, concern, and professional attention we have given you.

Comments: _____

_____

_____

Thank you for taking the time to answer these questions.

Pleasure Meeting You

FOR THE GREATEST IMPACT, MAKE THIS A HANDWRITTEN NOTE!

(Date)

Dear (Patient Name),

It was a pleasure to meet you today. If you have any questions about any of the dental treatment we discussed, please feel free to contact me. As I mentioned, during our discussion, I am enclosing with this note information relating to (subject discussed). I'm sure you will find it interesting and informative.

(Reiterate any specific information from the exam that will point out to patient the parts of the handouts that will be of most interest to the patient.)

(Mention, if possible, any personal conversation you might have had: e.g., the team both of your children are on, a helpful suggestion for your golf game, etc.)

If you have any friends or relatives who share your vision of wanting excellent oral health and are looking for a dentist, you can refer them here with confidence. I look forward to seeing you again.

Sincerely,

Thanks for Your Referral

THIS LETTER IS MOST EFFECTIVE WHEN HANDWRITTEN!

(Date)

Dear (patient name),

Thank you very much for your kind recommendation of _____ to our office. One of the highest compliments a patient can give a healthcare provider is the referral of friends and family. Your confidence in us is highly valued. One of our new patients has come to us because of your referral. You can be assured that we will give him or her the same care that prompted you to refer him or her to us.

Please accept the enclosed token of our appreciation. We hope you enjoy it.

Thank you again.

Sincerely,

Welcome to the Neighborhood

(EDIT THE ITALICIZED TEXT TO FIT YOUR SITUATION.)

Dear Neighbor,

Welcome to (community name). We have been in the area since (year) and find it a wonderful place to live and raise a family–qualities that we are sure prompted your final decision.

One of the most difficult decisions involved in any relocation is finding excellent health care for your family. We would like to help you find your new dentist. Let us introduce ourselves.

Enclosed are brief professional highlights of Dr. Stephen Candio and Beth Stolar Candio, BS, RDH, MA. We provide consistent and exceptional dental care for all ages. Through our prevention orientation, we strive to help you maintain your natural dentition. Our goal is for you to have functional, comfortable, good looking, and pain free teeth now and when you are 95 years old. Our main area of expertise is adhesive esthetic dentistry (bonding and conservative fillings). We have been engaged in original laboratory and clinical research in this area for years. We have actually worked with a manufacturer to develop many of the dental materials now used in dentistry. At our office we have two dental specialists: an orthodontist (braces) and periodontist (limited to treatment of diseases of the gums and oral bone). If you feel you need a consultation in either of these areas, they would be pleased to provide an evaluation.

For your health and benefit, we do not use nickel or base metals in any restoration we place. We do not use metal direct filling materials (silver amalgam). Our laboratory-processed restorations (inlays, onlays, or full crowns) are composed of ceramics, porcelains, processed resins, or high content gold alloy. If metal substructure is needed for crowns or bridges, only the highest quality gold or precious metal alloy is used.

Attached, you will find a listing of useful information that can help answer dental questions you may have. For the young children in the home, we have information that describes how to help children maintain decay-free teeth; when children should go to the dentist; at what age baby teeth and permanent teeth usually come in; systemic fluoride dosages *(Sparta does not have fluoride in the drinking water);* and protective sealants (quickly placed and painless plastic coatings that are placed on the biting surfaces of teeth to prevent decay). Whether or not you select our office for your dental care, we would like to offer you this *free* information on these and numerous other dental topics including: home tooth whitening, crowns, root canals, dental implants, and much more. Refer to the enclosure and check off what you would like to receive. Then either mail it back to us along with your name and address, drop it off at the office, or call and let us know which information you would like.

When you are ready, we would be happy to assist you in keeping your teeth in a healthy and beautiful state for your entire life. We have a unique dental office and would appreciate the chance to provide exceptional dental care to you and your family.

Sincerely,

Welcome to Our Practice

We are so pleased that you have selected our office for your dental care. Our goals will be to determine what dental treatment you need or want and deliver it in the most efficient manner with clinical excellence and courtesy. We will teach you how to combine regular interval professional dental evaluation with proper, routine daily oral self care to maintain optimum oral health for yourself for your entire life. We want you to have comfortable, pain free, good looking and functional teeth when you are 95 years old.

(In this space, type in short biography noting degrees/certification and other dental-related activities of dentist, hygienist, and/or other significant people at this office.)

Office hours are by appointment. When appropriate, we prefer to schedule longer appointments and complete as much dental treatment at a time as we can. This allows maximum efficiency and as little disruption to your daily schedule as possible.

Our office offers simple financial arrangements in order to avoid possible misunderstandings. Unless prior arrangements are made, payment in full is expected at the time treatment is provided. If you have dental insurance, for your protection, we will send a pre-estimate of dental treatment to your dental carrier. When the pre-estimate is returned (6 to 8 weeks), your portion of payment will be indicated. We ask that you pay that portion at the time treatment begins. If the treatment is extensive or will take several months to complete, partial payment can be made at appointments over that time span. For your convenience, VISA and MasterCard are accepted. For more involved procedures, an interest-free loan (up to 12 months) can be arranged.

You can expect to receive the best dental care we can provide. Dental technology has made remarkable strides. You may not be aware of some of the advances in diagnosis and treatment and how they can benefit you. If you have not been to a dentist recently, or have been in the care of someone who has not adopted these techniques, you will notice a difference the first moment you enter our office.

Once you have explained your dental concerns and a thorough dental examination and necessary radiographs have been completed, a treatment plan will be developed. Written and videotaped explanations of most procedures and problems are available and will be offered to you. Advantages and disadvantages of treatment, risks of treatment or no treatment, options and costs of treatment will be presented. Any questions you have will be answered before treatment begins.

We are committed to providing for each patient an initial appointment during which an exchange of patient concerns and dental desires can be addressed. We respect out patients' time. We do not double book. Unless an unexpected dental emergency arises, we make sure that patients are seen at their scheduled appointment time. We want each patient to feel comfortable, with adequate appointment time to address his or her dental concerns. Please allow adequate travel time to our office.

Enclosed you will find a medical and dental history form that you can complete before your first visit. Please bring it with you. Thank you for the opportunity to provide you with dental care.

(In this space, type in names of dentist, hygienist, and those mentioned above and have each sign above his or her name.)

Cancellation and No-Show Policy

Office hours are by appointment and we do value your time. This office is a private practice dental office and not a dental "clinic." Appointment time is reserved for you alone. Where appropriate, we prefer to schedule longer appointments so we can complete as much needed dental treatment as possible during one appointment. We feel this type of scheduling will cause minimal disruption to your daily schedule and will provide efficiency in completing your dental care. When you make an appointment, please be sure that you will be able to keep it. Morning appointments are best for more complicated procedures.

Emergencies and unforeseen patient treatment problems may arise, causing schedule changes. Emergencies are unexpected and seem to come at the most inconvenient times. If you have a dental emergency that needs immediate attention, we will always offer to see you at once. We expect that other patients who might be slightly inconvenienced by this will be understanding of the emergency situation. At some point, they may need the same courtesy too!

Unlike many offices, this office does not call to confirm your appointment. Please make a note of any dental appointments we have scheduled in a place where you will be easily reminded. If you cannot make an appointment as scheduled, please notify the office. There will be a charge of $25 per 30 minutes of scheduled time for a broken appointment or cancellation with less than 24 hours' notice for appointments before 4 p.m., weekdays. For appointments broken or canceled without 24 hours' notice after 4 p.m., weekdays or Saturdays, the charge is $50 per 30 minutes of scheduled time.

If our staff is successful in filling your appointment time with another patient, there will be no broken appointment charge.

If you have any questions about our appointment cancellation and no-show policy, please feel free to ask us.

Dental Emergencies

Regular dental care helps prevent inconvenient dental emergencies. However, dental emergencies can and do occur. Listed here are some of the more common dental emergencies and what you can do until you can get to our office. A good rule of thumb: if it hurts, do NOT wait to make an appointment. We will be happy to see you as soon as possible.

Toothache/Sensitive Teeth

A toothache or a sensitive tooth can be caused by several different types of problems. At times it is a sign of a dying nerve inside the tooth. Over-the-counter pain relief medication can temporarily relieve the pain. Contact us for an appointment as soon as you notice the problem. Slight pain, if left untreated, can progress into facial or oral swelling and severe pain. Commonly, tooth pain can be eliminated with endodontic treatment (root canal therapy).

A sensitive tooth may be due to exposed root, a leaking or defective filling, decay, a bite-related problem, or a dying nerve. See us as soon as possible for an evaluation.

Broken Tooth

Teeth with large fillings can easily break or fracture. Call us as soon as possible to have the tooth evaluated and restored. If the broken tooth is not treated, more serious problems can develop. Broken teeth may or may not be sensitive to air and temperature changes. Sensitivity and pain are not necessarily an indication of how badly the tooth is damaged.

Tooth Knocked Out

Place the tooth in water or a wet towel or cloth. **Do not try to scrub or wash the tooth**. Get the tooth and the patient to us immediately. The faster the tooth can be repositioned, the better the odds that the tooth can be saved. **Time is crucial.**

Object Stuck Between Teeth

Use dental floss to gently remove the object. **Do not use sharp or pointed objects to push or pry the object from between your teeth.** If the object does not come out easily, come to us for help.

Final or Provisional Crown/Bridge Falls Out

See us as soon as possible to have the crown recemented. If this is not possible, you can use a denture adhesive (FIXODENT®, for example) that can be purchased without a prescription. Place a small amount in the crown and reseat it. Do not try to force it into place. It should not be difficult to put into place. When you cannot put the crown in correctly, save it, and bring it with you to your appointment. We will do the cementation. The reason the crown came out may make it impossible for the dentist to recement the old crown. That decision will be made during your examination.

Broken Partial or Denture

Bring the partial or denture here for repair. **Do not try to glue the plastic yourself. Do not use CRAZY GLUE® or other similar materials.**

Orthodontic Problems

If the appliance is loose, take the patient to the orthodontist. If a sharp wire is exposed, cover it with a piece of wax, gum, a small cotton ball—anything to keep the sharp end from poking into the soft tissues.

Swollen Gums

Swollen gums are a sign of an infection. The infection may be caused by a dying nerve inside the tooth or a periodontal (gum) problem. Rinse your mouth with warm salt water. See us as soon as possible. The swelling may or may not be accompanied by pain. Either way, it needs immediate attention.

(In this space, type in dentist's name, address, and telephone number.)

How the Health Insurance Portability and Accountability Act (HIPAA) Will Affect Your Next Dental Visit

The U.S. Department of Health and Human Services has recently issued national health information privacy standards. The Health Insurance Portability and Accountability Act, a federally mandated law known as HIPAA, is designed to:

- provide protection for the privacy of certain identifiable health data (called *protected health information [PHI]*),
- ensure health insurance coverage when changing employers, and
- provide standards for facilitating electronic transfers of health care–related information.

While the privacy of your personal PHI will remain confidential, certain aspects of this law will permit disclosures of PHI to facilitate public health activities. The following charts review the types of health data disclosure allowed under HIPAA.

PHI can be disclosed with your authorization in the following categories.

You may request a limitation or restriction on the disclosure of this information. You have the right to:
- request a restriction or limit of any of the above disclosures used for treatment, payment, or office operations.
- inspect and copy information that may be used to make decisions about your care.
- request an amendment of this information if you feel it is incorrect or incomplete.
- an accounting of disclosures we have made that were not related to treatment, payment, or operations of this office.

These requests must be submitted in writing to the office manager and you will be informed of the specifics that are required for this request.

Treatment—PHI will be used to provide appropriate treatment either by this office or other healthcare providers, diagnostic or fabrication laboratories.

Payment—PHI will be used to facilitate payment for treatment rendered. Your health plan requires this information in order to bill, collect payments, or obtain approval prior to treatment.

Healthcare Operations—In order to ensure all patients receive timely and quality care, PHI will be used to facilitate the daily operations of our practice. These include, but are not limited to:
clinical/research studies to improve our practice
appointment reminders by phone calls or mailings
sign-in sheets used to notify us of your arrival
posted appointment schedules
information regarding your treatment options or related benefits and services
communications with family or friends that are involved in your care or payment for your care

---

PHI can be disclosed without your authorization in the following categories.

As Required by Law	Judicial and Administrative Proceedings	Oversight PHI can be disclosed to a health oversight agency as authorized by law for audits, investigations, inspections, and licensure.
Public Health	Lawsuits and Disputes	Workers' Compensation PHI may be released to workers' compensation or similar programs that provide benefits for work-related injuries or illness.
Public Health Risks	Law Enforcement	Military and Veterans
Health Research PHI disclosures are permitted when required by federal, state, tribal, or local laws.	Coroners and Medical Examiners Release of PHI to officials will occur: in response to a court order, subpoena, discovery request or summons; to identify a suspected fugitive, witness, or missing person; about a victim of crime if unable to obtain permission from the person; to identify a deceased person, determine cause of death, about a death that is believed to be the result of criminal conduct; criminal conduct occurring at the practice; in emergency situations.	National Security and Intelligence Activities

How the Health Insurance Portability and Accountability Act (HIPAA) Will Affect Your Next Dental Visit—cont'd

Abuse, Neglect, or Domestic Violence	Cadaver Organ, Eye, or Tissue Donations	Protective Services for the President and Others
PHI can be disclosed to prevent a threat to your health and safety or the health and safety of others.	PHI disclosure can be made to organ banks as necessary to facilitate organ or tissue donation and transplantation.	PHI may be released as authorized by law when requested by military command authorities, federal officials for national security, and protection of the president and other heads of state.

Dental Insurance Coverage

Responsibility for Payment

Your employer, management, or union has purchased dental insurance coverage from a selection of plans offered by an insurance company or broker. Each insurance company offers many different plans. The type of dental benefits that are covered relate to the dollar amount spent on the benefit package. Generally, the more money spent on a plan, the more services are covered. Most dental insurance covers only 50% to 80% of the cost of treatment. Major services (crowns, bridges, etc.), which are the most expensive dental procedures, are usually only covered at a 50% rate. For example, some dental benefit packages will not cover the fees for porcelain (tooth-colored material) crowns on teeth that are not visible when you talk or smile; they will only pay for a metal crown. Under this type of plan you must pay the full amount of the cost of the porcelain on those teeth. According to insurance companies, fillings in front teeth have both functional use and cosmetic components. They will pay for the functional part but not the full amount for the cosmetic restorations.

The fees charged for dental treatment reflect the many different parts of a particular procedure or procedures. Treatment for your particular needs may or may not fall within the limits set by your particular dental plan. Many dental procedures may not even be listed in your insurance's procedure/payment schedule. If your dental procedure falls into this category, you may not receive any insurance reimbursement for that procedure. **You are ultimately responsible for paying the entire fee for an accepted dental treatment, regardless of your insurance coverage.**

Choosing Treatment Options

Our goal through your examination, diagnosis, and treatment phases is to provide you with the best possible oral health. We do not allow the insurance company to tell us how to treat you. We recommend to you those treatments that we believe you need and we will discuss alternative plans with you. Whether or not the recommended treatment is a covered dental benefit is between you and your employer and the insurance carrier.

Submitting the Claim

We are happy to help you receive the maximum benefits you are allowed from your dental coverage. In order for us to submit your insurance claim, we will need an insurance form with your portion completed and signed. We deal with dental insurance companies on a daily basis; therefore, we have a great deal of experience submitting these claims to insurance carriers. We take great care in submitting claims properly the first time. There are three things we **cannot** do: 1) Alter the date of treatment; 2) Submit a claim for more than the actual fee; 3) Submit a claim for procedures that have not been performed. Because it is not at all uncommon for the insurance carriers to make a mistake, we would prefer to submit the claims ourselves, and then verify proper payment. Insurance carriers may respond to requests for payment of preauthorized treatment in as little as a week or as long as 45 days. Please be patient; we have no control over the post office or the speed with which the insurance carrier processes your claim.

Our office cannot negotiate with your insurance company for reimbursement of dental expenses. Only the purchaser of the plan (your employer) can negotiate better coverage. If you would like better or more coverage, you will need to talk with your plan purchaser about the features you want in your dental plan.

If you have any questions about your dental insurance coverage, please feel free to ask us.

Dental Insurance: Points to Consider

The following is a plain-language synopsis of most dental insurance contracts. Please read it carefully, and perhaps keep it for future reference.

✓ Dental insurance benefits do not work in the same way as medical insurance. There is ***almost always a co-payment*** due from the patient for ***almost every*** procedure.

✓ There are "deductibles" in all plans. At one time these deductibles were never taken out of preventive treatment ("cleanings"). Recently many carriers have begun to take deductibles out of preventive treatment.

✓ Insurance companies do not typically provide seminars or instruction books on the best method to obtain the highest financial reimbursement benefits for the patient.

✓ Irrespective of any dental insurance benefits that might exist, the patient is always legally responsible for the entire cost of dental treatment.

✓ The extent of dental coverage is solely dependent on the dental insurance plan purchased by the employer. The higher the premium the employer pays, the greater the dental insurance benefits.

✓ Even if there is a written predetermination of benefits returned from the insurance carrier, it is possible that after treatment is provided, there are no insurance benefits payable.

✓ We (the dental office) have absolutely no power or leverage to deal with the insurance carrier. Only the employee or the contract purchaser has power. Any complaints about benefits, payment, or coverage should be directed to Human Resources or the company owner.

✓ The letters *UCR* on insurance vouchers stand for *Usual, Customary, and Reasonable* fee. The dollar amount you see as UCR has no basis in reality. It is an arbitrary amount determined solely by the plan selected and insurance premium paid by the employee. There is no relationship to the actual dental office fee. The better the plan (i.e., the more premium paid), the higher the UCR will be.

✓ A single insurance carrier may have a dozen different UCR fees for the same procedure, same office, and same dentist.

✓ There is no universal coverage and payment schedule established. Just because an insurance code describing a dental service exists, it does not guarantee that it will be a paid benefit under your policy. There are many dental procedures that are necessary, and many of them are preventive, but are not covered benefits.

✓ Financial benefits cannot be saved and carried over into the next year.

✓ Your dental benefits almost always have a yearly maximum contribution level. This amount is the MOST your insurance carrier is contractually obligated to pay during a defined year (calendar or otherwise). When this amount is reached, there will be no further dental benefits payable until the next benefit year. If you have already begun some additional dental treatment prior to the maximum being reached, the insurance carrier has no payment obligation beyond that of the annual maximum.

Determination of Insurance Benefits

(Date)

Dear (patient name),

We have received the completed predetermination of benefits from your insurance carrier. You may also have received a copy of this predetermination of benefits form.

When you are ready to begin treatment, please call our office to review the treatment plan details and make the appropriate financial arrangements. Please note that your plan may have a limitation that requires treatment to begin within a set time period. When treatment does not begin within the set time period, the predetermination status may be canceled by your insurance carrier.

Sincerely,

Information Request

Date:

Dear (Patient):

In order to properly process and submit your dental insurance claim form for treatment provided on (date), we will need the following information (see below). For your convenience, a self-addressed stamped return envelope has been enclosed.

❑ Please fill out the entire enclosed form.
❑ Please fill out the entire patient portion of the enclosed form.
❑ Please sign the enclosed form in all places marked with an X.
❑ Please contact us concerning your claim form.

Thank you in advance for your prompt attention to this matter.

Sincerely,

Consent to Payment

Patient: _____   **Date:** _____

Account No:

I consent to authorize the indicated dental services (listed on Estimate of Fees form) to be performed. I understand that at any time I may terminate or postpone the proposed treatment. I have been informed of treatment alternatives that relate to my oral conditions, their respective advantages and disadvantages, the substantial risks and consequences of limited or delayed treatment or nontreatment. I have been informed of the costs of the dental treatment and alternative dental treatment. I have been informed of financial arrangements available to me. All questions have been answered to my satisfaction and I have read and understand the above directions and cautions.

Payment in full will be rendered at each appointment for dental treatment completed at that appointment. I will pay by
❑ MasterCard   ❑ VISA   ❑ Cash   ❑ Personal check at each appointment.

Payments are to be made for $_____ per month for _____ months.
Payment is due no later than the _____ day of the month.

Postdated checks or authorization of credit card for the balance of $_____ is to be
paid by _____ and the remaining balance of $_____ to be paid by _____ .

Coupon booklet: Payments to be received by the _____ day of the month for _____ months.
Monthly payment will be $_____ .

The estimate of fees for dental services is guaranteed for 90 days. If treatment is not begun within 90 days of the estimate date, cost of dental treatment could vary. Once dental treatment has begun, changes in the anticipated treatment plan may be required, depending on oral conditions encountered. I will be informed if this occurs and given the option of continuing treatment, changing treatment, or canceling treatment.

If my balance becomes 60 days or more overdue, the office reserves the right to interrupt or discontinue dental treatment and/or send my account to an attorney for collection. In the event that my account is sent for collection, I will be responsible for all costs and fees, including reasonable attorney's fees, incurred. If payment is not made within 30 days, my account will be charged at a rate of 1.5% per month. State dental regulations and standard-of-care legal options require that I be given treatment options, listed procedures, total fees for the procedures, and indicated financial arrangements. This is for the mutual protection of both the patient and the dentist.

Financial Coordinator:

_____   _____
Financial Coordinator's Signature   Date

_____   _____
Patient's or Guardian's Signature   Date

Estimate of Fees

Patient: _____   **Date:** _____

Insurance
Primary
Yearly maximum
Yearly deductible

Secondary
Yearly maximum
Yearly deductible

Tooth	Treatment	Ref#	Fee	Insurance Payment*	Your Co-Payment*

#Referral—This treatment is not provided by this dental office. You will be referred to a specialist for evaluation and treatment. They will inform you of exact treatment proposed, how long it will take, the cost involved, and answer any questions you may have. ***The fees for this treatment are not included in this treatment plan total.***

*This is *only an estimate* of your insurance payment. Insurance coverage for dental procedures varies tremendously among different carriers and different plans within the same carrier or employer. The actual insurance payment may be different than listed here. You will be responsible for the balance of the listed fee.

This treatment plan is designed with several goals: prevention of dental disease, minimal change to healthy tooth structure and gum tissue, and restoring teeth with materials that will last the longest with the fewest future problems. We want you to have teeth that are functional, a mouth that is pain-free, and an attractive smile for your lifetime.

Estimate of Fees

(BRIEF FORM)

Patient Name: _____   **Date:** _____

The following is a list of proposed dental treatment and an estimate of fees for that treatment.

Periodontal:
Total Fee: $ Estimated Insurance Payment: $ Patient payment: $

Restorative:
Total Fee: $ Estimated Insurance Payment: $ Patient payment: $

Endodontic:
Total Fee: $ Estimated Insurance Payment: $ Patient payment: $

Fixed Prosthetics:
Total Fee: $ Estimated Insurance Payment: $ Patient payment: $

Removable Prosthetics:
Total Fee: $ Estimated Insurance Payment: $ Patient payment: $

Cosmetic:

Total Fee: $ Estimated Insurance Payment: $ Patient payment: $

Financial Arrangements

Our goal in discussing financial arrangements relative to your dental needs includes:
- to inform you of treatment alternatives
- their respective advantages and disadvantages
- the consequences and/or risks of limited delayed treatment and/or nontreatment

We will discuss with you the costs of the dental treatment and alternative treatment. We will gladly answer your questions until you are completely satisfied.

Dental Insurance

We are happy to assist you in receiving your maximum dental insurance benefits. Dental insurance is a contract between your employer, who selects your coverage limits, and the insurance company. You (the subscriber) will receive the dental benefits as defined within this plan. Insurance payments received by this office will be credited to your account or refunded to you in the case of an overpayment. We cannot guarantee insurance carrier payments on office-generated insurance reimbursement estimates. You are responsible for all dental fees (charges) that your insurance company has not paid, for whatever reason, within a 60-day period from when treatment is begun. You will be expected to pay the full amount due.

Our office will accept assignment of dental insurance benefits directly to our office. Please bring your dental plan benefits booklet to our office to allow our staff to make a reasonable estimate of what the insurance company will pay for a given dental procedure. For an exact statement of benefits, a predetermination of benefits form can be sent to the insurance company. This process requires a dental insurance form with your section of the form completed to be used to request a predetermination of benefits from your insurance carrier. The insurance carrier will return the form stating their payment and your co-payment responsibility. You may need to bring in a completed insurance form for **each** appointment at which **new** treatment is begun.

Payment Options

In addition to accepting payments directly from your insurance carrier, financial arrangements need to be made for your co-payment. The co-payment is the difference between the treatment costs and the insurance payment. We offer a 5% courtesy discount for full payment prior to beginning treatment. Our financial coordinator can discuss monthly payment arrangements such as postdated checks, credit card authorization, and coupon booklets.

Fee Guarantees and Nonpayment Procedures

We are obligated by state regulations to be certain you understand your dental treatment needs, appropriate treatment and options, fees involved, and financial arrangements. This is for the mutual protection of both you and us.

The estimated fees we provide for dental services are guaranteed for 90 days. If treatment is not begun within 90 days of the estimate date, cost of dental treatment could vary. Once dental treatment has begun, changes in the anticipated treatment plan may be required, depending on oral conditions encountered. You will be informed if this occurs and given the option of continuing treatment, changing treatment, or canceling treatment.

If your balance becomes 60 days or more overdue, our office reserves the right to interrupt or discontinue dental treatment and/or send your account to an attorney for collection. In the event that your account is sent for collection, you will be responsible for all costs and fees, including reasonable attorney's fees, incurred. If payment is not made within 30 days, your account will be charged at a rate of 1.5% per month.

Preauthorization of Payment

I, (name of payer), authorize (name of dental office) to keep my signature on file and to charge my

❑ VISA   ❑ MasterCard   ❑ Other_____

the balance of charges not paid by dental insurance immediately on receipt of dental insurance co-payment or the balance of charges not paid within 30 days of completion of dental treatment and not to exceed $_____ for
  ❑ this appointment only
  ❑ all appointments this year.

Recurring charges for ongoing treatment or completed treatment of $_____ every
❑ week
❑ month
from (date) to (date). I assign my dental insurance benefits to the above-named provider.
I understand that this form is valid for 1 year from the date noted below unless I cancel authorization of the provider in writing.

Patient Name:
Cardholder Name:
Cardholder Address:
City, State, and Zip Code:
Credit Card Account #:   Expiration Date:

_____   _____
Cardholder Signature   Date

Schedule of Payment

Patient _____

Payment Arrangements

I understand the recommended dental treatment listed below or attached. The advantages/disadvantages of the procedures and alternate procedures, risks, and consequences of action or inaction have been explained to my satisfaction. I authorize the dentist or his or her authorized auxiliaries to perform the listed treatment. I am aware that I may delay or terminate treatment at any time. Treatment may be terminated for nonpayment of services performed. I have read the payment plan carefully and selected one of the payment options.

If I have dental insurance, the dental office will **estimate** what my cost will be. When the insurance payment is received, I will be immediately responsible for what is not covered. If the insurance coverage reimburses the office for more than what was estimated, I will be entitled to a credit or a refund, my choice. If I decide to prepay the entire estimated amount prior to beginning treatment, for any amount over $100, a 5% discount will be deducted from that amount. I understand cash, personal checks, and credit cards are accepted methods of payment.

❏ Payment in full at each appointment for treatment completed that day.

Date:_____	Appointment 1 $_____	Date:_____	Appointment 5 $_____
Date:_____	Appointment 2 $_____	Date:_____	Appointment 6 $_____
Date:_____	Appointment 3 $_____	Date:_____	Appointment 7 $_____
Date:_____	Appointment 4 $_____	Date:_____	Appointment 8 $_____

❏ Monthly payment of $_____ for _____ months.
   Initial payment of $_____ .
   A monthly payment coupon will be mailed to me.

❏ I will leave postdated checks to be deposited on the _____ day of each month.

❏ I will preauthorize payment by credit card: ❏ VISA   ❏ MasterCard
   My credit card will be charged $_____ on the _____ day of each month until fees are paid in full.
   Card # _____ Expiration Date: _____

I authorize payment directly to (name of dental office) of my dental benefits. I understand that I am solely responsible for all costs of the dental treatment. I authorize the dentist and dental staff to perform all diagnostic, preventive, and therapeutic procedures necessary for dental care. I permit the dentist to release any medical or dental information to other health practitioners or insurance carriers. My signature may be photocopied or the phrase "signature on file" may be used to help secure insurance benefits due.

Treatment Plan

Tooth # _____ Procedure: _____ Fee: $_____
This is an estimate only. Presenting conditions encountered when teeth are actually treated may require a change in fees. Treatment could be more or less extensive than originally determined. I understand that all efforts have been made by the dental office to estimate all dental procedure needs as accurately as possible. If a change occurs, I will be informed immediately, and treatment will not proceed without my approval.

Total fee for listed treatment: $_____

_____   _____
Patient's/Guardian's Signature   Date

Declination of Treatment

Patient Name: _____   **Date:** _____

The following dental treatment has been recommended by (dentist's name) to me on (date).

Advantages and disadvantages of treatment, risks of treatment and nontreatment, options, and fees have been disclosed. All of my questions have been answered to my satisfaction. I understand that in the future, a change in my oral health may make it impossible for the suggested treatment to be completed as explained today or may lead to a problem more expensive to repair. At this time, I decline to have the following treatment for me or for my child _____.

Periodontal:

Preventive:

Restorative:

Endodontic:

Prosthetic:

Oral Surgery:

_____   _____
Patient's/Guardian's Signature   Date

Dental Cosmetic Evaluation

Pupils: ❑ Horizontal   ❑ High Left   ❑ High Right

Nose: ❑ Centered   ❑ Left   ❑ Right

Lips at rest: ❑ Equal length left and right   ❑ Longer left   ❑ Longer right
   ❑ Horizontal   ❑ High Left   ❑ High Right

Dental midline centered: ❑ Under the nose   ❑ Under the lip
   ❑ In face   ❑ Over midline teeth #s 24 and 25

Left and right tooth symmetry/mirror image:

	8/9		7/10		6/11	
Length	❑ wnl	❑ no	❑ wnl	❑ no	❑ wnl	❑ no
Width	❑ wnl	❑ no	❑ wnl	❑ no	❑ wnl	❑ no
Vertical	❑ wnl	❑ no	❑ wnl	❑ no	❑ wnl	❑ no

Comments: _____

_____

Smile line: ❑ Low   ❑ Medium   ❑ High   ❑ Extended High
   ❑ Balanced   ❑ High Left   ❑ High Right

Smile extension: ❑ Normal   ❑ Forced/Artificial

Gingival Scalloping Architecture: ❑ "Classic" even   ❑ Irregular   #6   #7   #8   #9   #10   #11

Mirror Image Scalloping: 8/9   7/10   6/11
   ❑ yes ❑ no   ❑ yes ❑ no   ❑ yes ❑ no

Notes: _____

_____

Analysis of scalloping: _____

Evidence of abnormal wear–generated eruption:

	#7		#8		#9		#10	
	❑ yes	❑ no	❑ yes	❑ no	❑ yes	❑ no	❑ yes	❑ no

❑ **Orthodontic Consult**
❑ **Periodontal Consult**

Relative Dimension of Incisors:

	#6	#7	#8	#9	#10	#11
Length	_____	_____	_____	_____	_____	_____
Width	_____	_____	_____	_____	_____	_____

Problems with Relative Dimensions of Incisors: _____

Suggestions for Improvement: _____

Continued

Dental Cosmetic Evaluation—cont'd

Number of teeth visible at maximum smile width: _____ Maxillary _____ Mandibular

Incisal line: ❏ Horizontal "Normal"   ❏ Rises left–right   ❏ Rises right–left

Anterior/Posterior gingival line: ❏ Normal   ❏ Altered (describe) _____

❏ **Overbite** _____ mm   ❏ **Overjet** _____ mm   ❏ **Rotations,** tooth #s _____

❏ **Crowding,** tooth #s _____

❏ **Visible cementum,** tooth #s _____

❏ **Chipped teeth,** tooth #s _____

❏ **Visible toothbrush abrasions,** tooth #s _____

Attrition: Maxilla, tooth #s _____   Category: 1   2   3   4
                         Mandible, tooth #s _____   Category: 1   2   3   4

Lock and Key wear in:
❏ Direct   ❏ Protrusive   ❏ Right Lateral   ❏ Left Lateral   ❏ Right Oblique   ❏ Left Oblique

Stained Incisal Edges, tooth #s _____

Color of teeth   ❏ Uniform   ❏ Variable   Dominant hue _____

Striations   ❏ None   ❏ Present, tooth #s _____

White Spots   ❏ None   ❏ Present, tooth #s _____

Discolored restorations, tooth #s _____

Visible amalgams, tooth #s _____

Diastema acceptable to patient?   ❏ yes   ❏ no

Comments _____

_____

Suggestions for improvement _____

_____

Dental Hygiene Services: Dental Prophylaxis Visit

Patient Name: _____

Your dental prophylaxis visit on _____ included the following services:

- ❑ A review of your medical and dental history
- ❑ An oral cancer examination and soft tissue evaluation
- ❑ An oral self-care evaluation, including:
    - a. proper use of dental floss
    - b. toothbrushing technique
    - c. dental floss threaded technique
    - d. disclosing tablets/solution
    - e. evaluation of daily oral self-care habits
    - f. oral self-care product recommendation
    - g. other _____
- ❑ Intraoral radiographs
    - ❑ recare series   ❑ complete series   ❑ selected areas
- ❑ Periodontal evaluation, including:
    - a. measurement of sulcular depths (periodontal probing)
    - b. tooth mobility
    - c. furcation involvement
    - d. recession of gingival (gum) tissue
    - e. bleeding points
    - f. calculus deposits
- ❑ Dental caries (cavities) evaluation, including:
    - a. defective restorations
    - b. fractured teeth
    - c. decay
    - d. erosions and abrasions
    - e. attrition
- ❑ Ultrasonic removal of calculus (tartar)
- ❑ Root planing
- ❑ Subgingival irrigation of periodontal pockets with a medicated solution
- ❑ Prophylaxis and polish
- ❑ Topical fluoride application
- ❑ Sealant application on teeth numbers _____.
- ❑ Intraoral photographs/video
- ❑ Impressions for diagnostic study models and occlusal registration for model bite relation
- ❑ Vital/nonvital tooth whitening, tooth numbers _____.
- ❑ Application of root surface desensitizing agent on tooth numbers _____.
- ❑ Application of subgingival, site-specific medications, tooth numbers _____.

Hygienist's comments: _____

_____

_____

Examination/Consultation Overview

Patient Name:_____   **Date:**_____

Based on the comprehensive oral examination or consultation, the following areas of dental pathology or concern are noted. Please remember that this is **not** a specific treatment plan. It is a broad outline of what has been found, the proposed treatment, and the sequence of treatment. This will be followed by a detailed treatment plan listing specific services and fees. Some teeth may have more than one diagnosed problem; however, one dental procedure may be all that is needed to correct the condition.

Areas of Dental Pathology or Concern

Periodontal disease category:

Quantity of Teeth	UR	UL	LR	LL	
____	____	____	____	____	❏ Loose or hopeless teeth
____	____	____	____	____	❏ Broken teeth
____	____	____	____	____	❏ Decayed front teeth
____	____	____	____	____	❏ Decayed back teeth
____	____	____	____	____	❏ Teeth requiring endodontic treatment (root canal)
____	____	____	____	____	❏ Defective restorations in front teeth
____	____	____	____	____	❏ Defective restorations in back teeth
____	____	____	____	____	❏ Missing teeth to be replaced
____	____	____	____	____	❏ Poorly aligned teeth
____	____	____	____	____	❏ Crowns for front teeth
____	____	____	____	____	❏ Crowns/onlays for back teeth
____	____	____	____	____	❏ Toothbrush abrasions
____	____	____	____	____	❏ Attrition
____	____	____	____	____	❏ Cosmetic tooth whitening
____	____	____	____	____	❏ Cosmetic bonding (porcelain)
____	____	____	____	____	❏ Cosmetic bonding (resin)
____	____	____	____	____	❏ Replacement of discolored fillings
____	____	____	____	____	❏ Replacement of metal fillings
____	____	____	____	____	❏ Cosmetic plastic surgery

Overview of Treatment Sequence

_____	Periodontal treatment	Office:_____	Referral to specialist: _____
_____	Endodontics	Office:_____	Referral to specialist: _____
_____	Oral Surgery	Office:_____	Referral to specialist: _____
_____	Orthodontics	Office:_____	Referral to specialist: _____
_____	Operative (fillings)		
_____	Cosmetic		
_____	Prosthetics (crowns, inlays, onlays)		
_____	Replace missing teeth		
_____	Other: _____		

Medical History Update

Patient Name: _____

Has there been any change in your medical history since your last dental appointment?   ❑ Yes   ❑ No
   If yes, please explain: _____

Are you taking *any* medication? Be sure to include any NONPRESCRIPTION medicines you are taking.
   ❑ Yes   ❑ No   If yes, please list medications: _____
_____

_____   _____
Patient's or Guardian's signature   Date

Has there been any change in your medical history since your last dental appointment?   ❑ Yes   ❑ No
   If yes, please explain: _____

Are you taking *any* medication? Be sure to include any NONPRESCRIPTION medicines you are taking.
   ❑ Yes   ❑ No   If yes, please list medications: _____
_____

_____   _____
Patient's or Guardian's signature   Date

Has there been any change in your medical history since your last dental appointment?   ❑ Yes   ❑ No
   If yes, please explain: _____

Are you taking *any* medication? Be sure to include any NONPRESCRIPTION medicines you are taking.
   ❑ Yes   ❑ No   If yes, please list medications: _____
_____

_____   _____
Patient's or Guardian's signature   Date

Has there been any change in your medical history since your last dental appointment?   ❑ Yes   ❑ No
   If yes, please explain: _____

Are you taking *any* medication? Be sure to include any NONPRESCRIPTION medicines you are taking.
   ❑ Yes   ❑ No   If yes, please list medications: _____
_____

_____   _____
Patient's or Guardian's signature   Date

Has there been any change in your medical history since your last dental appointment?   ❑ Yes   ❑ No
   If yes, please explain: _____

Are you taking *any* medication? Be sure to include any NONPRESCRIPTION medicines you are taking.
   ❑ Yes   ❑ No   If yes, please list medications: _____
_____

_____   _____
Patient's or Guardian's signature   Date

Next Appointment Procedure

At your next appointment, the following procedures will be performed. If you have been told that you need to take a prophylactic antibiotic 1 hour prior to your appointment, please remember to take it. The appointment is scheduled for _____ minutes. It is possible that at the next appointment an unexpected situation may arise that will cause the anticipated treatment to be modified. If this happens, you will be informed immediately.

Periodontal
_____ Scaling and Root Planing
      Quadrant ❑ UR   ❑ LR   ❑ UL   Local anesthesia may be required.
_____ Periodontal surgery

Restorative
_____ Bonded, tooth-colored restorations
    ❑ Front teeth
    ❑ Back teeth
_____ Post
_____ Core
_____ Crown lengthening
_____ Preparation for crown _____ inlay _____ onlay
_____ Impression for crown _____ inlay _____ onlay
_____ Dental implant procedure _____
_____ Preparation for bridge
_____ Impression for bridge
_____ Try-in casting
_____ Provisional cementation
_____ Final cementation

Endodontics
_____ Begin root canal, tooth #_____
_____ Continue root canal, tooth #_____
_____ Finish root canal treatment, tooth #_____

Oral Surgery
_____ Extraction
_____ Other

Removable Prosthetics
_____ Preliminary impressions, registrations, face bow transfer
_____ Final impressions
_____ Try-in framework
_____ Try-in wax setup
_____ Delivery of full or partial denture

If you have any questions about any of the procedures or fees, please ask before you make your next appointment.

Patient Education Request

Please check off what you would like to receive. Then either mail this back to us along with your name and address, drop it off at the office, or call to let us know what information you would like to have sent to you.

CHILDREN

- ❏ A Child's First Visit to the Dentist — 203
- ❏ Prevention of Dental Disease in Infants and Children — 206
- ❏ Sealants — 207
- ❏ Eruption Patterns of Teeth — 205
- ❏ Orthodontics: An Overview — 198
- ❏ Care of Braces — 196

PERIODONTICS

- ❏ Prophylaxis (teeth cleaning) — 234
- ❏ Early Signs of Periodontal Disease — 215
- ❏ Gingivitis — 218
- ❏ Periodontal Disease — 221

RESTORATIVE PROCEDURES

- ❏ Bonded Resin Restorations — 118
- ❏ Defective Restorations — 293
- ❏ Crowns: An Overview — 252
- ❏ Bridges: An Overview — 262
- ❏ Implants: Options — 267
- ❏ Implants: Procedure Overview — 268
- ❏ Have Missing Teeth Replaced — 250

ENDODONTIC

- ❏ Endodontic Therapy: An Overview — 139
- ❏ Endodontic Therapy: Procedure — 140

COSMETICS

- ❏ Cosmetic Dentistry — 119
- ❏ The Perfect Smile — 125
- ❏ You Can Have Whiter Teeth — 127
- ❏ Tooth Whitening: Overview and Options — 126
- ❏ Replacing Unesthetic Restorations — 124
- ❏ Fluorosis, Mottled Enamel, and White Spots — 116

GENERAL

- ❏ Have the Dentistry You Need, Want, and Deserve — 149
- ❏ For a Lifetime of Great Oral Health — 160
- ❏ Treating the Adult Patient — 159
- ❏ Initial Oral Examination — 151
- ❏ Dental and Oral Anatomy — 148
- ❏ Radiographs (x-rays) — 164
- ❏ Bad Breath — 171
- ❏ How to Brush, How to Floss — 161
- ❏ Headaches: The Dental Connection — 179
- ❏ TMJ Dysfunction (TMD) Syndrome — 189
- ❏ Prevention of Decay — 163
- ❏ Reversing Decay — 165
- ❏ Supplemental Fluoride — 209
- ❏ Topical Fluoride — 167
- ❏ Junk Drink Alert — 162
- ❏ Sensitive Teeth — 187
- ❏ Wisdom Teeth—Third Molars — 192
- ❏ Sealants and Fluoride: Benefit to Adult Patients — 166

Your Name: _____

Address: _____

_____

City, State, Zip _____

Treatment Goals

Our goal in recommending the best treatment to meet your specific dental needs is to help you have the best oral health possible. Our treatment plan recommendation will be based on our many years of full-time clinical practice and research. When appropriate, we will also suggest treatment options from which you can make your selection. All options will be explained to you along with the advantages and disadvantages of each option. Using this information and knowledge of your own personal situation (such as the time you have available for treatment and financial considerations), together with our years of successful dental practice we can, together, choose the best plan for you.

We design treatment plans with several goals: prevention of dental disease, minimal change to healthy tooth structure and gum tissue, and restoring teeth with materials that will last the longest with the fewest future problems. Ultimately, we want you to have teeth that are functional, a mouth that is pain-free, and an attractive smile when you are 95 years old.

Insurance coverage for dental procedures varies tremendously among the many different insurance carriers, just as plans within the same carrier or employer can differ. The variations can affect deductible amounts, patient co-payments, and procedure coverage. At no time will we let any dental insurance coverage dictate your treatment. Whether you have no dental insurance, or some form of dental insurance, our recommendations will be the same.

While we will assist you with insurance submission for treatment you have had completed, you are responsible for payment not covered within 60 days (for any reason) by your insurance carrier. Payment plans for extensive dental treatment can be set up for you. Dental treatment for cosmetic improvement is rarely a covered dental benefit, regardless of the insurance plan you have. Several of the newer, innovative methods of restoring teeth, replacing missing teeth (dental implants), or regenerating bone or gum tissue may not be covered expenses. This is not because they are experimental procedures, but rather because coverage for them has not yet been purchased by your employer.

If you have any questions about your treatment and your insurance coverage, please feel free to ask us.

chapter 3

Insurance Narratives

Content at a Glance: Insurance Narratives

Keep the most commonly misunderstood procedures from becoming mired in the denial/appeal process by giving the appropriate supporting information and codes right from the start. These narratives allow the insurance company's dental consultant to see how and where various procedures fit into the benefit plan. All letters allow space at the top for your letterhead. Additional letters in this section can help solve other common insurance problems.

These items serve two purposes:
1. To maximize insurance reimbursement to patient.
2. To show patient, through patient copy, that you are trying the best you can to get proper reimbursement for him or her.

These may possibly generate better payment for a procedure, and they will surely help cement a stronger patient/dentist relationship.

Procedure Information Narrative
Documents are organized in three dental topic areas: Endodontics, Preventive/Periodontics, and Restorative Dentistry.

Problem Resolution
Changed Benefit Coding
Requests a review of codes that an insurance carrier has altered to restore them to a payable service.

Complaint to Insurance Commissioner
When the insurance company does not respond, engages in protracted delays, or keeps asking for information already sent, outside help can get things moving again. This letter is easy to individualize for your specific needs.

Information Narrative
Provides a form for specific procedure narration.

Predetermination of Benefits
Form for requesting a predetermination of benefits, with a space for specific narrative comments.

Radiographic Request Response
A response to an insurance carrier when radiographs have been requested but that will not add to the determination of disease and therefore appropriate treatment.

Request for Insurance Recoding
This letter requests reconsideration of a claim for a fixed bridge when it is not a policy benefit.

Apicoectomy

Patient:
Patient Soc. Sec. No.:
Patient ❑ **is** ❑ **is not** **the subscriber**

Insurance Carrier:
Group No.:
Employer:
Subscriber:

Re: ADA code #s:
- ❑ D3410 Apicoectomy Anterior Tooth, tooth #
- ❑ D3421 Apicoectomy Bicuspid First Root, tooth #
- ❑ D3425 Apicoectomy Molar First Root, tooth #
- ❑ D3426 Apicoectomy Each Additional Root, tooth #
- ❑ D3426 Apicoectomy Each Additional Root, tooth #
- ❑ D3430 Retrograde Filling, tooth #   , first root
- ❑ D3430 Retrograde Filling, tooth #   , additional root
- ❑ D3430 Retrograde Filling, tooth #   , additional root
- ❑ D3450 Root Amputation, first tooth #   , first root
- ❑ D3450 Root Amputation, first tooth #   , additional root

Date:

Dear Dental Consultant:

The following narrative will give further information about the treatment rendered to the patient on _____. Due to residual periapical pathology subsequent to endodontic treatment, the above indicated procedures were performed. The diagnosis was confirmed by:
- ❑ Chronic pain
- ❑ Fistula
- ❑ Tenderness to palpation/percussion
- ❑ Radiographic evidence of periapical pathology
- ❑ Endodontic-periodontic syndrome
- ❑ Calcified or severely dilacerated canals, unable to negotiate nonsurgically
- ❑ Separated instrument in canal, unable to remove nonsurgically
- ❑ Unable to remove existing endodontic filling material
- ❑ Other:

❑ Radiograph enclosed.

All customary postoperative appointments are included in the fee.

If you have any questions, please feel free to contact the office. Please apply the appropriate contract benefits to the procedures listed on the insurance form. If the listed procedures are not covered procedures and payment codes of your insurance company, please recode and apply alternate benefits as indicated.

Thank you.

Sincerely,

copy/(patient)

Nonvital Tooth Whitening

Patient: **Insurance Carrier:**
Patient Soc. Sec. No.:   **Group No.:**
Patient ❑ **is** ❑ **is not**   **the subscriber**   **Employer:**
                                                             Subscriber:

Re: ADA code #s:
    ❑ D3999 Nonvital whitening, endodontically treated tooth
    ❑ D9974 Internal whitening–per tooth

Date:

Dear Dental Consultant:

The following narrative will give further information about the treatment rendered to the patient. Tooth # _____ had been treated endodontically
    ❑ on _____,
    ❑ approximately _____ years ago, unknown completion date

The tooth has discolored significantly from the natural dentition. A nonvital whitening sequence was performed on this tooth. It involved removal of the coronal gutta percha obturation material and placement of a glass ionomer sealer over the canal opening.

❑ The whitening was accomplished by using an oxidizing whitening solution (hydrogen peroxide, 35%) and application of light/heat energy to activate the whitening chemicals.

❑ The whitening was accomplished by using an oxidizing solution in an office procedure of ___ minutes. The application of the bleach was repeated on ____ separate appointments made on the following dates: (Enter dates here).

❑ The whitening was accomplished by using a mixture of sodium perborate and Superoxol or water mixed to a paste consistency, followed by a provisional restoration to secure the access preparation. This procedure may have to be repeated several times before adequate color change is obtained.

❑ The fee for the initial preparation and glass ionomer/bonded restoration/restoration is $
❑ The fee for each whitening application is $
❑ The total whitening fee, exclusive of the final restoration is $

Comments:

Please apply the appropriate contract benefits to the procedures listed on the insurance form. If the listed procedures are not covered procedures and pay codes of your insurance company, please recode and apply alternate benefits as indicated, to fill your contractual liability with the purchaser of the contract.

If you have any questions, please feel free to contact our office. Thank you.

Sincerely,

copy/(patient)

Re-treatment of Endodontics

Patient:
Patient Soc. Sec. No.:
Patient ❏ **is** ❏ **is not** **the subscriber**

Insurance Carrier:
Group No.:
Employer:
Subscriber:

Re: ADA code #s:
- ❏ D3346 Re-treatment Endodontics, Anterior Tooth
- ❏ D3347 Re-treatment Endodontics, Bicuspid Tooth
- ❏ D3348 Re-treatment Endodontics, Molar Tooth

Date:

Dear Dental Consultant:

The following narrative will give further information about the treatment rendered to the patient on _____ .
Tooth # _____ required re-treatment of previously performed endodontics. The previously performed endodontics was completed approximately _____ years ago. The reason for the re-treatment is:
- ❏ Apical reinfection, noted by draining fistulous tract.
- ❏ Apical reinfection, radiographic radiolucent periapical area.
- ❏ Apical reinfection, noted by pressure/swelling/pain.
- ❏ Apical reinfection associated with endodontic-periodontic syndrome.
- ❏ Clinically unacceptable endodontic canal fill/condensation. No radiographic evidence of apical healing.
- ❏ Loose silver points in canals, silver point cement washout.
- ❏ This tooth exhibited a mechanical or natural obstruction that required more time to negotiate.

The re-treatment required greater technical skill and a longer treatment time in removing the existing endodontic filling material and negotiating the canal(s). It is more difficult to remove set endodontic sealer/cement and obturation materials than to initially treat any canal. A higher fee is appropriate for re-treatment endodontics.

Comments:

Please apply the appropriate contract benefits to the procedures listed on the insurance form. If the listed procedures are not covered procedures and pay codes of your insurance company, please recode and apply alternate benefits as indicated.

If you have any questions, please feel free to contact our office. Thank you.

Sincerely,

copy/(patient)

Bruxism: Full Arch Appliance

Patient: **Insurance Carrier:**
Patient Soc. Sec. No.:   **Group No.:**
Patient ❑ **is** ❑ **is not** **the subscriber**   **Employer:**
                                                                Subscriber:

Re: ADA code #:
     D9940 Occlusal Guard Appliance

Date:

Dear Dental Consultant:

This is a request for a predetermination of coverage liabilities.

This patient has been diagnosed as suffering from the effects of bruxing and/or clenching. The patient clinically exhibits clear evidence of an abnormally worn dentition. The wear is clearly pathologic and beyond what would be expected for a patient of this age. There ❑ are ❑ are not temporomandibular (TMD) syndrome symptoms.

Treatment will consist of upper and lower full-arch study models for occlusal analysis, followed by laboratory fabrication of a rigid, full maxillary bruxism appliance. It is not flat plane, but rather has been adjusted with indentations for all cusp tips and incisal edges. There is, where possible, exclusively canine-guided disclusion for left and right lateral excursions. In protrusive movements there is posterior disclusion. A final adjustment will be made with the patient in a supine and seated position.

Fees for this procedure include the following: study models, occlusal analysis, bruxism appliance fabrication, final adjustment prior to delivery, delivery, follow-up appointments, and readjustments as needed.

With proper patient compliance, the prognosis is good. The wear rate of the natural dentition should decrease to normal physiologic levels. If the bruxing/clenching continues in the presence of the appliance, it is expected that a new appliance may have to be made in the future.

If you have any questions about the diagnosis or treatment of this patient with respect to this procedure, please contact our office. Thank you.

Sincerely,

copy/(patient)

Bruxism: Tension Suppression System

Patient:
Patient Soc. Sec. No.:
Patient ❏ **is** ❏ **is not** **the subscriber**

Insurance Carrier:
Group No.:
Employer:
Subscriber:

Re: ADA code #:
    D9940 Occlusal Guard Appliance

Date:

Dear Dental Consultant:

This is a request for a predetermination of coverage liabilities.

This patient has been diagnosed as suffering from the effects of bruxing and/or clenching. The patient clinically exhibits clear evidence of an abnormally worn dentition. The wear is clearly pathologic and beyond what would be expected for a patient of this age. There ❏ are ❏ are not temporomandibular (TMD) syndrome symptoms.

Treatment will consist of the fabrication of a tension suppression system intraoral device that will be custom fabricated in the dental office.

Fees for this procedure include the following: occlusal analysis, bruxism appliance fabrication, delivery, follow-up appointments, and readjustments as needed.

With proper patient compliance, the prognosis is good. The wear rate of the natural dentition should decrease to normal physiologic levels. If the bruxing/clenching continues in the presence of the appliance, it is expected that a new appliance may have to be made in the future.

If you have any questions about the diagnosis or treatment of this patient with respect to this procedure, please contact our office. Thank you.

Sincerely,

copy/(patient)

Desensitization: Entire Dentition

Patient: **Insurance Carrier:**
Patient Soc. Sec. No.:   **Group No.:**
Patient   ❏ **is**   ❏ **is not**   **the subscriber**   **Employer:**
                                                               Subscriber:

Date:

Dear Dental Consultant:

❏ This adult patient was treated with office-applied topical desensitization medication fluoride (D9910) subsequent to adult prophylaxis procedures (D1110). This was done with iontophoresis, tray application, or a combination of both modalities. These clinical procedures have been shown, in numerous studies, to reduce and possibly eliminate the pain elicited by thermal changes in the affected sites. The procedure was performed to reduce moderate to severe tooth sensitivity, probably caused by age-related migration of gingival tissues, mechanical/inadvertent abusive oral self-care, or purposeful surgical repositioning of the marginal gingival tissues.

If you have any questions about the services rendered, please feel free to contact the office.

Sincerely,

copy/(patient)

Desensitization: Site-Specific

Patient:
Patient Soc. Sec. No.:
Patient   ❑ **is**   ❑ **is not**   **the subscriber**

Insurance Carrier:
Group No.:
Employer:
Subscriber:

Re: ADA code #s:
   ❑ D9910 Application of Desensitizing Medication
   ❑ D9911 Application of Desensitizing Resin for cervical and/or root surface, per tooth

Date:

Dear Dental Consultant:

The patient has experienced extreme dentinal sensitivity of tooth #s _____. This sensitivity to hot and cold manifests when the patient eats or drinks anything that is above or below the normal oral cavity temperature.

Each tooth was individually isolated and treated with:
   ❑ Enamel/dentin bonding agent and/or restorative resin
   ❑ Fluoride
   ❑ Iontophoresis
   ❑ Desensitizing solution

Following the application of the desensitizing material on _____, the discomfort to thermal change was reduced or eliminated. I expect the material to be retained for several months. If the sensitivity returns, the material will be reapplied.

If this procedure is a covered benefit, please remit the appropriate compensation. If the procedure is not coded correctly for your reporting purposes, please recode according to the details supplied in this narrative and apply for the proper dental benefit.

If there are any questions, please feel free to contact our office. Thank you.

Sincerely,

copy/(patient)

Dental Hygiene Appointment

Patient: **Insurance Carrier:**
Patient Soc. Sec. No.:   **Group No.:**
Patient ❑ **is** ❑ **is not** **the subscriber**   **Employer:**
                                                       Subscriber:

Date:

Dear Dental Consultant:

The following narrative will give further information about the treatment to the above named patient on this date.

❑ D1330 Oral Self-Care Instruction
   The fee of $ _____ is a one-time fee, charged at the time of the first appointment only. All other oral self-care instruction will not be
   a separate charge.

   This patient is receiving periodontal therapeutic treatment for diagnosed periodontal disease, periodontal disease type_____ . It is not a
   Preventive Periodontal Prophylaxis, ADA 01110. The fee for oral self-care instruction includes demonstration and instruction of proper
   toothbrushing, use of dental floss, periodontal cleaning aids, disclosing of plaque, the use of appropriate rinses, instruction in the use of
   subgingival irrigation where required, and video presentations.

   The patient has demonstrated an understanding of and can successfully perform these functions.

   The patient will have these oral self-care instructions repeated during each of the anticipated_____ appointments in this treatment sequence.
   Total time spent in oral self-care instruction will be approximately_____ minutes.

❑ D1110 Adult Prophylaxis
   An additional fee of $ _____ has been charged to this patient for the adult prophylaxis. Although the diagnosis of gingivitis has been
   made, ❑ extra time ❑ extra appointments have been scheduled. Length of extra time needed:_____ minutes per appointment.
   Number of extra appointments needed:_____ .
   The reason(s) for the extra fee is:
      ❑ Length of time since last prophylaxis appointment. The patient's last prophylaxis appointment was completed on_____ .
      ❑ Excessive accumulations of calculus, which required extra time to remove.
      ❑ Excessive stain present, which required extra time to remove.
      ❑ The patient presented a management problem and therefore required more time for treatment and/or oral self-care instruction.

Please apply the appropriate contract benefits to the procedures listed on the insurance form. If the listed procedures are not covered procedures and
pay codes of your insurance company, please recode and apply alternate benefits as indicated, to fill your contractual liability with the purchaser of
the contract.

If you have any questions, please feel free to contact the office. Thank you.

Sincerely,

copy/(patient)

Periodontal Diagnosis

Patient:
Patient Soc. Sec. No.:
Patient ❏ **is** ❏ **is not** **the subscriber**

Insurance Carrier:
Group No.:
Employer:
Subscriber:

Date:

Dear Dental Consultant:

This letter provides supplemental information to aid in your review of this claim for dental benefits.

The following are the American Academy of Periodontology's definitions of the case types as used for diagnosis identification.

   I. **Gingival Diseases:** An inflammation or lesion of the gingiva characterized by changes of color, gingival form, position, surface appearance, and presence of bleeding and/or exudate.

  II. **Chronic Periodontitis:** An inflammation of the periodontium associated with plaque and calculus. The rate of progression is impacted by local, systemic, or environmental factors. It can be further classified as localized or generalized.

 III. **Aggressive Periodontitis:** Rapid rate of periodontal disease progression in an otherwise healthy individual, in the absence of large accumulations of plaque and/or calculus. It can be further classified as localized or generalized.

  IV. **Periodontitis as a Manifestation of Systemic Disease:** Periodontitis associated with hematologic or genetic disorders.

   V. **Necrotizing Periodontal Diseases:** Ulcerated and necrotic papillary and marginal gingiva. It can be further classified as necrotizing ulcerative gingivitis or necrotizing ulcerative periodontitis.

  VI. **Abscesses of the Periodontium:** A localized purulent infection of the periodontal tissue.

 VII. **Periodontitis Associated with Endodontic Lesions:** Localized deep periodontal pocket extending to the apex of the tooth, preceded by pulpal necrosis.

VIII. **Developmental or Acquired Deformities and Conditions:** Gingival disease or periodontitis initiated by localized tooth-related factors that modify or predispose to plaque accumulation or prevention of effective oral self-care measures.

Treatment at this time consisted of periodontal evaluation, periodontal pocket charting, scaling, root planing, medicated irrigation of periodontal pockets, polishing, oral self-care instruction, and reevaluation of periodontal condition. Treatment required _____ appointments.

Enclosed, please find   ❏ radiographs   ❏ claim form   ❏ charting   ❏ other:

Sincerely,

copy/(patient)

Periodontal Prognosis

Patient: **Insurance Carrier:**
Patient Soc. Sec. No.:   **Group No.:**
Patient ❑ **is** ❑ **is not** **the subscriber**   **Employer:**
                                                      Subscriber:

Re: Prognosis of periodontal related treatment

Date:

Dear Dental Consultant:

At this time, the prognosis for the areas involved in treatment for correction of periodontal pathology is classified as:
❑ I Gingival Disease
❑ II Chronic Periodontitis
❑ III Aggressive Periodontitis
❑ IV Periodontitis as a Manifestation of Systemic Disease
❑ V Necrotizing Periodontal Disease
❑ VI Abscesses of the Periodontium
❑ VII Periodontitis Associated with Endodontic Lesions
❑ VIII Developmental or Acquired Deformities

Condition, except as otherwise noted, is generally:

❑ excellent   ❑ good   ❑ fair   ❑ guarded   ❑ poor   ❑ hopeless

Comments:

Please note that the prognosis for this case can change at any time. Some of the factors affecting the prognosis are treatment results, healing, patient's motivation, patient's daily self-care routine, patient's systemic health, and the preventive maintenance care (D4910) interval.

As of this date, the active periodontal therapy has:
❑ not started   ❑ started   ❑ been completed

Future treatment (if the active phase of treatment has been completed) involves periodontal maintenance procedures (code D4910) on a _____ month interval, periodontal charting and evaluation at each appointment, and continued oral self-care instruction.

If you have any questions about any aspects of this case, please feel free to contact our office.

Sincerely,

copy/(patient)

Scaling/Root Planing

Patient: **Insurance Carrier:**
Patient Soc. Sec. No.:   **Group No.:**
Patient ❑ **is** ❑ **is not**   **the subscriber**   **Employer:**
                                                          Subscriber:

Re: ADA code #s:
   ❑ D4341 Root Planing and Scaling by Quadrant
   ❑ D4342 Root Planing and Scaling, 1-3 teeth per Quadrant

Date:

Dear Dental Consultant:

The following narrative will give further information about the treatment rendered to the patient on this date. The patient had root planing and scaling performed for his or her ❑ UR ❑ UL ❑ LR ❑ LL quadrants. These quadrants had at least five remaining natural teeth. The reasons for completing two full quadrants of root planing and scaling in one appointment were:

   ❑ The patient comes from a long distance to this office and time constraints with respect to the patient's employment or family situation were evident. It was easier for the patient to spend several long appointments receiving treatment rather than many more shorter appointments. Actual treatment time was not decreased.

   ❑ The appointment today was a double appointment, 2 hours in length. This is exactly the same total amount of time that would be spent for the code 4341 procedure if two quadrants were completed on different dates of treatment. The patient should not suffer financial loss of contracted dental benefits because the ❑ UR ❑ UL ❑ LR ❑ LL quadrants were completed on the same day.

Enclosed and attached, please find the initial periodontal charting and diagnosis and a copy of the complete and exact treatment services provided, by quadrant.

Please apply the appropriate contract benefits to the procedures listed on the insurance form. With the information I have provided, I would expect full benefit payment for the code 4341 procedures thus far completed. If this is not to be done and the patient's benefits are to be decreased from the maximum permitted, I ask that the dental consultant speak to me personally to explain.

If you have any questions, please feel free to contact our office. Thank you.

Sincerely,

copy/(patient)

Site-Specific Therapy

Patient: **Insurance Carrier:**
Patient Soc. Sec. No.:   **Group No.:**
Patient ❑ **is** ❑ **is not**   **the subscriber**   **Employer:**
                                                    Subscriber:

Re: ADA Code #:
   D4381 Localized delivery of chemotherapeutic agents via a controlled-release vehicle in diseased reticular tissue per tooth, by report.

Date:

Dear Dental Consultant:

Tooth #s _____ have been treated with:

   ❑ Arestin®   ❑ Atridox®
   ❑ Periochip®   ❑ Other _____

This therapy includes the cost of the material, placement of the material into the diseased pocket, oral self-care instruction, removal of material (if required), and necessary follow-up appointments to evaluate the results of the treatment.

Scaling and root planing of the treated area were previously completed as a primary therapeutic procedure. This material was placed because this site was unresponsive to the conventional therapy. This patient has a history of prior periodontal therapy.

The above-noted material was placed into the diseased periodontal pocket due to the following recorded depths:

Tooth # _____ MB   B   DB   Tooth # _____ MB   B   DB
                  ML   L   DL   ML   L   DL

Enclosed please find:
   ❑ Periodontal chart
   ❑ Radiographs

Please note that because of the location of the treated area, it is possible that the existing bone loss and/or probable pocket depth may not be evident and may only be able to be detected clinically.

If you are unfamiliar with the material or technique, or have questions about the treatment rendered to this patient, please contact our office.

Sincerely,

copy/(patient)

Splinting

Patient:
Patient Soc. Sec. No.:
Patient ❏ **is** ❏ **is not** **the subscriber**

Insurance Carrier:
Group No.:
Employer:
Subscriber:

Re: ADA Code #s:
   ❏ D4320 Provisional Splinting, Intracoronal
   ❏ D4321 Provisional Splinting, Extracoronal

Date:

Dear Dental Consultant:

The following narrative will give further information about the treatment rendered to the patient on _____ .

❏ Splinting of the teeth is required **prior to periodontal treatment** due to tooth mobility.

❏ Splinting of the teeth is required **after the periodontal treatment** due to tooth mobility in order to aid in the healing of the soft and hard periodontal tissues.

Enclosed, please find: ❏ Preoperative radiograph   ❏ Preoperative photograph

Please apply the appropriate contract benefits to the procedures listed on the insurance form. If the listed procedures are not covered procedures and payment codes of your insurance company, please recode and apply alternate benefits as indicated.

If you have any questions, please feel free to contact our office. Thank you.

Sincerely,

copy/(patient)

Subgingival Irrigation

Patient: **Insurance Carrier:**
Patient Soc. Sec. No.:   **Group No.:**
Patient ❑ **is** ❑ **is not   the subscriber**   **Employer:**
                                                               Subscriber:

Re: ADA code #s:
   ❑ D9630 Other Drugs and/or Medications
   ❑ D4999 Unspecified, by Report

Date:

Dear Dental Consultant:

The patient   ❑ has undergone   ❑ will undergo subgingival medication with the following medication(s): chlorhexidine gluconate 0.12%, sodium fluoride 2.0%, hydrogen peroxide 1.7%, zinc chloride 1.0%. This procedure was done for tooth #s_____; or the   ❑ UR   ❑ UL   ❑ LR   ❑ LL quadrant(s). The purpose of the subgingival irrigation is to deliver the medicated solution to the area so that pathogenic bacteria might be killed and removed. The worst type of plaque has been proven to be unattached plaque that resides in the pathologic periodontal pocket. This type of plaque is more virulent than supragingival attached plaque, and removal of the subgingival plaque by irrigation will benefit the patient's periodontal health. Subgingival irrigation has also been proven, in numerous studies, to reduce or eliminate bleeding and other signs of periodontal infection/inflammation from areas of increased sulcular depth.

The subgingival irrigation procedures to be completed will be done by:
   ❑ tooth #s: _____
   ❑ quadrant (defined as five teeth or more per quadrant) number and location of quadrant:
   ❑ arch

If subgingival irrigation or application of a medicated solution is a covered benefit for the patient under his or her dental benefits contract, please ensure proper treatment coding for the procedure according to your payment code schedule.

If you have any questions, please contact me personally. Thank you.

Sincerely,

copy/(patient)

Topical Fluoride Treatment in the Presence of Active Caries

Patient: **Insurance Carrier:**
Patient Soc. Sec. No.:   **Group No.:**
Patient   ❑ **is**   ❑ **is not**   **the subscriber**   **Employer:**
                                                      Subscriber:

Date:

Dear Dental Consultant:

❑ This adult patient was treated with a topically applied fluoride (code D9630 Other Drugs and Medications by Report) with an intraoral tray delivery. The reason for the fluoride application was either the discovery of active carious lesions that are to be treated or a recent past history of active carious lesions. Application of the topical fluoride is intended to either slow the progression of the caries process and/or reduce the severity and incidence of this disease.

If you have any questions about the services rendered, please feel free to contact our office.

Sincerely,

copy/(patient)

Crown Lengthening

Patient: **Insurance Carrier:**
Patient Soc. Sec. No.:   **Group No.:**
Patient ❏ **is** ❏ **is not** **the subscriber**   **Employer:**
                                                      Subscriber:

Re: ADA code #s:
   ❏ D4249 Crown lengthening, by report
   ❏ D4211 Gingivectomy

Date:

Dear Dental Consultant:

A crown lengthening procedure   ❏ was   ❏ will be performed on tooth #s_____
The reason for the crown lengthening is:
   ❏ Removal of hyperplastic and/or redundant tissue.
   ❏ Removal of edematous tissue.
   ❏ Exposure of deep or extensive subgingival decayed tooth structure, removal of healthy tissue.
   ❏ Exposure of deep or extensive existing subgingival restoration margin, removal of healthy tissue.
   ❏ Exposure of margin fracture site, removal of healthy tissue.
   ❏ To obtain correct clinical length for adequate crown retention, removal of healthy tissue. The clinical crown(s) was too short for adequate retention of the cast restoration(s).
   ❏ A direct placement restoration.
   ❏ A laboratory-processed cast restoration.
   ❏ Other: _____

The crown lengthening procedure is **not** part of the usual and customary services for the completed restorative or prosthetic dental procedure. Crown lengthening is a completely separate clinical procedure, used only when inadequate crown height exists. At no time is crown lengthening considered part of the restorative or prosthetic dental procedure.

If you have any questions, please contact our office.

Sincerely,

copy/(patient)

Inlay/Onlay: Metallic

Patient:
Patient Soc. Sec. No.:
Patient ❑ **is** ❑ **is not**   **the subscriber**

Insurance Carrier:
Group No.:
Employer:
Subscriber:

Re: ADA code #s
- ❑ D2510 Metallic Inlay (1 surface)
- ❑ D2520 Metallic Inlay (2 surfaces)
- ❑ D2530 Metallic Inlay (3 or more surfaces)
- ❑ D2542 Metallic Onlay (2 surfaces)
- ❑ D2543 Metallic Onlay (3 surfaces)
- ❑ D2544 Metallic Onlay (4 surfaces)

Date:

Dear Dental Consultant:

This is a request for ❑ payment   ❑ for predetermination for tooth # _____ of the above indicated restoration. Clinical examination of the tooth indicates that a direct placement restoration is contraindicated because of:
- ❑ Undermined cusps
- ❑ Inadequate dentin thickness to support enamel
- ❑ Extent of damage/prepared tooth structure
- ❑ Preparation was 2/3 or more the distance up the cusp slopes from the primary occlusal groove.

According to current dental science operative textbooks, the inlay/onlay and the capping of cusps are mandatory to protect the weak underlying cuspal structure from fracture and to remove the occlusal margin when subjected to heavy stress.

A direct placement restoration, whether amalgam or bonded resin, would be neither clinically acceptable nor the standard of care. Because of the unsupported nature of the tooth without the laboratory-processed occlusal coverage restoration, it is expected that weakened portions of the tooth would fracture under normal occlusal loading. The subscriber may have an "alternative materials or restoration" clause in the benefits contract. This should not be used as justification for changing benefits or codes from that of the submitted insurance form. While the extent of the necessary preparation may not be evident on the submitted radiograph, it is clinically observable.

If you have any questions about this restoration, please contact our office. Thank you.

Sincerely,

copy/(patient)

Inlay/Onlay: Porcelain

Patient: **Insurance Carrier:**
Patient Soc. Sec. No.:   **Group No.:**
Patient ❑ **is** ❑ **is not** **the subscriber**   **Employer:**
                                                          Subscriber:

Re: ADA code #s
   ❑ D2610 Porcelain/Ceramic Inlay (1 surface)
   ❑ D2620 Porcelain/Ceramic Inlay (2 surfaces)
   ❑ D2630 Porcelain/Ceramic Inlay (3 or more surfaces)
   ❑ D2642 Porcelain/Ceramic Onlay (2 surfaces)
   ❑ D2643 Porcelain/Ceramic Onlay (3 surfaces)
   ❑ D2644 Porcelain/Ceramic Onlay (4 or more surfaces)

Date:

Dear Dental Consultant:

This is a request for ❑ payment ❑ for predetermination for tooth #_____ of the above indicated restoration. Clinical examination of the tooth indicates that a direct placement restoration is contraindicated because of:
   ❑ Undermined cusps
   ❑ Inadequate dentin thickness to support enamel
   ❑ Extent of damage/prepared tooth structure
   ❑ Preparation was 2/3 or more the distance up the cusp slopes from the primary occlusal groove.

According to current dental science operative textbooks, the inlay/onlay and the capping of cusps are mandatory to protect the weak underlying cuspal structure from fracture and to remove the occlusal margin when it is subjected to heavy stress.

A direct placement restoration, whether amalgam or bonded resin, would be neither clinically acceptable nor the standard of care. Because of the unsupported nature of the tooth without the laboratory-processed occlusal coverage restoration, it is expected that weakened portions of the tooth would fracture under normal occlusal loading. The subscriber may have an "alternative materials or restoration" clause in the benefits contract. This should not be used as justification for changing benefits or codes from that of the submitted insurance form. While the extent of the necessary preparation may not be evident on the submitted radiograph, it is clinically observable.

If you have any questions about this restoration, please contact our office. Thank you.

Sincerely,

copy/(patient)

Inlay/Onlay: Resin

Patient:
Patient Soc. Sec. No.:
Patient ❑ **is** ❑ **is not   the subscriber**

Insurance Carrier:
Group No.:
Employer:
Subscriber:

Re: ADA code #s
- ❑ D2650 Resin Inlay (1 surface)
- ❑ D2651 Resin Inlay (2 surfaces)
- ❑ D2652 Resin Inlay (3 or more surfaces)

- ❑ D2662 Resin Onlay (2 surfaces)
- ❑ D2663 Resin Onlay (3 surfaces)
- ❑ D2664 Resin Onlay (4 or more surfaces)

Date:

Dear Dental Consultant:

This is a request for ❑ payment ❑ for predetermination for tooth #_____ of the above indicated restoration. Clinical examination of the tooth indicates that a direct placement restoration is contraindicated because of:
- ❑ Undermined cusps
- ❑ Inadequate dentin thickness to support enamel
- ❑ Extent of damage/prepared tooth structure
- ❑ Preparation was 2/3 or more the distance up the cusp slopes from the primary occlusal groove.

According to current dental science operative textbooks, the inlay/onlay and the capping of cusps are mandatory to protect the weak underlying cuspal structure from fracture and to remove the occlusal margin when subjected to heavy stress.

A direct placement restoration, whether amalgam or bonded resin, would be neither clinically acceptable nor the standard of care. Because of the unsupported nature of the tooth without the laboratory-processed occlusal coverage restoration, it is expected that weakened portions of the tooth would fracture under normal occlusal loading. The subscriber may have an "alternative materials or restoration" clause in the benefits contract. This should not be used as justification for changing benefits or codes from that of the submitted insurance form. While the extent of the necessary preparation may not be evident on the submitted radiograph, it is clinically observable.

If you have any questions about this restoration, please contact our office. Thank you.

Sincerely,

copy/(patient)

Sealants

FOR INSURANCE PLAN ADMINISTRATOR AT PLACE OF EMPLOYMENT

Patient: **Insurance Carrier:**
Patient Soc. Sec. No.:   **Group No.:**
Patient ❑ **is** ❑ **is not**   **the subscriber**   **Employer:**
                                                                Subscriber:

Re: ADA code #:
    ❑ D1351 Sealants

Date:

Dear Plan Administrator:

It has come to my attention that your dental benefits plan does not include payment for the application of "sealants" (ADA code D1351). I have recently placed sealants on the permanent teeth of one of your employee's children, and there was no payment made to the subscriber.

I would suggest that your plan needs review in this area. It has not kept pace with accepted preventive practices available since the late 1960s. You are doing both your subscribers and your company a disservice by not having dental sealants included as a payable benefit. Sealants are a cost-effective preventive treatment—much less costly than the need to place restorations, which sealants actually prevent. Your plan does pay for the more expensive procedures needed as the problems arise.

The fact that sealants are not included as a payable benefit indicates that you may be unaware of what they are and what they do. Despite systemic and topical fluoride applications to teeth, and despite adequate oral self-care, the occlusal (biting) surfaces of teeth are the first areas to become decayed. These surfaces are characterized by pits and fissures that are smaller than the diameter of a toothbrush bristle. They cannot be easily cleaned. Bacteria colonize the bottoms of the pits and fissures and begin the decay process. There is little or nothing a patient can do at home to prevent these lesions from beginning. The sealant is a noninvasive, quick-to-place, painless plastic coating that fills the pits and fissures, thus preventing the colonization of bacteria and subsequent decay. In fact, studies have clearly shown that active decay in these areas can be effectively sealed and prevented from causing more damage. The only other alternative to the sealants is a filling. The tooth is drilled, permanently damaged, and condemned to more drilling and filling as the patient ages. These fillings can be expensive. Endodontic therapy and full-coverage restorations might be needed. These can cost 25 times that of the sealant. Sealants are safe and effective.

Sealants can remain on the teeth for years. A 5-year retention rate is not uncommon. I have personally placed sealants that are still performing after almost 20 years of service. You do not cover sealants costing $_____, yet you cover cast restorations costing $_____. You also pay to have these castings redone every 5 years.

Sealants are endorsed by the American Dental Association, National Institute for Dental Health, and (in 1984 and 1994) the Surgeon General. If you are concerned with control of healthcare costs for your employers, I strongly advise that you immediately make sealants a payable benefit in your dental plan. Your employees benefit, you benefit. Consider this action a sound business practice, one that has a wonderful cost/benefit ratio.

Sincerely,

copy/(patient)

Veneers: Indirect

Patient: **Insurance Carrier:**
Patient Soc. Sec. No.:   **Group No.:**
Patient   ❑ is   ❑ is not   the subscriber   **Employer:**
                                                               Subscriber:

Re: ADA code #s:
   ❑ D2961 Resin Veneer
   ❑ D2962 Porcelain Veneer

Date:

Dear Dental Consultant:

The following narrative will give further information about the treatment rendered to the patient on _____ .

❑ Due to the extensive nature of the fracture/decay of the incisal edge of tooth #_____, a direct bonded resin restoration would not prove to be clinically successful.

❑ Because there have been repeated failures of directly placed, chairside-fabricated resin restorations, only a laboratory-processed restoration of this tooth is clinically indicated.

Please apply the appropriate contract benefits to the procedures listed on the submitted insurance claim form. If the listed procedures are not covered procedures and payment codes of your insurance company, please recode and apply alternate benefits as indicated, to fill your contractual liability with the purchaser of the contract.

If you have any questions, please feel free to contact our office. Thank you.

Sincerely,

copy/(patient)

Veneers: Placed to Correct Discoloration

Patient: **Insurance Carrier:**
Patient Soc. Sec. No.:   **Group No.:**
Patient ❑ **is** ❑ **is not**   **the subscriber**   **Employer:**
                                                     Subscriber:

Re: ADA code #s:
- ❑ D2960 Resin Veneer, Direct
- ❑ D2961 Resin Veneer, Indirect
- ❑ D2962 Porcelain Labial Veneers

Date:

Dear Dental Consultant:

The patient anticipates the placement of _____ veneers, of the type indicated above on tooth #s_____. These teeth show evidence of ❑ moderate ❑ severe tetracycline discoloration.

The teeth appear ❑ blue ❑ gray ❑ purple ❑ brown in color and ❑ are or ❑ are not banded.

The condition is extremely disfiguring, causing the patient great mental anguish. The patient has exhibited problems interacting with others in normal daily social and work-related activities. The patient has a reduced self-image and reduced self-esteem because of the unusual and undesirable coloration of the teeth.

Documentation from the physician who prescribed the tetracycline medication is
       ❑ attached ❑ unavailable. Diagnostic photographs are also available on request.

Please advise this office whether full-coverage porcelain/metal crowns or bonded porcelain veneers to correct this situation is a covered benefit for this patient. You may refer to the attached completed predetermination form for the details of the fees to be charged.

Thank you for your prompt attention to this matter.

Sincerely,

copy/(patient)

Changed Benefit Coding

Patient: **Insurance Carrier:**
Patient Soc. Sec. No.:   **Group No.:**
Patient   ❑ **is**   ❑ **is not**   **the subscriber**   **Employer:**
                                                               Subscriber:

Date:

Dear Benefits Coordinator:

It has come to our attention that you have changed a procedure code submitted for treatment for this particular patient to a procedure code that does not reflect necessary therapy for this patient. You have determined by radiographs that this procedure could be done in a simpler/different fashion.

The question of appropriate treatment can only be determined by the treating dentist at the time of the diagnosis and treatment planning. Unless your dental consultant examines the patient, you should not dictate or suggest treatment possibilities different from that of the treating dentist.

If the patient is not appropriately reimbursed according to the definition of the contract, I will recommend to the patient and insured that:

■ The insured/patient contact the State Board of Dentistry concerning the manipulation of treatment codes by your insurance company and the conduct of your dental consultant.

■ The insured contact the State Insurance Commissioner with respect to this particular matter and file a formal complaint against your insurance company.

■ The insured contact his or her attorney and seek direct compensation from the insurance company or individual responsible for altering the legal document of the submitted dental insurance claim form as filed.

Sincerely,

copy/(patient)

Complaint to Insurance Commissioner

To: Insurance Commissioner, State of _____

Re: Delay in processing dental insurance
  ❏ Predetermination
  ❏ Request for payment

Date:

Dear Insurance Commissioner:

A dental insurance claim form has been filed with: (name of insurance company)
Located: (address of insurance company)
All information necessary for the processing of the claim has been sent   ❏ one   ❏ two   ❏ three times.

❏ The insurance company has requested resubmission of information that has already been supplied.

❏ The insurance company has arbitrarily delayed, beyond any reasonable time frame, the processing of this claim.

❏ I would like to file a formal complaint against the insurance company.

❏ Please refer to the attached information regarding the claim.

Thank you for your attention to this matter.

Sincerely,

copy/(patient)

Information Narrative

Patient: **Insurance Carrier:**
Patient Soc. Sec. No.:   **Group No.:**
Patient ❑ **is** ❑ **is not** **the subscriber**   **Employer:**
                                                                Subscriber:

Re:

Date:

Dear Consultant,

The following narrative will give further information about the treatment rendered to the patient on _____.

(Write narrative here.)

Please apply the appropriate contract benefits to the procedures listed on the insurance form. If the listed procedures are not covered procedures and payment codes of your insurance company, please recode and apply alternate benefits as indicated, to fill your contractual liability with the purchaser of the contract.

If you have any questions, please feel free to contact our office. Thank you.

Sincerely,

copy/(patient)

Predetermination of Benefits

Patient: **Insurance Carrier:**
Patient Soc. Sec. No.:   **Group No.:**
Patient ❑ **is** ❑ **is not** **the subscriber**   **Employer:**
                                                    Subscriber:

Date:

Dear Dental Consultant:

Cast restorations are not being placed for cosmetic reasons, to restore/alter the vertical dimension, or for periodontal splinting.

❑ Single unit   ❑ Abutment teeth   ❑ Pontic

Missing maxillary tooth #s: _____
Missing mandibular tooth #s: _____

	ADA Code	Tooth #s	Initial Placement Date	Prior Placement Date (Prior restoration)
Single unit				
Abutment				
Pontic				

Dates of extraction of teeth being replaced by pontic:

Reason for replacement of existing cast restorations:
    ❑ Open margins
    ❑ Defective restorations, tooth #s: _____
    ❑ Decay in tooth #s: _____
    ❑ Fractures/cracks not visible in plane of x-ray
    ❑ Teeth previously restored with large direct placement materials that cannot be adequately restored without cast restorations
    ❑ Undermined cusps or incisal edges, tooth #s: _____
    ❑ Teeth previously treated endodontically, tooth #s: _____
        Date of endodontic treatment: _____

Comments:

Enclosures: ❑ Preoperative radiographs or thermal prints   ❑ Insurance form   ❑ Photographs

Delay in processing this predetermination claim could be deleterious to the patient's oral health. It could necessitate further, more costly dental procedures or loss of teeth. The patient and I both thank you for your prompt attention to this matter. If you have any questions, please contact our office.

Sincerely,

copy/(patient)

Radiograph Request Response

To: Dental Claims Review

Date: _____

Re: _____ Request for Dental Radiographs

_____ Pre-estimate Radiographs

Patient:

Patient Soc. Sec. No.:

Patient ❑ **is** ❑ **is not** the subscriber

Insurance Carrier:

Group No.:

Employer:

Subscriber:

Tooth #_____

ADA Code _____

Numerous dental pathologies (soft and hard tissue) or problems do not lend themselves to radiographic diagnosis. Dental tooth and soft tissue problems that are not able to be routinely diagnosed from dental radiographs include (but are not limited to):

- abfraction, attrition
- toothbrush abrasion
- chemical erosions (gastric reflux, etc.)
- incipient to medium-sized occlusal carious lesions
- class V facial and lingual decay
- fractured restorations
- facial and lingual overhangs
- buccolingual width of restorations
- unsupported cusps
- cracked-tooth syndrome
- fractured and missing cusps (especially if there is a large existing metal restoration)
- cracks in enamel and dentin radiating from an amalgam restoration that has absorbed water and expanded
- rough surfaces
- inadequate remaining tooth structure for clinically acceptable ferrule
- sensitive teeth (hot, cold, sweets)
- leaking restorations, restorations with clinically unacceptable margins
- recession of gingival tissues
- hyperplastic or edematous gingival tissues
- bleeding on probing
- facial or lingual bone loss and increased pocket depths
- traumatic occlusion
- tooth mobility
- irreversible pulpitis
- teeth with an adverse reaction to pressure or palpation
- gingivitis
- facial or lingual calculus
- sulcular exudate
- recurrent decay under crowns and in a mesial or distal orientation with respect to metal restorations and the plane of the x-ray source and image capture device

Diagnosis requires physical examination. Sound and accurate diagnosis of a dental problem does not necessarily require dental radiographs. Diagnosis should not be made from radiographs alone or a conversation with the patient. In many of the above-mentioned dental abnormalities, diagnosis can be made from clinical examination alone. Use of dental radiographs may be contraindicated, unnecessary, and in fact, expose the patient to harmful nondiagnostic ionizing radiation that, in the professional clinical judgment of the treating dentist, has no potential to change or modify the diagnosis. The patient has been informed of the nature of the problem and understands that preoperative radiographs would add nothing to the diagnosis or change the proposed treatment plan.

Preoperative radiographs for this proposed dental treatment may not or cannot demonstrate the nature or the extent of the problem. If there are any questions, please have the dental consultant call me. Thank you.

Phone Number _____

Sincerely,

copy/(patient)

Request for Insurance Recoding

Patient: **Insurance Carrier:**
Patient Soc. Sec. No.:   **Group No.:**
Patient ❑ **is** ❑ **is not**   **the subscriber**   **Employer:**
                                                   Subscriber:

Date:

Dear Dental Consultant:

Enclosed, please find a   ❑ pretreatment estimate or   ❑ request for payment. If our submitted claim form indicates a cast porcelain to gold/noble metal bridge and the insured's policy does not permit payment for either the bridge or the pontics, please review the claim and recode for payment for teeth designated abutment teeth, ADA code # D6750; single-unit cast restorations, ADA code # D6250.

If a fixed bridge is not a payable benefit to this subscriber, please refer to the following supportive documentation. Reason for full coverage of abutment teeth if fixed bridge is not a payable benefit (please refer to radiographs):

     ❑ Large existing defective restorations that cannot be restored with direct placement materials, tooth #s: _____
     ❑ Unsupported cusps or incisal edges, tooth #s: _____
     ❑ Fractured tooth #s: _____
     ❑ Decay, tooth #s: _____
     ❑ Fracture lines, cracked not visible in plane of radiograph, tooth #s: _____
     ❑ Tooth previously treated endodontically, tooth #s: _____
     ❑ Abutment teeth were previously restored with full-coverage cast restorations that are being replaced because of recurrent decay.

Additionally, if fixed bridge is not a payable benefit to the insured, please recode, evaluate, and apply benefits for a removable partial denture to replace the missing tooth or teeth.

Comments:

If you have any questions, please contact our office. Thank you for your prompt attention to this matter.

Sincerely,

copy/(patient)

chapter 4

Referral Letters and Forms

Content at a Glance: Referral Letters and Forms

These referral letters make patient referrals smooth and precise. They give the specialist both business and dental information that will keep treatment on schedule. Complete with necessary evaluation/treatment requests and enclosure check boxes.

Referral/Consultation Letters
Medical Consultation Request

Dental treatment may affect or be affected by other aspects of a patient's medical condition. Let your patient's other healthcare providers know just what dental treatment you propose and encourage them to answer promptly with pertinent recommendations.

Patient Referral to Dental Specialist

Use to inform your patient of the specifics he or she needs to contact the required specialist, the treatment you propose, and when he or she should seek this treatment.

Specialty Referrals

Dental specialty referral and consultation documents outline requested services and posttreatment follow-up.

    Endodontic Referral
    Oral Surgery Referral
    Orthodontic Referral
    Periodontal Referral

Requests
Radiograph and Records Request

Request a patient's radiographs and dental records from another healthcare provider.

Send per Patient Request

Cover letter for patient records being sent to another office at the patient's request.

Medical Consultation Request

(Name and address of
doctor to be consulted)

(Date)

Dear Doctor:

Our mutual patient, (patient's name), has been examined and needs the following dental treatment:

❑ Oral surgery [extraction(s)]

_____
_____

❑ Restorations

_____
_____

❑ Endodontic Treatment

_____
_____

❑ Periodontic Treatment (cleaning/scaling/prophylaxis)

_____
_____

❑ Periodontic Treatment (surgical treatment)

_____
_____

❑ Fixed prosthesis (bridgework)

_____
_____

❑ Full or partial dentures

_____
_____

❑ Other

_____
_____

Would you please inform me of any special recommendations you have regarding this proposed treatment, especially premedications needed by the patient before dental treatment and/or contraindications to the dental treatment. If you require that the dental treatment be delayed, please let me know when you believe treatment might be resumed.

If you have any questions, please contact me. The patient is not currently scheduled for any dental treatment and will only be scheduled for further treatment after your reply.

Please answer on the lower portion of this letter and return it to my office. The patient and I both thank you for your prompt attention to this matter.

Sincerely,

Patient Referral to Dental Specialist

Patient:_____   **Date:**_____

You are being referred to the following specialist for dental evaluation and/or treatment. Noted are the details of what we want the specialist to evaluate. When you call the specialist's office for an appointment, please read these instructions to them.

Prior to your appointment, we will speak with the specialist and/or send a letter outlining the technical aspects of your dental needs.

Once the specialist's examination is completed, they will inform you of the exact treatment they propose, how long the treatment will take, the cost involved, discuss postoperative details with you, and answer any questions you have.

Before you return to our office for further treatment, please see the specialist for:
❑ Evaluation only
❑ Evaluation and treatment

Any time during treatment in our office, please see the specialist for:
❑ Evaluation only
❑ Evaluation and treatment

As soon as possible, please see the specialist for:
❑ Evaluation only
❑ Evaluation and treatment

❑ **Endodontist** (root canal):

❑ **Periodontist** (gums, implants):

❑ **Oral Surgeon** (extractions, implants):

❑ **Orthodontist** (braces):

Endodontic Referral

Patient:_____   **Date:**_____

Referred to:_____   **Referred by:**_____

Dear Doctor:

❑ The above-named patient was referred to you on (date).
❑ The patient was given your phone number and instructed to call for an appointment.
❑ The patient would like you to call to set up an appointment.   Home phone:_____
                                                                    Work phone:_____

Please   ❑ Evaluate   ❑ Treat   ❑ Re-treat   ❑ Apicoectomy
Tooth #s: _____

Proposed final restoration:

Other:_____

_____

❑ Please refer the patient back to us when treatment has been completed.
❑ Please call our office if the patient has not contacted you by: (date)
❑ Please call me to discuss this case after your examination and before your treatment begins.
❑ Please send a written report on your:
    ❑ initial findings
    ❑ treatment plan
    ❑ final recommendations

❑ The patient is presently appointed at this office on (date) for:_____.
❑ The patient has been told to schedule no further appointments at this office until seeing you.
Comments:_____

_____

Enclosed: ❑ PA   ❑ BW   Date:_____

Sincerely,

Copy/(patient file)

Oral Surgery Referral

Patient:_____   **Date:**_____

Referred to:_____   **Referred by:**_____

Dear Doctor:

❑ The above-named patient was referred to you on (date).
❑ The patient was given your phone number and instructed to call for an appointment.
❑ The patient would like you to call to set up an appointment.   Home phone:_____
                                                                                                    Work phone:_____

Please: Evaluate   Treat
                    ❑   ❑   Extraction, tooth #_____
                    ❑   ❑   Biopsy of_____, tooth #_____
                    ❑   ❑   Frenectomy, tooth #_____
                    ❑   ❑   Tuberosity reduction   ❑ L ❑ R
                    ❑   ❑   Apicoectomy, tooth #_____
                    ❑   ❑   Implant, tooth #_____
                    ❑   ❑   Other:_____

Proposed final restoration:

Remarks:_____
_____

❑ Please refer patient back to our office when treatment has been completed.
❑ Please call me to discuss this case after your examination and before your treatment begins.
❑ Please send written report on your:
   ❑ initial findings
   ❑ treatment plan
   ❑ final recommendations
❑ Please take a panoramic x-ray and send a copy to our office.
❑ The patient is presently appointed at our office on (date) for_____.
❑ The patient has been told to schedule no further appointments at our office until you have
   completed your   ❑ Exam   ❑ Treatment

Enclosed: ❑ PA (Date)   ❑ BW (Date)   ❑ Radiographs (Date)

Special considerations:_____
_____

Sincerely,

Copy/(patient files)

Orthodontic Referral

Patient:_____   **Date:**_____

Parent/Guardian:_____   **Referred by:**_____

Referred to:_____

Dear Doctor:

❑ The above-named patient was referred to you on (date).
❑ The patient was given your phone number and instructed to call for an appointment.
❑ The patient would like you to call to set up an appointment.

Home phone:_____
Work phone:_____

Please   ❑ Evaluate   ❑ Treat for the following conditions:

Complete orthodontic evaluation:

Upright:_____
Intrude:_____
Extrude:_____
Other:_____

The patient has had all operative dentistry completed and has been advised to have 3-month hygiene continuing care intervals while under active treatment. The patient has been instructed to use a daily topical fluoride treatment while under active treatment.

❑ Please call me if the patient has not contacted you by (date).

❑ Please call me to discuss this case after your examination and before treatment begins.

❑ Please send a written report on your:
   ❑ initial findings
   ❑ treatment plan
   ❑ final recommendations

The patient is presently appointed at this office on (date) for_____.

We appreciate the care you and your staff take in reinforcing proper daily oral self-care and the 3-month hygiene recare interval.

The patient has been told to schedule no further appointments at this office until seeing you.

Comments:_____

_____

Sincerely,

Copy/(patient files)

Periodontal Referral

Patient:_____   **Date:**_____

Referred to:_____   **Referred by:**_____

Dear Doctor:

❑ The above-named patient was referred to you on (date).
❑ The patient was given your phone number and instructed to call for an appointment.
❑ The patient would like you to call to set up an appointment.   Home phone:_____
                                                                        Work phone:_____

Please   ❑ Evaluate   ❑ Treat for the following conditions:

❑ Periodontal disease classifications:
   Quadrant   ❑ UR   ❑ LR   ❑ UL   ❑ LL
   Sextant   ❑ UR   ❑ LR   ❑ UL   ❑ LL
   Tooth #:_____
❑ Implant evaluation, tooth #:_____
   Proposed final restoration:_____
❑ Crown lengthening, tooth #:_____
❑ Furcation, tooth #:_____
❑ Other:_____

At this time the patient has received and completed the following indicated periodontal services:
                              Date
❑ Scaling and root planing   _____
❑ Subgingival irrigation   _____
❑ Oral self-care instruction   _____
❑ Polishing   _____
❑ Site-specific therapy #:_____ with (product) _____

❑ Please send written report on your:
   ❑ initial findings
   ❑ treatment plan
   ❑ final recommendations
❑ The patient is presently appointed at our office on (date) for_____.
❑ The patient has been told to schedule no further appointments at our office until you have completed your
   ❑ Exam   ❑ Treatment
❑ Please appoint the patient for alternate hygiene maintenance appointments between offices.
   Interval:_____
❑ Please call me to discuss your findings after your examination and before your treatment begins.
❑ Please inform me in writing whether the patient accepts or declines treatment recommendations. If treatment is accepted, please send updates of progress, anticipated completion date, and restorative recommendations. Advise of long- and short-term prognosis of the teeth and recommended intervals of professional hygiene maintenance.

Enclosed: ❑ Periodontal charting (Date)   ❑ Radiographs   ❑ PA   ❑ BW   ❑ FMS (Date)

Sincerely,

Copy/(patient files)

Radiograph and Records Request

(Name of doctor who has records)
(Address of doctor who has records)
(City, state, zip code of doctor who has records)

(Date)

Dear Doctor:

At the request of (patient's or guardian's name), please forward the most recent radiographs and dental records for (patient's name). Please forward the requested materials to:

    (Name of office where records are to be sent)
    (Address of office where records are to be sent)
    (City, state, zip code where records are to be sent)

Thank you for your assistance in this matter.

Sincerely,

Copy/(patient file)

Send per Patient Request

(Name of office where records are to be sent)
(Address of office where records are to be sent)
(City, state, zip code where records are to be sent)

(Date)

Dear Doctor:

Enclosed, please find the dental records and most recent radiographs of (patient's name). Our records indicate that this patient was last seen in our office on (date). These records are being forwarded to your office at the patient's request.

Sincerely,

Copy/(patient file)

part two

Patient
Education

Cosmetic Dentistry

Content at a Glance: Cosmetic Dentistry

Congenital Conditions
Altered Passive Eruption: Soft Tissue
Defines altered passive eruption in relation to appearance and explains treatment options with soft tissue. Describes how tooth and gum ratios and lip lines affect appearance.

Altered Passive Eruption: Hard Tissue
Defines altered passive eruption in relation to appearance and explains treatment options for hard tissue. Describes how tooth and gum ratios and lip lines affect appearance.

Congenitally Missing Teeth: Closing Spaces Between Teeth
Alerts patients to the problems associated with congenitally missing teeth and the treatment needed.

Diastemas
Defines how and why diastemas may occur. Offers an overview of treatment possibilities.

Fluorosis, Mottled Enamel, and White Spots
Describes fluorosis, mottled enamel, and white spots and the treatment options available.

Peg Laterals
Describes peg laterals and how available treatment options depend on extent of malformation and patient's age.

Cosmetic Procedures
Bonded Resin Restorations: Tooth-Colored Fillings for Posterior Teeth
Explains the use of, advantages, and disadvantages of bonded resin restorations for posterior teeth. Assumes these restorations will be in place of silver amalgam restorations.

Cosmetic Dentistry
Overviews and lists the many possibilities and procedures available in cosmetic dentistry.

Cosmetic Tissue Recontouring
Advises how periodontal surgery can improve the appearance of teeth and gum architecture. Includes treatment options.

Enamel Recontouring
Relates the use of enamel recontouring, particularly in relation to other possible procedures.

Porcelain and Resin Veneers: Bonding
An overview of veneers: indications, advantages, and disadvantages of each type.

Porcelain Inlays and Onlays
Explains when porcelain inlays and onlays are used. Also gives advantages, disadvantages, and treatment timing.

Replacing Unesthetic Restorations
Points out conditions that would make replacement of older restorations desirable, even when the restorations are still functional, with cautions on waiting too long.

The Perfect Smile
Gives patients insight into the role the gingiva plays in the perfect smile.

Whitening
General Information
Tooth Whitening: Overview and Options
Important considerations of tooth whitening and available treatment options are reviewed.

Content at a Glance: Cosmetic Dentistry—cont'd

You Can Have Whiter Teeth!

Introductory information on the at-home and in-office methods of tooth whitening.

Specific Procedures

At-Home Tooth Whitening Options

Comparison of the custom tray, Whitestrips, and brush-on gels for patient-applied whitening.

At-Home Tray System: Tooth Whitening Instructions

Information, specific directions, and fees for home mouthguard tooth whitening.

In-Office Power Whitening Technique without Light Activation

Details of the power whitening technique without light activation are explained.

In-Office Power Whitening Technique with Light Activation

Details of the power whitening technique with light activation are explained.

In-Office Tooth Whitening Postoperative Instructions

Postprocedural instructions for the in-office power whitening technique.

Nonvital Tooth Whitening Options

Discusses the walking whitening and power whitening techniques: indications, procedures, and results to be expected, both in the short and long terms.

Tetracycline-Discolored Teeth: Options for Cosmetic Improvement

Description of tetracycline-discolored teeth and the possibilities for cosmetic improvement.

Altered Passive Eruption: Soft Tissue

Esthetic Concerns

Attractive smiles are in no small part determined by the amount of tooth structure visible when you smile. Teeth are composed of two basic parts—the root portion (below the gumline) and the crown (above the gumline).

That ratio is approximately 1.6:1, length to width. That is teeth should appear longer than they are wide, or a ratio of the tooth length (1.6:1) to the width (1). Teeth that do not have this approximate ratio appear less attractive to our culture.

Altered Passive Eruption

Teeth that appear short and "stubby" may actually be covered with gum tissue. The correct height to width ratio is present, but the gumline simply rests too far down on the crown of the tooth to appear attractive. This condition is termed *altered passive eruption*. While the exact cause of altered passive eruption is unknown, we do see this condition in early teen years. The good news is, it is treatable through a minor surgical procedure. Small amounts of gum tissue can be removed with a laser or electrosurgical device; many times, suturing and extensive postoperative care are not required.

Lip Lines

A complicating factor to altered passive eruption can be a high lip line, or one that exposes more tooth and gum when the patient is smiling. A low lip line would effectively "hide" the gum tissue covering the crowns. As the lip line appears higher, the attractiveness of the smile goes down.

Smile Lines

Occasionally, it may be necessary to slightly reshape the biting edges of one or more teeth to help form an attractive smile line. More extensive smile redesign can include the actual fabrication of thin outer covering veneers that are slipped over the reshaped front teeth and cemented into place, or a crown of porcelain may be the best treatment.

You can have the stunning smile you want and deserve. Following a comprehensive examination, we will recommend the best treatment plan to help you achieve that goal.

If you have any questions about altered passive eruption, please feel free to ask us.

Altered Passive Eruption: Hard Tissue

Teeth are composed of two basic, visible parts—the root portion and the crown (enamel-covered) portion. The term *crown* does not refer to the type of tooth replacement fabricated by a dental laboratory. Rather, it is the part of the tooth that is normally seen when you speak.

The present-day esthetic dental philosophy, demonstrated by people who have beautiful teeth and smiles, shows that there must be a certain amount of enamel-covered tooth visible for an attractive smile. That ratio is about 1.6:1, length to width. Teeth that are shorter than this look progressively less attractive. They look short and stubby. If they are actually worn down from a clenching or grinding problem, this is a different type of problem. But it may not be that the teeth themselves are too short. It could be that there is not enough of the crown of the tooth that can be seen. The remainder that should be seen is covered with gum or gum and bone tissue. This is known as *altered passive eruption*. It is not entirely clear why this happens. It may become obvious as early as age 14. The teeth may have a pleasing color and be very straight, but they still leave something to be desired, because they are too small and too much gum shows when you smile.

This can be a severe cosmetic problem when coupled with the type of lip line that frames the teeth. A low lip line will probably hide most or all of the gum covered part of the tooth, so there is less of a need to correct the defect. A medium or high lip line, especially a high lip line, will show all of the tooth and gum. As the lip line gets higher, the attractiveness of the smile goes down. The situation can be so severe that the patient will train his or her muscles to artificially hold the upper lip stiff or cover the mouth with a hand when smiling. In this way, the short teeth or the great expanse of gum tissue will be hidden from view. It can cause significant psychological problems.

The solution can be easy or complicated, depending on the exact nature of the problem. If there is only a small amount of gum tissue to be removed from a single tooth, or multiple teeth, and there is a medium lip line, then the tissue is easily removed with a laser or electrosurgical cutting device. Scalpels and stitches are not needed in small cases. As more gum must be removed and more tooth exposed, there may be some underlying bone that must be reshaped. Bone removal will be followed, about 2 months later, by the soft tissue removal mentioned earlier. The first surgery must heal long enough for the tissue to reach its final position before the second can be completed. Remember, you are looking at differences of several millimeters to a fraction of a millimeter that will cause the case to be a success or failure. A two-step procedure is better than a one-step procedure.

The biting edges (enamel and/or dentin) of one or more teeth may be reshaped if there is a need not only to lengthen the teeth but also to make it appear that they have actually been placed higher in the smile line. This is for top teeth, of course. If a great deal of tooth must be reshaped to accomplish the desired effect, root or dentin may be exposed, making the tooth sensitive. These teeth will need to be covered with porcelain veneers or crowns to achieve the proper esthetics. Even if only a little amount of tooth is reshaped, the veneers or crowns may be indicated to get the exact appearance you want. We will discuss this with you before you begin treatment. It is important that you know what is being done, how long it will take to complete, and what you will look like when it is finished.

We will make the veneers or crowns and reshape the teeth. We will determine what can be done. We may also do the soft tissue recontouring. This is most common. For procedures that involve a reshaping of the bone, you may be referred to a periodontist (gum specialist). Since we will do the restorative treatment, we know exactly where the soft tissue should be. We are the cosmetic specialists. We will establish the final position of the gum line. In extreme cases, the problem will be corrected with a combination of the above-mentioned procedures and orthognathic surgery to reposition the jawbone and teeth. This is done by an oral surgeon. With a comprehensive examination, we can tell you what is appropriate for you. You do not have to live with an unattractive smile because you have short-looking teeth due to showing too much gum tissue. These problems can be corrected. Let us know what you do not like about your smile or teeth. More than likely, the smile you now have can be made into something you will like to show off.

If you have any questions about altered passive eruption, please feel free to ask us.

Congenitally Missing Teeth

Some of us will have 32 teeth develop during our lifetime. This has been considered a normal complement of teeth. More often than not, however, we do not develop a full set of 32 teeth. It is quite common for people to be missing one or more of the third molars (wisdom teeth). And as the jaw sizes of modern human beings have decreased in size, it is not unusual that there is no room for the proper placement of the third molars in a mouth, and they must be extracted.

Not as common, but not at all unusual, is a condition in which certain permanent front teeth never develop. When permanent teeth don't develop, they are considered to be congenitally missing. The term for this condition is *congenitally missing teeth*. When this happens, it is frequently one or both of the upper lateral incisors, which are the smaller teeth on either side of the two top front teeth. Less often, the permanent eyeteeth (canines) or premolars don't develop.

The problem that results from congenitally missing teeth involves the space where the tooth (teeth) should have been. The teeth nearest the space shift into different positions to fill in the gap, often resulting in a crowded smile—when in fact, some teeth are missing!

The problems resulting from missing permanent teeth can be reduced or eliminated with early detection and a plan for future treatment. The usual treatment involves orthodontics to move the permanent teeth into better position or keep the permanent teeth in the correct location. Because we treat missing lateral incisors so often, the treatment routine is well established. The best esthetics, the most natural look, will be achieved by leaving the adjacent permanent central incisors and canine teeth in their customary places.

When there are missing lateral incisors, it is likely that we will recommend moving the eyeteeth (canines) into their positions. This will keep the bone in the missing tooth space at the proper level. We will then recommend moving the eyeteeth back into their proper positions. This may sound like extra treatment, but it is needed to keep the bone at the proper height for future tooth replacement treatment.

The sequence of treatment is orthodontics as early as necessary to maintain the space. The further the teeth have shifted from this original position, the more orthodontic treatment will be necessary. Then, while the child and mouth are growing, a removable replacement tooth is made. This appliance is worn until the teeth are ready to receive the implant or bridge, after age 18 or so when the mouth and dental structures are more mature.

When the permanent teeth further back in the mouth are missing, it is common for baby teeth to be retained in these spaces. Sometimes the baby teeth can last for years, but they do not have the root structure to remain stable over a lifetime. Because the retained baby teeth are meant for a small mouth, they do not have the right size, shape, or function as the permanent teeth. When lost, they can be replaced with implants or a bridge. Your own particular situation will determine the best course of treatment.

If you have any questions about congenitally missing teeth, please feel free to ask us.

Diastemas: Closing Spaces Between Teeth

The Cause

A diastema is space between teeth, that is, adjacent teeth that do not touch. There are a number of reasons why spaces may exist between teeth. The two most common are an arch length discrepancy (teeth are too narrow for the arch that supports them), or because there are congenitally missing teeth. The remaining teeth then either shift or merely don't touch the next available tooth. The spaces between the teeth can be just a fraction of a millimeter wide or so wide that a straw can easily fit between the teeth.

The missing teeth can and often do cause a cosmetic problem. In the present culture of the Western world, spaces or gaps between teeth are not regarded as being desirable or attractive.

Treatment Options

There are several options available to treat a diastema. Most of these options work well whether the spaces are large or small or whether there are several spaces or just one space between two teeth.

Orthodontics can be used to move the teeth into a more pleasing alignment. This could be done with a retainer or fixed bands and wires. Clear Invisalign orthodontic aligners are often used to close these spaces. The advantage is that complex restorations are usually unnecessary and you have no worry about the restoration chipping or breaking after years of service. The disadvantage of orthodontics to close a diastema is the time needed to move the teeth, which can range from a few months to 18 months.

The other option is to have the teeth restored with bonding. The bonding can be done with either resin or with porcelain. The resin will be less expensive and work well to close small diastemas. The porcelain takes an additional visit, is more expensive, and is more appropriate for larger cases in which a more significant appearance modification is needed. This would include changing the color of the teeth, the length of several teeth, or the alignment of several teeth. As a rule of thumb for small spaces, a bonded resin will work well; for larger spaces, orthodontics and porcelain must be considered. Porcelain and resin both can be made to exactly match your existing tooth.

Each situation must be individually examined and evaluated before treatment. Often, we will require study model impressions to be made so we can make measurements of the tooth length, width, and amount of separation between teeth. Using this method, we can show you how you can look through the use of a diagnostic "wax up" showing the new shape of the teeth.

An important point to remember is that if you also want a whiter appearing smile, we should complete the whitening process before the bonding process. Teeth can be whitened, but dental materials such as porcelains and resins cannot be whitened. The restorations are placed to match your tooth color at the time they are placed, so whitening has to come first.

Afterwards

After the teeth are moved orthodontically or reshaped with porcelain or resin, your appearance will change! Not only that, but also your teeth will feel different to you. Your lips will be supported differently. Air will be deflected from your teeth in a different fashion. Depending on the amount of change, you may even need to make slight adjustments to your speech. The good news is that all the adjustments take only several hours to a few days to make. Very quickly, additions and changes become natural for you and you don't even notice that they were done, except that people will compliment you on how lucky you are to have been born with such beautiful teeth!

If you have any questions about diastema closures, please feel free to ask us.

Fluorosis, Mottled Enamel, and White Spots

Fluorosis and Mottled Enamel

Fluoride is the dental marvel of our lifetime and a definite benefit to the oral health of our nation. But too much of a good thing can cause problems! Fluorosis of the teeth and mottled enamel can occur when there is too much fluoride uptake by the teeth while the teeth are forming. Prescription fluoride vitamins of the proper dosage are normally given to children. But a child can get too much fluoride if it's available from multiple sources. Children with access to a public water system containing fluoride may also be prescribed fluoride supplements or they may swallow fluoride-containing toothpastes, mouthrinses, or certain fruit drinks, which may increase their fluoride intake above recommended levels. Fluorosis is a condition in which teeth form with unsightly dark spots on them. Some medications and illnesses can also cause a similar problem. These dark spots, most often seen on the permanent teeth, are not more prone to decay, just unattractive. One, several, or all of the teeth can be affected. The color change (usually brown/orange or flat/opaque white) can be mild, moderate, or severe.

Treatment Options

Generally speaking, three solutions are possible. Sometimes the stain is very superficial and can be merely polished off. It does not return. There is no pain involved in this procedure. The enamel is simply polished and made smooth again.

Many times it is quite easy to whiten the brown spots to match the surrounding tooth color. This is most often an in-office procedure (as opposed to whitening yellow teeth, which can be done at home with custom-made tooth-whitening trays). Strong whitening chemicals are placed on the dark area and activated by light or heat or both. Several applications (in the same visit) are done, and the spot usually disappears in one visit!

If the spot is very dark or goes deep into the enamel, the whitening may work, but not enough to remove the total discoloration. In this instance, a combination of whitening and a bonded composite tooth-colored restoration will solve the problem. The tooth is whitened, and then the remaining dark area is prepared (drilled) to receive a bonded-type filling. The natural color of the tooth is matched and a resin is bonded into the prepared section. The color match can be nearly perfect, and patients see a big improvement over what was there before.

White Spots

White spots on teeth can also be caused by too much fluoride, illness, medication, or an interruption of the proper enamel formation. The spots may be barely visible, or they may contrast with the surrounding tooth. If the teeth dry out, as in the case of a patient who routinely breathes through his or her mouth, the white spots become quite prominent. Most of the time, these spots can be simply polished off. If they go too deep into the tooth, however, they must be restored with tooth preparation and bonding of a tooth-colored material. Once removed, they do not return. White spots affect the permanent teeth more than baby teeth. While they cannot be bleached out, as can fluorosis discolorations, whitening of all the teeth may make them less noticeable.

The best solution to your problem will be discussed with you during your examination.

If you have any questions about fluorosis, mottled enamel, or white spots, please feel free to ask us.

Peg Laterals

At times, for several reasons, the maxillary lateral incisors do not form properly. Maxillary lateral incisors are the smaller teeth on either side of the top two front teeth. This malformation of the tooth is genetically determined. The malformation can take on several different appearances, and both teeth or only one of the teeth may be affected. The teeth can be shorter in height or lesser in width or a combination of the two. This type of deviation from the normal shape of the tooth is called a *peg lateral incisor*. The solution to this cosmetic problem can be simple or complicated, depending on what shape the tooth has when it is diagnosed and treatment is begun.

Restorative Possibilities

If the peg tooth (or teeth) is just slightly more narrow than normal and there is a space available on either side or both sides of it, the tooth can be bonded with a directly placed composite restoration. This is the most common treatment. The results are very positive and can last a long time. An excellent color match is not difficult to obtain. The procedure is similar to closing a diastema (a naturally occurring space between teeth).

If there is not enough space on either side to place the composite material, orthodontics might be required to provide room for the bonding. Diagnosed early, this is not a problem to do. If the patient waits until adulthood for the orthodontics, shifting of the teeth may have forced the peg tooth out of line, and more extensive orthodontics may be needed.

If the peg tooth is too small in both height and width and there is adequate space remaining, the tooth can still be rebuilt with a composite. However, if the patient is older and there is a significant amount of tooth to be replaced, a porcelain restoration may be more appropriate. This restoration is made in a laboratory with excellent esthetic results. It will last a very long time. It is more expensive to accomplish and will not be placed until the mouth is fully developed and the teeth and gum tissue are in their "adult" position—sometime after age 18.

In brief, restoration of a peg lateral can be done with composite resin (in all ages) or porcelain (after age 18). Size and position of the teeth will determine what is done and when. As soon as it is noted, plans should be made for eventual restoration. It is important to make sure there is sufficient space for the proper length and width bonding. This spacing may happen naturally or need orthodontic assistance.

If you have any questions about peg laterals and their restoration, please feel free to ask us.

Bonded Resin Restorations: Tooth-Colored Fillings for Posterior Teeth

Tooth-colored fillings have been used in dentistry for many years, especially to restore front teeth. The newest tooth-colored filling materials (resins) are quite successfully used to restore cavities in back teeth. These tooth-colored materials are especially useful when the restoration will be visible when you talk or smile. These posterior (back) tooth-colored resins can be expected to last for several years. A reasonable estimate at this time is approximately 10 to 12 years or more. The length of time the resin fillings (and silver filling) last depends on the position and size of the filling, the care the patient gives it, and the foods the patient eats.

Resin restorations in back teeth require less drilling than for silver fillings; and the less the dentist must drill your tooth, the better off you are and the fewer dental problems you will develop in the future. When a tooth is prepared (drilled), it becomes weaker; restoring it with a bonded resin material will help make it strong again. Advantages of the resin restorations include a natural finished appearance similar to that of your real tooth and the most conservative removal of tooth structure. They require only one appointment for completion.

Disadvantages of tooth-colored fillings in posterior teeth include the difficulty in their placement. They also cost about 50% more than silver fillings. They can be used only rarely in patients who have a grinding or bruxing (clenching) habit, they cannot be easily used in areas where there is not a sufficient amount of original tooth structure, and they require more time to finish.

Resin restorations are among the most conservative restorations in dentistry today. They require the least amount of drilling. The smaller any filling can be, the longer it will last. They are best for small to medium fillings. In areas where the display of metal from a silver filling would be unsightly, they are of great cosmetic importance.

If you have any questions about bonded resin restorations, please feel free to ask us.

Cosmetic Dentistry

The goal of cosmetic dentistry is to enhance, improve, or change the appearance of your teeth. In today's society, appearance is very important. While judgment based solely on appearance may be superficial and not reflective of who you really are, it can still affect how people think of you. When you talk, people focus on your face, your eyes, and teeth. People notice a natural looking mouth, teeth, and smile. An unsightly mouth due to visible cavities, defective fillings, gum disease, or crooked or misshapen teeth is noticed, too. People will often form opinions of you based on what they see.

You can get an objective look at how other people see you. Get about 18 inches away from a mirror. This is about as close as most people get to you when you speak with them. If you get any closer to the mirror, the light will not be right and you will not get a true picture of how your teeth look. Smile, talk, laugh, and observe which teeth are visible and what they look like. Then ask yourself, "If I could wave a magic wand over my teeth and change anything I don't like, what would I change?" Write it down, then read on.

Many people think of dentistry as fixing cavities, root canals, false teeth, caps, and gum disease. But you will be fascinated by what we can do to improve your appearance. Here is just a partial list of dental procedures that can improve the way your teeth look:

- ❑ Replace discolored fillings in front teeth
- ❑ Whiten teeth to a lighter color
- ❑ Straighten crooked teeth with orthodontics or recontouring your natural enamel
- ❑ Close up spaces between teeth
- ❑ Porcelain or resin veneers to change the shape and alignment of teeth (bonding)
- ❑ Place tooth-colored fillings in back teeth (instead of silver/metal fillings)
- ❑ Porcelain or resin inlays or onlays for back teeth
- ❑ Cosmetic periodontal surgery to even out gum tissue that is crooked
- ❑ Restoration of worn and short teeth to their proper shape
- ❑ Fill in toothbrush abrasion notches
- ❑ Cover missing gum tissue due to recession with soft tissue grafts
- ❑ Replace missing teeth with bridges or implants
- ❑ Replace defective and unsightly crowns (caps)
- ❑ Cover stained root surfaces
- ❑ Remove stained fracture lines from enamel
- ❑ Restore chipped teeth (bonding)
- ❑ Make teeth appear longer
- ❑ Make teeth appear shorter

Costs for these cosmetic procedures vary according to the extent of treatment. Tell us how you wish your smile looked. Then we can tell you what we can do, how long it will take, and what it will cost. Most of the time, people are pleasantly surprised to find that the cost is not as much as they thought. If you have dental insurance, you may often find that some of the procedures are a part of your benefit package.

If you have any questions about improving your appearance by cosmetic dentistry, please feel free to ask us.

Cosmetic Tissue Recontouring

It is not uncommon for us to suggest to a patient who has absolutely no signs of periodontal (gum) disease to seriously consider having elective periodontal procedures performed. In these cases, the procedures are almost always needed to improve appearance. Sometimes they are suggested to promote future periodontal health or attend to a potential problem that might develop.

When you smile or talk, your teeth are framed by your lips and the visible gum tissue. People looking at you notice your teeth. People notice missing teeth, tooth alignment, gum color, discolored fillings, silver fillings, tooth color, and how much of your teeth actually show. If everything is integrated well and looks natural, people say you have a nice smile. If something does not look natural, it may be easy to define, such as crooked, stained, or yellow teeth; periodontal disease shown by red-colored gum tissue; or discolored fillings. Or it may be something not as readily to determine. It's just that something does not look right.

That "something" may be related to the teeth and gum architecture. The position of the gums where they meet the teeth is esthetically important. If the teeth look too short, there may be more gum tissue covering them than is considered attractive. You may show too much gum tissue when you smile. There may be a difference in height of the gum of one tooth versus an adjacent tooth or its partner on the other side of the mouth. This could be caused by recession from brushing too hard; gum disease; poor or defective restorations, especially crowns; or just a problem with the way the tooth erupted into place. All of these things can detract from your appearance.

Several different periodontal procedures, simple to accomplish, can correct most of these routine problems. Some involve removal of unwanted tissue; some involve grafting of tissue. Orthodontics might be helpful in some cases. The more extensive procedures will require referral to specialists.

In one common type of cosmetic periodontal plastic surgery, the gum tissue is reshaped and recontoured without the use of sutures (stitches). This procedure is done in the office. One tooth or several teeth may benefit from treatment. Postoperative discomfort is usually minor. There may be tooth sensitivity when gum tissue is removed, but this usually disappears. The improvement generated by this type of procedure can be startling.

We will show you and describe in detail how you can benefit from cosmetic periodontal procedures. In many cases, the cosmetic periodontal surgery will complete the treatment you need. In some cases, it will be part of a larger treatment plan including crowns, veneers, or bonded restorations.

If you have any questions about elective cosmetic periodontal surgery, please feel free to ask us.

Enamel Recontouring

Most people want straight, beautifully aligned, white teeth. Unfortunately, most people are not that lucky. When teeth are in poor alignment, rotated, tilted, and/or crowded, the obvious way to correct the problem is by orthodontics (braces or Invisalign aligners). However, there are situations in which it may not be possible or desirable to use braces to straighten teeth. You might feel that you are too old (although this is rarely the case), the cost of the orthodontics may be beyond your current means, you may not want to wear braces, or perhaps there are only a few areas that need attention and full orthodontics are simply not indicated.

In certain select cases, the appearance of your top and bottom teeth can be slightly or dramatically improved by recontouring the enamel. The four top and four bottom incisors and canines can be routinely altered. Sometimes teeth further back in your mouth can also be cosmetically improved. Recontouring is useful when there is slight to moderate overlapping of the front teeth, uneven wear, or teeth that do not have their biting and incising edges in harmony, creating an uneven "picket fence" look.

Enamel recontouring is usually a painless procedure and no local anesthetic is needed. The enamel that is overlapping or poorly shaped is removed, recontoured, and polished. Depending on your individual needs, one or several teeth may require some reshaping. Different amounts of enamel may be removed from different teeth. The recontoured teeth do not become more prone to decay, are not made more sensitive to temperature changes, and they are not made significantly weaker or damaged by the procedure.

Many times, the recontouring is all that is necessary to significantly improve your appearance. Other times, when the poor alignment is more pronounced, it may be done in conjunction with bonding of resin or porcelain to teeth. Your treatment will depend on your present conditions and on what you would like to see changed.

The procedure is not difficult for the patient and can often be done in only one appointment. The change is immediate and permanent. It does take an artistic flair on the part of the dentist to see what possibilities for change exist. We need to determine what enamel needs to be removed, where we must add, and where orthodontics is the treatment of choice. The fees are reasonable and depend on the extent of the treatment.

If you have any questions about enamel recontouring, please feel free to ask us.

Porcelain and Resin Veneers: Bonding

When people speak of "bonding" their teeth to make them look better, they are usually referring to either porcelain or resin veneers. Veneers cover only the outside portion of the tooth, the part that shows when you smile or talk. In fact, all tooth-colored dental restorative materials are bonded, whether the restoration is in a front tooth or a back tooth. Strictly speaking, in dentistry, *bonding* refers only to adhesive joining of two dissimilar materials. Silver fillings can be bonded, as can crowns (caps).

Porcelain and resin veneers are placed in order to correct slight or severe defects in tooth alignment, shape, or color. They are also placed when teeth have been moderately restored and the teeth have been weakened. This is done when there is still enough enamel left for the bonding to be successful. If the teeth are in very poor alignment or there is insufficient enamel remaining, bonding to improve the appearance is not possible. At that point orthodontics or full-coverage crowns must be considered. The most common use for bonding veneers, either porcelain or resin, is to improve the cosmetic appearance of the patient.

Without question, porcelain veneers look the best and last the longest. They are indicated when the teeth are in fair to good alignment or when a more pleasing tooth color is desired. They are not usually placed in a patient under 16 years of age. The procedure usually requires some slight to moderate tooth preparation (drilling). Local anesthesia is usually necessary. The procedure requires two separate appointments, approximately 10 days apart to complete. This is because the veneers are constructed in an offsite laboratory. Once bonded into place, the porcelain veneers become very strong. The success rate is high, and they can last up to 12 or more years. Anything that will break your natural teeth can break the porcelain veneers, for example, hard candy or frozen candy bars. Veneers are highly stain resistant. They are a good treatment choice when all the front teeth are being restored. They are more expensive than resin veneers, but they last longer and look better than resin. Porcelain biting surfaces can cause more rapid wear of opposing natural teeth.

Resin veneers are also available. They are placed by the dentist in one office visit. Resin veneers are used in similar situations to porcelain veneers. However, they last only half as long before requiring repair or replacement. They are advised for patients who are still growing. They look very good but are not as good as porcelain. While repairs to the resin veneers are not too difficult, they have a tendency to chip more than porcelain veneers.

Basically, porcelain looks better, lasts longer, is stronger, more expensive, and requires two dental appointments to complete. Resin veneers are less expensive, easier to repair, and better for children, or if there are financial considerations.

It is very important to come in for regular recare appointments for cleaning and examination if either type of veneer is placed. This way, we will be better able to quickly correct any problems that develop. A 3- to 4-month interval between appointments is customary.

If you have any questions about porcelain and resin veneers, please feel free to ask us.

Porcelain Inlays and Onlays

Porcelain

When a tooth has been moderately to extensively destroyed by decay, previous drilling, or fracture but there is still sufficient enamel remaining, one innovative way it can be restored is with a porcelain inlay or onlay. An inlay is a restoration in which a portion of occlusal (biting) surface is replaced with porcelain. An onlay will restore a larger portion of the biting surface of the tooth. These are considered very conservative restorations. The porcelain allows an excellent esthetic result. It is attached to the tooth using a bonding procedure, allowing it to become very strong. It can be used with wonderful results in small, medium, and even large restorations lasting more than 12 years, relatively trouble-free.

A dental laboratory is involved in the construction of the restoration. There is a 2- to 3-week delay while the inlay or onlay is being made, so the tooth must have a temporary restoration in place during that time.

They have some disadvantages. They are moderately expensive to very expensive to make and place. They take two appointments to complete. They must be adjusted and polished well or they can cause wear of the opposing enamel, similar to a porcelain fused to metal crown. Of course, we make sure they are adjusted and polished well to begin with. Porcelain biting surfaces can cause more rapid wear of opposing natural teeth, especially in the posterior areas where a metal biting surface may be advised.

Advantages include the excellent esthetics, high strength, predicted longevity, and conservative preparation, that is, less drilling than a crown. If the porcelain does chip, it can be repaired. However, you should not chew ice cubes, "jaw breakers," or any other hard candy with these or any other type of restoration.

For those who want the strongest, longest-lasting, conservative restoration that very closely matches a tooth, porcelain is possibly the best choice. Once it is finished, the tooth, if cared for properly, should not have to be restored again for years. It does allow the conservation of most of the natural tooth.

Resin

Resin inlays and onlays are used in the same areas as the porcelain inlays and onlays. They are very natural in appearance and, like porcelain, are bonded into place. They are considered an extremely conservative restoration. Two appointments, approximately 2 weeks apart, are required to fabricate the resin inlay/onlay. The tooth will be protected with a temporary filling while the final restoration is being made. The wear of the resin is similar to that of enamel. So unlike porcelain, it will not have a tendency to wear the opposing natural tooth structure.

The resin may be considered slightly "weaker" than porcelain. However, porcelain is more brittle and more difficult to repair. The difference in strengths is not significant. The resin is more forgiving and is more easily finished or repaired and resin is easier to work on.

With both types of materials, porcelain or resin, you can develop decay on unrestored surfaces, so excellent oral self-care is required. Neither material is advised for patients who have a bruxing (grinding) or clenching habit unless a protective mouthguard is constructed for you.

Unless you have a preference, we will select the most appropriate material for your dental needs. Cost of each is comparable. Both types are excellent choices and are considered highly conservative in the amount of drilling needed.

If you have any questions about porcelain or resin inlays and onlays, please feel free to ask us.

Replacing Unesthetic Restorations

Everything has a life expectancy, even dental filling materials. Dental materials appear to have two different types of life spans—a functional life span and an esthetic life span. The better the original dental restorative material and the skills of the operator, the longer the restoration will last. Lab-processed materials will generally last longer than direct placement materials.

The *functional life span* is defined as the length of time a material will last before it fails to function properly. This failure will either (a) weaken the tooth or (b) permit decay or gum disease to begin. For example, when a piece of the filling breaks off (or often in the case of an amalgam [silver metal] filling, it causes a piece of the tooth to break off), the tooth requires a new restoration.

An *esthetic life span* is somewhat different. In the case of bonded and tooth-colored restorations, it means that the material, while possibly still able to function, has begun to degrade. A filling may have matched the tooth beautifully when placed, but over time, the change in color of the filling material, as well as actual tooth color changes, cause an obvious mismatch between tooth and filling material. Since the restorative material does not have the same properties as tooth enamel, it will wear a little differently. The shape will change over time, too. Luckily, it is a very slow process.

With lab-processed restorations, crowns and bridges, the crown may still be working well, but age and changes in your mouth make it and the surrounding soft tissues look less acceptable than it was when first placed. Again, this happens slowly, over many years.

Other esthetic problems that can be corrected include notches in fillings or under crowns caused by improper brushing (or decay), recession of the gum tissue that exposes darker root surfaces around crowns or fillings, porcelain crowns (caps) that no longer match the adjacent teeth, and metal margins of crowns that are visible due to gum recession (and this is quite common).

When you can see these types of changes, you can be sure that others who look at you when you are speaking or smiling will see them too. If you place a high value on your personal appearance, this is the time to consider having the restorations replaced with newer materials. Newer dental restorative materials look better, last longer, are more color-stable, and more wear-resistant than older-generation bonded materials. You can expect them to look good for many years.

In our opinion, silver metal fillings never look "good." Even at their best, polished and shined, they do not represent a picture of health. As the metal ages, it corrodes, pits, and darkens. Its constant expansion and contraction due to hot and cold foods we eat weakens the tooth. The darkening of a filling can cause a darkening of the tooth itself. After time, the tooth will become permanently dark gray. The wider your smile is (and the more teeth you show when talking and smiling), the more of a problem this can be.

Broken, stained, worn, and visible fillings detract from your appearance. When you look at a tooth (from about 2 feet away) that has been restored, you should not see the filling. While these types of problems are, of course, not life-threatening, consider attending to them before they get worse—and difficult and expensive to correct.

In our office, we place a high value on the appearance of your teeth and how you feel about your smile. We want you to look your best. We use the best materials and techniques available in dentistry today to ensure a healthy smile. We will be happy to evaluate your particular condition and discuss options with you.

If you have any questions about replacing unesthetic restorations, please feel free to ask us.

The Perfect Smile

Almost anyone can have the perfect smile they dream about. But there is a great deal more to the perfect smile than white teeth. Most people who look at a smile will look at the color and the alignment of the top and bottom teeth and notice whether teeth are crooked. A filling or a crown that doesn't match natural tooth structure may also be noticed. But the teeth are only one of three equally important components of a perfect smile. The human mouth is a stage and is framed by the lips and the soft tissue (gums) that surround the teeth. If either of these deviates from the accepted norm, even if the teeth are straight and white, the smile may appear to be unsightly.

Your lips frame your gums and teeth. There is not much a dentist can do about the muscles and attachments of the lips. But the lips have a dominant role in your perfect smile. The lip line is divided into three types—low, medium, and high. A *low* lip line means you show little or no tooth structure when you talk or smile. In the United States today, this is regarded as being the appearance of an older person. The skin and muscles of the human face drop about 1 mm every 10 years, beginning at about age 40. This is due to gravity and a loss of tissue elasticity. As the muscles and skin drop, less tooth structure is seen, which contributes to an older appearance, of a low lip line. The older you are, less of the top teeth will be visible and more of the bottom teeth will be visible. A *medium* lip line is one where the whole tooth shows when talking or smiling. The line of the teeth generally follows the lower and upper lip lines. This appearance, coupled with dominant front teeth, is considered as being the most desirable type of smile. A *high* lip line is one where all of the front teeth and gum tissue above the top front teeth are visible. It can range from a little gum to a large amount of gum tissue visible. This is considered a less pleasing appearance.

The gum tissue surrounds the teeth. The gum tissue should fill in the space between teeth that touch so that all you see is gums and teeth—no spaces. Where the tooth appears to come out of the gum, the gum should have a scalloped (wave-like) look. The gum should be situated higher on the central incisors (front two teeth), lower on the lateral incisors (smaller two side teeth), and higher again on the two eyeteeth. Usually, the gum tissue is higher around the eyeteeth than the front two teeth. And, of course, the left and right sides should be a mirror image of each other. This scalloping should follow the upper lip line. Correct appearance here is of primary importance in developing a perfect smile. If the height of the gum is too low or too high around a specific tooth or several teeth, even if the teeth are straight, they will look "wrong." Gum position defects can be (and should be) corrected before any major front tooth restoration. Treatment may be minimal or major, depending on the number of teeth and type of problem present.

The teeth themselves should generally follow the lip line from left to right. They should be proportional to each other and themselves. Most often, a length to width ratio of 1.6:1 is desirable. Adjacent teeth also follow a similar proportional ratio when viewed straight on. If individual teeth are too long, wide, not in proportion to each other, or not mirror images left to right, esthetic problems result.

We can recognize these problems and offer suggestions for improved esthetics. You may look and not know what is wrong with your smile, but you know that you do not have the smile you want. It may not be the teeth alone. The framing of the teeth by your lips and the architecture and position of the gums surrounding your teeth are two variables in a three-part equation for a perfect smile—yours!

If you have any questions about your perfect smile, please feel free to ask us.

Tooth Whitening: Overview and Options

You have expressed an interest in making your teeth whiter. The following are important considerations for you in determining which method is best for you:

- Ninety-seven percent of patients who whiten their teeth have successful results.
- The process does not damage the teeth.
- It is impossible to predict the degree of whitening prior to treatment.
- Active gum disease, decay, or dental pathology must be corrected prior to beginning the whitening process.
- The teeth must be clean. If it has been more than 3 months since your last professional dental cleaning, we advise that this be done first. The cleaner the teeth are, the better they will lighten.
- If you have tooth-colored restorations (fillings), porcelain crowns (caps), or a removable partial denture with teeth that are visible, note that these materials **will not** change color as your teeth will. It is possible that these restorations will need to be replaced or modified after the whitening is completed. This should be done after allowing 1 month for the color to stabilize.
- The more yellow your teeth are initially, the more color change (lighter/whiter) will be noticed after whitening. The whiter/lighter your teeth are to begin, less color change will be noticed.
- Research indicates that teeth can only get "as white as they can get." The color is a function of the physical properties of the teeth. Further whitening beyond that point will not have a noticeable effect.
- Teeth with tetracycline discolorations will probably need multiple whitening treatments.
- If you have whitened your teeth before (with professional solutions and trays), there will be a less noticeable color change.
- The difference between in-office and at-home tray tooth whitening appears to be only in how long it takes to achieve the color change. The in-office procedure is faster; the at-home technique is slower (and requires more time commitment on your part). The in-office process uses more concentrated whitening solution than the at-home solutions.
- The lightening process continues for 2 days after the in-office whitening. You should not drink tea, coffee, cola beverages, or smoke for those 48 hours.
- There is a "rebound" color change possible after the whitening is completed. It is between one-half and one shade as noted on the commonly used shade color guides. In the combination in-office/at-home tray technique, this rebound is minimized or eliminated.
- Some people experience sensitivity after the procedure. This sensitivity is not permanent and will quickly disappear. Fluoride gels may be prescribed in this event.
- The color change remains satisfactory for approximately 3 to 7 years. Your eating/drinking habits contribute to future yellowing of the teeth.
- Teeth can have the whitening process repeated when they again darken.

There are three possible whitening combinations available at this office:

1. In-office technique alone. Involves 6 to 10 top and bottom front teeth; 12 to 20 total. Total number of teeth whitened depends on the presenting conditions. Although the teeth are isolated and soft tissues are protected, it is possible some of the whitening solution can contact the tissues. The tissues may temporarily turn white and be sensitive. This will go away in a few hours at most. This procedure is completed in one appointment. Some postoperative color rebound is possible.
2. At-home tray system tooth whitening alone. Trays cover all top and bottom teeth. One box of whitening solution (possibly two) is usually needed. Trays can be worn while sleeping or during the day. This technique can take several weeks to complete. Trays can be kept and used in the future, with only a syringe of whitening gel to "touch up" teeth before important events. Food and drink will yellow teeth over time.
3. A combination of in-office and at-home tray whitening. This is the fastest, most effective, and best value. The in-office whitening is done in one appointment. The trays stabilize the color, reduce rebound, and are available for the future.

Option 1 fee: $ Option 2 fee: $ Option 3 fee: $

You Can Have Whiter Teeth!

The least damaging and most conservative way of making your teeth lighter is with the use of a whitening solution. Contrary to what you might think, brushing your teeth harder with an abrasive toothpaste will not make your teeth whiter, but rather may darken them faster. The tooth-whitening concept has been around for many years, and the techniques have become easier and less expensive to accomplish. Tooth whitening was noted in the dental literature in the 1920s. The technique has become easier and the cost has decreased. Today, there are two convenient methods to whiten dark teeth: At-Home Whitening and In-Office Whitening.

Why Do Teeth Get Yellow?
The intrinsic (normal) color of your teeth is related to the color and thickness of the enamel and dentin, as well as the types of foods and liquids you ingest. The thinner the enamel, the darker the underlying dentin; the more coffee, tea, cola beverages, and red wine you drink, the darker your teeth will be. Cracks that are commonly found in the enamel of your teeth may provide a pathway for discoloring fluids to reach the underlying dentin.

If you have a yellow, brown, or orange shade to your teeth, in most cases it can be made lighter by the whitening procedure. Whitening works very well in removing age-related darkening of your teeth. This age-related darkening is most likely due to years of drinking the darkening beverages, or other environmental factors, rather than genetics. No drilling or anesthesia is required for whitening. Your teeth will not become weaker. Because the mineralization of teeth varies so much from person to person, there is no way to determine how many office visits it will take to effect the color change or how white the teeth will get. The darker your teeth are, the more time required for the change and the more distinctive the color change will be.

The whitening procedure will also work to a lesser degree on teeth with tetracycline discoloration. We have seen several fair to good results from both in-office and at-home whitening. It does take more time to achieve good results on this type of stain, and unfortunately, sometimes the change is minor.

Two Available Techniques
There are two types of whitening available. One is done by the patient at home, and the other is done by us during an office visit. They can be done separately or in conjunction with each other. The at-home technique involves using a soft, thin, comfortable mouthguard-like tray. An impression is made of your teeth, and custom whitening trays are fabricated. Then at home, you place the whitening solution in the trays and wear them for an hour or two each day or sleep with them in place all night. With in-office whitening, you come to the office for 1 or 2 hours, and a stronger whitening solution is applied by us and activated for that time. Usually only one visit is required.

The color change should last for 3 to 7 years in most people. The color change you see immediately after the whitening is completed will regress one shade over the course of 1 to 3 months, with most of the change taking place in the first week. If you drink a lot of coffee, tea, cola beverages, red wine, or if you smoke, the teeth may begin to turn darker again. When this happens, the whitening process can be repeated.

The possible side effects include temporary white discoloration of the gum tissue if the office whitening solution comes into contact with the gum. This goes away quickly. The teeth may become slightly sensitive to temperature changes for a short time. This also goes away quickly. There is **no** damage to the tooth enamel, dentin, or pulp from the whitening process. Fillings and crowns do not whiten. When your teeth change to a lighter color, you may need to have those fillings and/or crowns redone. We will let you know whether this is a possibility before we whiten your teeth. There are no other adverse effects known.

The teeth that show when you talk, smile, or eat are the teeth that would benefit your appearance most if whitened. Usually the top teeth are whitened because they are much more visible than the bottom teeth, but both arches can be successfully whitened. The lower teeth take about three times as long to reach the color change of the top teeth.

If you have any questions about whiter teeth, please feel free to ask us.

At-Home Tooth Whitening Options

Selecting one of the many different tooth-whitening systems available today can be very confusing. There are whitening toothpastes, whitening gums, nonprescription whitening kits to be used with trays, whitening strips, whitening gels, professional mouthguard-like tray whitening systems, and professional in-office whitening procedures. To simplify all of these, we have narrowed the field to three very different and practical options—Crest Professional Strength Whitestrips, custom-made tray home whitening systems, and over-the-counter gels. All have advantages and disadvantages and all have the potential to whiten your teeth. The following discussion should give you a fair overview of each type and help you to make an informed decision about which system is right for you.

At-home mouthguard tray tooth whitening has been around the longest. It is most appropriate for those 18 years of age and older. Impressions are made of your teeth (both upper and lower), stone models are made from the impressions, and a mouthguard is molded that exactly matches your teeth. The whitening solution is supplied to you in syringe containers. You will dispense a slight amount into the mouthguard tray at each tooth and place the tray over your teeth. Only a small amount of whitening material is needed. The trays are worn for about one hour daily. A color change can be noticed in 3 to 5 days, but the complete process can take 2 to 3 weeks, depending on the original color of the teeth.

The teeth will stay white for 12 to 24 months and you can keep the new color longer by "touching up" with a one- or two-day application of bleach once a year. The ideal time to touch up is after having your teeth professionally cleaned. We have touch-up tubes of bleach available for purchasing. This process does not harm the teeth in any way. The disadvantage to this technique is cost. The total cost of the impressions, models, custom mouthguard trays, and the initial supply of bleach is $ _____.

Crest Professional Strength Whitestrips are a new whitening option. Clear strips containing the whitening solution are placed over the upper and lower teeth twice a day for 30 minutes a day, for 21 days. The professional kit also contains a toothbrush and whitening toothpaste. The professional version is 42% more effective than the over-the-counter Whitestrips. The Crest Professional Strength Whitestrips are useful for those with financial concerns and for teenagers. The cost of Crest Professional Strength Whitestrips is quite affordable at $_____ a kit. The disadvantages are that the strips are not custom-made so that they do not cover as many teeth or fit as well or as comfortably as the tray system. The strips work best for teeth in good straight alignment. They may need to be rewhitened at 6-month intervals according to the manufacturer; we have found the whitening to last satisfactorily for a longer time.

New over-the-counter gels are available that can be painted onto the tooth surface. Colgate Simply White, Crest Night Effects, and Go Smile ampules are a few of the products currently available. These clear gel formulas are applied to the teeth twice a day for 2 weeks. The gels will effectively work to whiten your teeth until it is washed away by your saliva. Because there is no way to determine and compare the salivary flow of patients, we cannot determine how effective the brush-on gel will work for you. This method is ideal for teenagers to young adults who may desire only a slight change in color. These over-the-counter gels are the least costly of all the methods but will also produce the least dramatic whitening results.

Any of the described systems can work. The degree of color change will depend of the original color of your teeth and how faithful you are to adhering to the treatment process. The custom trays are the most reliable of the methods, with the color change lasting a long time, but they are the most expensive of the three methods. The Crest Professional Strength Whitestrips can also produce results, but the color change may not last as long and may require more frequent touch ups, but they are inexpensive.

At-Home Tray System: Tooth Whitening Instructions

Patient Name:_____   **Date:**_____

A technique is now available for whitening your teeth at home. The whitening procedure works best for teeth that have a yellow shade, although it can work to a lesser extent with teeth that have a gray shade or tetracycline discoloration. A mouthguard will be constructed from an impression that is taken of your teeth. This will hold the whitening solution against your teeth. The general instructions for mouthguard tooth whitening are as follows. They may be slightly modified by us to suit your particular needs.

1. Before using the tooth whitening gel, brush and floss your teeth. Rinse your mouth.
2. As demonstrated, place a small amount of whitening gel into the mouthguard in each tooth to be whitened.
3. Insert the mouthguard as instructed, allowing the excess material to extrude. Spit out the excess solution. If there is much to spit out, place less bleach in the tray at the next application.
4. Wear the mouthguard as instructed. Keep the mouthguard in place for 1 to 2 hours. Follow this routine each day until the whitening gel we supply is finished. You may wear the trays with the whitening solution during the day or you may choose to wear the trays while you sleep. Diminished salivary flow while sleeping will keep the whitening gel active for a longer period. How long or how much you can wear the tray depends entirely on your comfort. If there is no tooth sensitivity, you can wear the trays as often as you want. If you start to develop tooth sensitivity, **stop** wearing the trays until the sensitivity is gone (a day or two at most), and then begin again.
5. Do not eat or drink for 30 minutes after you have removed the mouthguard and finished the whitening session. After each use, rinse the mouthguard out with water, dry it, and store it in a safe place.
6. Return to the office to have the whitening progress evaluated after _____ days of whitening.
7. Note any changes you might see in your gums and be sure to bring this immediately to our attention. Any sensitivity or alteration in their appearance is temporary.
8. **Home mouthguard whitening must only be done under the supervision of a dentist.**
9. Because the mineralization of teeth is so variable from person to person, there is absolutely no way to determine how much color change can be expected or how long it may take to achieve the color change. Expect that it can take as little as 2 to 3 hours and as long as 6 weeks for teeth that are especially dark. This time frame, of course, depends on how often you wear the trays filled with whitening gel. If you do the procedure for 1 hour every other day, it will take twice as long to finish as if you do it for 1 hour every day. If you skip a few days, it will not affect the final result. The ultimate color change will be the same whether you take 1 week or 1 month or longer. The important aspect in this is the contact time of the tray and gel with the teeth to be lightened.
10. The lighter tooth color you see immediately after the whitening process is finished will regress one shade darker over 1 to 3 months, with most of the regression evident after the first week. Lower teeth may take longer to whiten than top teeth.
11. Your eating and drinking habits and resident chromogenic bacteria will determine the duration of the whitening effect. Most patients maintain a satisfactory result for 3 to 7 years. If you smoke, drink a lot of tea, coffee, colas, red wine, etc., your teeth will, over extended time, darken again. **Keep your whitening trays in a safe place.** At some point you may decide to "touch up" your teeth, by whitening for a short duration. Touch ups do not take as long or require as much whitening product.
12. If you are going to have fillings replaced, you should wait at least 2 weeks after the whitening is completed for the tooth color to stabilize before new restorations are placed.

Other Instructions:
The cost for the **mouthguard whitening** is $_____ for one arch; $_____ for both arches.

If you have any questions about mouthguard tooth whitening, please feel free to ask us.

In-Office Power Whitening Technique without Light Activation

Front teeth, the 6 to 10 teeth most easily seen when you talk or smile, are the teeth that can benefit most from an in-office "power" tooth whitening. Just as with back teeth, if there are medium- to large-sized fillings in the teeth, it is probably better if these teeth were protected with crowns. The in-office power whitening procedure is one of the most conservative and least expensive methods to attempt to lighten tooth color back to a more acceptable appearance.

The procedure involves isolating the teeth to be whitened and protecting the gum tissues and lips. A whitening solution is then mixed and applied to the teeth. The type of application and number of appointments depends on the type of whitening system we believe will be best in your situation.

Most patients show great improvement after only one treatment. Since the protective biofilm that normally covers the tooth enamel is removed during the whitening procedure, you should avoid smoking and drinking pigmented liquids (coffee, tea, red wine) for about 24 hours after the whitening is completed. After 24 hours, the biofilm is usually back in place. The final color will usually regress one shade in the first 1 to 3 months, with most of the change coming in the first week. Some teeth may need a second appointment (or a combination of in-office and at-home tray system whitening) to achieve the desired result. The degree of whitening for any tooth is variable and impossible to predict. However, recent studies show that 97% of all patients who whiten their teeth are happy with the result. The color change should be satisfactory for 3 to 7 years.

If you have dental restorations (crowns, bonding), the plastics and porcelain will not change color. You may need to have some of those fillings redone once your teeth are lightened. We will let you know whether you can expect to have some fillings replaced due to the color change. If you are going to have fillings replaced, you should wait at least 2 weeks after the whitening is completed for the tooth color to stabilize before new restorations are placed. Some postoperative sensitivity is possible, but it usually disappears quickly. The tooth enamel or dentin is not damaged by the whitening process.

We will discuss your particular needs and make the appropriate treatment recommendations.

If you have any questions about in-office power whitening, please feel free to ask us.

In-Office Power Whitening Technique with Light Activation

Front teeth, the 6 to 10 teeth most easily seen when you talk or smile, are the teeth that can benefit most from an in-office "power" tooth whitening. Just as with back teeth, if there are medium- to large-sized fillings in the teeth, it is probably better if these teeth were protected with crowns. The in-office power whitening procedure is one of the most conservative and least expensive methods to attempt to lighten tooth color back to a more acceptable appearance.

The procedure involves isolating the teeth to be whitened and protecting the gum tissues and lips. A whitening solution is then mixed and applied to the teeth. A special light will be placed over each individual tooth for several minutes. The light will provide the energy for the chemical reaction to take place. This procedure will be repeated about three times for each tooth during the 60- to 90-minute appointment.

Most patients show great improvement after only one treatment. Since the protective biofilm that normally covers the tooth enamel is removed during the whitening procedure, you should avoid smoking and drinking pigmented liquids (coffee, tea, red wine) for about 24 hours after the whitening is completed. After 24 hours, the biofilm is usually back in place. The final color will usually regress one shade in the first 1 to 3 months, with most of the change occurring in the first week. Some teeth may need a second appointment (or a combination of in-office and tray system whitening) to achieve the desired result. The degree of whitening for any tooth is variable and impossible to predict. However, recent studies show that 97% of all patients who whiten their teeth are happy with the result. The color change should be satisfactory for 3 to 7 years.

If you have dental restorations (crowns, bonding), the plastics and porcelain will not change color. You may need to have some of those fillings redone once your teeth are lightened. We will let you know whether you can expect to have some fillings replaced due to the color change. If you are going to have fillings replaced, you should wait at least 2 weeks after the whitening is completed for the tooth color to stabilize before new restorations are placed. Some postoperative sensitivity is possible, but it usually disappears quickly. The tooth enamel or dentin is not damaged by the whitening process.

We will discuss your particular needs and make the appropriate treatment recommendations.

If you have any questions about in-office power whitening, please feel free to ask us.

In-Office Tooth Whitening Postoperative Instructions

Patient Name:_____   **Date:**_____

You have just finished "power" whitening your teeth. You should have very few postprocedural problems. Here are some things to remember:

- Please avoid smoking or drinking heavily pigmented beverages (coffee, tea, colas, red wine) during the next 24 hours.
- The final color change will regress about one shade in the next 1 to 3 months, with most of the change occurring in the first week after whitening.
- You may experience some postprocedural sensitivity from the heat and chemicals used in the power whitening process. This will disappear after a few days at most. If you wish, you can use a desensitizing toothpaste. We can also prescribe a fluoride toothpaste that works well in this situation.
- Since your lips were stretched for about 60 to 90 minutes, expect them to feel sore or different for a few hours.
- Although great care was taken to prevent the whitening solution from contacting your gum tissue, it is not uncommon for a few spots of gum tissue to have had whitening material on them. In those spots, the gums will turn white for a few hours. They may be slightly sore. Both the whiteness and the soreness are temporary and will go away after a short time.
- You may use any nonabrasive toothpaste to clean your teeth and remove superficial stains. If you wish to use a whitening toothpaste to help maintain the color, feel free to do so.
- If you have decided to use the combination in-office power whitening/at-home tray system whitening technique, use the mouthguard as instructed.
- If you are going to have fillings replaced, you should wait at least 2 weeks after whitening is completed for the tooth color to stabilize before new restorations are placed.

If you have any questions about these instructions, please feel free to ask us.

Nonvital Tooth Whitening Options

When a nerve in the tooth dies, the tooth needs endodontic treatment (root canal). The tooth that has been endodontically treated can, however, slowly darken over time. The color change can range from light gray to dark black. This color change is not cosmetically pleasing.

For the back teeth, molars, and premolars, this color change may not be objectionable. The tooth might not be visible when you speak or smile. Usually, a back tooth will be protected and covered with a ceramic or porcelain to metal crown. The crown color is made to match your natural tooth color.

Front teeth, or teeth easily seen when you talk or smile, benefit the most from nonvital tooth whitening. Just as with back teeth, when a medium- to large-sized filling is present, it is probably better to protect the tooth with a crown. However, many times the front teeth that have had root canal therapy have smaller-sized restorations. When these teeth turn a darker than normal color, a cosmetic problem results. The nonvital whitening procedure is the most conservative and least expensive method to attempt to change the unwanted color to a more acceptable appearance.

The procedure involves gaining access to the original preparation made for the root canal and removing part of the filling and any other debris that remains. A small portion of the existing root canal filling is removed to allow a new sealer material to be placed over the remaining root canal filling to protect it from the whitening solution. Depending on your particular situation, the tooth may then be whitened internally, externally, or both at the same visit. As a rule, the longer a tooth has been dark, the longer it will take to whiten.

There are three methods available to whiten the endodontically treated tooth: power whitening, walking whitening, or patient-applied whitening.

Power whitening involves the application of a whitening solution to the outer surface and internally (where the filling has been partially removed). Most patients show great improvement after only one treatment.

Walking whitening involves placing the whitening solution into the opening in the tooth and temporarily sealing it in place. It will remain there for about 1 week. At that time, the color of the tooth is reevaluated and the need for another application of the whitening solution is determined.

The patient-applied process will require that you place the whitening solution into the access opened in your tooth. It will be held in place by a cotton pellet. You will remove the cotton and solution after about 1 hour. You will repeat this process daily until the tooth has reached the desired shade.

Some teeth may not be at all responsive and will need porcelain veneers or full crowns to be made attractive again. The degree of whitening for any tooth is impossible to predict. It is possible that after some time, the tooth may start to turn dark again, and the whitening process may need to be repeated.

There is a fee associated with the initial access opening of the tooth and cleaning and sealing of the internal portions of the teeth.

In many cases the improvement of the appearance of the darkened tooth is quite noticeable. It is certainly the simplest and most cost-effective manner of correcting this type of problem.

We will discuss your particular needs and make the appropriate treatment recommendations.

If you have any questions about nonvital tooth whitening, please feel free to ask us.

Tetracycline-Discolored Teeth: Options for Cosmetic Improvement

When the permanent teeth are forming in a young child's jaw (before they come through the gum tissue and can be seen), they can be positively affected by controlled systemic fluorides (made stronger and more resistant to dental decay). They can be adversely affected by high fevers, malnutrition, and prescription medications, most notably, the antibiotics in the tetracycline class. Tetracyclines are given to children who have shown a reaction to penicillin or who have a medical problem that can be treated best with the tetracyclines.

Depending on the age of the patient, the stage of development of the permanent teeth, and the type and dosage of the medication, the change in the tooth color (both dentin and enamel) can be slight, moderate, or quite disfiguring. The color of the teeth can change from the normal homogeneous yellow/white to light or dark gray, brown, yellow, or even purple/blue. Most often, the color is not uniform throughout the tooth. There may be horizontal bands or stripes of color that are visible. If you have ever seen a photograph of the planet Jupiter, with the brightly colored horizontal bands that mark the different wind zones, it would be similar to the tetracycline bands and colors seen on the permanent teeth.

Improving the Appearance of the Teeth

The color change due to tetracycline staining is not a superficial or surface problem. The dentin (the layer of tooth underlying enamel) is usually darker than the enamel and gives the tooth its color. Brushing harder or using a whitening toothpaste will not improve the color. Today the appearance of discolored teeth can be improved through tooth whitening, bonded porcelain or ceramic veneers, resin veneers, or full crowns.

What Is Right for You

What is right for you depends on the amount and type of discoloration, the speed with which you want them improved, and your finances. For mild to moderate discolorations, a whitening process can significantly improve the appearance of the teeth. A combination of in-office and at-home whitening works well. In the in-office "power" whitening process, a solution is applied to your teeth. The solution is activated by light energy and allowed to remain on each tooth to be whitened for several minutes. If we believe it is appropriate for you and you will need even more whitening, we may suggest that you continue the whitening process at home with a mouthguard whitening technique. In this technique, special mouthguard-like trays are custom fabricated to fit your teeth. You will be given a whitening solution to place in the trays and wear nightly until the desired color change occurs. The time required to achieve the desired effect depends on the degree of discoloration. Usually the at-home whitening procedure will need to be done nightly for 6 months at least to be effective. This is the least invasive and least costly method for improving the tooth color.

Custom porcelain veneers require preparation of the tooth and processing by a dental laboratory. Veneers are much quicker but more costly and maintenance requirements are more involved. Veneers can be expected to last 8 to 15 years, perhaps longer. Direct resin veneers are placed onto the teeth in one visit. They are less expensive than laboratory-processed veneers. Direct resin veneers can look almost as nice as laboratory-processed resin but are not as natural looking as porcelain. They will last about 5 years before needing replacement or touch up. If you are considering veneers, we may still recommend some degree of tooth whitening before they are made because the darker the teeth are, the harder it is to opaque or mask out the underlying color, which is the point of placing the veneers in the first place. The veneer that can transmit some underlying tooth color tends to look better than a fully opaque veneer. Alternatively, more tooth preparation can be made to permit an opaque layer to be covered by thicker esthetic porcelain. Each case is different, but an improved appearance is possible. In the case of the darkest discolorations, the only effective cosmetic solution may be full-coverage crowns.

If you have any questions about treating tetracycline-discolored teeth, please feel free to ask us.

chapter 6

Endodontics

Content at a Glance 136

Content at a Glance: Endodontics

Apicoectomy
Explains indications and procedures for apicoectomy. Includes postoperative information for the patient.

Endodontic-Periodontic Syndrome
Describes endodontic-periodontic syndrome, its diagnosis, and treatment options.

Endodontic Therapy: An Overview
Explains endodontic therapy, why it may be needed, and what the procedure entails.

Endodontic Therapy: Procedure
Takes the confusion out of endodontic therapy. Presents what the fee for the endodontic procedure covers.

Re-treatment of Root Canals
Explains why a tooth may require endodontic re-treatment, the procedure, and possible problems that may arise during re-treatment.

Root Hemisections and Root Amputations
Reasons and procedures for root hemisections and amputations are explained.

Apicoectomy

Indications

Although endodontic treatment has an extremely high rate of success, it is not 100% effective. Some teeth may not respond as expected to the root canal therapy. Sometimes, it is clear from the beginning that the root canal is not working as planned. Other times, it may be years later that the need for other treatment arises. The first and most desirable method of solving the problem is to re-treat the root canal at one or more roots. In other words, the root canal treatment is redone in a method similar to the original therapy. If it is possible to re-treat the root canal with this nonsurgical approach, this is best. If not, a different form of treatment, an *apicoectomy,* must be considered.

Teeth that have narrow, curved roots, "blockages" of the canal, root resorption, persistent infection, fractures, a wide open apex, and associated cysts are some of the problems that can be corrected with an "apico." There may be reasons not to perform the apico, such as surgical inaccessibility, poor or lack of bone support, short roots, or vertical fracture of the root.

The Procedure

The root or roots that are to receive the apicoectomy are measured with radiographs, and the approximate location of the root tip is estimated. The area to be treated is anesthetized with a local anesthetic. An incision of the gum is made over the root tip area and the gum is moved to the side. Access is made through the bone, and the tip or apex of the root can then usually be seen through this "window" in the bone. The infection is visualized and cleaned out. The tip of the root is usually removed, and a sealing filling is placed in the remaining tip opening. The tissue is then sutured back into place. The tooth does not lose significant stability from this procedure.

There is no pain during the surgery. Postoperative discomfort will be eliminated with antiinflammatory and analgesic medication. There is usually some slight swelling of the surgical site. The swelling is temporary and will disappear after a few days.

When the "apico" is begun and the tooth can actually be seen, another type of problem may be noted. A fractured root may be the problem, and an apico would not work and the tooth would have to be removed.

This procedure can be completed by a general dentist, but it is most often referred to an endodontist (root canal specialist) for evaluation and treatment.

If you have any questions about apicoectomy, please feel free to ask us.

Endodontic-Periodontic Syndrome

Endodontic-periodontic syndrome is a combination dental problem. The term *endodontic* refers to the inside of the tooth, and the term *periodontic* refers to the tissues and bone around the tooth. In this particular dental problem, the nerve in a tooth is dead or abscessed and bone destruction has occurred around the tooth.

Decay or trauma to a tooth can cause the nerve in a tooth to die. Severe periodontal (gum) disease and significant bone loss can expose an accessory nerve of a tooth, also causing nerve death. Most often, a dead nerve in a tooth is the cause of the endodontic-periodontic syndrome. You may or may not experience any symptoms with any of these conditions.

This type of bone destruction is characterized by a drainage tract between the abscessed root and sulcus (space between the gum and the tooth). The sulcus of a tooth can be pictured as a collar of tissue around the tooth where the tooth and gum visibly meet. It is normally only about 3 millimeters deep. An abscess forms at the root tip and this infection can spread, moving up the root toward the crown of the tooth. The infection can drain into the sulcus and enter your mouth. You might even notice a bad taste in your mouth when this happens.

Once the draining tract is established, and there is no pressure buildup from the abscess, the tooth can be symptomless. You may not even experience a bad taste in your mouth.

Diagnosis and Treatment

Endodontic-periodontic syndrome is diagnosed by the use of radiographs and a periodontal probe. The treatment will first involve traditional endodontic treatment (root canal therapy) to eliminate the cause of the infection. Antibiotics may be prescribed to help eliminate the infection. This should be started as soon as possible.

Following completion of the root canal, the drainage tract should begin to disappear and the bone starts to fill in. This process can take from 3 to 4 months. The longer the infection was active before it was treated, the longer it will take for the bone to fill in. In severe circumstances, the bone may not fill in and the tooth may need to be removed.

If the bone is not filling in well, another evaluation will be done. This evaluation may be done by a periodontist (a specialist who treats problems associated with the gums and supporting bone). The periodontist may suggest additional treatment to fill in the damaged bone areas. If the bone fill procedure is not successful, or if the infection returns, it may indicate additional problems with the tooth. A hairline crack of the root, extra canals that cannot be visualized or filled, or microscopic accessory canals that are untreatable may be the reason. In these cases the tooth may not be able to be saved.

The endodontic-periodontic syndrome is not uncommon in dentistry. It can occur around any tooth. When treated in a timely fashion, the problem is usually resolved in a satisfactory manner. When left untreated for a long time, the tooth may become unsalvageable.

If you have any questions about endodontic-periodontic syndrome, please feel free to ask us.

Endodontic Therapy: An Overview

ROOT CANAL

The pulp of your tooth, which contains the nerve and tiny blood vessels, can become infected. The pulp has a limited ability to heal itself. This infection can be caused by a deep cavity that reaches the center of the tooth causing the pulp to die, a traumatic injury to the tooth, or an extensive preparation (drilling) of the tooth. The extensive preparation may have been done to prepare the tooth for a crown (cap) or other large preparation for a restoration. The pulp may or may not abscess immediately in these cases. It may take years for a problem to develop. The infected pulp tissue may or may not be painful. It may or may not be visible on a dental radiograph. A tooth with this type of an abscess is not usually extracted because the infection can be treated with endodontic therapy on the tooth. This routine procedure can save the tooth and enable you to avoid the harmful effects of tooth loss. It is successful in more than 90% of the teeth in which the treatment is completed.

Endodontic treatment can take from one to three appointments to complete. Teeth can have one to four canals that need to be treated. An opening is created to access the nerve, and the abscessed nerve is removed from the root or roots. The canals where the nerves had been located are then cleaned and shaped and a medication may be placed in the canal to promote better healing.

When it has been determined that the canals are free of infection, they are filled with a special rubber-like material and sealed with a cementing medium. The abscessed area associated with the tooth will then begin to heal. It may take several months before healing is completed and for the tooth to become asymptomatic, that is, for any soreness in the area to disappear.

Once the endodontic therapy has been completed, the tooth is usually restored with a cast crown or onlay. This is done to protect the tooth and prevent it from fracturing. Failure to follow through with mandatory restorative procedures after endodontic therapy on a previously uncrowned tooth can result in a vertical fracture. If there is very little tooth structure remaining, we may also advise the use of a post and core to further help the tooth retain its final restoration. We will discuss with you the exact type of restoration that you will need.

Please note that this infection may cause discomfort between root canal appointments. This is normal and usually not a cause for any concern. Contact the office if there is pain and/or swelling. Remember to avoid biting down on the tooth until the root canal is completed and the final restoration has been placed. You may have had no discomfort from the tooth prior to the root canal treatment or have been unaware that you even had an abscess. However, you may experience pain or swelling after the root canal treatment has begun.

If we have prescribed antibiotics for the abscess, be sure to fill the prescription and take it until it is finished. It is important that you do this in order to quickly control the infection. If you do not take the prescribed medication, the resolution of the abscess may be delayed and problems with the postoperative pain are more likely.

If you have any questions about the root canal procedure or the final restoration of the tooth, please feel free to ask us.

Endodontic Therapy: Procedure

Although we make a great effort to explain specific treatment and related fees, we find that concerning endodontics (root canal therapy) in particular, there sometimes remains some confusion. Please carefully read the following so you know what is included in the fees for the procedure and where other fees might be warranted.

Endodontic Treatment (Root Canal)

The fee for endodontic treatment for each individual tooth includes:

❑ All radiographs
  - the initial diagnostic radiographs
  - working and measurement radiographs
  - radiographs of the completed root canal for your records and, where indicated, for insurance carrier verification of treatment
❑ All necessary anesthesia (local) to "numb" the tooth
❑ Access into the tooth
❑ Removal of the nerve tissue
❑ Cleaning and shaping of the canals
❑ Irrigation of the canals with medicated solutions
❑ Placement of medicated dressings where needed
❑ Filling the canals with root canal filling materials
❑ A temporary filling in the access opening between appointments or at completion of the root canal
❑ Any emergency visits necessary during treatment of the root canal for the tooth being treated
❑ One year of postoperative checkups and necessary radiographs. The fee does NOT cover:
  - Prescription medication (we will write a prescription that must be filled at a pharmacy)
  - The final restoration, which is always a separate fee

The final restoration you will need after the root canal is completed will depend on which tooth is being treated and on how much natural tooth remains and how strong it appears. You will be informed of the probable restoration you will need and its cost, before the root canal is started. Again, this fee is separate from the root canal fees.

If you have any questions about what is included in fees for endodontic therapy, please feel free to ask us before treatment begins, if possible.

Re-treatment of Root Canals

Endodontic treatment is one of the most successful forms of dental therapy that is available today. But approximately 10% of the teeth that are treated will never heal completely or will develop problems later on. You have a situation that falls into that 10%.

There are several possible indications that there is a problem. You may experience pain or sensitivity on the treated tooth when you bite or put pressure on it. There may be either slight or severe swelling in the treated area. A fistula (drainage tract) may develop or never fully close. This drainage site will have pus that can be expressed through it. Or you may feel nothing at all. The problem may be something that was discovered through a postoperative radiograph. The bone around the tooth may not have grown back, or there may be more bone destruction seen.

These problems occur for a variety of reasons. The pre-existing infection, the reason for the root canal in the first place, may have left residual effects that never disappeared entirely and have begun to act up again. It is also possible that the original root canal filling was not clinically ideal. This happens due to any of several factors such as severely twisted or curved roots; small, extra canals; separated root canal instruments; cement washout; and others. Sometimes, no clear reason can be seen for the root canal failure. It just happened.

Even if the problem has not been noticed by you, it is not wise to leave an active infection in your body. A nonsurgical retreatment procedure will remove the root canal filling materials, clean and refile the root canal, then refill the canals. The re-treatment is usually more difficult and time consuming than the first root canal. It is harder to remove condensed, cemented root canal material, cemented posts, and bonded resins or cements in order to re-treat the canals. Attempts to remove these materials may cause the tooth to fracture and become hopeless. It may not be possible to re-instrument the tooth, based on what is in it. This may not be known until the treatment is begun. It is also possible that re-treatment will not work at all.

Despite these possible problems, re-treatment is the most conservative approach and usually the least expensive approach. When the situation arises, it is the method of choice. It is performed on a tooth that you need to keep. If the re-treatment cannot be done, the problem must be addressed surgically or the tooth will have to be extracted. A surgical endodontics procedure, called an *apicoectomy,* may be required if the re-treatment does not work.

If you have any questions about re-treatment of root canals, please feel free to ask us.

Root Hemisections and Root Amputations

Indications

At times, a portion of a molar is hopelessly damaged, but there is still sound tooth available. Depending on the individual problem, it may be possible and desirable to retain the good part of the tooth and remove the damaged portion. Back teeth have two (in the lower) or three (in the upper) roots. One of the roots may be severely decayed, periodontally involved, or split. Most commonly, if it is a split root, the tooth has already had endodontic therapy (root canal treatment). If the problem is decay, there may be no root canal on that tooth and it will need a root canal on the roots that will be retained.

Procedure

A root amputation is the removal of part or all of an individual root. A root hemisection is the dividing of the tooth through the middle to make two separate roots and two separate teeth out of what was once a single tooth with two joined roots. This procedure is most often performed on lower molars.

The procedure for either is similar. If a root canal was not completed, it is started and finished on the root or roots that will remain. The area is then surgically accessed to view directly and the hopeless root section is removed, or the tooth is divided. Usually, the removal of the root is not too difficult to accomplish. Sectioning of the root is done with a standard, high-speed dental handpiece.

The area is then closed, sutured, and left to heal for 6 to 8 weeks. When sufficiently healed, the remaining root is finally restored. Nearly 100% of the time, the tooth will need a cast restoration. For a root resection, in which the molar tooth has been divided into two premolar-sized portions, the roots will receive a post and core, and then splinted crowns. If necessary, other teeth may be crowned too and added to the hemisected molar for additional support. In a tooth that has had a root amputated, a single crown may be placed, or it may be attached to another tooth for support. Your individual needs will dictate which is best for you.

The critical aspects for the success of these procedures are the diagnosis and execution of treatment. Posts and cores might be necessary. Often, the treated teeth must be splinted to adjacent teeth. The roots and cast crowns must be shaped just right to ensure that the remaining parts can be easily and thoroughly cleaned with a toothbrush and dental floss.

In many cases, the advent of successful implant procedures has replaced root hemisection and amputation. Your particular situation may indicate which procedure is best for you.

If you have any questions about root hemisection or amputation, please feel free to ask us.

chapter 7

General Dentistry

Content at a Glance: General Dentistry

General
These documents include general information regarding procedures and concepts in general dentistry.

Before Treatment Begins
Helps to clarify the treatment goals, the time and financial commitment, and oral self-care requirements for the patient prior to initiation of treatment.

Dental and Oral Anatomy
Helps patients to understand the parts of the oral environment and how they work together.

Have the Dentistry You Need, Want, and Deserve
Helps patients understand why there may be treatment options, written from a financial point of view.

Infection Control Procedures
Eases patients' concerns about the dental office as a source of infection by explaining sterilization procedures.

Initial Oral Examination
Prepares patients for the initial oral examination with this overview of the procedures involved. Informs patients of the extent of the examination process.

Prescription Medication
Reminds patients of the need to take prescription medication exactly as prescribed. Includes a brief description of drugs likely to be prescribed by an oral healthcare professional.

Sample Patient Handout
A sample patient education handout for penicillin V potassium.

Prophylactic Antibiotics for Premedication
Assure patient cooperation with reasons for premedication and a brief description of drugs likely to be used in this capacity.

Smile (Lip) Line
A discussion on how the lip contributes to the overall esthetics of the patient's smile and ways in which this component can be altered.

Staying Well: How to Keep Your Mouth Healthy
Suggestions on how patients can have great oral health for a lifetime.

Treating the Adult Patient
General information on changes in dental needs of adult patients. Includes discussions about aging, restorations, endodontic therapy, tooth fracture, and problem prevention.

Prevention
Detailing concepts of prevention, these documents outline key concepts as cornerstones of practice.

For a Lifetime of Great Oral Health
Point-by-point recommendations for maintenance of great oral health in patients.

How to Brush! How to Floss!
Description of brushing and flossing technique, used to remind patients of what they learned during their hygiene appointment.

Junk Drink Alert
Notifies patients of a possible new threat to their oral health and recommends solutions to the problem.

Prevention of Decay
Addresses bacterial causes of infection and its prevention in both infants and adults.

When Radiographs Are Necessary
The necessity of radiographs and safety measures used are covered.

Content at a Glance: General Dentistry—cont'd

Reversing Decay
Reviews the process of demineralization and ways to halt or reverse the process.

Sealants and Fluoride: Benefit to Adult Patients
Adult need for sealants and topical fluoride is explained.

Topical Fluoride: At Home and in the Dental Office
Urges patients to take advantage of both in-home and/or in-office fluoride delivery. Includes specific instructions for fluoride tray procedures.

Problems: Causes and Cures
Each document discusses a specific dental condition and possible treatment options.

Abfraction: A New Dental Term
Explains abfraction, its causes, and possible treatment options.

Acid Reflux (Gastroesophageal Reflux Disease)
Explains gastroesophageal reflux disease and the impact on the oral cavity.

Attrition and Abrasion
Covers why teeth abrade, grinding and clenching habits, dentin abrasion, and treatment options.

Bad Breath
Discusses prevention and treatment of chronic halitosis.

Cracked Tooth Syndrome (CTS)
Overview of cracked tooth syndrome, its causes, diagnosis, treatment options, and nontreatment consequences.

Cracked Tooth Syndrome (CTS): Postoperative Instructions
Postoperative instructions for treatment of cracked tooth syndrome by occlusal adjustment, replacement of restoration, or placement of provisional crown.

Dentin Decay
Explanation, detection, and treatment of dentin decay, with prevention information.

Enamel Dysplasia
Enamel dysplasia is defined, and causes and corrective procedures are explained. Also, information on enamel decalcification, which patients may confuse with enamel dysplasia, is provided.

Excessive Wear
An alternative document on abrasion, which concentrates on abrasion only, as well as its causes, consequences, and treatment.

Extraction
Short overview of reasons for extraction as well as what patients can expect postoperatively.

Extraction: Postoperative Instructions
General and specific follow-up care for patients after a dental extraction.

Headaches: The Dental Connection
Explains the important causal relationship between headaches and temporomandibular joint dysfunction (TMD).

How to Encourage Tooth Decay (Humor)
A humorous review of the best way to encourage tooth decay.

Impacted Teeth
An explanation of impaction and which teeth are commonly affected.

Metal Filling–Induced Cracks in Enamel
Discusses possibility of removing amalgams where alloy is causing cracks in enamel. Possible precursor to cracked tooth syndrome.

Continued

Content at a Glance: General Dentistry—cont'd

Metal Sensitivity
Explains metal sensitivity detection and the accommodation of metal-sensitive patients.

Occlusal (Bite) Guards
The fabrication and uses of antibruxing/antigrinding appliances are clarified.

Pericoronitis
A description of the infection commonly associated with third molars and possible treatment options.

Root Surface Caries
Factors contributing to root decay, treatment, and prevention are discussed.

Sensitive Teeth
Describes causes and treatment of sensitive teeth.

Temporomandibular Joint Dysfunction (TMD) Questionnaire
Questionnaire for the healthcare professional to use in diagnosis of temporomandibular joint dysfunction.

Temporomandibular Joint Dysfunction (TMD) Syndrome
Describes the temporomandibular joint dysfunction syndrome and possible treatment options.

Toothbrush Abrasion: Preventing Tooth Destruction
Helps patients comprehend the effects of improper toothbrushing.

Traumatic Occlusion: Occlusal Equilibration or Bite Adjustment
Cause and treatment information on traumatic occlusion.

Wisdom Teeth (Third Molars)
Reassures patients with an understanding of wisdom teeth, why we have them, the troubles they can cause, and reasons for extraction.

Xerostomia: Dry Mouth Syndrome
Explanation of xerostomia, its consequences, and prevention of these consequences are discussed.

Before Treatment Begins

As you consider having extensive dental treatment, it may be beneficial for you to review the following points:

- *Time Commitment.* Because of the nature of dental appointments, it may be necessary for you to take some time off work. A few longer appointments are generally more efficient and less inconvenient than many short appointments. This will minimize your time in the office. Usually, the best time to have a long appointment is in the morning. Once the treatment has begun, it needs to be completed in a timely fashion. If treatment is delayed or missed, it could change the proposed treatment plan. This could adversely affect the total cost to you.
- *Dentistry is both an art and a science.* In complicated and technically difficult cases, and because of our high standards, it may prove necessary to redo a portion or go back and retake impressions or remake crowns, etc.
- *Make certain you are aware of what treatment is required and the goals of treatment.* If you do not understand why we have made a particular recommendation or treatment sequence, or the length of treatment required, please ask us for clarification before treatment begins. It is possible that previously undetected dental problems will be discovered once tooth preparation has begun. When this occurs after the treatment plan has been developed, you will be immediately informed.
- *You should be comfortable with all financial arrangements before any treatment is begun.* Pre-estimates sent to insurance carriers can help approximate your out-of-pocket costs. Establish your dental budget. This will determine how much and how quickly treatment can proceed. Understand that you, and not your insurance carrier, are ultimately responsible for the total cost of treatment. If you would like to have more treatment than you can easily afford at one time, the dental procedures can be done in phases over months or years. This will also allow you to use your insurance benefits to the maximum permitted. Payment is expected as work is completed.
- *Thorough oral self-care is very important, both at the beginning of treatment and afterward.* The better your oral health is, the easier the restoration process will be. You may be asked to use an antimicrobial prescription mouthrinse from 2 weeks before we begin treatment until after all restorative treatment is completed. Please follow these instructions.
- *While dental restorations function well for years of service, nothing lasts forever.* Not us, not dental restorations. We use the best available dental materials and techniques, but the reality is that some restorations simply last longer than others. With today's longer life span, the restoration might even wear out! The better you maintain your dental restorations, the longer they will last. Just as with anything else, proper maintenance is required.
- *Before beginning treatment, understand clearly what will be required of you for daily oral self-care, your periodic professional dental hygiene recare appointments, and the limitations of the restorations and dental prostheses you will receive.* This means that you must brush and floss your teeth as instructed every day. When extensive dentistry is completed, a 3- to 4-month interval for periodic dental hygiene recare appointments is strongly advised.
- *Dental restorations are subject to the same physical abuse as natural teeth.* Whatever oral habits will break a natural, undrilled, undamaged tooth—such as chewing ice, biting fingernails, hard objects, etc.—will probably be able to break a restoration as well. Expansion and contraction for hot liquids and cold foods can cause damage, as can the wet, dark, bacteria-filled oral environment of the oval cavity.
- *If you have ever considered whitening your teeth, the time to do it is before dental restorations are placed in teeth that are visible when you talk or smile.* If you are interested in tooth whitening, ask us now!

Dental and Oral Anatomy

The Anatomy of Teeth

Crown: the portion of the tooth that is visible above the gumline

Root: the portion of the tooth that is not normally visible and is below the gumline

Enamel: the outer covering of the tooth crown

Teeth are one of the body's hardest naturally occurring substances. They are strong enough to adequately resist normal wearing that occurs over a lifetime of chewing food. Teeth are composed of several different parts—enamel, dentin, cementum, and pulp (nerve) tissue. The enamel is the outside covering of the tooth. It is the part of the tooth that you normally see when a person smiles. Yet, while enamel is very hard, it is also very brittle. It is mostly inorganic in nature. When fluoride is incorporated into the enamel (systemically when the enamel is forming, topically when the tooth is in the mouth), it becomes more resistant to acid attack and decay. The enamel of the tooth covers the inner layers of the crown portion of the tooth.

Dentin: the layer beneath the enamel

Dentin is not normally visible. Only when a tooth breaks or is worn can it be noticed. Dentin is darker in color, softer, and more resilient than enamel. Small nerve fibers running from the dentin to the pulp can make the tooth sensitive to temperature changes or other stimuli when dentin is exposed to the oral cavity. If a tooth is sensitive, many times, exposed dentin is the reason. Dentin, when exposed to the oral cavity, will wear away faster than enamel, and this can lead to other dental problems.

Pulp: the innermost tooth layer

The pulp of the tooth is composed of soft, highly organic material—mostly nerve fibers and blood vessels. When the pulp becomes damaged from deep decay or other dental problems, it can become abscessed and must then be treated with endodontic therapy (root canal) or be extracted.

Cementum: the outer covering of the root of the tooth

The root of a tooth is normally not seen. It is surrounded and covered by bone and gum tissue. The root is covered by a thin layer of cementum. Cementum is similar to dentin in composition and can decay or wear away if exposed in the mouth. Fibers that attach the tooth to the bone are embedded in the root cementum and serve as shock absorbers during normal functioning, such as chewing.

Bone: the structure that makes up the jaws

The bone that surrounds each tooth is less dense in the upper jaw and more dense in the lower jaw. As with bone elsewhere in the body, it can undergo resorption and repair. The spaces in which the teeth rest, called *sockets*, provide the pathways for a rich supply of blood and nutrients and other vital fluids to reach the teeth.

With proper care and attention, your teeth will serve you well for a lifetime. Brush and floss correctly, daily. See us for periodic examinations and dental hygiene (cleaning) preventive recare appointments three times a year. Research indicates that a 3- to 4-month interval will promote **prevention** of oral disease more effectively than a twice-a-year schedule. Your goal and our goal is to prevent disease.

If you have any questions about dental and oral anatomy, please feel free to ask us.

Have the Dentistry You Need, Want, and Deserve

You have been given verbal and written information describing in detail your dental problems and the treatment alternatives available to you to eliminate these problems. You need this information in order to base your decision on fact. As your dentist we must, by law, inform you of your dental problems and the alternative treatments we can provide. You must also understand the financial responsibility involved, because you will have to make financial arrangements to pay for all procedures.

How to Know What Is Best

One way to determine the best way to proceed in restoring your mouth to optimum oral health is to decide how long you want the restorations to last before they have to be replaced. It is a fact of life that almost anything a dentist makes for you (any type of filling or restoration placed) will eventually need to be replaced. Laws of physics and chemistry simply cannot be suspended. All filling materials are subject to fatigue. When the fatigue reaches a certain point, the filling breaks and the tooth must be restored again.

You have great control over the interval at which the fillings must be replaced. In short, you get what you pay for. The restorations that will last the longest and protect the tooth will cost the most initially. If we examine this option over the long term, you will wind up paying less money for the tooth to be filled because the same restoration will not have to be replaced and paid for again and again.

Less expensive restorations can work very well, but usually for a shorter length of time. Most of the less expensive restorations will need to be replaced in at least 5 to 12 years. Laboratory-processed or fabricated crowns, bridges, and porcelain or gold inlays and onlays can last much longer. It is not unusual for a gold inlay to last 25 or more years. But, again, this type of restoration will cost more initially.

The expertise of the dentist, as well as the quality of the materials, is an important aspect to consider in making your treatment decisions. But the best dentist cannot make a less expensive, direct placement material last as long or protect the tooth as well as the more expensive laboratory-processed material.

Our Recommendation

What we recommend is that the best possible, longest-lasting material or restoration be placed first. Do it right the first time and it will not have to be done over again as soon. If your financial situation and the amount of dental treatment dictate that you cannot have all the desired dentistry completed immediately, then the treatment can be phased over weeks, months, or years. This way, over the course of time, you can afford to have the dentistry you need, want, and deserve.

We will make suggestions indicating what we think is the best course of treatment for you. We will also advise you of alternative courses of treatment and we will tell you advantages and disadvantages of the possibilities. The final decision is yours. While we will not force recommendations on you, we do want to provide you with the best, longest-lasting, most protective restorations that dentistry has to offer, even if they cannot all be done at one time.

If you have questions about your dental needs, please feel free to ask us.

Infection Control Procedures

If you have been a patient of record at this office for any length of time, you know that we have been concerned with proper infection control procedures long before it became a regulation for dentistry. We wear gloves for every patient. The gloves are used once and then discarded. Since the 1970s, we have used eye protection, gowns, and masks for procedures during which there may be an aerosol spray or splatter of potentially infectious materials. That was a long time before it became a requirement. We have worn clinic gowns for years. We change from our street clothes when we enter the office and change out of clinic attire when we leave. If you are new to the office, please know that we have always taken infection control and your safety, as well as our own, seriously.

All instruments that are to be reused are properly cleaned according to the most current infection control protocol appropriate to dentistry. Instruments are then placed in pouches and sterilized. The pouches are opened in the presence of a patient only as they are needed for a dental procedure. We have been sterilizing instruments this way for years, long before any governmental regulations.

When possible, we purchase single-use only, disposable items, which are properly discarded after one use. The cost of disposable items is greater than the cost of reusable dental products and instruments.

The dental handpieces have always been disinfected and sterilized according to the manufacturers' directions. All handpieces are sterilized after each use. Each year, we spend thousands of dollars on new handpieces and on repairing handpieces damaged by the sterilization process.

We have always been concerned with proper sterilization: this is not new for this office. What is new is the cost. With the greater demand for sterilization and disinfection products universally, the cost to us has risen dramatically. Calculations show that sterilization procedures add considerable cost to a patient visit—between 8 and 15 dollars **per patient visit.** This cost estimate covers sterilization and disinfection supplies, increased cost of more frequent purchases and repairs of dental handpieces, and the cost in time (approximately 12 to 15 minutes) to properly clean the treatment room after each use. There is also the cost of the salary paid to the dental team members who spend more time with mandated infection control procedures and, therefore, less time with the actual dental treatment of the patient. These added costs are considerable. Dental insurance carriers have not yet increased payments to reflect the increased costs.

We are unwilling to compromise your health and our health by not following proper infection control guidelines. We follow Occupational Safety and Health Administration (OHSA) guidelines (for the employee and workplace) and Centers for Disease Control (CDC) guidelines (for the patient). Other than the newly required mountain of paperwork, our office did not have to make any changes to meet the CDC guidelines; we were already following all the proper infection control guidelines and procedures.

If you have any questions about infection control procedures, please feel free to ask us.

Initial Oral Examination

Possibly one of the most important parts of successful dental treatment is the complete **initial oral examination**. In order to make an accurate diagnosis and an appropriate treatment plan for you, we must know the exact nature of any pathology (disease) present in your mouth. Even if there is no dental disease present at the time of the initial oral examination, it is extremely important to record the normal appearance of your mouth, so that in the event of a change, we can make a proper diagnosis. This baseline record makes it possible to more accurately judge the progress and severity of change that has occurred.

The initial oral examination includes inspection of your head, neck, and facial structures and palpation of the lymph nodes of the neck. We examine your temporomandibular joint (jaw joint or TMJ) for proper function. We note the condition of your lips, insides of your cheeks, tongue, glands and gland duct openings, muscle attachments, and hard and soft palates. This all occurs before we even look at your teeth and gums.

When examining your teeth, we chart how many are present and which teeth are missing. We look at tooth alignment and status of decay. In addition, we chart the existing restorations and record which restorations might be broken or defective and need replacement. If you have replacement teeth present, either partial dentures (which are removable) or fixed crowns, we assess their present condition and function. If you are missing teeth, we begin to determine whether it is in your best dental health interest to consider their replacement.

We also look at the appearance of your teeth, the position of your teeth, how you look when you smile; in short, how other people see your teeth. We note irregularities in the tooth alignment and discolorations in teeth and fillings that might detract from your appearance.

We examine the support for your teeth, the gums and bone. We look at the color, contour, texture, and consistency of the gum tissue surrounding the teeth. We carefully determine whether there is bleeding of the gums. We note any recession of the tissue where the gum tissue has pulled away from its original position against the tooth. We use a periodontal probe to help measure and quantify the health of your gums, as we check for increased sulcular depth (periodontal pockets) around the teeth. The mobility of the teeth is also checked. Signs of gum disease include, but are not limited to, bleeding of the gums spontaneously or when probed, recession of the gums, redness and swelling, exudate (pus), and mobility of teeth.

To be complete, the examination must also include an evaluation of recent radiographs (x-rays) of diagnostic quality. Depending on the condition of your mouth, we may need from 14 to 20 recent radiographs. From the radiographs, we can more directly examine the health of the bone that ultimately supports the teeth. We look for unerupted or impacted teeth, decay that may be present under old fillings or in between teeth, and areas of infection around roots that might require endodontic therapy (root canal treatment). An estimated bone height around teeth and abnormalities that might exist is also noted. While a complete diagnosis cannot be made without this vital diagnostic tool, we take only the necessary number of radiographs of your teeth. We are well aware of hazards posed to the patient and the person making the radiographic exposures. Safe radiographic practices are extremely important to us.

For certain types of treatment, we may also need to take intraoral photographs, video pictures, impressions for study models of the teeth and bite (arch) relationships.

Some parts of the exam will be completed and recorded by trained and licensed dental auxiliary personnel such as dental hygienists and dental assistants.

Using the results of the diagnostic findings and your expressed concerns, we will arrive at a diagnosis of your dental condition. We can then formulate treatment plans with appropriate options that will address all of your needs. Only when this is done will your dental treatment begin.

Due to the many facets of a complete initial oral examination, you can see that it cannot be adequately done in 10 minutes. The more your mouth deviates from the ideal (all teeth in place, perfect alignment, no decay, no restorations [fillings], and no gum disease), the longer the examination will take. If your mouth has been neglected or improperly cared for, the examination could take more than an hour to complete. We want to provide you with the best oral care possible and that begins with a thorough dental examination.

If you have any questions about the initial oral examination, please feel free to ask us.

Prescription Medication

The Correct Dose Is Important

The most important part of taking prescription medication is making absolutely sure you take it as directed. Do not diagnose and treat yourself by deciding that you do not need to continue taking your medication (especially antibiotics) as you begin to feel better. The medications are designed to be taken in specific doses for specific lengths of time to cure or alleviate specific problems. Changing either the amount you are taking or the length of time you are taking the prescribed medication could negate its effect.

Keep Your Dental Team Informed

It is also important for your dental team to be informed of all of the medication you are currently taking. Drugs do interact and the interaction could be undesirable. We should also be told of any problems you have had in the past with prescription medication. These can include, but are not limited to, allergic reactions, upset stomach, rashes, hives, trouble breathing, nausea, and itching.

Analgesics   **Nonopioids**
acetaminophen (Tylenol)
aspirin (Zorprim, Ascriptin)

Analgesics   **Opioids**
acetaminophen with codeine (Tylenol with Codeine No. 2, 3, or 4)
meperidine (Demerol)
propoxyphene hydrochloride (Darvon)
propoxyphene napsylate (Darvon-N)

Antianxiety/Sedative-Hypnotics
diazepam (Valium)

Anti-infectives
erythromycin (Erytroderm)

Antiviral (topical)
penciclovir (Denavir)

Antiulcerative
amlexanox (Aphthasol): used to treat aphthous stomatitis

Cephalosporins
cefaclor (Ceclor)
cephalexin (Keflex)

Fluoroquinolones
ciprofloxacin (Cipro)

Nonsteroidal Antiinflammatory Drugs (NSAIDs)
celecoxib (Celebrex)
diflunisal (Dolobid)
etodolac (Lodine)
ibuprofen (Motrin)
naproxen sodium (Anaprox)
rofecoxib (Vioxx)

Penicillins
amoxicillin (Amoxil)
penicillin V potassium (V-Cillin K)

Tetracyclines
doxycycline (Atridox, Periostat, Vibramycin)
minocycline (Minocin, Arrestin)
tetracycline (Achromycin)

Please refer to the next two pages (pp. 153–154) to see a sample patient education handout for V-Cillin K. The accompanying CD-ROM provides patient education handouts for **all** of the above listed medications that can be customized for your office. To access patient education handouts for additional drugs prescribed to dental patients, please refer to the CD-ROM that accompanies Gage TW, Pickett FA: *Mosby's Dental Drug Reference,* ed 6, St. Louis, 2003, Mosby, Inc., or visit **www.mosby.com/dental** for purchasing information.
Technical information obtained from *Mosby's Drug Consult 2003,* Online. Internet, **www.mosbysdrugconsult.com** and Gage TW, Pickett FA: *Mosby's Dental Drug Reference,* ed 6, St. Louis, 2003, Mosby, Inc.

Please inform us of any medication you are taking (including nonprescription medication) so it can be checked for possible drug interactions before a prescription for a new medication is written.

Sample Patient Handout

Name:_____

This medicine is prescribed for:_____

Dose and time to take:_____

Generic ID #: d001971

_____

_____

_____

Form—Oral

Generic Name

Penicillin V Potassium (pen-i-sill'-in vee poe-tass'-ee-um)

Brand names
Pen-Vee K
V-Cillin K

What is Penicillin V Potassium?
Penicillin V is used to:
- Treat many different kinds of infections (including infections of the ear, nose, throat, skin, and respiratory tract).
- Prevent rheumatic fever or chorea in people who have had these problems before.

How Do I Use Penicillin V Potassium?
- Take this medicine by mouth.
- Take this medicine about the same time every day.
- If you forget to take a dose, skip that dose and take the next dose at the regular time.
- Take this medicine until it is all gone, even if you feel better.
- Measure the liquid form of this medicine using a measuring spoon or dropper, not a kitchen spoon.

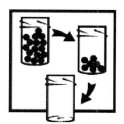

Take this medicine until it is all gone, even if you feel better.

Side Effects
Tell your doctor about any side effects that happen to you.

Possible Side Effects
- Vomiting
- Loose bowel movements
- Stomach pain
- Black hairy tongue

Rare/Severe Side Effects
- Hives
- Itching

Seek immediate medical attention if any of these side effects happen to you.
- Trouble swallowing
- Wheezing
- Trouble breathing
- Feeling lightheaded or fainting
- Dizziness when standing up
- Dizziness when sitting up

Continued

Sample Patient Handout—cont'd

Do take this medicine exactly as your doctor tells you to.

Do

- Do take this medicine exactly as your doctor tells you to.
- Do talk to your doctor or pharmacist if you have any questions or concerns about this medicine.
- Do tell your doctor if you have had a reaction to this medicine or any other medicine.
- Do keep this medicine in a cool, dry place away from sunlight.
- Do keep the liquid form of this medicine in the refrigerator.
- Do always shake the liquid form of this medicine well before using.
- Do rinse the measuring spoon or dropper after using the liquid form of this medicine.
- Do throw away any liquid medicine that is left after 14 days.

Don't

- Don't take more than one dose at a time.
- Don't increase the amount of the dose unless directed by your doctor.
- Don't start taking any new medicine (including birth control pills) without first telling your doctor or pharmacist.
- Don't keep this medicine in the bathroom because of the heat and moisture.

This leaflet does not contain all the possible uses, actions, precautions, side effects, or interactions of this drug and is intended as a summary of information only. Please contact your physician or pharmacist directly, if you have any questions or concerns.

Special instructions

Prophylactic Antibiotics for Premedication

Certain health conditions can lead to a sluggish valve on your heart. If bacteria are introduced into your blood stream, there is a chance these bacteria can lodge on that sluggish valve and cause an inflammation of the lining of your heart. This is a serious condition called *infective endocarditis,* which can have significant health consequences for you. **For that reason, if you have been diagnosed with any of the following conditions, you will need to be premedicated before some or all types of dental treatment:**

- medical history of a mitral valve prolapse with valvular regurgitation and/or thickened leaflets
- prosthetic heart valve including bioprosthetic and homograft valves
- replacement joints such as hips or knees
- complex cyanotic congenital heart disease
- rheumatic heart disease
- hypertrophic cardiomyopathy
- replacement grafted animal tissues
- subacute bacterial endocarditis
- intravascular access devices (for chemotherapy, hemodialysis, hyperalimentation)
- cerebrospinal fluid shunts

Before we can begin treatment in some cases, we must consult with your physician to determine which premedication is recommended for your specific condition. When it has been determined that you need to be premedicated prior to dental procedures, we will ask you before each dental appointment whether you have taken the premedication.

When your physician, surgeon, or cardiologist determines that it is best for you to be premedicated prior to certain dental procedures, you must take the premedication. Your physician may prescribe an antibiotic different from those listed below.

If you have not taken it as prescribed, we will not be able to perform any dental treatment. There are no exceptions. The result could be a serious illness with a prolonged hospital stay.

Recommended Standard Regimen for Prevention of Endocarditis
Adults

Situation	Agent	Regimen
Standard general prophylaxis	Amoxicillin	2.0 g orally 1 hour before procedures
Unable to take oral medication	Ampicillin	2.0 g intramuscularly (IM) or intravenously (IV) within 30 minutes before procedure
Allergic to penicillin	Clindamycin	600 mg orally 1 hour before procedure
	or	
	cephalexin[†] or cefadroxil[†]	2.0 g orally 1 hour before procedure
	or	
	azithromycin or clarithromycin	500 mg orally 1 hour before procedure
Allergic to penicillin and unable to take oral medications	Clindamycin	600 mg IV within 30 minutes before procedure
	or	
	cefazolin	1.0 g IM or IV within 30 minutes before procedure

[†]Cephalosporins should not be used in individuals with immediate-type hypersensitivity reaction (urticaria, angioedema, or anaphylaxis) to penicillins.

Continued

Recommended Standard Regimen for Prevention of Endocarditis—cont'd
Children

Situation	Agent	Regimen*
Standard general prophylaxis	Amoxicillin	50 mg/kg** orally 1 hour before procedure
Unable to take oral medication	Ampicillin	50 mg/kg** IM or IV within 30 minutes before procedure
Allergic to penicillin	Clindamycin	20 mg/kg** orally 1 hour before procedure
	or	
	cephalexin† or cefadroxil†	50 mg/kg** orally 1 hour before procedure
	or	
	azithromycin or clarithromycin	15 mg/kg** orally 1 hour before procedure
Allergic to penicillin and unable to take oral medication	Clindamycin	20 mg/kg** IV within 30 minutes before procedure
	or	
	cefazolin†	25 mg/kg** IM or IV within 30 minutes before procedure

*Total children's dose should not exceed adult dose.
**Kilograms to pound conversion: 1 kg = 2.2 lb.
†Cephalosporins should not be used in individuals with immediate-type hypersensitivity reaction (urticaria, angioedema, or anaphylaxis) to penicillin.

If you have any questions about prophylactic antibiotics for premedication, please feel free to ask us.

Smile (Lip) Line

How many teeth you show when you smile or speak and how much of each tooth (length) is displayed when you smile broadly or (at the opposite end of the spectrum) when your lips are at rest are functions of where your upper lip attaches to your face and how old you are.

There are three classifications of "lip line" that dentists use—low, medium, and high. A *low* lip line is one in which very little of your teeth are visible when you talk or smile. Someone with a low lip line will show, at the most, a millimeter or two of the edge of the biting edge of the tooth. A *medium* lip line will allow most of the tooth, up to and including a millimeter or two of the gum tissue, to be visible. A person with a *high* lip line will show all the top front teeth and a significant amount of gum tissue when speaking or smiling.

Dentists (and plastic surgeons) have not been very successful in surgically changing the low, medium, or high lip line. There are some dental "tricks" that can be used in limited situations to reduce the amount of gum display evident with a high smile line. Most of the corrective procedures to improve the esthetics of the situation require significant investments of both time and money. Periodontal (gum) surgery, alone or in conjunction with porcelain veneers or ceramic crowns, is more likely. In extreme cases the only option may be to surgically reposition the entire maxilla (with or without orthodontics). Conversely, the appearance of showing no teeth when talking or smiling is regarded as one associated with advanced aging.

There is another component to how much of your teeth show when your lips are at rest, and it has to do with gravity and time. Your face and lips are composed of soft tissue that is under a constant gravity challenge. Gravity always wins, given enough time. The skin and subskin tissues drop over the years. If, with your lips at rest, you showed about 3 mm of the biting edges of the top two front teeth when you were 20 years old, by the time you are 40, you may show only 2 mm of edge. Someone 50 years of age would show 1 mm, and at 60 years, maybe no tooth is seen when the lips are at rest. The tissues of the human face will drop about 1 mm every 10 years, beginning around age 40. As the facial tissues lose elasticity, they slowly drop. Obviously, some lucky people have better genetics and their faces will stay tighter and the tissue drop will be slower. Correcting the age-related facial tissue drop can be done with plastic surgery—the common face lift.

Genetics or Gravity? If you are reading this, then you have either asked questions about your smile and lip line or this issue has been addressed in the broader context of cosmetic dentistry procedures you require. After a thorough examination, we will explain what situation you have and what corrective measures are possible.

If you have any questions about your smile line, please feel free to ask us.

Staying Well: How to Keep Your Mouth Healthy

Congratulations! You have completed all dental treatment necessary up to this point. If you follow the listed suggestions, you will have the best chance of maintaining that optimum oral health for the longest time. If you are unsure about any aspect of what you should be doing, please ask us for further instruction.

Brush, floss, and use recommended dental cleaning aids correctly, at least once each day. Use a fluoride-containing mouthrinse (not a prescription medication) at least once each day.

PLEASE come to the office for recare hygiene appointments at the specific intervals we recommend. This is very important. Every mouth is different. Based on the number of dental restorations you have, the number and alignment of your teeth, your apparent ability at this time to keep your teeth clean, and your medical history, we recommend that the interval be no longer than ____ months. With this interval, there is the best opportunity to prevent disease or correct problems found early when they are small, easier, and less expensive to treat.

Each time you come in to have your teeth cleaned and examined, make your next hygiene recare appointment before you leave the office. This way you will stay in the "system" and not get lost. But please try to remember when you are due for an appointment. No matter how attractive we make our reminder cards, they seem to have a habit of getting mixed up in junk mail and being discarded without being noticed.

If you have followed our advice, we have used the best and most appropriate procedures and materials for you. You should receive years of successful service from them. Natural teeth and restorative materials are subjected to great stress on a daily basis. Please do not put things in your mouth that do not belong there. This will tremendously shorten the effective life span of your teeth and restorations.

Do not chew on ice or frozen candy bars, bite on hard candy, or keep hard candy or breath mints in your mouth on a routine basis. Any sugary food that you keep in your mouth for a long time (as it dissolves) can easily and quickly cause tooth decay.

If you smoke, stop. If you can't stop, remember that smoking has a negative effect on your gum tissue and on your general health.

Smoking and drinking coffee, tea, and cola beverages will have a tendency to stain or darken your teeth over time. This can be reversed with your regular recare dental hygiene and, if necessary, noninvasive tooth whitening procedures.

If you are having your dental treatment "phased" for time or financial reasons, please make a note to yourself to continue at the time we have discussed.

If you have had a protective mouthguard made (to protect your new restorations or reduce the effects of a bruxing/grinding habit), please wear it as instructed.

We have used the most appropriate diagnostic and treatment knowledge, procedures, and materials available for your treatment. Like any piece of machinery, service on a routine basis is necessary if the machine (or your teeth and restorations) are to last you the longest possible time. Teeth and restorations can break from excessive force or trauma. If you take care of your car, it will last longer than if you never change the oil, fluids, etc., and will cost you much less to keep in operation. Your teeth and gums need regular care too. No individual treatment you received cost as much as your car, but with adequate care, you will probably still have your restorations long after the car is history. Thanks for giving us the opportunity to serve you, and we hope to see you soon.

Treating the Adult Patient

Age Affects Needs

Dental treatment needs change as you age. From our years of dental experience, we have found that dental needs of adult patients fall into two distinct categories: those who have not had a history of many restorations (fillings) and those who have had their teeth drilled and filled repeatedly over the years.

The first group is fortunate. While new decay can begin at any time, the older you get, the less likely you are to get new cavities. When those adults who have had few fillings brush and floss their teeth properly to prevent periodontal disease, they will probably develop few new dental problems. Old restorations need infrequent replacement (especially if the fillings are only small fillings). The need for crowns (caps), bridges, implants, or endodontic treatment (root canal therapy) is also minimal.

Multiple Restorations

Those who have had numerous fillings over the years will probably experience more dental treatment needs than the first group. Large, existing restorations have a tendency to break more often than small fillings. When a tooth contains a large filling, there is correspondingly less natural tooth left, which can lead to fractures. Silver fillings are held in place by the surrounding tooth. When there is insufficient tooth left, the silver fillings will not last a long time. The second group can expect to have heavily filled teeth break over and over until a cast restoration (crown or inlay) is needed to restore the tooth.

Cast Restorations

Cast, laboratory-processed restorations will last longer than direct placed materials (silver fillings). In fact, it would be wise to consider placing the cast restorations (when indicated) sooner rather than later. This can eliminate further drilling and aggravation to the patient.

Endodontic Therapy

The adult patient who has had a history of moderate to severe decay and large restorations may also require more endodontic treatment (root canals) than an adult who has few fillings. Larger restorations are likely to have been placed very near to the nerve of the tooth. Over time, a tooth nerve can die when a restoration is placed very near the nerve or occasionally becomes apparent when the tooth is prepared for a crown or cast restoration. The only alternative to endodontic treatment is to extract the tooth—not a solution we recommend.

Tooth Fracture

Any tooth that has been drilled and filled could also be subject to fracture. The older and larger the filling, the more likely it is to fracture. If the gum has receded due to improper brushing habits or periodontal disease, sensitive roots or root surface decay may become evident. Root surface decay can damage a tooth much faster than enamel decay.

Prevention Remains a Key Element for Sound Oral Health

There is a bright side. Many problems can be prevented or quickly resolved with proper treatment. Proper treatment includes your good oral self-care habits, appointments with us for periodontic examinations and prophylaxis (cleaning) at intervals based on your individual needs (not based on dental insurance benefits), and prompt attention to developing problems.

Prevent the problem from starting: **brush and floss**. Once you notice symptoms, get the problem diagnosed and treat the area of concern when it is small. **See us at the recommended intervals.** Fix the problem so that it stays fixed for the longest time and does not cause more problems. **Less drilling is better than more. The longest-lasting restoration may be the restoration of choice.**

If you have any questions about dental treatment for the adult patient, please feel free to ask us.

For a Lifetime of Great Oral Health

Prevention is the key to great oral health. Better diet, medical care, and other factors are allowing us to live longer lives. Unfortunately, our teeth have not adapted to our longer life span and need help to last as long as we do. If you want to have your teeth for your whole life, here is what to do:

- Brush, floss, and use recommended dental aids correctly, at least once a day. Use a fluoride-containing mouthrinse daily.
- Come to the office for the recare hygiene appointments at the intervals we recommend. Let us provide a prescription-strength topical fluoride treatment at **every** recare appointment.
- Let us take radiographs when we believe they are necessary.
- Teeth age and wear, just like the rest of your body. The outer covering of hard enamel can get thin, break off, or wear through and expose the softer dentin. Dentin erodes very quickly. When we see exposed dentin, let us get it covered and protected.
- Have sealants placed on all teeth that can benefit from them.
- Don't ask us to "patch" anything. Patchwork dentistry is contrary to the concept of keeping your teeth trouble-free for a lifetime. If small repairs are possible and appropriate, we will tell you.
- Choose the procedure or restorative material that will last you the longest. All dental materials have a life expectancy, after which time they fail and must be replaced. Each time a tooth is redrilled, it gets weaker. Only solid, yellow gold could last for your entire life. Tooth-colored ceramics and porcelain may last as long. It is your choice.
- Bonded restorations (current state-of-the-art) require less drilling than silver fillings. Less drilling is good. The tooth retains more strength and the restoration lasts longer. Let us use the good stuff.
- Gum disease can start at any time. Genetics, diet, oral self-care, medications, and general health can all have an influence. Gum disease is both site-specific (most often starts in a localized area) and episodic (can begin at any time). It is also painless in its early stages. We will tell you as soon as we spot gum disease. It will need to be treated properly and immediately.
- Our treatment recommendations are always based on your needs, not on what your insurance company wants or its bottom line. There are dozens of common dental procedures that are not part of benefit packages. Dental insurance carriers are in business to make money. They want to pay out as little as possible as late as possible. An attitude of "If my insurance company doesn't pay for it, I don't want it," only hurts you and YOUR oral health.
- We have listened to what you want, examined your mouth, and know your dental needs. Most patients can have all the best dentistry they want and deserve. It just takes a little planning. We can help with that, too. If you want all of your teeth, all of your life, follow the above recommendations and do it right the first time.

How to Brush! How to Floss!

An old humorous expression says, "You don't have to brush all your teeth every day. Only the ones you want to keep!" And while we laugh at these words, the message could not be more correct. To maintain good oral health, teeth must be thoroughly cleaned each and every day. One good method of brushing is called the *modified Bass technique*. It is easy and quite effective. We can instruct you on how to brush properly. It is certainly easier to see it done than to read and imagine. But this will help you get started.

Use a multitufted, soft, nylon-bristled toothbrush. Hard-bristled toothbrushes can easily damage your teeth and gums. Soft-bristled toothbrushes last about 3 months before they need to be replaced. Don't keep a toothbrush for an extended period of time. When the toothbrush bristles become worn, they will not give you the best possible performance. Medium and hard brushes will last longer, but almost everyone brushes too hard to use these brushes. If you use medium and hard brushes or brush improperly with any toothbrush, you can cause permanent damage to your gum tissue, causing it to wear away. This can also wear notches into the tooth itself, exposing the dentin. In both cases, severe tooth sensitivity could develop.

The Bass Method
- The bristles of the brush should be angled toward the area where the tooth meets the gum, approximately a 45-degree angle.
- The bristles of the brush should be able to gently slide under the gum tissue. Gently move the brush back and forth so that there is a vibrating motion, **not a scrubbing motion.** The brush head should be able to cover and clean about two teeth at a time.
- Brush each area for about 10 seconds, then roll the bristles to the biting surface. Move the brush head so that it overlaps a small portion of the tooth just brushed and the next teeth. Repeat until all teeth are brushed.

Brush all teeth. Start on the cheek side of the back teeth, at one corner of your mouth, brushing as you move across to the opposite corner. Then switch to the inside (tongue or palate side) and again brush from one corner to the other. Brush both upper and lower teeth using the vibrating back-and-forth motion.

Some areas will require you to switch the brush to a different angle such as the inside (tongue and palate side) of the top and bottom front teeth. Using the tip or small end of the brush will help brush around this curved area. Use the same type of vibrating motion with the brush, moving up and down against the tooth.

Brushing the biting surfaces of the teeth is easy. Place the bristles on the biting surface of the teeth into the grooves and brush back and forth. Be sure to brush the biting surfaces of left side and right side, upper and lower teeth.

Use of Dental Floss
Start with a 14- to 16-inch piece of floss. Any type of floss is okay to use. Nonshredding is easiest to use. It's thinner and most people find it easier to use. Lightly wrap the floss around the forefingers of each hand until there is a length of about 1 to 1.5 inches available between the fingers. Don't wrap it so tightly that you cut off circulation and your fingers turn blue! Using your thumbs and forefingers, position the floss over the spot where two teeth meet. With a **gentle** buffing motion, back and forth, move the floss between the teeth and slide it first under the gum around one of the teeth in a U shape. Move the floss up and down a few times, then reverse the U and floss the other tooth. The floss needs to get under the gum. Then remove the floss and place it between the next two teeth. Holding the floss taunt between your fingers will give you more control, and flossing will be easier.

When you are able to perform these daily procedures effectively, you will significantly reduce your risk of gum disease and decay, and the associated expenses of treatment. There are other flossing aids available if you have problems using your hands. Let us know about these problems. Electric or mechanical toothbrushes can also be used. Again, talk to us about these devices. Keeping your teeth healthy for the rest of your life can be accomplished—one day at a time.

If you have any questions about how to brush or floss, please feel free to ask us.

Junk Drink Alert

We have recently noticed a developing and serious decay problem. What we are seeing in our dental practice is tooth decay that progresses much more quickly than we are accustomed to seeing. This decay is seen around the margins of restorations (fillings) and crowns (caps) where the tooth and restorative material meet. In some individuals these restorations were only placed a short time ago. From discussion with the patients who exhibited this extreme and unusual type of decay, there seems to be two common factors. First, by far and away, the majority of these people are female, and second, they drink diet beverages, mostly soda and bottled iced tea. Their brushing and flossing habits appear to be adequate. They are taking no special medication. The age range is from 12 to 55 years. All seem to be concerned with their weight, which is why they are consuming the diet drinks.

Years ago, this type of decay was seen in patients who kept candy, mints, or other edible breath fresheners in their mouths for hours on end, causing decay at the gumlines of teeth. Although another factor or factors may be the actual or contributing causes of this problem, the only currently detected causes are the diet beverages—soda and artificially sweetened bottled iced tea.

Sugar in food and drink feeds the bacteria present in dental plaque, allowing the bacteria to produce lactic acid. The lactic acid breaks down the minerals in the tooth enamel, which causes cavities. Although diet drinks are sugar-free, they are also very acidic. This acid also breaks down the minerals in the tooth enamel, causing cavities. By the time the saliva dilutes these acids enough to bring the mouth back to its proper acidity, new or additional decay may already be in progress. Or worse, before the mouth does recover its proper acid balance, the patient is already uncapping another bottle of that diet drink!

Suggestions for the reduction or elimination of this type of decay include reduction or cessation of the drinking of these diet drinks, rinsing your mouth with water as soon as possible after the beverage contact, use of fluoride mouthrinses, and stronger prescription topical fluoride treatments both in the office (four times each year) and at your home. We may even need to recommend the use of special fluoride delivery trays to increase the time that fluoride can remain in contact with the teeth. This will help make the enamel of the teeth stronger to resist the acid attack that starts decay. It will also promote a better equilibrium in the constant enamel demineralization/remineralization process that occurs in everyone's mouth. Decay lesions in the very beginning stages can be stopped and even reversed in this way.

Though most of us could stand to lose a few pounds, be aware that some of the things you put in your mouth, in the hope of losing weight, may actually have an adverse effect of losing teeth.

If you have any questions about this accelerated decay, please feel free to ask us.

Prevention of Decay

Dental Decay

Dental caries (decay) is a bacterial infection, first of the enamel, then of the dentin of the tooth. The tradition in dentistry has been to surgically remove the diseased portion of the tooth by "drilling" out the decay and then filling the resulting hole in the tooth with some inert material. As most adults know, this procedure will be performed over and over again when new decay begins or when the filling (often silver) breaks or the tooth fractures.

Would it not be better to eliminate the cause of the infection and thus not be forced to have big holes drilled in the teeth? We believe the bacterial cause of the infection should be addressed.

Preventing the Risk of Dental Decay

There are several positive steps that you can take to reduce your risk of dental decay. First, all the active decay in your mouth should be treated immediately. Next, all teeth that would benefit from **sealants** (see additional handout) should be treated. This will prevent bacteria from reaching into the pits, fissures, and grooves that normally exist on the occlusal (biting) surfaces of teeth. Any stray bacteria that may still be in the sealed area are effectively cut off from their source of food and become inactive. Although sealants are most effective on teeth that have not been previously restored, they can be successfully placed on teeth filled with bonded fillings.

The infection can be treated with antimicrobials. We believe that the use of a fluoridated mouthrinse twice daily or use of a prescription fluoridated dentifrice as directed provides a great advantage. Not only is fluoride effective against bacteria but it also creates an environment that promotes remineralization of slightly damaged enamel. The decay process is reversed and the tooth may not have to be drilled. We may also prescribe a chlorhexidine mouthrinse, an antimicrobial oral rinse that has a great effect on *Streptococcus mutans*.

Your diet and oral self-care are important in dental decay prevention. When you eat junk food and drink sugary liquids, your teeth are more prone to decay. The more frequently you snack, the more prone your teeth will be to decay. If your brushing and flossing are not effective, your teeth will be more prone to decay. When you can't brush after a meal, at least rinse your mouth with water within 15 minutes to dilute the acids forming from the ingested food or drink. If you have a diminished salivary flow, take frequents sips of water during the day to help dilute the acids produced by the bacteria.

If you have a continuing problem with active decay, we recommend more frequent preventive recare appointments. It has been repeatedly shown that patients who have good oral self-care and maintain a recare interval of 3 to 4 months have many fewer dentally related (cavities or gum disease) problems.

The routine 6-month recare interval is no longer our recommended schedule. I personally would be happy if I never heard that "see your dentist every six months" phrase again. That recare interval was based on a 50-year-old philosophy that never had any scientific basis! Times have changed. Present dental practice is based on proven scientific information. You might need to have your teeth cleaned by the hygienist twice each year or you may need to be seen more frequently.

For certain individuals, we also suggest testing the oral bacterial levels to determine the magnitude and presence of a *Streptococcus mutans* infection and to determine your risk level for future dental disease.

If you have any questions about the prevention of dental decay, please feel free to ask us.

When Radiographs Are Necessary

We only take necessary radiographs at this office. A necessary radiograph is one that is used to diagnose the extent of a dental problem that we already know exists, such as a broken tooth, a cavity, or an abscess. We also must use radiographs as part of an initial or periodic oral examination. In these examinations, radiographs are used to determine whether there are problems in a beginning stage that cannot be seen merely by looking at the tooth or area.

We can only see about 50% of your oral conditions without radiographs. Radiographs allow us to see, among other things, in between the teeth, at and below the margins of fillings and crowns, and the location and density of bone that supports your teeth. With this information we can make a full diagnosis, treating little or hidden problems before they become really big problems. Radiographs are **not** considered a preventive measure. However, they do allow us to diagnose and treat a problem early, thus preventing it from becoming worse.

Sometimes we must take several radiographs of one particular area. Radiographs are only a two-dimensional, black and white representation of a three-dimensional, colored tooth and bone. Radiographs taken from different angles give a more three-dimensional and therefore truer look at various anatomic features. We will have a much clearer picture of kind, size, and location of any problems.

The healthier your mouth is and the more unremarkable your dental history, the fewer radiographs we need to advise. The more dental problems you have had, the more monitoring and therefore the more radiographs we will need. However, if we don't take the radiographs, the problem will grow undetected and even more radiographs than originally advised may be necessary.

Radiation Safety

We are very concerned with radiation safety. Appropriate protective lead shields are **always** provided to you. We work in the office around the radiograph units all day, every day. We have a vested interest in taking only necessary radiographs for both your health and ours. Be assured that the only radiographs we recommend are those we need in order to accurately diagnose and treat.

If you have any questions about radiographs, please feel free to ask us.

Reversing Decay

If you were asked to describe a cavity, you would probably say the process was similar to rust—something that happens on the outside of the tooth that makes the tooth soft and creates a hole that would eventually be visible. You might even have the notion that bacteria are involved. And, you would be right in both cases.

The process of decay is a complicated interplay of an acidic and basic balance of chemistry in the mouth. Salivary flow and content, the presence of decay-causing bacteria, the age of the teeth, diet, and the level of plaque all play a role in the decay (demineralization) as well as the rebuilding (remineralization) process involved in tooth decay.

Demineralization

At the very earliest stage of the decay process, there is not an actual "hole" in the tooth. There is, however, an alteration of the mineral content of the enamel. This stage of decay is completely invisible to the eye. It cannot be detected by an x-ray. It is a microscopic change where, due to the level of acid in the immediate area, the building blocks of enamel (calcium and phosphate) begin to dissolve on a microscopic level. When the acid environment is left unchecked (plaque is allowed to accumulate undisturbed against the tooth surface), more and more of the bonds between calcium and phosphate dissolve. This is a process called *demineralization*. If the acid challenge becomes severe and more of the underlying structure of the tooth begins to dissolve, the outer surface becomes unsupported. It is at this time that the actual hole, or what you call a *cavity*, appears.

Remineralization

When the outer surface of the enamel is still intact, with no break detectable, there is an opportunity for the bonds between calcium and phosphate to become re-linked through a process termed *remineralization*. And the great news is that dental science discovered that in the presence of fluoride, these bonds actually become stronger than they were initially. It is in this way that an early cavity can be reversed. When this happens, the tooth does not need to be drilled and filled.

The process of demineralization and remineralization can be seen as a tug of war on the molecular level of all surfaces of all your teeth, all the time!

How You Can Promote Remineralization

There are several steps you can take on a daily basis to help ensure that you are promoting remineralization. These are:

- Control your diet: watch the type of decay-promoting foods you eat and the quantity
- Improve your oral self-care by brushing and flossing daily
- Use topical fluoride on a daily basis
- Use antimicrobials and other anticaries agents as directed on a regular basis
- Maintain your dental hygiene recare schedule

The early stages of dental decay CAN be reversed with no loss of tooth structure, and you can help promote a healthy mouth by following just a few simple rules.

If you have any questions about the process of decay, please feel free to ask us.

Sealants and Fluoride: Benefit to Adult Patients

Dental decay can develop at any time, regardless of a person's age. A change in diet, change in lifestyle, change in oral self-care habits, the use of prescription medications, or a change in systemic health due to the normal aging process can all affect the caries (decay) susceptibility. Few people remain completely free of decay. Proper oral self-care on your part and properly spaced dental hygiene prevention appointments will go a long way to reduce the opportunity to have new decay to begin.

As you age, it is possible that some of your gum tissue will recede, exposing the root surfaces of your teeth. This gum recession can occur from improper brushing (brushing too hard with a hard toothbrush) or as a result of past periodontal problems. The more a tooth and root are exposed, the greater is the surface area you will have to keep clean. Sometimes the teeth with exposed roots are very hard to keep clean. These roots may be sensitive to temperature changes and are often times uncomfortable to brush. Decreased salivary flow helps to create a breeding ground for bacteria to accumulate on the enamel and especially on the root surface. And root decay usually progresses quite quickly!

Goal of Prevention

Your goal should be to keep the dentist from drilling your teeth. Any reasonable preventive measure that is available should be seriously considered. When the dentist drills, you lose. When the dentist does not drill, you win.

Dental Sealants

Please refer to the **sealant** handout. Although sealants are primarily designed for children, adults who have a history of active decay should consider having sealants placed on the posterior (back) teeth where indicated. We will tell you where it is possible to place the sealants. Even if you have not had a cavity for a long time, consider the application of a sealant as an inexpensive insurance policy for your teeth. Perhaps you would never get decay on the unsealed surfaces. But, just as you insure your home against destruction by fire, a sealant insures the tooth surface from decay. Preventive measures may allow you to avoid having your teeth drilled. You win!

Topical Fluoride

For a similar reason, we advise the use of topical fluoride treatments for adults. The effectiveness of systemic and topical fluoride in preventing decay is well documented. When a cavity first starts, an application of fluoride might (depending on when it is used) reduce or eliminate the need for drilling.

An alternative to the fluoride treatment we can provide in our office is a daily rinse. If you can rinse with an over-the-counter mouthrinse containing fluoride **every night** as directed on the rinse label, you do not need the office topical fluoride treatment. If you cannot rinse **daily** as instructed, you will need the benefit from the stronger office-applied topical fluoride treatment. Your oral health will benefit most from small increments of fluoride that are applied **daily** rather than one larger concentration every 6 months. However, only you know whether you will be faithful in your rinsing routine. When in doubt, let us do it here.

You have selected our office to administer to your dental needs. If you have been a patient here for any length of time, you know that we stress **prevention** of dental disease above all else. Sealants and topical fluoride treatments are two of the more important preventive dental measures that we believe will significantly enhance your oral health.

If you have any questions about sealants and fluoride, please feel free to ask us.

Topical Fluoride: At Home and in the Dental Office

Why Topical Fluoride

Everyone is familiar with the dental advantages of fluoride supplements, systemically administered to children while their teeth are forming. Research on this type of fluoride treatment shows a 35% reduction in tooth decay. The use of fluoride to reduce and eliminate decay is one of the most highly studied and documented public health measures yet. In this office, we have recommended this 4-minute tray-type fluoride delivery at least twice a year, usually after your periodic dental hygiene recare appointment. We have found that this type of preventive aid does four things:

- Reduces the solubility of enamel to acid attack, making the teeth more resistant to decay
- Aids in remineralizing the tooth enamel where decay has just begun
- Longer-term, daily use reduces tooth sensitivity to temperature changes
- Reduces the surface tension of the enamel so that plaque does not easily adhere to the tooth

Recent research has also shown that you can benefit from a nonprescription topical fluoride rinse, especially if you use it faithfully every day. There is, in addition, a reduction in decay seen if you have the stronger concentration topical fluoride that we use in this office. It is applied four times each year. Decay reduction can be as high as 30%! If you have had recent active decay, no matter what your age, we will recommend this routine for you.

Special Fluoride Applications

Another option for topical fluoride is available to patients with tooth or root sensitivity, higher and chronic decay levels, root decay, or dry mouth syndrome (xerostomia). If you have been diagnosed with any of these dental problems, we will make custom fluoride trays for you. We will then either prescribe or dispense a high-concentration fluoride gel product for you to use nightly in the tray.

The instructions are simple. Dry your teeth as much as possible, either with a gauze square or washcloth or by sucking air through your teeth. The fluoride will work better if the teeth are not quite so wet. Since trays fit closely to the teeth, place a small amount of fluoride gel into the tray every few teeth, and then place the trays into your mouth. Spit out the excess. If you notice an excess of fluoride, place a smaller amount in the trays at your next application. Leave the trays in place for _____ minutes. Then, take the trays out. Spit out the saliva and fluoride that remains. **Do not eat or drink for _____ minutes.**

The number of weeks that you will need to apply tray fluoride in this manner depends on your oral condition. If diminished salivary flow has caused an increase in your decay rate, you will need to follow this procedure until saliva flow returns to normal. In the case of sensitive teeth, you will need to follow this procedure until the sensitivity is reduced. However, please note: sensitivity reduction is usually a gradual process; do not expect overnight improvement. Root desensitization may also require that additional materials be placed over the area as an adjunct procedure.

If you have any questions about the use of topical fluorides in the home or dental office, please feel free to ask us.

Abfraction: A New Dental Term

Abfraction—A new term for an "old" problem

You probably have not heard this dental term before because it is relatively new to dentistry. It describes a newly recognized problem that has been commonly mistaken for abrasion in the past. Until recently, *abfraction* was thought to be caused by improper toothbrushing techniques.

An abfraction lesion is now known to be the loss of tooth structure seen clinically on the cheek side of a tooth near and often under the gumline. It is identified by its sharply demarcated horizontal notch-like appearance. While a cavity may develop in the area due to the exposed dentin, the decay process is not responsible for the abfraction.

The Cause

Abfraction is caused when two opposing teeth—one top and one bottom tooth—meet improperly during chewing and nonfunctional clenching or tooth grinding habits, etc. At that point of stress, the tooth will "flex" very slightly. When a bite relationship is not correct, teeth undergo forces of compression and tension from the opposing teeth. In this way, the tooth is flexed slightly every time the teeth fully close.

This chronic flexing of the tooth causes a loss of tooth substance (enamel and dentin) at the gumline where the enamel is the thinnest. Enamel is brittle and cannot easily bend. As the tooth is moved back and forth (because the bite is off or because you grind your teeth), pieces of enamel fracture. The dentin, or underlying tooth structure, is more elastic and can bend slightly. The bending of the tooth will slowly damage the tooth, and a notch will eventually become visible.

One characteristic of abfraction that can make diagnosis difficult is that it may be partially or entirely under the gum tissue. At one time, it was thought that this type of tooth notching was caused by improper brushing habits, such as forcefully scrubbing back and forth against the neck of the tooth. While it is true that you can actually wear a notch in the tooth by brushing too hard in a see-saw fashion, the first tissue to wear away under those conditions is the gum tissue. Unlike abfraction, abrasion occurs above the gumline. In contrast, an abfraction occurs many times under the gum, or is partially covered by gum tissue.

Treatment Options

Your occlusion (bite) must be checked and adjusted so that your teeth meet properly in all jaw movements. This bite adjustment may require more than one appointment to successfully complete, depending on the specific nature of the occlusal problem.

Second, the notch in the tooth must be treated. The missing enamel and underlying exposed dentin need to be replaced and covered. Dentin is not designed to be exposed to the oral environment; that's why it is naturally covered with enamel. Even when the factors that initially caused the notch have been eliminated, the exposed dentin may continue to abrade because dentin is soft. This exposed dentin may decay. The tooth may also become sensitive to temperature changes. It can become weaker.

A tooth-colored, bonded resin material is often placed to restore the notched tooth, and is a relatively easily restoration to accomplish. If the notch extends deep under the gumline, the tissue may have to be removed to expose the extent of the notched area in order to restore it.

If all procedures are successful, the abfraction notch will be restored to exactly match the natural tooth structure and the bite will be adjusted so that the teeth meet properly. Please be aware that if the teeth shift slightly, or if you continue to grind your teeth, the restored tooth may begin to flex again and the restoration could be forced out. Or, other teeth may begin to exhibit the same type of enamel loss. If this occurs, the bite can again be adjusted and a new restoration can be placed.

If you have any questions about abfraction, please feel free to ask us.

Acid Reflux (Gastroesophageal Reflux Disease)

Teeth are so hard you would think they would be indestructible and that they would not be adversely affected by anything. Due to the strength of enamel and bone, they should remain the same from the day the teeth come into the mouth to the day they are no longer needed. Unfortunately, this is far from true. While we would like to think of teeth as being strong and unchanging, most people know that teeth can be damaged by tooth decay–causing bacteria. We know, too, that teeth can be damaged by mechanical means—attrition caused by tooth grinding and clenching and abrasion caused by improper toothbrushing. However, few people know that there is a third factor that can destroy teeth—chemical erosion.

Chemical erosion is caused by excess acid coming in contact with a tooth for extended periods of time. The acid attack can be self-inflicted (bulimia) or more commonly from a problem with acid reflux. In acid (gastric) reflux, the acidic and partly digested contents of the stomach are returned back into the throat and oral cavity. Normally, the lower esophageal sphincter muscle (LES), connecting the esophagus with the stomach, closes once food passes into the stomach. This closure prevents the stomach contents from flowing back up into the esophagus. Acid reflux occurs when this sphincter does not work properly and allows acidic fluid to return to the esophagus and higher—the mouth.

This condition can actually be noted by a dentist long before it is acknowledged by a patient or physician. The dentist will see a characteristic smooth and circular erosion of the cusp tips of the lower first molars. The cusp tips (bumps on a tooth) lose their peak, flatten, and become concave. Soon the enamel cover is broached and the underlying dentin is exposed. Because dentin is "softer" than enamel, the erosion can progress more quickly. This acid erosion has a very different appearance from tooth loss due to a mechanical etiology. Attrition and abrasion have a very sharp, edged, and well-delineated look. Chemical erosion has a softer and more rounded presentation and is localized first to lower first molars (lower first molars are the first permanent molars to erupt into the mouth) so that the permanent teeth have the longest potential exposure. When the acid refluxes (returns) to the mouth, it pools mostly around the lower first molars. This is the site of the most erosive features.

A significant portion of the population experiences acid reflux at least once a month. About 25% of those who are affected are unaware of their problem. Infants and young children can be affected, and there may be a genetic component to this disease. Early diagnosis from erosion of the permanent lower first molars can be made as early as 7 or 8 years of age. A hiatal hernia may weaken the LES and cause reflux. Diet and lifestyle contribute to acid reflux. Chocolate, peppermint, citrus, tomatoes, fried or fatty foods, coffee (especially acidic coffee), alcoholic beverages, garlic, and onions are foods to avoid. Weight gain (also weight gain associated with pregnancy) and smoking (by relaxing the LES) may be contributing factors. Further information may be obtained from the Internet by going to a search engine and typing in "acid reflux," "gastric reflux," or "gastroesophageal reflux disease (GERD)."

As is true with most medical and dental problems, the earlier the diagnosis is made, the easier it is to treat. If we have brought this condition to your attention, we ask that you speak to your physician. Variable factors include the nature and severity of the problem, as well as frequency and type of fluid that refluxes from the stomach. Change in diet, eating habits, and/or medication (over-the-counter or prescription) can be effective. Dentally, once the enamel is broached and the dentin becomes visible, it is recommended that the affected areas be protected by covering them with an enamel replacement—a tooth-colored bonding material. This material not only protects the dentin and enamel but it also may be more resistant to the acid than is naturally occurring dentin. Many times, drilling preparation is not needed.

If you have any questions about acid reflux, please feel free to ask us.

Attrition and Abrasion

Why Teeth Abrade

The natural friction of teeth moving against each other produces wear of the enamel. It is considered a natural process and happens over many years, so the changes are very gradual. Attrition (wear or loss of tooth substance) of the biting surfaces of teeth occurs one out of every four adults in the United States, or approximately 25% of the population.

You may notice these types of changes by observing that your front teeth appear to be chipping. These teeth might look shorter and the biting edges may appear discolored, especially on the lower front teeth. This process can occur more rapidly when you have a nonuseful or nonpurposeful biting, grinding, or clenching habit that can cause teeth to be in contact longer and more forcefully, either in waking hours or when sleeping.

Grinding and Clenching Habits

Grinding and clenching habits are most usually a physical expression of psychological physical or emotional stress. Many times, patients are completely unaware of their clenching, grinding, or biting habits. Most typically, this destructive habit occurs during sleep, and patients commonly deny knowing that it occurs. These habits can occur during periods of high stress or at times of high personal demand. Whenever nonfunctional wear of the teeth occurs, the enamel will wear much more quickly than can be normally expected. When this happens, the underlying dentin of the tooth is exposed, and this creates a problem.

Dentin Attrition

Enamel is quite hard and resistant to wear. Dentin, on the other hand, has a higher organic component and does not handle the frictional forces of grinding, biting, and clenching very well. Consequently, once the outer covering of the tooth (enamel) is worn away, the underlying dentin will begin to wear faster, exposing even more of the dentin to the oral cavity. The tooth can chip and fracture. The dentin also has a tendency to show more stain from smoking, food, and drink. Coffee, tea, cola drinks, and red wine are noted for causing the unsightly brown/orange stain on the dentin.

Even when you eliminate the offending habit, once the dentin is exposed, it will continue to wear more quickly than the surrounding enamel. This will cause a dish- or donut-shaped area that progresses into a larger defect. At the very least, it is best to restore the areas as soon as possible (even if they are not yet cosmetic problems) to prevent further deterioration of the tooth structure.

Treatment Options

There are several possible solutions to attrition and abrasion problems, depending on the level of tooth wear. You can elect to do nothing. Your teeth will probably continue to wear down, stain, and become increasingly unsightly as they lose their proper shape, break, chip, and/or discolor. They may become more sensitive to temperature changes. Excessive wear may even require endodontic treatment (root canal therapy). In the most advanced cases, the back teeth are actually worn flat and the jaw relationships change to the extent that the jaw joint (temporomandibular joint [TMJ]) does not function properly, resulting in pain.

- A mouthguard or bite guard can be made, which prevents your teeth from coming into contact when you clench or grind. It is worn at times of high stress when you are most prone to clenching and grinding.
- Fractured and worn posterior (back) teeth can be restored. Cast restorations can be used to restore and maintain a proper jaw relationship. Cast gold is usually the material of choice for patients who suffer from clenching and grinding habits. The final decision on materials will be made on an evaluation of each individual situation.
- Exposed dentin on front teeth can be restored with a tooth-colored resin material bonded directly to the areas.
- Identify and eliminate the cause of your stress.

Unfortunately, once the tooth has been worn away, it will not grow back. It can only be repaired. It is much better to stop the progression of attrition. When is the best time to begin treatment for the bruxing and grinding habit? As soon as the problem is diagnosed.

If you have any questions about attrition or abrasion, please feel free to ask us.

Bad Breath

At one time or another, everyone experiences bad breath. The occasional meal—heavy with garlic, onions, or spices—may leave a lingering odor, but it is a temporary problem. Chronic bad breath is another problem entirely. It can be caused by periodontal disease, decay in teeth, decay under fillings or crowns, as well as digestive system or sinus problems. Foul breath odor caused by any of these conditions needs to be corrected by your dentist or physician.

Although there can be medical and/or systemic problems that cause the breath odor, most of the time bad breath is the result of things left on and around your teeth. Your mouth is warm, moist, and dark—the perfect place for bacteria to grow and decompose. When this happens and the teeth are not cleaned properly on a daily basis, a chronic odor can result. Bad breath can be eliminated fairly easily, or at least controlled, by removal of food debris, plaque, or calculus; replacement of broken fillings causing a food trap; restoration of areas of decay; and/or eliminating gum disease. Plaque that accumulates at or along the gumline can also find its way into the deep recesses on the top surface of your tongue, contributing to mouth odor.

Toothbrushing, tongue cleaning, and flossing correctly, at least once a day, are the best prevention and cure for bad breath. Not only will these procedures prevent periodontal disease and decay by removal of bacteria but they will also remove all food debris. Manufacturers of toothpastes, toothbrushes, floss, tongue scrapers, and mouthrinses do make claims to help prevent bad breath and may provide temporary relief of that symptom. No matter which product you use, be sure to thoroughly remove the bacterial plaque on a daily basis.

The key to preventing dental problems and preventing bad breath odor is to clean your teeth and tongue properly every day. The best way to learn how to clean your mouth is by visiting us. You have the ability to take good care of your mouth; it is just a matter of practicing the right hand skills best suited to your unique oral conditions. Whether you have many fillings, crowns or bridges, removable partial or full dentures, implants, braces, or other appliances in your mouth, there is a method or tool that will work for you.

Also, to ensure fresh breath, have your teeth cleaned professionally, by us, on a regular basis. The goal here is not only to correct any disease-related problems but also to prevent any problems from beginning in the first place.

Your bad breath problem does not have to be a chronic source of embarrassment. Most often it is a sign of a dental problem. The sooner it is treated, the easier and less expensive it will be to fix.

If you have any questions about bad breath, please feel free to ask us.

Cracked Tooth Syndrome (CTS)

CTS Defined

When teeth have been heavily filled, it is not unusual that they develop a cracked (or split) tooth syndrome (CTS). Symptoms include a sharp pain when you bite down into something hard. When you open your mouth and the teeth are no longer touching, the pain goes away.

The most common sites of occurrence of CTS are the premolars and molars, back teeth that grind and crush food. Often the tooth has an extensive filling (usually silver amalgam) that has been in place for a long time. Occasionally, CTS occurs in a tooth that has recently been drilled and a great amount of tooth structure has been lost. However, split-tooth syndrome can also occur in teeth that only have a small silver filling. In most instances, the filling has weakened the tooth just enough so that when you chew or bite, the tooth and filling separate slightly (flex), causing immediate and sometimes severe pain. The pain does not usually linger after the biting action is finished.

The fact that you feel pain when pressure is applied to the tooth means that the nerve is being affected. If the problem is not solved quickly, the nerve may die and the tooth will then require endodontic treatment (root canal).

Treatment

Treatment will involve at least one x-ray to assist in the diagnosis to help rule out other causes. We will try to find the section of the tooth that is causing the problem by pushing on the various sections of the tooth or having you bite on a hard object. When the section of the tooth that is cracked is found, it makes treatment easier. First, the tooth is anesthetized and the old filling is removed. Then we carefully inspect the area to determine whether the cracked section can be seen. Very often it is visible at this point. The next step is to see whether the split area can be fixed with a direct filling (bonded). This is the ideal situation if the crack is small. Unfortunately, this rarely occurs. More often (over 95% of the time), the biting surfaces of the tooth must be entirely covered and protected first with a provisional (temporary) onlay or crown. If this is successful in eliminating the pain (we usually wait for a few weeks to be sure the problem is resolved), an impression for a laboratory-fabricated casting—either a porcelain or resin onlay or a crown—is made. If adequate tooth structure remains, a partial coverage restoration—an onlay—is preferred. If the tooth has been badly cracked or if not much tooth remains, then a crown will be necessary. The purpose of either type of cast restoration is to unite all sections of the tooth so it cannot move or separate under normal biting forces. If the provisional restoration is successful in eliminating the pain, we expect that the final cast crown or onlay will correct the problem.

Delaying Treatment

What happens if CTS is not treated quickly? The best you can hope for is that the tooth continues to hurt only when you chew or bite. This does not often happen. Usually, the broken section of tooth gets weaker and weaker until it fractures off. Additionally, if the crack gets deeper into the tooth, the nerve will die and the tooth will need endodontic treatment before the crown or onlay is placed. Sometimes the nerve is immediately affected by the initial split and dies. This may occur quickly or may take years before it is evident. Every case of CTS is unique. If it is any consolation, the cracked tooth is not your fault. It is a result of your teeth being drilled and filled with big silver fillings when you were younger. We see this particular dental problem mostly in patients who are between 25 and 45 years old.

Unfortunately, cracked teeth do not go away. Many times, they only hurt when you bite on them from one particular angle. If the fractured segment is not stressed, the tooth feels normal. You might also be able to "train" yourself to chew on different teeth and avoid the cracked tooth. At best, you only postpone necessary treatment while the nerve may be slowly dying.

If you have any questions about cracked tooth syndrome, please feel free to ask us.

Cracked Tooth Syndrome (CTS): Postoperative Instructions

Patient:_____   **Date:**_____

❏ Your tooth has been diagnosed with **"cracked tooth syndrome."** Because of the nature of the clinical appearance of the fracture, we have attempted to lessen the symptoms by adjusting your occlusion (bite) on the tooth. This may be the only treatment you will need. **If the discomfort you feel when you bite is not eliminated within one week, please call our office and let us know**. If the split is still present, a different approach must be tried. Give the tooth a few days to "calm down" before you try to bite down on hard foods.

❏ The split tooth has been treated by removing the old restoration and placing a bonded filling in its place. If the split is small, this may eliminate the problem. Do not bite down hard on the tooth for a few days, then gradually place more pressure on the tooth. **Call our office in one week and let us know how it feels.** If the split is still causing a problem, a different approach must be tried. If left untreated, the tooth may split further and you may need endodontic treatment and a crown. If the tooth splits severely, it may have to be extracted.

❏ A temporary crown has been cemented onto the cracked tooth with a temporary cement. Because the crack was so severe, we will use this procedure to determine whether or not the tooth can be treated without performing a root canal. **Please give the tooth several days of rest before you try biting down on hard foods**. Expect the tooth to be sensitive for a few days after the temporary is placed. This is normal. Gradually apply more force when you bite into foods, and gradually try to eat harder foods. Expect the temporary crown to remain in place for several weeks, until it can be determined whether or not the problem is solved.

The earlier a split tooth is diagnosed and treated, the better success there is in treating it. If the split is severe, a root canal may be necessary to save the tooth. Depending on the symptoms you describe, we may choose to treat it as a bite adjustment, small filling, or larger preparation for an onlay or crown. If these do not work, the treatment plan will be modified. If left untreated, the tooth may eventually be lost. It is also possible that the initial split of the tooth may be such that it cannot be saved, despite our best efforts.

If you have any questions about these postoperative instructions for cracked tooth syndrome, please feel free to ask us.

Dentin Decay

Usually, dental decay is fairly easy to detect. When a cavity is just beginning, it is typically identified by a brown or white color or a change in the translucency of the enamel of the tooth. The dentist or dental hygienist uses a special dental instrument called an *explorer* to feel the suspect area and check its hardness. If the area is hard, in other words, if no break in the enamel layer is detected, we feel there is not a cavity present. If, however, the surface feels soft and the explorer "sticks" in the suspect site, we feel a cavity is present.

Because of the widespread use and availability of fluoride in our drinking water, foods, and oral care products, we are seeing a different decay pattern. The appearance is different from the typical pattern of decay and more difficult to detect. As the outer surface of the enamel absorbs fluoride (from toothpaste, for example), the enamel becomes very resistant to demineralization and eventual decay. If there is a small break in the integrity of the enamel, a pit or groove where decay-causing bacteria can live, the bacteria can dissolve the enamel in such a way that the hole in the enamel cannot be detected. Once the decay-causing bacteria reach the underlying dentin, the acids eat away at that substance and quickly make a large cavity—but one that still cannot be easily seen or detected. In this way the enamel becomes undermined. A dentist looking at such a small cavity would think it very easy to restore. However, once the decayed portion of the enamel is removed and the dentin becomes visible, the true extent of the damage becomes obvious. The small cavity becomes a big cavity.

Detection and Treatment

One of the major problems with decay that appears to occur only in the dentin is in the detection. If a radiograph is taken as part of the periodic examination process, we may be able to see dentin decay if it is moderate to extensive. Decay seen on radiographs is typically two to seven times greater in the tooth. Modern high-speed radiographic film and reduced x-ray exposure makes it more difficult to detect early decay on radiographs.

Prevention

The conscientious application of a source of topical fluoride, through either an over-the-counter dentifrice or a prescription fluoride product, and thorough plaque removal are essential. Bonded **sealants** are also an effective protection against dentin decay. **We strongly advise these procedures.** Periodic examinations at intervals recommended by the dentist catch decay at the earliest possible time. This is the only way to keep small problems from developing into larger problems.

If you have any questions about dentin decay, please feel free to ask us.

Enamel Dysplasia

Definition
Enamel, the first word in the title, is probably familiar to you as the hard outer covering of the tooth crown. The second word, *dysplasia*, is probably less familiar. *Enamel dysplasia* is a dental term that discusses a number of dental problems, both cosmetic and structural. The condition may affect only the tooth surface and appear as small pits in the enamel or as a gross malformation of the enamel and shape of the tooth. Enamel dysplasia can range from slight to severe with all grades in between.

Causes
The causes of the dysplasia are numerous, but occur during a critical stage of enamel/tooth formation. Fever, illness, medication, change in nutrition, or prescription medication have all been cited as causes.

Corrective Procedures
Rarely do these conditions make the tooth weaker or more prone to decay. Teeth with dysplasia are not "soft." In fact, many times these affected teeth exhibit less incidence of decay than teeth that have normal shape, color, contour, and texture!

Everyone agrees that enamel dysplasia is unsightly and correction of the problem is needed. The solution depends on the type of defect and the extent to which the teeth are involved. If the blemish is superficial, many times it can be polished off the tooth, and it never returns. This is done either with a drill or with special polishing compounds, or both. Sometimes a whitening agent is also used. Local anesthetic is not required because there is no pain involved. A restoration (filling) is not necessary to correct a superficial dysplasia.

When the defect is deeper in the tooth, the defect may have to be mechanically removed (drilled) and a bonded, tooth-colored restoration will be placed. Sometimes an injection of a local anesthetic is needed to correct a deeper defect. The filling should last for many years before it needs to be replaced. The color match is usually perfect.

Smoothing the enamel defect or replacing the area with a small filling is often all that is needed. When the defect is more severe, however, reconstruction of the tooth with bonded onlays or crowns is necessary. We will tell you what is indicated after examining your mouth and determining the extent of your problem.

Enamel Decalcification
There is one type of white spot or line that forms on a tooth that is not really a dysplasia of the enamel but it looks like one. This appears as a white line along the gumline and is caused by a decalcification of the enamel because of plaque or debris sitting on the tooth. In short, the area is not being brushed properly and a cavity has started to form. When a patient has orthodontic braces, cleaning the space between the orthodontic band and the gumline can be a problem. Proper oral self-care is a must for patients undergoing orthodontic therapy.

Treatment, other than some treatment with topical fluoride, may not be necessary if the enamel decalcification is discovered in the early stage. When the white line is soft or the decalcification has invaded the underlying dentin, drilling and restoration will be needed.

If you have any questions about enamel dysplasia, please feel free to ask us.

Excessive Wear

TOOTH-TO-TOOTH CONTACT

When two surfaces are rubbed against each other, the surfaces will eventually wear away. How fast this occurs and how much surface area is lost depends on the hardness of the surface (resistance to abrasion) and how long the force (abrasive action) continues.

How Abrasion Occurs

Enamel is an extremely hard substance. In fact, few substances are harder. Because of the hardness, enamel can resist wear and last throughout a lifetime of chewing food. It protects and covers the underlying and much softer inner tooth substance, dentin, and nerve tissue.

While enamel is very resistant to abrasion, it does occur. Here's how: The most common abrasion we see is when bottom front teeth rub against top front teeth. The enamel on the biting surfaces of these teeth is moderately thick, up to approximately 2 mm. Over the course of a person's life, these teeth will come in contact and enamel will slowly be lost. Normally, this happens quite slowly. This type of wear is not of concern. The problem with excessive wear begins when a patient grinds or clenches, putting more force on the teeth or working them together for long periods of time. Although the enamel is very hard, if it is "abused" long enough, it, too, will wear away. Wear occurs more quickly when a natural tooth opposes a porcelain crown. Porcelain is much harder than enamel and may actually wear the enamel away even under normal use. In this case it is critical that the bite be properly adjusted to reduce this possibility.

Consequence of Abrasion

Why is the accelerated wear of enamel a problem? Although the wear continues on all teeth, it is most visible on the lower front teeth. Lower front teeth may be the most important teeth in your mouth, since they control the bite relationships of your top and bottom jaws.

Once the enamel is worn away, two undesirable things can happen. First, the exposed dentin can become sensitive to air or temperature changes. Secondly, when not supported by resilient dentin, the enamel can break off and the tooth will become smaller. As this happens, the natural movement of the tooth pushes the tooth further out of its socket. The now shorter tooth stops only when it meets its opposing tooth. Additionally, the dentin tends to stain more readily than enamel, so there will be a distinct and disagreeable cosmetic appearance that will become excessive as time goes on.

Treatment of Abrasion

The treatment of excessive wear depends on how much tooth is missing. If only the enamel is affected, a protective mouthguard is recommended. If a small to moderate amount of dentin is exposed, it can easily be covered with a bonded, tooth-colored resin. The resin, although not as resistant as the original enamel, is still much harder than the dentin. If you still continue to grind or clench your teeth, the resin will be the only tooth structure now affected. In extreme cases of excessive wear, porcelain veneers or full crowns may be the only means of restoration.

Excessive wear is difficult to diagnose in the early stages. It may take months and years for it to become evident. It does not happen overnight. When noted, it is best treated early when there is the least amount of tooth loss and the highest chance for a long-lasting, conservative solution.

If you have any questions about excessive wear, please feel free to ask us.

Extraction

Reasons for Recommending Tooth Extraction

Teeth may need to be extracted for several reasons, including but not limited to:

- severe periodontal disease
- irreversible damage to the nerve tissue inside the tooth (and the patient decides against saving the tooth)
- failed endodontic therapy
- extreme fracture or decay of the tooth structure
- improper positioning of the tooth or for orthodontic purposes

To a great extent, the reason for the extraction will influence the amount of discomfort you might experience subsequent to the procedure. When the tooth is to be extracted for periodontal reasons, there will be reduced bone support for the tooth and the tooth might be removed more easily than if there were full bone support. In this case there might be lessened discomfort following the extraction.

Following the Extraction

We will tell you the reason for the extraction and let you know what to expect following the procedure. Please follow the instructions given to you. If antibiotics are prescribed, take them until the prescription is *completely* finished. If pain medication is prescribed, *take it only if necessary*. If the medication prescribed contains a narcotic component, such as codeine, do not drive a motor vehicle or operate machinery that could prove dangerous to yourself or others. **Expect some bleeding to occur from the extraction site for the first 24 hours.** Remember, there is now a hole in your jaw from which the tooth has been removed, and the hole can be quite large. Some bleeding is to be expected.

Some infrequent complications of routine oral surgical procedures include (but are not limited to):

- fracture of adjacent teeth or restorations (which of course would mean that these affected areas must be restored to normal function after the healing of the extraction site)
- separated root tips or root fragments
- temporary or permanent nerve damage to the area, resulting in anesthesia or paresthesia (numbness)
- incomplete healing, resulting in severe pain—a "dry socket"
- fracture of the surrounding bone

If you have any questions about reasons for dental extraction, please feel free to ask us.

Extraction: Postoperative Instructions

Patient:_____   **Date:**_____

If these instructions are not followed, the extraction site may not heal properly and the time needed for proper healing will be increased.

- Keep your mouth closed firmly on the gauze for_____ minutes. At that time, remove the gauze.
- Do not change the gauze unless instructed to do so by the dentist.
- Do not spit, rinse, or smoke for 24 hours.
- Do not drink through a straw for 24 hours.
- It would be a good idea not to brush near the extraction site for a day or two.
- When you brush and floss the area, be gentle!
- For 24 hours after the extraction, try to chew food away from the extraction site.
- Some slight swelling in the area is to be expected, especially if the extraction was difficult.
- If sutures are placed, return to have them removed.
- If medication has been prescribed for possible post extraction discomfort, take it as directed.
- If prescription medication has NOT been given, you may take your usual over-the-counter pain reliever, as directed.
- Return in_____ weeks so the dentist can evaluate the healing of the extraction site.

Please notify us if:

- There is extended bleeding from the extraction site. Slight bleeding for several hours is normal.
- Anything other than slight swelling occurs.
- Discomfort continues for more than 24 hours, especially if it is not relieved by over-the-counter pain relievers.

Special instructions:_____

_____

Tooth #(s) to be extracted: **,** commonly known as

Comments:_____

_____

I have read and understand this information on dental extraction and consent to have the procedure performed in this office. I have no further questions about the procedure or postoperative care.

_____   _____
Patient's or Guardian's Signature   Date

Headaches: The Dental Connection

You probably remember the old song "… the knee bone's connected to the leg bone; the leg bone's connected to the hip bone…. etc." Your (lower) jaw bone actually is connected to your "head bone"—and it is connected by muscles, ligaments, and tendons. This area is known as the *temporomandibular joint* or the *TMJ*. When the lower jaw lines up perfectly with the upper jaw and everything functions normally, everything is fine. If the lower jaw does not line up properly or, perhaps more importantly, if there is abnormal stress present when the lower jaw contacts the upper jaw, problems can occur. The abnormal stress is usually clenching or grinding of the teeth and it can occur any time, day or night, awake or asleep. When this happens, a person can develop regular, chronic, or migraine headaches; muscle pain or tenderness in the jaw joint muscles; or the temporomandibular joint dysfunction (TMD). Forty-four million Americans suffer from chronic clenching and grinding, resulting in tooth damage, and 23 million suffer from migraine headache pain.

While mouthguards have been used with some success to treat TMD patients, a new FDA-approved device seems to offer a higher success rate in eliminating TMJ problems. This device has an additional advantage in that it was designed to reduce the clenching habits that often lead to chronic and migraine headaches. This device prevents the upper and lower teeth from coming into contact. By preventing high-intensity clenching (and the muscular irritation that leads to migraine pain, TMD, and chronic headaches), studies have shown that 82% of migraine and headache sufferers had a 77% reduction in the migraine incidents. In short, the frequency and intensity of headache episodes and muscle tenderness can be reduced with the use of a mouthguard.

A tension suppression system is another effective form of mouthguard that can treat TMD. This small removable device, made in the office, can be worn day and/or night and has been shown to reduce clenching intensity by 66%. It takes advantage of a naturally protective reflex that suppresses the powerful chewing muscles active in clenching. For those concerned about insurance coverage, the cost of this device is submitted first to medical insurance for evaluation of benefit coverage. Most insurance carriers do consider this device a payable benefit.

How important is the reduction of the clenching stress? Try this simple demonstration. Put a pencil between the last top and bottom molars on one side and bite hard. Remember how hard you were biting. Then take the pencil and place it between the top and bottom front teeth and bite down hard again. You will not be able to bite down as hard when just biting on the front teeth. You should be able to detect a great difference between biting (clenching) on back teeth only and front teeth only. Try another test: lightly place your fingertips on either side of your head in the temporal area (above and in front of the ears). Clench your teeth and feel the muscles on either side of the head bulge out. Then take a pencil, place it between the top and bottom front teeth, and bite down again. You will easily feel that the temporal muscles do not (cannot) bulge out as much, meaning that not as much clenching compression is possible.

If you have any questions about the connection between headaches and your teeth, please feel free to ask us.

How to Encourage Tooth Decay

A PRIMER ON HOW TO GET ALL THE DECAYED TEETH YOU WANT AND DESERVE...

Decay starts on teeth in specific locations in a fashion that is almost entirely dependent on what you do. This primer will describe the different types of cavities and what YOU can do to ensure that you get all the rotten teeth you want.

1. Cavities can start on the biting surfaces of teeth. In order to get decay in these areas, do the following:
    a. Whether a child, teenager, or adult, do not get protective, painless sealants on your teeth.
    b. Daily and as often as possible, eat and drink foods that have high sugar content.
    c. Eat sticky candy as often as possible.
    d. DO NOT brush your teeth daily. DO NOT use a fluoride-containing mouthrinse.

2. Cavities can start between teeth. These are called *nonflossing cavities*. To get this specific type of decay:
    a. DO NOT floss your teeth properly every day. Rationalize and find excuses not to floss your teeth. If this proves difficult, only floss the teeth you want to keep.
    b. DO NOT use a fluoride-containing mouthrinse on a daily basis.

3. Cavities can start along the gumline (where the tooth appears to exit the gum tissue). These are a special type of cavities. They can progress very quickly to the point where you might even need a root canal! To get quick and large cavities in these areas (especially back teeth):
    a. Be sure to suck on sugar-rich hard candies, cough drops, and breath mints. Do this often during the day.
    b. Do not brush your teeth properly. Make sure the toothbrush bristles do not come in contact with the tooth-gum junction. If you find this proves hard to do, let the dental hygienist show you how to do it properly and then do the opposite of what is said.
    c. DO NOT use a fluoride-containing mouthrinse.

4. If you are missing teeth:
    a. DO NOT get them replaced in a timely fashion. The remaining adjacent and opposing teeth will then be able to move to new areas that are difficult to clean and be more prone, not only to decay, but to gum and chewing problems as well.

5. DO NOT see the dentist and dental hygienist on a routine basis (2-4 times per year, depending on your individual situation) to have your teeth checked and cleaned. If you do go, the dental professionals may find and treat decayed teeth when the decay is minimal. They are not inclined to let the cavities grow properly. In fact, if we find the decay when it is really small, we may be able to treat and remineralize the incipient (beginning) decay without even using a drill or having to give an injection!

Under no circumstances use sugar-free gum or mints. Some of these products have an additive (RECALDENT) in them that has been shown to make enamel stronger and more decay-resistant. The RECALDENT promotes enamel remineralization. This could slow down the decay process or even keep some cavities from forming.

If you adhere strictly to the above rules, you will ensure that you get the most and biggest cavities you possibly can.
The responsibility for growing cavities is yours alone.

Impacted Teeth

An impacted tooth is a tooth that has not erupted (emerged fully into the oral cavity). The impacted tooth can be totally surrounded by bone (a full bony impaction), can be partially surrounded by bone (partial bony impaction), or be only surrounded by soft gum tissue (a soft tissue impaction).

Traditionally, the term *impacted teeth* usually refers to the wisdom teeth (the third molars, the teeth furthest back in the mouth). Both top and bottom wisdom teeth can be impacted. Many times if they appear to be causing no problems for the patient, they are left alone. If they are positioned in a fashion that they appear to be pushing up against the roots of the second molars (the next teeth forward) or if they are causing periodontal (gum) problems, they will need to be removed. While most general dentists are comfortable removing teeth, patients with impacted teeth are usually referred to a specialist (oral surgeon) for their removal.

Wisdom teeth are not the only teeth that can be impacted. Every permanent tooth can be impacted. If the impaction does not appear to affect adjacent teeth, no treatment may be required. If it affects other teeth, it may be need to be removed.

It is not uncommon for "eye" teeth (canine teeth) to be impacted. This is usually discovered early in life, and recommendations for orthodontic treatment (braces) will be made accordingly. Most often, these impacted teeth are not removed, but rather surgically exposed and orthodontically moved over several months into their proper position. Early detection and diagnosis is important to the successful treatment of this situation.

Normally, there is bone separating tooth roots from adjacent teeth. If the impacted tooth, because of its angle and position, gets too close to the roots of the next tooth, the bone between the two teeth will dissolve. If this happens, it is possible that a deep, pathologic periodontal pocket may form. Further deterioration of the periodontal tissues surrounding the tooth in normal position could compromise its health and lead to additional dental treatment. To prevent this from happening, the impacted tooth is removed. If the impaction is deep and difficult to approach, and if there are four wisdom teeth to be removed at the same time, the dentist may elect to perform the procedure in a hospital or surgical center setting.

The more bone that surrounds the impacted tooth, the more difficult it is to remove. The position of the tooth near other teeth or nerves and the manner in which the impacted tooth is angled in the bone also affects the difficulty level of the extraction. The younger the patient is, the better and easier the healing appears to be. If there is a great deal of bone that is removed to allow the impacted tooth to be removed, the dentist may choose to place some "bone fill" material in the place the tooth used to be (the socket) to promote better healing of the bone.

If you have any questions about impacted teeth, please feel free to ask us.

Metal Filling–Induced Cracks in Enamel

You have been diagnosed with cracks in one or more teeth that were previously restored with a silver amalgam (metal) filling material. We may have shown you, with the intraoral video camera, some of the teeth that have these cracks and where on the teeth the cracks are located. Usually, the cracks pick up stain readily and are easily seen.

While tooth enamel is normally hard and brittle, over time very small microcracks will appear in the enamel. This is thought to be due to the thermocycling of the enamel from items you eat and drink that are hotter or colder than room temperature. Again, over time, the expansion and contraction of the enamel causes the cracks to appear. This is not considered a dental problem and is not usually treated. However, teeth that are restored with metal fillings are a different story. Silver amalgam (metal) fillings are composed of not only silver, but also other metals, too. One of the metals is mercury. Most filling materials are at least 30% and some are as high as 50% mercury. Besides being classified as a heavy metal, mercury is a liquid at room temperature (although it is not a liquid in the filling material) and rapidly expands and contracts when its temperature is raised and lowered.

How Cracks Occur
Your mouth is at a temperature of about 98.6 degrees. When you drink hot coffee, followed by eating cold ice cream, the temperature of your mouth will rapidly cycle up 20 or 30 degrees, then down 60 or 70 degrees, then back up to 98.6 degrees. This happens every time you eat or drink something that is not the same temperature as your mouth. Because of the expansion of the mercury component and other metals of the filling material, this expansion and contraction of the filling will cause an outward pressure on the enamel and dentin. The larger the filling is in the beginning and the thinner the enamel is, the more prone the tooth will be to developing cracks. Cracks also provide an avenue for the ingress of fluids and bacteria, a pathway for a cavity to start deep in the tooth. If this were not bad enough, the metal will absorb some of the moisture present in your mouth, and as time passes, will increase in volume. As it expands, it will put outward pressure on the walls of the original filling preparation. This also promotes development of cracks in the tooth.

There are two different paths by which the metal filling can break teeth. You can see for yourself that the fillings are changing. The once smooth and shiny metal becomes black, dull, pitted, and rough. There is metal fatigue. The older the filling, the more likely this has happened. You may also have some tooth sensitivity from fluids or sweets. This is an additional indication that the filling may be leaking and failing. If the filled tooth hurts when you bite down, the tooth may be split and nerve damage may have occurred, or it may be a different, more serious problem altogether. Directly placed metal fillings are an antiquated technique with a material that has been essentially unchanged for almost 180 years.

Treatment Options
You have a choice. You can wait until the cracks become serious and painful and then do even more extensive restorative work, or you can begin, right away, to replace the metal fillings where the cracks are evident. Sometimes, cracks do not get bigger or cause problems; however, many cracks do. During the years, the metal fatigues more and more, and the crack enlarges. In most cases a tooth-colored, bonded direct resin can be used to replace the metal. It seals better to your tooth and has not shown that it cracks the teeth as the metal fillings do. If the existing crack or filling is moderate to large, a gold, resin, or ceramic inlay/onlay will be recommended for the replacement material.

If you have any questions about metal filling–induced cracks in enamel, please feel free to ask us.

Metal Sensitivity

It has become clear that many people can develop sensitivity to some of the metals commonly used in dental restorations. This may or may not have been the case in past years. Perhaps patients were not as sensitive to metals then, or may be the sensitivity was not recognized and diagnosed properly. There are many different kinds of metals used in dentistry. We in this office have, for years, limited your exposure to possible problems by using either materials that have fewer combinations of metals or metals that have a very low potential for sensitivity reactions.

Women appear to have more reactions to metals than men. Studies indicate that at least one woman in seven has an adverse reaction to metals. It may be related to the costume jewelry that women wear, especially earrings for pierced ears. The posts can be made of stainless steel that contains nickel. You might then notice, after some time wearing the jewelry, that your earlobes get red, dried out, or itchy. It can also be seen any place that jewelry comes into contact with your skin—wrist, neck, fingers, etc. If this is your case, you are having a metal sensitivity reaction. If you have any of these problems, it is probably advisable that you limit contact with the problem metals. This can include metals used in restoring your teeth.

At times, you could even notice a metallic taste in your mouth. This can come from silver amalgam fillings that are commonly used. Some studies show leakage of metal through the tooth into the tooth supporting structures (periodontal ligament) from the posts bonded into the tooth after the root canal treatment. These posts are entirely surrounded by tooth or restorations and are not at all in contact with the oral environment. Other oral signs of metal sensitivity include gum tissue that remains chronically red and swollen or bleeds easily where it comes into contact with the metal crown or filling.

Which metals are used in dentistry? Silver fillings (available since approximately 1816) can contain copper, silver, zinc, mercury, and other metals. At this time, we know that several countries have mandated reduced use of silver fillings because of health concerns. Crowns are composed of gold, silver, platinum palladium, and others. A post used to strengthen a tooth after a root canal is either stainless steel or titanium. Sensitivity to each of these metals has been exhibited— some more than others. Gold and titanium rank low. Titanium has been used for years for joint replacements. Pure gold is too soft to be used in dental restorations and titanium is too brittle. If you have a metal sensitivity and need a crown, it may be better to use a metal that is only gold and platinum—or perhaps a bonded ceramic material. While these options may prove to be more expensive than others, metal sensitivity should be avoided.

Nonmetal Options

Options to metal restorations include bonded resins, ceramics, and porcelain. While it is possible that you could have sensitivity to some of the bonding materials, these types of sensitivities are not at all common. The advantages of silver fillings are that they are quick to place and comparatively inexpensive. Advantages of cast metal used under porcelain crowns is similar; the metal/porcelain crowns are less expensive to make and easier to place than full ceramic varieties.

We would prefer not to use silver/mercury fillings, especially for children and women planning to have children. Bonded tooth-colored resins significantly reduce the need for drilling a tooth. They look better and help keep the tooth stronger than silver fillings. If you have a proven metal sensitivity, we will automatically choose materials with less potential for causing you problems.

If you have questions about metal sensitivity, please feel free to ask us.

Occlusal (Bite) Guards

Making a Bite Guard Appliance

The appliance constructed to eliminate or reduce the adverse effects of a bruxing and/or grinding habit(s) is made of a rigid plastic. It is custom-made to fit your mouth exactly. It will take two visits to complete. It can only be inserted one way; it will not stay in place if it is inserted improperly. At the first visit we will make impressions of your upper and lower teeth and record the occlusal (bite) relation of your jaws. After the bite guard is made, you will return for a second visit a week or two later for adjustments and delivery. At the second appointment, the appliance will be adjusted so that your teeth properly meet the plastic. The appliance fits just around the biting surfaces of the teeth of the top jaw. It will not cover the roof of your mouth.

After the appliance has been delivered, you will be expected to return in a few weeks with the appliance for observation and possible further adjustments. You should at no time have any pain or soreness in muscles or joints around your face or ears, whether or not you are wearing the bite guard. It is meant to protect your natural teeth (enamel and dentin) from unnatural, pathologic wear caused by the bruxing or grinding habit. Since the plastic of the appliance is "softer" than your remaining enamel, the plastic will wear when you brux or grind. Expect the plastic to last about 2 years—longer if you do not have a severe problem, shorter if the habits are very abusive.

Wearing Your Appliance

After you receive the protective guard, please wear it as instructed. If you grind or brux at night while sleeping (very common), wear the guard while you sleep. If you brux or grind during the day, try to identify when during the day you have the problem (stuck in traffic, talking on the phone, working at a desk) and wear the guard at that time. Becoming aware of the times of day or stresses that cause you to clench or grind may help you to break the habit.

If at any time, you develop soreness of the muscles around the temporomandibular joint, or TMJ (jaw joint), stop wearing the bite guard and call the office. The TMJ is the hinge joint in front of each ear; you can feel them when you open and close your mouth. Do not wear the bite guard again until we have had a chance to evaluate your situation.

Length of Treatment

How long must you wear the protective appliance? It all depends on the nature of your problem. If this application is being used to prevent stress-related abnormal wear of your teeth, then you will need to wear it until you are no longer burdened by heavy stress. When the source of the problem is eliminated or resolved, the problem may disappear and you will no longer need to wear the appliance. We will periodically evaluate your condition.

When you are not wearing your bite guard, it should be cleaned with a soft toothbrush and water to remove any plaque and stored in a dry place.

Please bring your bite guard with you when you come in for your routine dental hygiene prophylaxis appointment so that we can check the appliance and make sure that it is functioning well. Always stay on the recare interval that we have designated for you. When dental problems are diagnosed in the very early stages, the treatment is usually easier (and less expensive).

Keep the bite guard clean. When you are finished wearing the appliance, brush it with a toothbrush and toothpaste, rinse it, dry it, and store it in the provided container. If it cannot be brushed immediately, at least rinse it under clean water to remove any saliva or debris.

If you have any questions about antibruxing/antigrinding appliances, please feel free to ask us.

Pericoronitis

Pericoronitis is an inflammation (infection) of the soft gum tissue that surrounds the coronal portion (enamel-covered part) of a tooth. It can be associated with the eruption of a tooth, but most often is related to the mandibular (lower) wisdom teeth. The pericoronitis around the lower wisdom teeth is the subject of this short explanation.

Over thousands of years, the diet humans eat has been getting softer and requires less chewing. Our decreasing jaw size and lessened need for wisdom teeth reflects this trend. Unfortunately, our jaws are shrinking faster than our wisdom teeth are disappearing. As a result, particularly in the lower jaw, the wisdom teeth do not have enough room to fully grow (erupt) into the mouth. Although many do find their way into proper position and cause no trouble, all too often the wisdom teeth appear partially covered with gum tissue. This causes a situation in which it is difficult, if not impossible, for the wisdom tooth and surrounding gum to be effectively cleaned on a daily basis. There is a high potential for recurring gum infections. If the tooth and gum cannot be cleaned daily, debris builds up under the gum tissue that partially covers the wisdom tooth. The debris and by-products deteriorate and cause an inflammatory response in the surrounding gum. The gum becomes infected and swollen. If it swells enough, you may even unavoidably bite down on it each time you try to chew food or even swallow.

These infections can be mild, moderate, or severe in nature. They can happen just once or be a continuing problem. There may be little pain or so much pain that you cannot even open your mouth. You may run a fever, have a sore throat, or have swollen glands down the side of your neck.

There are several possible solutions to this problem. You can have the wisdom tooth extracted, and the problem will never occur again. Depending on the position of the teeth, it might be done in this office or you might be referred to a specialist. If you decide to not have the tooth extracted, we can irrigate the area around and under the gum with a medicated solution and clean out the debris with special instruments. Then we will prescribe a specific mouth rinse for you to use postoperatively for several days. If the infection is not too severe, this will often resolve the immediate situation. However, it can recur! In some people, recurrence is frequent; in others, it is just the one time and never happens again. It is very difficult to predict. The better able you are to effectively clean the area, the less likely you are to have the infection again.

After an evaluation of your problem, we will suggest the appropriate option to you. Please remember that the better you can follow our specific recommendations on daily brushing and flossing of your teeth and keeping the time intervals between your periodic hygiene recare appointments, the less likely you will be to have any pericoronitis problems.

Today the following procedures were performed:

❑ Extraction of tooth #_____ with local anesthesia.
❑ Irrigation of the affected tooth/infected pocket with_____ .
❑ Hand and/or ultrasonic instrumentation of infected pocket.
❑ Prescription for　❑ Antibiotic:_____　❑ Analgesic_____　❑ Peridex rinse_____
❑ Referral to an oral surgeon for extraction of tooth #_____

If you have any questions about pericoronitis, please feel free to ask us.

Root Surface Caries

Causes

In a normal mouth, a small portion of the enamel is covered with gum tissue. The root section of the tooth (that part not covered by enamel) is embedded in the bone and covered by gum tissue. As you get older, the gum tissue recedes from the crown portion of the tooth, and the root structure becomes exposed. This may occur due to improper brushing technique, gum disease, periodontal surgical repositioning of the gum tissue, decay, or just aging.

The enamel of a tooth readily absorbs fluoride and becomes hard and resistant to the attack of decay-causing acids. The root, however, is covered with cementum and/or dentin. Both are very soft compared with enamel. With the receding of the gums, the cementum and dentin become unprotected from the attack of acids and are prone to decay. There are additional problems. The root covering is not as thick as the enamel, allowing the decay to start closer to the nerve. This increases tooth sensitivity and the opportunity for nerve death, leading to the need for root canal therapy. Root decay can lead to lack of support for the crown portion of the tooth, resulting in fracturing if the tooth has metal fillings. If the tooth starts to fracture, it may require a laboratory-prepared crown.

Other factors can contribute to root decay: poor oral self-care, root exposure, and diminished salivary flow, which can be due to many factors such as medications, radiation therapy, the natural aging process, and chemotherapy. Saliva provides chemicals that remineralize teeth after exposure to acid and can buffer against destructive acid concentrations. Without normal salivary flow, root decay has a higher potential for beginning.

Treatment

Treatment for root decay involves removing the decayed portion and restoring the tooth. We may use a tooth-colored filling material that actually slowly releases fluoride. More serious root decay may require treatment with endodontic therapy and a cast crown.

Prevention

Preventive measures include thorough oral self-care. This may include use of a fluoridated toothpaste, either over-the-counter or a higher fluoride level prescription toothpaste, daily nonprescription topical fluoride rinses, medication, and nightly use of a fluoride tray. A topical fluoride application and more frequent hygiene recare appointments are also appropriate preventive measures.

If you have any questions about root decay, please feel free to ask us.

Sensitive Teeth

Teeth can become sensitive for many reasons. Sometimes the sensitivity is an indication of a potentially serious problem. Other times, the dentally related problem may be small but the effects (the sensitivity) are extremely aggravating. A tooth can become sensitive after it has been prepared (drilled) for a restoration (filling). You may have been anesthetized during the procedure, so you did not feel any discomfort when the nerve in the tooth reacted to the heat generated by the drill. The closer the drill comes to the nerve, the more likely it is to cause a sensitivity problem. The high-speed rotation of the bur in the drill generates heat, and the response of the nerve to heat is inflammation. This inflammation is felt by you as a "sensitivity." If the decay, fracture, or drilling was not too deep, this sensitivity will decrease over time. A week to a month or two is not an unusual length of time for the sensitivity to disappear. A good sign is the continued decrease of sensitivity. However, if the occlusion (bite) is off after the restoration has been placed, the tooth may either become sensitive or may stay sensitive. Once the bite is adjusted, though, the sensitivity should disappear.

Additional reasons for single sensitivity are decay, a defective restoration, or a fractured tooth. When a tooth is decayed, temperature changes and sweets will make it sensitive. If a filling is defective or failing, leakage around the filling may cause the tooth to become sensitive. In both of these cases, the solution can be as simple as removing the decay or defective filling and placing an appropriate restoration. If the tooth is fractured, you may be sensitive to temperature changes, or when chewing food. This fracture condition may be hard to diagnose. If you think you might have this type of sensitivity, please ask for the separate handout that explains the "cracked tooth syndrome" in much greater detail.

Tooth sensitivity can also be caused by a dying nerve. This can be the result of a deep cavity. Commonly, the sensitive tooth holds an old large filling. The nerve may have been damaged during drilling and the nerve has been dying gradually ever since. If this is the problem, the tooth will need endodontic treatment.

Two other reasons for tooth sensitivity are related. One is an inadvertent notching of the tooth surface and/or recession of the gum tissue (exposing the root surface of the tooth) caused by improper brushing: either brushing too hard, brushing with a toothbrush that is too hard, or using an improper brushing technique. This sensitivity can range from mild to extreme; the degree of sensitivity does not appear to be related to the size of the root exposure or notch. Finally, purposeful repositioning of the gum tissue during gum surgery can also lead to tooth sensitivity. While recession from brushing is slow, gum recession following gum repositioning occurs very quickly. The portion of the tooth once covered with gum and bone may now be exposed. Root sensitivity in these instances can be quite severe and immediate. It can sometimes last for months or years if not treated.

Treatment Options

Treatment in these last two instances is similar. If there is a notch in the tooth or the shape of the defect is appropriate, the defect is restored (filled in) with a bonded material. This can give immediate relief—sometimes partially, sometimes fully. When there is no defect to be restored, the exposed and sensitive root surfaces are covered with a dentin-bonding or other material. This material is invisible and has very little thickness, so you do not notice any change in the appearance of the tooth; but it works. It may have to be reapplied after several months because the bonding material has worn away by toothbrushing.

If you have any questions about tooth sensitivity, please feel free to ask us.

Temporomandibular Joint Dysfunction (TMD) Questionnaire

Patient: _____

Date of examination: _____

Patient's chief complaint: _____

	Yes	No
Do you have difficulty opening your mouth?	❏	❏
Is it painful for you to open your mouth wide?	❏	❏
Do you notice any clicking, popping, or other noises when you open?	❏	❏
Do you have frequent headaches?	❏	❏

Where are they located? _____

_____

	Yes	No
Do you have frequent earaches or neck pain?	❏	❏
Do you have difficulty chewing hard foods?	❏	❏
Do you have difficulty chewing soft foods?	❏	❏
Has your jaw ever locked in the open position?	❏	❏

Please explain: _____

_____

	Yes	No
Do you clench your teeth?	❏	❏
Do you grind your teeth?	❏	❏
Daytime?	❏	❏
While sleeping?	❏	❏
Do you ever wake up in the morning and find that your jaw muscles are sore or tired?	❏	❏

Please explain: _____

_____

For the doctor:

Range of motion: Vertical _____ Horizontal _____

Deviation on opening: Left _____ Right _____ Degree _____

Maximum occlusal opening: _____

Tenderness to palpation: _____

Diagnosis: _____

_____

_____

Temporomandibular Joint Dysfunction (TMD) Syndrome

Causes and Symptoms

Temporomandibular joint (TMJ) dysfunction, or TMD, can be a complicated and complex problem. The TMJ is located in front of each ear and is responsible, with the associated ligaments, tendons, disks, and muscles, for all jaw movements. Problems with the joint are referred to as *TMD*. They can be manifested in a variety of ways including headaches, earaches, ringing in the ears, problems with jaw opening or closing, tenderness of the jaw muscles, popping or clicking noises when the jaw is opened or closed, neck pain, and upper back pain.

When the jaw joint does not function properly, there can be pain and muscle spasms. However, it should be noted that muscle spasms and resulting pain may have nothing to do with the jaw joint. The TMJ is essential to all movements that involve the jaw. The pain can be slight, moderate, or severe. It can be sporadic or constant and even debilitating. It is common for a TMD patient to have difficulty chewing hard foods or opening the mouth wide without discomfort. Some of the patients may have a problem chewing soft foods. Normal function of the joint can be affected by trauma (accident), improper positioning of the teeth, disease (arthritis), and stress-related habits such as clenching and grinding.

TMJ dysfunction has been called *The Great Imposter* because it mimics other problems. Sometimes it is hard to diagnose. Sometimes it is easy to determine. Many times, special radiographs are absolutely necessary to see the nature of the problem.

Treatment Options

Once the problem is diagnosed, possible treatments are considered. The usual method of treatment is very conservative: mouthguards and various appliances specifically constructed for you. They permit the joint area to rest and give it a chance to heal. These therapies are relatively inexpensive. Time of treatment varies considerably among patients. Some may get relief in a few days; others may need months. Some may have to wear the appliances all the time; some, just at night. Other treatment may include prescription medication, habit-breaking appliances, TMJ orthodontics, physical therapy, biofeedback and counseling, and orthodontic corrective surgery.

Depending on the exact nature of your TMD problem, we may decide to treat you here or send you to a dentist who specializes in this treatment. Early treatment may help you to a better chance for a successful result. This is especially true if the nature of the problem is degenerative, and not related to clenching or grinding. Although diagnosis of TMD problems may often be easy, the exact nature of the treatment needed to obtain relief may be difficult.

If you have any questions about temporomandibular joint dysfunction (TMD), please feel free to ask us.

Toothbrush Abrasion: Preventing Tooth Destruction

The Cause

Brushing improperly (especially with a hard-bristled toothbrush) can cause erosion/abrasion of your tooth or teeth. This is a very common problem. It begins as a small V- or U-shaped area of wear near the gingival (gum) tissue right next to the tooth, usually where the tooth and gum meet. Improper brushing causes the gum tissue to recede; and the tooth may become sensitive to heat, cold, or air stimulation. With time, more enamel wears away and a small horizontal notch is seen on the tooth at the gumline. This is not an area of decay, but a mechanical "cavity" cut in the tooth. Eventually the enamel is worn completely through and the dentin becomes exposed. When that occurs, some people experience severe tooth sensitivity. It may be so severe that it is painful to drink cold fluids, breathe in air, or just brush your teeth. However, others experience little to no extra tooth sensitivity.

Once enough of the gum is brushed away, the root of the tooth becomes exposed. The root surface is not covered with enamel and is much softer than the enamel. It can also be unsightly to have the tissue recede. Since the root surface is not protected by hard enamel, if the improper brushing continues, the root cementum will be worn through and a notch will be made in the dentin. This notch will increase in size, weaken the tooth, and sometimes make the area more prone to decay.

Tooth Sensitivity

Some patients with very little loss of tooth structure experience extreme sensitivity. This problem can usually be corrected with the application of a dentin-bonding material or other desensitizing chemicals. The sensitivity problem is often completely cured. The treatment can last (depending on your brushing habits) for 6 months or longer. If necessary, the tooth can be re-treated if the sensitivity returns.

Some patients with a tremendous loss of tooth structure notice very little tooth sensitivity. Whether or not the teeth become sensitive, it is advisable to correct the brushing problem to slow down or eliminate the wear process. It is also recommended that the notches be restored with a tooth-colored filling material. This will restore the appearance of the tooth and protect the previously exposed dentin. In this way, even if you continue to brush improperly, the tooth will be protected.

In cases of minor sensitivity, we might recommend the use of desensitizing toothpaste as a low-cost alternative to the placement of bonded materials. Some cases might also be managed through the use of topical fluoride applications.

Preventing Abrasion

The problems of improper toothbrushing are easily and inexpensively corrected when they are diagnosed in the early stages of development. If allowed to progress, the tooth damage will increase, as will the cost to repair it. The best solution is **prevention!**

Brush your teeth thoroughly but not abusively. Do not scrub them or cross brush them (an exaggerated horizontal brushing motion). We will select a method of toothbrushing that will best meet your needs and teach you to care for your mouth. Use a soft toothbrush. Change to a new brush every 3 months. But if it happens that you are creating the problem of toothbrush abrasion, get it corrected as soon as it is diagnosed.

If you have any questions about toothbrush erosion or abrasion, please feel free to ask us.

Traumatic Occlusion: Occlusal Equilibration or Bite Adjustment

The Normal Bite Relation

In the normal, healthy mouth, teeth should meet without extra stress being placed on any individual tooth. Teeth that mesh and meet properly are similar to two metal gear wheels that, when rotating together, have the projection (or *tooth* as it is called) of one gear fit perfectly and smoothly into the depression of the other gear. If for some reason the teeth of the two gears do not meet exactly, the projections on both gears will hit and there will be an unwanted interference. This interference could make portions of the gear teeth chip, fracture, or wear abnormally causing wear facets in the metal teeth. If the interference continues for a longer period of time or the interference is severe, the gear teeth will be more likely to break, and the break could be more severe. The gear wheels themselves could also loosen on their axis and begin to wobble when rotating.

Even though teeth are not made of metal, similarities to the meshing of gears do exist. The outside surface that normally contacts the opposing tooth is made of enamel—hard but brittle. Your teeth are held in place and supported by the bone that surrounds the teeth. When your occlusion (bite) changes, preventing your teeth from meshing in unison, the enamel could begin to chip or wear. When these teeth have been restored, these restorations could fracture. In the most severe cases, the teeth will become loose. You may also find that the enamel wears away abnormally quite quickly and the teeth change shape and become shorter.

Traumatic Occlusion

All of the above problems could be a sign of traumatic occlusion. The teeth that meet improperly can be damaged every time you close your mouth. One tooth or all of your teeth may be affected. Very often, you don't know that a problem exists because you experience little or no pain until it reaches a very advanced stage. If you have teeth that have compromised bone support because of active or past periodontal disease, the teeth will have a tendency toward slight movement that could place them in traumatic occlusion. The "bite" doesn't have to be off by very much before a problem occurs. Movement from the proper position no more than the thickness of a piece of paper is often sufficient to cause a problem. If you have a clenching or grinding habit related to stress, you can induce a traumatic occlusion.

Treatment

Once the problem has been diagnosed, it should be treated quickly. Treatment can be simple or complex. It will involve determining which teeth are not meeting correctly when you close your teeth together. If only one tooth is in a poor position, it may be able to be corrected with one appointment. If more than one tooth is involved or if teeth are looser, several appointments may be needed to correct the problem. Your teeth may be slightly sensitive to temperature changes for a time after the occlusal adjustment is completed.

If you have any questions about traumatic occlusion, please feel free to ask us.

Wisdom Teeth (Third Molars)

Human beings have more teeth than they actually need: four more teeth, to be exact. The third molars (wisdom teeth) are the last teeth on each side and in each arch of the mouth. If we don't need them, why do we have them? Hundreds of thousands of years ago, our ancestors didn't look a great deal like we do today. They had smaller bodies but larger and more powerful jaws. Their diet dictated this jaw structure and number of teeth. Our ancestors ate a tougher and more abrasive type of food. It wasn't cooked well, and it wasn't ground up well. There were a lot of hard grains and foods that required lots of chewing. Big jaws were capable of holding more teeth for this chewing.

Today, we don't need the heavy grinding capacity that early humans had. Food is easier to eat, less abrasive, and much softer. Evolution is reacting (slowly) to this fact by decreasing the size of our jaw bones and chewing muscles. The human jaw that once comfortably held 12 molars (32 teeth total) is now often only large enough to hold eight molars (28 teeth total). Unfortunately, our jaws are getting smaller faster than our wisdom teeth are disappearing. The wisdom teeth often do not have enough room to grow properly. Eventually, thousands of years from now, humans will not have wisdom teeth. They have lost their function and are gradually disappearing, just like the appendix.

Since the jaw is too small (for most people) to accommodate the third molars, they come into the mouth partially, poorly positioned, or not at all. They can be fully erupted, partially erupted, a soft tissue impaction, partial bony impaction, or full bony impaction. If teeth come in well and you are able to keep them clean, we leave them alone. If they are crowded or poorly positioned and cannot be kept clean, they are like an accident waiting to happen. Decay and gum infection are likely to result. These teeth are usually removed—ideally before they begin to cause big problems with the second molars that are directly ahead of them. Teeth that are partially erupted should always be removed: there is too much opportunity for gum infection to begin. If the teeth cannot be cleaned, chronic painful inflammation may occur (pericoronitis). The earlier they are removed, the better your healing will be.

Less complex extractions (fully erupted teeth or partial soft tissue impactions) can be done by a general dentist. We will refer difficult extractions to an oral surgeon for treatment. Depending on the type of extraction and the medical history of the patient, the extractions may be done in an office or in the hospital. This will be determined after viewing radiographs of the teeth. Having all four wisdom teeth out at the same time is a common practice. Postoperative discomfort can be minimal to extreme—in the case of difficult full bony impactions. Antiinflammatory and pain relief medications are prescribed appropriately.

We do not need wisdom teeth to eat well. If they need to come out, it is better they come out (1) before they cause problems with the adjacent teeth that you really need and (2) when you are younger and heal well. If you need to have one wisdom tooth taken out, also have the opposing wisdom tooth removed. When a tooth does not meet an opposing tooth, it "super erupts" or continues to grow out of the normal position. When left for some time, the remaining tooth can develop decay and gum disease and cause the same thing to happen to the tooth in front of it.

If you have any questions about your wisdom teeth, please feel free to ask us.

Xerostomia: Dry Mouth Syndrome

Xerostomia (dry mouth) is not a condition everyone should expect. You may notice it as you age due to a change in hormones, medication, and/or radiation therapy in the head and neck region.

Why Xerostomia Is a Problem

Saliva is important to oral health for several reasons. The flow of saliva helps clear debris from the oral cavity. It provides minerals necessary to support the process of remineralization. Tooth enamel daily undergoes acid attack that removes inorganic minerals from teeth. This is called demineralization. Remineralization is the opposite of demineralization. It occurs when inorganic molecules flow into a region of weakened enamel and make it stronger.

When the salivary flow is reduced, a chain of events occurs. The natural cleansing action is diminished, as are the buffering action and remineralization properties of saliva. People with diminished salivary flow experience a very fast rate of decay, many times faster and over several teeth. This type of dental decay is typically noted along the gumline, around existing dental work, and on exposed root surfaces.

Prevention

You can help prevent dental decay that can result from xerostomia.

- Brushing and flossing correctly at least once each day becomes very important.
- Frequent sips of water during the day can help moisten the mouth and can help clear debris.
- Daily use of a mouthrinse containing fluoride can help remineralize the teeth.
- Use a toothpaste containing sodium fluoride.
- We recommend a daily brushing with a prescription, high-concentration sodium fluoride gel or paste. We will either dispense this or give you a prescription for it.
- Chew sugarless gum or a rubber band to help stimulate salivary flow.
- In moderate to severe cases, special fluoride delivery trays can be made for you to use at home. These will keep the high-concentration fluoride in a position to "soak" your teeth with fluoride for several minutes at a time.
- We recommend that you have your teeth cleaned, polished, and an office-applied topical fluoride treatment every 3 months while the condition persists.

Dry mouth can have serious dental consequences and must be treated accordingly.

If you have any questions about xerostomia, please feel free to ask us.

chapter 8

Orthodontics

Content at a Glance: Orthodontics

Care of Braces
Discusses proper oral self-care including a checklist of recommendations for the individual patient.

Congenitally Missing Teeth
Alerts the patient to the problems associated with congenitally missing teeth and the treatment needed.

Fixed and Removable Orthodontics
Compares both methods of orthodontic therapy, highlighting benefits of each.

Orthodontics (Braces)
Overview of the need for orthodontia, timing, and oral self-care during the active phase.

Uprighting Tilted Molars
An explanation of the changes in tooth alignment possible as a result of nonreplaced extracted teeth.

Care of Braces

If you are undergoing orthodontic treatment, you probably feel that you have many "things" in your mouth. Dentistry has names for the different types of orthodontic hardware: bands, brackets, arch wires, ligatures, elastics, etc. What it means to you is that any type of orthodontic appliance cemented and/or bonded to your teeth makes it more difficult for you to properly clean your teeth. You will find that you have more food debris caught around your teeth and orthodontic hardware than ever before. It is harder and more time-consuming to clean the debris away.

It is very important to keep your teeth immaculately clean while the braces are on. The extra food that can be easily trapped around the band, brackets, and wires will decompose over time and can cause gum decay and possibly gum disease. It is pretty devastating to see braces removed from newly straightened teeth and find that the teeth are all decayed or disfigured. It is even more depressing to have restorations placed in these nice straight teeth. Fortunately, this can be avoided with proper oral self-care and maintenance.

We will spend as much time as you need in showing you how to keep your teeth clean and your gums healthy. There are dental cleaning aids available to help maintain proper oral self-care while undergoing active orthodontic therapy. We will demonstrate their use and either provide them for you or tell you where you can purchase them.

We advise that you return to the office **every three months** while the braces are on in order to have your teeth cleaned by the dental hygienist and receive a topical fluoride treatment. We find that with this preventive recare interval, you have less chance of developing periodontal (gum) problems around the braces and decay under and around the orthodontic appliances.

Listed below are several additional tips for caring for your braces:
- ❑ Use a toothpaste containing fluoride when you brush your teeth.

- ❑ Use a dental floss threader as instructed and demonstrated to clean under the arch wires every night.

- ❑ Rinse with a fluoride-containing mouthrinse at least once each day. Follow the instructions included with the mouthrinse. Use of the fluoride mouthrinse will help reduce the possibility of decay or decalcification (white or soft spots in the enamel) under the cemented or bonded bands and brackets. We consider it to be a very important prevention aid.

- ❑ Use an oral irrigator as demonstrated to help remove debris from around the braces. **This is in no way a substitute for proper brushing and flossing.** It is an adjunct oral self-care aid.

- ❑ Use an electric toothbrush as instructed.

Take proper care of your teeth while your braces are on. You will be glad you did.

If you have any questions about orthodontic and preventive dental care, please feel free to ask us.

Congenitally Missing Teeth

Some of us will have 32 teeth develop during our lifetime. This is considered a normal number of teeth in an adult. However, as human beings evolve, we are seeing fewer adults with a full set of 32 teeth. It is common for people to be missing one or more of the third molars, also called *wisdom teeth*. The jaw sizes of modern humans are such that there often is simply not enough room for the proper placement of the third molars in a mouth, and they usually have to be extracted. We have all known people who have had impacted wisdom teeth that needed to be removed.

Not as common, but not at all unusual, is a person who never develops some other permanent teeth. When this happens, it is frequently one or both of the upper lateral incisors, which are the smaller teeth on either side of the two top front teeth. Less often, the permanent eyeteeth (canines) or premolars will never develop.

The problem that results from congenitally missing teeth is due to the space where the tooth (teeth) should have been. This is a very serious cosmetic problem. The other teeth around the space will shift into different positions.

The problems that can result from missing permanent teeth can be reduced or eliminated with early detection and a plan for future restoration. The usual treatment involves orthodontics to move the permanent teeth into better position or keep the permanent teeth in the correct location. We see missing lateral incisors so often that the treatment routine is well established. The best esthetics, the most natural look, will be achieved by leaving the adjacent permanent central incisors and canine teeth in their customary places. The maintenance of proper tooth positioning is very important for the future appearance of the replacement.

The sequence of treatment is orthodontics as early as necessary to maintain the space. If the tooth has moved too much, more orthodontic treatment will be necessary. Then, while the child and mouth are growing, a removable replacement tooth is made. This is worn until the teeth are ready to receive the implant or bridge, after age 18 or so.

The permanent teeth further back in the mouth are less often missing entirely. It is common for baby teeth to be retained in these areas when the permanent teeth do not come in. Sometimes the baby teeth can last for years, but they do not have the root structure to remain stable over a lifetime. If they are decayed and filled, they become weak and more prone to fracture. If you are lucky, they have enough root to function and look better through the use of bonding resins and porcelain. Because the retained baby teeth are meant for a small mouth, they cannot function in the same ways as permanent teeth. When lost, an over-retained baby tooth can be replaced with an implant or a bridge. Your own particular situation will determine the best course of treatment.

If you have any questions about congenitally missing teeth, please feel free to ask us.

Fixed and Removable Orthodontics

The traditional and stereotypical movie, television, and commercial vision of orthodontic treatment is one of yards of metal wire tied down to teeth so covered with silver bands and brackets that the whites of the teeth are barely visible. With today's advanced dental technology, this picture is far from accurate.

Changes in tooth alignment can be accomplished in several different ways. When appropriate, upper and lower arch expanders can be used to increase the curvature of the tooth-bearing supporting structures. These expanders are usually cemented into place and are not able to be removed by the patient. The expanders are often a prelude to fixed metal bands. They can be cemented to the teeth as well as longitudinal arch wires and springs and still be used to move teeth.

Some time ago, the desire of patients to show less metal resulted in the development of bonded tooth-colored and clear brackets (as opposed to the metal bands that completely surround a tooth). These brackets cover only about 25% of the tooth surface and are bonded into place. The trade-off with the more esthetic bonded brackets is a higher percentage of dislodgement of the bracket, requiring additional office visits for repair and replacement. The wires and springs are changed periodically to accomplish the various stages of movement. The metal components stay in place until the tooth movement is finished. Some dental conditions mandate the use of this traditional orthodontic process.

It is not always necessary to use fixed devices to move teeth. Less aggressive tooth movement can additionally be done with patient-removable appliances. Some are made of a gum-colored pink acrylic material with metal wires and springs embedded in them. These are worn by the patient except when he or she is eating, brushing, and flossing. The metal and plastic appliances do not show as much metal so they are somewhat more acceptable. The trade-off with removable appliances is that they only work when they are in the patient's mouth, making proper patient compliance a big issue. If you do not wear them, the teeth will not move as planned. The metal and plastic appliances are used in what is called *minor* tooth movement. Many orthodontic cases are not appropriate for removable appliance therapy.

Several years ago, a new type of removable appliance therapy was developed and patented. Align Technology has a product called *Invisalign®*. Clear, thin plastic aligners (positioners) are sequentially placed to move the teeth in a precise fashion. The aligners are left in the mouth as much as possible and removed only for eating, drinking, and cleaning the teeth. Again, if you do not wear them, the teeth will not move. The aligners are almost invisible when in place and are extraordinarily acceptable esthetically. They are indicated for adults and patients older than 14 years who have all permanent teeth in including fully erupted second molars. They can be used to treat simple to fairly extensive misalignment problems. Most cases are completed in about 12 months. Research is still in progress to determine the limits of this process.

The doctor who will be performing the orthodontic treatment will take these different modalities into consideration and develop a treatment plan best suited to your needs. Age of the patient, number of teeth involved, and extent of movement are primary factors in the decision-making process. Please be sure to ask why or why not one technique rather than another was suggested.

If you have any questions about your orthodontic treatment, please feel free to ask us.

Orthodontics (Braces)

If your teeth are in poor alignment, you could be facing a functional or cosmetic problem. Orthodontics (braces) can eliminate that problem for you. One of the first things people notice about you is your smile and how your teeth look. You don't have to be a dentist to notice poorly positioned, crooked teeth. In today's culture, crooked teeth are not regarded as attractive or desirable. Most people, when asked, say that they would like to have straight teeth. Straight, white teeth are the cosmetic dental improvements patients most request.

The need for orthodontics is best discovered when you are young. A dentist will have a good indication of whether or not your teeth will be straight when he sees you as a child 6 to 8 years of age. Most treatment would not begin until a patient is 8 years old, although in some cases, orthodontics can be started earlier.

It is easier to direct the movement of teeth in a child. Early tooth guidance is a very important phase of orthodontic care, which can take place even though all the permanent teeth are not yet in place. Certain problems are much easier to correct at this stage of a "mixed dentition" of baby and permanent teeth. When more treatment than simple early tooth guidance is required, an average case can last from 18 to 24 months.

While orthodontic therapy is admittedly easier in the child patient, you are never too old to begin orthodontics. The number of adults seeking orthodontic treatment has risen dramatically during the past decade. As long as you have healthy bone support for your teeth, you can have orthodontic therapy. Most adult cases take 18 to 24 months to complete.

Once the braces are removed, it is usually necessary to wear a retainer. This retainer will maintain the new tooth alignment until the teeth have had a chance to become firmly set in their new positions. This retainer may be either removable or fixed in place.

While the orthodontic treatment is in the active phase, that is, while the braces are on your teeth, you must be very diligent about keeping your teeth clean. This will be more difficult than and somewhat different from cleaning your teeth without braces. You will be instructed in the use of any cleaning aids needed. These may include dental floss threaders, an oral irrigator to flush out debris, proper brushing habits, fluoride mouthrinses, and periodontal aids. You **must** follow your proper oral self-care routine each night to prevent decay, decalcification of the teeth, and gum disease.

Braces may also be suggested to correct a specific dental problem that only affects one or several teeth. This is not a cosmetic tooth repositioning, but rather a functional tooth movement. Occasionally, in order to properly finish an orthodontic case, the orthodontist may ask the dentist to adjust the enamel of some teeth or bond a resin to some teeth to improve the occlusion (bite alignment) or to enhance cosmetics. This will be discussed with you as soon as it becomes apparent.

In summary, remember that you are never too old to begin orthodontic treatment.
- It may be easier and less expensive to be treated at a young age (about 8 years old).
- You must follow your proper oral self-care routine every night.
- Get your teeth cleaned professionally by a dental hygienist every three months to reduce the occurrence of decay and gum disease.

Orthodontics can make a dramatic improvement in your appearance, your life, and how you feel about yourself.

If you have any questions about orthodontics, please feel free to ask us.

Uprighting Tilted Molars

One of the most common conditions in an adult who has experienced an early loss of an anterior molar or premolar is the drifting and tilting forward of first or second molars. This drifting or tilting will cause the teeth to move off their normal vertical and horizontal positions. Teeth move at a very slow pace, so it may take many years for this movement to become noticeable to you. Teeth are normally held in position by the contact with the adjacent and opposing teeth. When this contact or occlusion is changed because of an extraction, the teeth will migrate toward the front of the mouth. Because of the forces of occlusion, they will begin to tilt and move into the space created by the extraction. Because of the change, the tooth that has moved will be more prone to having decay start between it and the one behind it. There will also be a tendency for an adverse change in the position of the bone and gum architecture, and the change is not for the better. Because of a change in the way food deflects off the tooth and different actions and forces on the root, pathologic periodontal pockets can and usually do develop. As one tooth begins to move, the other teeth around it begin to change position too. The closer they are to the tooth next to the space, the more they move. Three, four, five, or more teeth can easily be affected.

Since this is not normally a stable or good situation, we advise that you consider having it corrected. The easiest solution when there is one tooth missing and only one tooth that has moved forward and tilted is to orthodontically upright the malpositioned tooth. This can often be done in a matter of several months. Once the tooth has been moved back into position, you must stabilize it so that it will not drift back into the space again. If the tooth can be moved forward so that it is in contact with the more anterior tooth, stabilization might include some type of night retainer for several months. If there is a space anterior to the moved tooth, that is, if the tooth was moved backward in the uprighting process, you should consider replacing the missing tooth with a conventional fixed bridge, a bonded bridge, an implant, or a removable partial denture. All of these options should be considered and the choice should be made before the orthodontic treatment begins.

If more than one tooth has moved, the orthodontic correction will become more complicated and involve more time and more teeth. Some teeth may be moved forward, and some, backward. Opposing teeth may have extruded into the space and need to be intruded back into the socket. As with the movement of only one tooth, the final prosthetic plan must be determined before any work begins. Stabilization and restoration must be begun as soon as possible after the teeth have been correctly moved, or they will move again.

Prevention is the best treatment. Dentists recommend saving teeth. If you have had a tooth removed, get it replaced as soon as possible, thus preventing future improper movement and misalignment. But if you are unlucky enough to have had a back tooth removed at an early age and the teeth are beginning to move, consider orthodontics to upright and reposition the teeth. If you do not, you can expect future problems with decay and your periodontal supporting tissues. Continued movement may even cause the loss of more teeth!

If you have any questions about uprighting teeth, please feel free to ask us.

chapter 9

Pediatric Dentistry

Content at a Glance: Pediatric Dentistry

A Child's First Visit to the Dentist
Explains to parents when and how to prepare their child for the child's first visit to the dentist.

Early Childhood Caries
Explains "baby bottle tooth decay" and provides suggestions for prevention.

Eruption Patterns of Teeth
Informs parents of how and when teeth are formed and eventually erupt in children.

Prevention of Dental Disease in Infants and Children
Specifies suggestions for preventing dental disease in infants and children.

Sealants
Sealants for the prevention of oral disease are discussed.

Sealant Warranty
Assures your patients of the need for and integrity of sealants with a sealant warranty.

Supplemental Fluoride
Makes sure that children receive the right amount of fluoride with a chart for fluoridated water.

Topical Fluoride: At Home and in the Dental Office
Urges patients to take advantage of both in-home and in-office fluoride delivery. Includes specific instructions for fluoride tray procedures.

A Child's First Visit to the Dentist

Getting Ready

A child's first visit to the dentist should be at a much earlier age than most parents think—and for a different reason. The first dental visit should occur in infancy, as teeth are beginning to erupt. During this visit, we will let you know how to care for your child's teeth and what preventive measures you should be taking for your infant at this early stage. Many dental problems can be intercepted when we have the opportunity to examine your child and visit with you in the early developmental stages.

The first cleaning for your child (pedodontic prophylaxis) should be done at about 2 to 2½ years of age, depending on the child's behavior. Importantly, this should not be the first time the child visits our office. Before this visit, we would like the child to come in with a parent who is getting a routine preventive prophylaxis. We have many toys, coloring books, and children's movies that can be shown. In this way, children come to know the dental office as a very pleasant, nonthreatening experience. Hopefully, by the time they come for their own prophylaxis, they have been to the office several times. They know the dentist, the dental hygienist, and the way the office and dental equipment looks. They will have a good idea of what will be expected of them. They will have had only good experiences with all of these people at this location. Usually, children introduced to dentistry in this manner are very excited about having their own dental appointments.

It is important for parents to always talk positively about going to a dental appointment as well as after the dental appointment has occurred. Children are very smart. They may not know what some of the words mean, but they can understand how you feel about it. You should try not to use any words around them that might have an unpleasant connotation: toothache, drill, pull, hurt, pain, unhappy, etc. Always talk about how happy you are to go to the dentist and what a great experience it was. If your appointment wasn't great, talk about it in private where children cannot overhear. If necessary, and if your child asks, tell him or her about how glad you are that the dentist is making your mouth feel good again, without mentioning any of the discomfort.

It is also important that the children are not threatened by the dentist and to avoid making the dentist appear to be the "heavy." Don't tell children, for example, that if they eat candy, they will have to go to the dentist to get their teeth drilled and filled. Children will then think of the dentist's office as a place where you get punished for doing something bad. We want children to be completely comfortable and to not worry when it is time for a dental appointment.

The Visit

The first time the child has a dental procedure performed, at the age of 2 to 2½ years, it will usually be very simple, quick, and entirely painless. Of course, we assume you have followed all the preventive suggestions we have given you: fluoride vitamins, if appropriate, brushing the child's teeth, nothing in a night bottle but water, and so forth.

First, we will spend a little bit of time with the child in a show-and-tell mode. We will show the child the various instruments: polishers, mirrors, "Mr. Thirsty" (saliva ejector), the water gun (air/water syringe), and so on. The dental hygienist will also begin to instruct the child in proper brushing techniques. At this young age, children do not manipulate dental floss and a brush properly. This is a project for the parent. Since children admire and try to imitate their parents, your good example of brushing and flossing each day will help tremendously in this area. Children will see that it is something you do, which they will then try to imitate.

Also during this visit, the dentist will "count" the child's teeth, while looking for decay or other problems. Then the dental hygienist will "tickle" (clean and polish) the teeth. Stains and plaque that might have accumulated will be easily removed. It is very unusual for a child to have major periodontal problems.

If the child is prepared correctly, the first treatment visit at the dentist will be anticipated with no anxiety, proceed smoothly, and make the child excited about coming again. What you do at home in preparation for this first visit is most important to its success. Good luck!

If you have any questions about your child's first visit to the dentist, please feel free to ask us.

Early Childhood Caries

What is Early Childhood Caries?

Early childhood caries, which used to be called "baby bottle tooth decay" and "nursing caries," is a severe form of dental decay found in very young children who presumably are put to sleep with any liquid other than water in a bottle. Children who have experienced prolonged breastfeeding will have the same type of tooth decay patterns. Many times, the decay is very advanced before the parent notices the problem. This is another reason that we want to see your child for his or her first dental visit while those new teeth are still in the eruption phase.

How Does Early Childhood Caries Develop?

The teeth most affected by early childhood caries are the upper front teeth. As the child falls asleep with a bottle containing any liquid other than water (or at the breast), pools of the sugared liquid collect against the tooth surfaces. These sugars feed the bacteria found in bacterial plaque to produce an acid, which starts the decay process. When the demineralization process is not stopped through proper prevention, the crowns of the teeth can be destroyed to the gumline; abscesses can develop, and the child can experience severe pain and discomfort.

What is the Best Prevention?

When oral bacteria are fed liquid sugar for a prolonged period of time, the resulting acid can be very damaging to tooth structure. Similarly, when oral bacteria are fed little bits of sugared liquid, nonstop, over a day's time, the results can be quite damaging to tooth structure.

We believe the best prevention for this type of problem begins with an understanding of the decay process, and how you can stop it before it even starts. We recommend that you bring your children to the dentist when they are in the infant stage so that we can perform an infant oral examination and discuss with the child's oral self-care, including:

- Children should not be put to sleep with a sugared liquid in a bottle. No milk. No juice. No soda. Plain water only.
- Children, including infants, require daily oral cleansing. If no teeth are present, the gums should be gently wiped with a wet cloth.
- When teeth are present they should be brushed with fluoridated toothpaste, but only with a *very small amount*—about the size of a pea, or less.
- Liquid sugars and other easily fermentable carbohydrates such as white bread, cakes, cookies, or crackers should be given with meals and not as "snacks."
- The proper level of systemic fluoride should be in place by the time your child is 6 months of age. We will discuss with you the fluoride regimen specific to your location and the age of your children.

If you have any questions about early childhood caries, please feel free to ask us.

Eruption Patterns of Teeth

Teeth begin forming in children very early in life, as early as the first month of the second trimester of pregnancy. That is why it is so important for pregnant women to follow a proper diet. It is not only to have a healthy baby but also to ensure the proper formation of the teeth. When the hard tissue (the future enamel) of the tooth is forming, minerals and nutrients are taken up by the teeth and incorporated into the structure of the enamel. Good nutrition makes the teeth stronger. Poor nutrition can interfere with proper enamel formation. Eat wisely. Consult your physician about needed vitamin supplements and before taking any medications.

This reference will help you know when baby teeth, also called *deciduous teeth*, are due to come in and eventually fall out, as the permanent teeth come in. Girls' teeth usually come in before boys' teeth. There is a 6 to 8 month leeway that is considered a normal variation on either side of the age the teeth come into the mouth. Some children might get teeth even earlier or later than that. It depends on their growth patterns. We hope to see teeth come in later, rather than earlier. If the teeth come in later, there is a good chance the mouth will be bigger so the teeth have the necessary room to come in straight. The older a child is when he gets a tooth, the more hand skill he will have for brushing and flossing the tooth to keep it clean and disease-free.

The normal child dentition will have 20 baby teeth. Adults typically have 32 teeth, although there is evidence that many adults do not have tooth buds for the 4 wisdom teeth.

Primary Teeth

Primary teeth start forming at 4 to 6 months in utero, the second trimester of pregnancy. After the baby is born, the teeth continue to grow and erupt into the mouth.

lower central incisors	6 months
lower lateral incisors	7 months
upper central incisors	7.5 months
upper lateral incisors	9 months
lower canines and eyeteeth	16 months
lower second molars	20 months
upper second molars	24 months

Permanent Teeth

The enamel of the permanent teeth actually begins forming at 3 to 4 months of age. If your water is not fluoridated, make sure your baby receives the necessary fluoride supplements. Permanent teeth come in under the baby teeth. Pressure from the upward movement of the permanent tooth causes a resorption of the root of the baby tooth. When the root disappears, the tooth gets loose and eventually falls out. If the permanent tooth does not come in directly under the baby tooth, the baby tooth root will not resorb and not loosen. The second tooth will come in either in front of or behind the baby tooth. This is common. When it happens, see the dentist to determine whether the baby tooth should be removed to permit the proper positioning of the permanent tooth.

lower central incisors	6-7 years
lower first molar	6-7 years
upper first molar	6-7 years
upper central incisors	7-8 years
lower lateral incisors	7-8 years
upper lateral incisors	8-9 years
lower canines	9-10 years
upper first premolars	10-11 years
lower first premolars	10-12 years
upper canines	11-12 years
lower second premolars	11-12 years
lower second molar	11-13 years
upper second molar	12-13 years
wisdom teeth	17-22 years

Be sure to remember the sealants for the molars and premolars!

If you have any questions about the formation of teeth, please feel free to ask us.

Prevention of Dental Disease in Infants and Children

There are a number of positive steps that you can take to ensure that your child has few, if any, cavities and dental-related problems. A daily routine of proper and effective oral self-care (toothbrushing and dental flossing) is the most important part of prevention. Scheduled visits with the dentist and dental hygienist for examinations and prophylaxis (cleaning) procedures are also very important for your child's dental well-being. These suggestions will help keep your child's teeth and gums disease-free.

1. Clean your infant's teeth daily with a wet washcloth or a wet two-inch-square gauze pad.

2. Floss your child's teeth daily until the child can develop the ability to do it alone. This may not be an easy transition, but it is well worth the effort.

3. Once the teeth can be seen breaking through the gum tissue, night bottles should contain only water. Fluids from night bottles pool behind the teeth while the infant sleeps. Night bottles containing milk, juice, punch, soda, etc. can cause **extensive** decay.

4. If you do not live in an area with fluoridated water, the infant should be given a fluoride vitamin supplement. Dosage will depend on the age and weight of the infant. This should continue until the child develops wisdom teeth—well into the teen years. Your pediatrician or your dentist can write a prescription for these very important systemic fluoride vitamins.

5. Children do not develop the dexterity to properly brush and floss their own teeth until about age 6 or 7. You must make sure that the job is done well, even if it means doing this oral self-care for them. Your own good example of brushing and flossing your teeth daily will greatly enhance your child's willingness and abilities in this area.

6. Your child's first visit to the dentist should be as an infant, as teeth are just beginning to erupt. During this visit we will give you guidelines as to what you can expect in terms of oral development and what type of nutrition and oral self-care tips are appropriate for your child.

7. Your child's first treatment visit to the dentist should take place at 2½ years of age. An examination, cleaning, and fluoride treatment will be completed at this time.

8. The topical fluoride treatment given at the time of the child's regular cleaning appointment is important. It helps make the teeth that are already in the mouth stronger and more resistant to decay and plaque accumulation. Systemic fluoride vitamins strengthen the enamel of unerupted teeth. Topical fluoride takes over after that.

9. A plastic coating known as a *sealant* can be placed on the chewing surfaces of the back teeth. This sealant can reduce the incidence of decay on the treated surfaces by 90%. It should be placed on most back teeth, both premolars and molars, as soon as it is possible to keep these teeth dry enough for bonding the sealant in place. It is sometimes placed on baby teeth in special situations. A separate handout is available that will cover this topic in more detail. Sealants are usually applied when children are about 6 years old. The dentist or hygienist will advise you as to when he or she believes the sealant can be successfully placed.

10. When your child can understand and perform the "rinse and spit" routine, it is time to begin using a fluoridated mouthrinse. This is not a mouthwash used to cover bad breath. It is actually a nightly supplement to the topical fluoride treatments your child receives at the dentist's office. However, it is not nearly as strong as the office version. This is not a prescription medication.

By faithfully following these suggestions, your child may never develop any decay. If decay should begin, it will be small and easy to treat. Nothing replaces thorough daily brushing and flossing or good eating habits. Routine dental examination and cleaning appointments are vital. You will find that following these instructions will prove to be very effective in helping your child to maintain optimal dental health.

If you have any questions about dental disease prevention, please feel free to ask us.

Sealants

Why Sealants?

Decay on back teeth, premolars, and molars usually begins in the grooves and fissures that normally exist on the biting surfaces of the back teeth. Dental sealants, available since the 1960s, are clear plastic coatings that can be placed on the biting and grinding surfaces of posterior teeth. These sealants prevent the formation of decay on the treated surfaces. Sealants can even be placed on teeth with small areas of decay known as *incipient carious lesions*. The sealants will stop the customary progress of tooth destruction. It can remain on the tooth from 3 to more than 20 years, depending on the tooth, type of sealant used, and the eating habits of the patient. It can only be placed on teeth that have not been previously restored.

The sealant is placed on the tooth through a chemical/mechanical bonding procedure. There is no drilling or local anesthesia required for the sealant application procedure. It is entirely painless.

We, at this office, are dedicated to the prevention of oral disease. It is clear that if the initial decay is prevented from beginning or is small enough to use a sealant, there is a great savings in time, money, discomfort, and tooth structure. Decayed teeth must have the decay removed by drilling, then they must be filled. This drill and fill may have to be done several times over the patient's lifetime as the filling ages and needs replacement. We strongly suggest that patients who have teeth that can be successfully protected with a sealant material consider having this procedure performed as soon as possible.

Sealants and Prevention

We especially advise that children have the sealant applied to their teeth as soon as the teeth break through the gum and the biting surfaces of the teeth are no longer covered with gum tissue. If the teeth cannot be totally isolated from the moisture in the mouth during the bonding process, it is likely that the sealant will not remain on the tooth for as long a period of time as expected. The sealant is most often applied to permanent teeth, but sometimes a situation arises in which it would be beneficial to have the sealant applied to a primary tooth.

A study completed in 1991 found that one application of sealant reduced biting surface decay 52% over a 15-year period. Another study, completed in 1990, showed that decay on biting surfaces could be reduced 95% over 10 years if 2% to 4% of the sealants were routinely repaired each year. We expect sealants to last many years. Replacing or repairing sealants, as needed, on an ongoing basis will give the best protection.

A sealant is not meant as a substitute for proper brushing and flossing habits. The effectiveness of the sealant is reduced if oral self-care is neglected. Also, cavities can still form on untreated surfaces. Therefore, a topical fluoride treatment remains an essential and necessary preventive aid.

In both 1984 and 1994 sealants have been recommended by the U.S. Public Health Service and the Surgeon General of the United States, among others. We know that sealants are one of the most important treatments available for prevention of dental decay.

If you have any questions about sealants, please feel free to ask us.

Sealant Warranty

Patient Name:_____   **Date:**_____

We believe that sealants are one of the most important preventive dental procedures you can have. This is true for children and adults. Cavities can start in almost anyone at almost any age.

Placement of a sealant does not require drilling. The cost of a sealant is less than half the cost of a tooth that needs to be prepared and have a restoration placed. When the sealant is placed by this office and you follow a few simple and beneficial instructions, we guarantee that if the sealant ever needs to be replaced, we will (as long as Dr._____ is in active dental practice) replace the sealant at no additional charge to you or your insurance carrier. The reason we do this is to give you a further incentive to have the sealant placed.

This warranty will be in force as long as you live in the area and visit this office at the recommended intervals for a periodic examination and prophylaxis (teeth cleaning). For most patients this interval is every 6 months.

Tooth #(s) sealed:_____

Date sealant placed:_____

Material used:_____

Placed by:_____

_____

(Dentist's name, credentials)

If you have any questions about the sealant warranty, please feel free to ask us.

Supplemental Fluoride

There are two methods by which you or your child can receive fluoride. The most common method is a topical application. This includes fluoride contained in mouthrinses, toothpastes, and professionally applied fluoride treatments (tray delivery) in the dental office. Each of these fluoride-containing items is meant to work on the exposed, superficial, developed enamel of the tooth that is already in place in the mouth. The fluoride makes the enamel harder and provides the building blocks for remineralization. Fluoride can also inhibit the growth of bacteria. In topical oral self-care products, the fluoride concentration is low, but the repeated and daily application of the fluoride can help ensure that your teeth have fewer cavities. This type of fluoride is not meant to be swallowed.

Before teeth can be seen, while they are still developing under the gums, the teeth can also be made stronger and more resistant to decay with the use of fluoride. Systemic fluorides are dispensed by prescription and are swallowed. They make developing teeth stronger. We strongly recommend that your children receive the benefits of this proven decay fighter.

The dosage for systemic fluoride recommended by the American Dental Association (ADA) was lowered in May of 1994. The use of fluoride vitamins (systemic), in conjunction with young patients swallowing fluoride toothpastes and mouthrinses, proved to be too much of a good thing. Many dentists had noticed a higher incidence of small white spots forming on front teeth. While not a dental problem, these white spots could be unsightly. Although the white spots are often easily removed, the rationale for the dosage change is to reduce their incidence of formation.

The new recommendations are as follows:

Fluoride Concentration in Drinking Water (parts per million [ppm])			
Age	Less than 0.3 ppm	0.3-0.6 ppm	More than 6 ppm
6 mos. - 3 yrs.	0.25 mg	0	0
3 yrs. - 6 yrs.	0.50 mg	0.25 mg	0
6 yrs. - 16 yrs.	1.0 mg	0.50 mg	0

If your children fall into the above age groups, **and if you are not on a fluoridated water supply,** they should be taking supplemental fluoride. Systemic fluoride makes the enamel stronger and better able to resist acid attack from bacteria and less susceptible to decay. It is one of the most important preventive actions you can take for your children. In our opinion, even one cavity is too many. The best way to preserve teeth is to keep them undrilled and unfilled. This requires serious preventive measures: brushing, flossing, good diet, and fluoride supplements.

If you have any questions about supplemental fluoride, please feel free to ask us.

Topical Fluoride: At Home and in the Dental Office

Why Topical Fluoride?

Most of us are familiar with the dental advantages of fluoride supplements systemically administered to children while their teeth are forming. Research on this type of fluoride treatment shows a 35% reduction in tooth decay. The use of fluoride to reduce and eliminate decay is one of the most highly studied and documented public health measures yet. In our office, we recommend a 4-minute tray-type fluoride treatment at least twice a year, usually after a periodic dental hygiene recare appointment. We have found that this type of preventive aid does four things:

- Reduces the solubility of enamel to acid attack, making the teeth more resistant to decay.
- Aids in remineralizing the tooth enamel where decay has just begun.
- With long-term daily use, reduces tooth sensitivity to temperature changes.
- Reduces the surface tension of the enamel so that plaque does not easily adhere to the tooth.

Recent research has also shown that you can benefit from nonprescription topical fluoride rinses, especially if you use them faithfully every day. You can expect an additional reduction in decay when we also apply a topical fluoride in the office. It is applied four times each year. Decay reduction can be as high as 30%! If you have had recent active decay, no matter what your age, we will recommend this fluoride routine for you.

Special Fluoride Applications

Another option for topical fluoride is available to patients who experience tooth or root sensitivity, higher and/or chronic decay levels, root surface decay, or dry mouth syndrome (xerostomia). If you have been diagnosed with any of these dental problems, we will make custom fluoride trays for you. We will then either prescribe or dispense a high-concentration fluoride gel product for you to use nightly in the tray.

The instructions are simple. Dry your teeth as much as possible, either with a gauze square or washcloth or by sucking air through your teeth. The fluoride will work better if the teeth are not quite so wet. Since trays fit closely to the teeth, place only a small amount of fluoride gel into the tray every few teeth, and then place the trays into your mouth. Spit out the excess. If you notice a lot of extra fluoride after the treatment is completed, simply cut down on the amount you place in the tray. Leave in place _____ minutes. Then take the trays out. Spit out the saliva and fluoride that remains. **Do not eat or drink for __minutes.**

The number of weeks that you will need to do this fluoride tray procedure depends on your specific condition. If you have diminished salivary flow with increased decay or the possibility of increased decay, you will need to follow this fluoride routine until saliva flow returns to normal. In the case of sensitive roots or teeth, you will need to follow this routine until the sensitivity is reduced. *Note:* Sensitivity reduction is usually a gradual process: do not expect overnight improvement. Root desensitization may also need other materials placed over the area as an adjunct procedure.

If you have any questions about the use of topical fluorides at home or in the dental office, please feel free to ask us.

chapter 10

Periodontics

Content at a Glance 212–213

Content at a Glance: Periodontics

Evaluation and Diseases
Classification of Periodontal Disease
Use to inform the patient of his or her type of periodontal disease using descriptions from the American Academy of Periodontology.

Early Signs of Periodontal Disease
Describes to the patient how to recognize the changes in tissue that signify periodontal disease and how the office routinely screens for these early signs.

Furcation Involvement
A description of the furcation, bone loss, and the implications in periodontal disease.

Gingival Hyperplasia
Discusses how gingival hyperplasia occurs, treatment options, and prevention.

Gingivitis
Provides information on the characteristics, consequences, and treatment of gingivitis.

Insufficient Attached Gingiva
Defines insufficient attached gingiva and the oral problems that can result.

Necrotizing Periodontal Disease
Explains what ulcerative gingivitis is, how it develops, and the professional and self-care steps in treatment.

Periodontal Disease
Gives an overview of periodontal disease, etiology, progression, and prevention.

Periodontal Disease and Systemic Health
Stresses the aspect of gum disease as an infection and the correlation to systemic health.

Periodontal Treatment Recommendations: Initial Therapy
Lists the classification of the patient's periodontal disease, number of expected office visits, procedures and fees involved, with checkboxes.

Pocket Depth Measurement
Describes the periodontal charting method and how the numbers relate to levels of oral health.

Smoking and Adult Periodontitis
Emphasis on the link between smoking and the occurrence of periodontal disease.

Treatment Options
Cosmetic Elective Periodontal Plastic Surgery: Tissue Recontouring
Advises how periodontal surgery can improve the appearance of teeth and gum architecture and possible treatment avenues.

Electrosurgery
Describes electrosurgery procedures and their use in dentistry.

Flap Procedures
Indications and procedures for the periodontal flap surgical procedure are discussed.

Gingival Grafts
A description of conditions requiring a gingival graft and a review of the procedure.

Gingivectomy and Gingivoplasty Procedures
Indications and treatment are explained for these two procedures.

Content at a Glance: Periodontics—cont'd

Gross Debridement
Explains what gross debridement is and what will happen both during and after the procedure.

Osseous Surgery
Discusses the indications and procedures associated with periodontal osseous surgery.

Periodontal Surgery
Gives patients a general understanding of periodontal surgery and the probable results.

Prophylaxis
An explanation of the importance of the dental prophylaxis visit and the factors used to determine the recommended intervals.

Ridge Augmentation
Explains indications and possible treatment options for ridge augmentation.

Root Hemisections and Root Amputations
Reasons and procedures for root hemisections and amputations are explained.

Scaling and Root Planing
The purpose and procedures involved in scaling and root planing are discussed.

Scaling and Root Planing: Postprocedure Instructions
A checklist to customize posttreatment instructions for the patient.

Scaling and Root Planing: Reevaluation
The purpose and importance of reevaluation after scaling and root planing are discussed.

Soft Tissue Management
Information on initial periodontal therapy: why it is necessary, what is involved, and what can be done to prevent the need for it in the future.

Splinting Teeth
Information on the need for and procedures involved in the splinting of teeth.

Chemotherapeutics
Chlorhexidine Gluconate Oral Rinse 0.12%
An overview of the prescription rinse, chlorhexidine gluconate, and its uses and precautions.

Oral Rinse Protocol
Instructions for an adjunct rinse protocol procedure for patients who decline conventional periodontal surgery.

Periostat: Systemic Submicrobial Dose of Doxycycline
Review of systemic submicrobial dose of doxycycline as an adjunct to scaling and root planing.

Site-Specific Antibiotic Therapy
Describes the use of site-specific antibiotic therapy, the procedures involved, and the types of products available for this therapy.

Subgingival Irrigation
Introduces subgingival irrigation as a modality used with various other procedures.

Classification of Periodontal Disease

Any periodontal disease is undesirable and, if left untreated or ignored, can lead to a number of serious dental problems. If you wish to maintain your teeth and gums (gingiva) in a healthy and disease-free state, it is important that you brush properly and use dental floss daily. Do these procedures as we have instructed. Return for continuing dental hygiene care at the time intervals that we have recommended. These time intervals for your cleaning appointments have been established specifically for your existing dental condition. The intervals can and will fluctuate according to your ability to take care of your teeth and gums. A periodontal infection is site-specific and episodic in its nature. Any delay in your office-related routine dental hygiene recare appointments could prove detrimental to your oral health.

The following is a brief overview of the American Academy of Periodontology's classification of the types of periodontal disease.

Type I.
   Gingival Diseases: An inflammation or lesion of the gum characterized by changes of color, gingival form, position, surface appearance, and presence of bleeding and/or pus.

Type II.
   Chronic Periodontitis: An inflammation of the supporting structures of the teeth associated with plaque and calculus; the rate of progression is affected by local, systemic, or environmental factors. It can be further classified as localized or generalized.

Type III.
   Aggressive Periodontitis: Characterized by a rapid rate of periodontal disease progression in an otherwise healthy individual in the absence of large accumulations of plaque and/or calculus. It can be further classified as localized or generalized.

Type IV.
   Periodontitis as a Manifestation of Systemic Disease: Periodontitis associated with blood or genetic disorders.

Type V.
   Necrotizing Periodontal Disease: Ulcerated and necrotic gums between the teeth and at the tooth margins. It can be further classified as necrotizing ulcerative gingivitis or necrotizing ulcerative periodontitis.

Type VI.
   Abscesses of the Periodontium: A localized pus-forming infection of the periodontal tissue.

Type VII.
   Periodontitis Associated with Endodontic Lesions: Localized deep periodontal pocket extending to the tip of the root of the tooth involving pulp death.

Type VIII.
   Developmental or Acquired Deformities and Conditions: Gingival disease or periodontitis started by localized tooth-related factors that modify or predispose to plaque accumulation or prevention of effective oral hygiene measures.

Due to the nature of the disease, most classifications will involve both a generalized and a localized diagnosis.

If you have any questions about the classification of your periodontal disease, please feel free to ask us.

Early Signs of Periodontal Disease

The early warning signs of every disease occur at a microscopic level. The early warning signs cannot be seen, felt, touched, diagnosed, or discovered. They cannot be noted by their symptoms. The early changes might be able to be detected by sophisticated chemical or biologic analysis, but not by normal diagnostic measures.

By the time you notice that your gums are bleeding (gingivitis), the disease has already been present for some time and it is not in its earliest stage. It is not unusual to hear, "My gums have always bled like this," but treatment is not sought. Yet if our eyes started to bleed when we washed our faces, we would generally rush to seek medical treatment! Bleeding gums are not normal and healthy. Luckily, at this stage the periodontal disease is fairly easy to treat and is reversible. When the disease has progressed past the bleeding gum stage, you may notice some pain, gum recession, loosening of teeth, and bad breath. If you have ignored your bleeding gums (possibly the earliest sign of gum disease) because you think it is normal to have a little "pink" on your toothbrush, you will likely have additional symptoms and conditions associated with disease progression. At this point the bone and gum support for the teeth may be permanently altered and diminished.

It is recommended that you adhere to the suggested time intervals for your dental cleaning appointments. We will examine your gums during your periodic dental cleaning appointments for early signs of periodontal disease. While we clean your teeth, we will note areas where it is difficult for you to remove plaque or where calculus forms and areas of gum tissue inflammation and will record probing depths, which will measure your gum tissue for signs of periodontal disease. We can then demonstrate effective oral self-care to prevent these areas from progressing into periodontal disease.

We want to stress prevention. Don't wait for the warning signs of gum disease to occur before you schedule your dental hygiene appointment. If you have very few fillings, have not lost any permanent teeth (other than wisdom teeth), and have very thorough oral self-care daily, a yearly cleaning and exam by the dental hygienist and dentist may be adequate. If you have had a great deal of dental work performed (bridges, crowns, fillings) or if you have missing teeth that have not been replaced and you don't spend time with adequate oral self-care, visiting the dental office three or four times a year might be necessary. We will let you know what is appropriate for your individual oral condition.

Furcation Involvement

The roots of the teeth are covered and surrounded by bone and gum tissues when they are in their normal state and have been disease-free. Only the crown portion is visible. Some teeth toward the back portion of your mouth have two or three roots extending into the jaw bone from the crowns of the tooth. This "V-shaped" area where the tooth branches or forks into two or three roots is called the *furcation* or *furca*. The furca is also covered with bone and is attached to the tooth by periodontal ligament fibers.

As long as the furcation of a multirooted tooth is covered with the normal amount of bone and gum, everything is fine and the furca holds no exceptional interest for the dentist or dental hygienist. When there is an alteration in the density of the furca bone, or it actually starts to resorb (disappear due to some type of dental pathology), the furca area becomes important and interesting. Continued loss of bone would lead to loss of the tooth.

The loss of the bone in the furca area could be related to periodontal disease (gum disease). The periodontal pathology in the furca could be part of a localized problem—only present at that one site—or a sign that there is a more widespread problem that needs attention. The breakdown of bone in the furcation could also indicate that the nerve inside the tooth is dying, and the tooth will need a root canal (endodontic treatment).

If the breakdown is specific to the site on that one tooth, treatment would be localized. The type of therapy recommended would depend on the severity of the breakdown. Minimal disease might be treated by a dental prophylaxis (cleaning) and reinforcement of personal oral self-care. Treatment of a more extensive breakdown could involve aggressive periodontal procedures including but not limited to periodontal surgery and bone augmentation. You may be referred to a periodontist for these procedures.

If the furca breakdown is a sign of more widespread periodontal disease, the whole mouth will be evaluated and specific treatment recommendations will be made.

There are many very small nerves that exit through various portions of the tooth, and a localized furcation problem could indicate that the nerve in a tooth is dead or dying and the tooth may require a root canal.

You may think that teeth are difficult to floss and brush when tooth alignment and gum position are ideal. When there is bone loss in a furca, daily oral self-care becomes more complicated. A furca is a difficult area to clean—the more bone loss, the more difficult. In extreme cases, there is no bone or gum left in the furca, and a patient could actually place an interdental cleaning aid completely between the roots of a two-rooted tooth. For a three-rooted tooth with a furcation involvement, the cleaning process is even more of a problem.

You have been diagnosed with a furcation involvement problem. After careful examination, a treatment recommendation will be made. Our recommendation will be based on not only treating your furcation problem but also preventing further exposure of the furcation area.

If you have any questions about a furcation involvement, please feel free to ask us.

Gingival Hyperplasia

Predisposing Factors

Gingival hyperplasia is an increase in the size of the gum tissues caused by an increase in the number and normal arrangement of the cells. It is characterized by inflammation of the soft tissues surrounding the teeth. The gum tissues will appear shiny and swollen and dark red to bluish purple in color. The predisposing factors in this inflammation can include but are not limited to systemic factors (diabetes mellitus), antiepileptic medications (such as Dilantin®, Mysoline®, and Depakene®), immunosuppressant drugs (cyclosporine), calcium channel blockers (Procardia®, Calan®, Cardizem®, and Bayotensin®), select other medications, hormonal changes associated with pregnancy, oral contraceptives, or the types of hormonal changes younger teenagers experience during puberty. We commonly see hyperplasia associated with pregnancy, oral contraception, and puberty.

These conditions **do not** necessarily cause the gums to become inflamed or enlarged, but rather in the presence of only slight amounts of plaque and/or calculus, the response of the gum tissues can be out of the ordinary. Hyperplasic gingivitis can also occur just because of a large presence of bacterial plaque without any of these factors being present.

Indications

If you have any of these predisposing factors or take certain drugs, there is a potential for gingival hyperplasia. Unfortunately, gum disease does not hurt until it is too late. If you have gingival hyperplasia, and if you are lucky, you will probably notice that your gums bleed when you brush and floss. Bleeding is always a sign of disease or infection.

Elimination and/or Prevention

To eliminate or prevent these problems, your oral self-care must be thorough. You must brush and floss and do whatever other oral self-care procedures you have been instructed to do every day. This may clear up the problem entirely. If not, you will need to adjust the interval between recare appointments with the dental hygienist. A time frame of 2, 3, or 4 months between cleanings, depending on the severity of the problem, will be more appropriate for prevention of hyperplasia. This will be necessary for as long as the predisposing factors exist. If medication is the factor, you will have to see the hygienist at the interval recommended.

If you are pregnant, gingival hyperplasia could persist until the hormonal changes associated with pregnancy revert back to normal. Until then, you need to schedule your oral recare appointments with the dental hygienist as recommended. Similarly, if you take oral contraceptives and notice signs of recurring gum infections (bleeding when brushing and flossing), assuming that your oral self-care is thorough, a more regular recare schedule may be necessary.

Gingival hyperplasia in young teens is generally seen where oral self-care in not adequate. A 3-month interval is best in this circumstance. Some teenagers have inadequate oral self-care habits. Junk food and sugary drinks (even juice) coupled with almost nonexistent brushing and flossing cause serious gum disease, bad breath, and decay. Generally, the hormonal change stabilizes and the acute problem resolves. For this age group, social issues of wanting to be more attractive many times will influence oral self-care habits when all the dental attention in the world cannot!

These recommendations are designed to prevent gum problems. Prevention is better and much less expensive than any cure. If you have dental insurance, it will probably **not** cover the additional necessary dental treatment. While you do need them to maintain your oral health, these situations are considered unusual by the carrier and are not generally covered procedures.

If you have any questions about gingival hyperplasia, please feel free to ask us.

Gingivitis

Almost everyone knows what a cavity is. Because of the far-reaching effects of advertising by toothpaste and oral rinse manufacturers, by 2004 almost everyone has heard of **gingivitis**. What may not be quite clear to you, however, is exactly what gingivitis is. You may recognize it as a problem but not know why and how serious it might be. You may even know that it is a type of gum (periodontal) disease. You may also know that it is somehow related to plaque and tartar (calculus) on teeth. But why should you be concerned about having it?

Gingivitis is an infection of the gum tissues surrounding the teeth. It is a very common infection and affects almost 95% of the world's population. This infection can be characterized by redness, swelling, and bleeding of the gums around the teeth. This gum infection absolutely needs to be treated as soon as possible. Gum infections are almost always preventable with sound daily oral self-care.

Gingivitis is the mildest form of periodontal disease and is reversible. By definition, there is no loss of bone that supports the tooth. If treated early, gingivitis can be eliminated. If left untreated, it can progress into the more serious form of periodontal disease called *periodontitis*. In its more serious form, the bone and gum tissues can be permanently affected. Bleeding gums, one of the signs of gingivitis, are a sign of infection in the mouth. Your gum tissues should never bleed. It is not normal for blood to appear on your toothbrush when you have finished brushing. Gingivitis does not generally hurt, so you may not even know that you have it. It can be localized (around a few teeth) or generalized (around most or all of the teeth). Gingivitis is seen most often in patients who do not brush and floss well daily, but it can also be related to medication. Bad breath can be another sign of gingivitis. If you are using a mouthwash to get rid of bad breath, you may need dental attention. While bad breath can be related to some medical problems, most often it is just debris that is not cleaned properly from your teeth, gums, and tongue that is decomposing in the dark, warm, and moist environment of your mouth—a perfect place to breed germs.

If you have bleeding gums, you should be concerned. Healthy tissue anywhere in our bodies does not bleed. So what can you do to stop the bleeding?

We can help you eliminate the gingivitis. It involves a good professional cleaning and good oral self-care habits. Plaque (soft debris made up of bacteria) and tartar (calculus or hardened debris) must be removed before the gum tissues can heal and the infection can be eliminated. If it has been some time since you had your teeth cleaned properly, it may take more than one appointment to get you back into shape.

Get your teeth and gums cleaned on a regular basis. Keep them clean with daily brushing and flossing. The infection you have will be eliminated. If you keep your teeth and gums clean, they can be healthy and trouble-free for your whole life.

If you have any questions about gingivitis, please feel free to ask us.

Insufficient Attached Gingiva

If you were to view a cross-section of the tooth and jaw, you would see, from the tip of the tooth toward the gingiva (gum), the following: the enamel-covered portion of the tooth getting wider, then constricting as it approaches the gingival area; the margin of the gingival tissue (which just abuts the tooth); the gingival tissue that is firmly bound down to the underlying bone and cannot be moved, perhaps with a pebbly appearance; and smoother looking gingival tissue, which is very movable and not tightly bound down to the underlying bone. The last area may be redder in color than the other described gingival tissue and leads to the cheeks and lips.

The focus of this topic is on the zone of attached gingiva. As part of your periodontal exam, we use a periodontal probe to measure and record the depth of the sulcus. The sulcular depth is the depth of the space between the marginal gingiva and the tooth. The periodontal probe used to measure this sulcus is gently inserted into the margin of the gingiva and placed into the sulcus until it is stopped by the gingival tissue, which is more tightly bound to the bone. This measurement helps to determine your periodontal health. Hopefully, the sulcular depths measured were 3 millimeters or less. This tightly attached zone of gingival tissue surrounding the tooth is quite important.

This zone of attached gingiva needs to be intact and of adequate width to protect (by separating) the tissue around the tooth. If it is not sufficient, improper (too hard) brushing or a muscle attachment that is not in a proper position can pull on the attached gingival tissue. If it pulls enough, the 1-3 millimeter normal depth can increase to 4 millimeters, or even 6 millimeters or more. This will not be a stable or healthy change in your periodontal health. The normal gingival margin (gumline) is scalloped (like small, regular waves). If there is insufficient attached gingiva, the scalloping will be altered, and the gingiva will turn red and bleed easily. The pulled area will be more prone to trapping bacterial plaque and food debris, will be harder to clean, and will always be more inflamed and infected. If you have this problem, you might have even seen this yourself. It can lead to early tooth loss. Insufficient attached gingiva is not good and needs to be corrected.

Once diagnosed, the correction is relatively easy. It will require minor periodontal surgery. Usually, a periodontist (gum specialist) will be asked to perform this procedure. You will receive a local anesthetic to numb the area, and the problem tissue area will be reshaped and formed to give back the correct width of attached gingival tissue.

While this is a relatively common problem, patients do not commonly recognize it. If you have it diagnosed, get it fixed as soon as possible. You will save yourself from many future problems.

If you have any questions about insufficient attached gingiva, please feel free to ask us.

Necrotizing Periodontal Disease

Necrotizing periodontal disease is an acute inflammatory destructive disease of the gum tissues. Other names that have been used to describe this disease process are *trench mouth*, *Vincent's disease* or *infection*, *necrotizing ulcerating gingivitis*, and *necrotizing ulcerating periodontitis*.

Symptoms
Necrotizing periodontal disease can occur at any age. However, it is usually seen in young people between the ages of 15 and 30. Often, it is seen in high school or college students under stress, studying for examinations. Poor dietary habits and lowered resistance to infection are significant predisposing factors. Signs of necrotizing periodontal disease may include:
- sudden onset
- pain and soreness to the extent that normal chewing is difficult
- bleeding is spontaneous on even the slightest of pressure
- metallic or unpleasant taste
- slight fever
- swollen lymph glands

Causes
Necrotizing periodontal disease is an infectious disease caused by a specific complex of microbes that develop and increase once the body's defenses have been lowered. Major predisposing factors are smoking, stress, very poor oral self-care, and poor nutrition.

Treatment
Treatment for necrotizing periodontal disease involves both our dental team and you. Treatment consists of careful evaluation of your personal habits: what you eat and how you care for your mouth. We will remove the accumulated dead bacterial cells and decomposing food from those infected areas and instruct you in oral self-care habits that will help get rid of the disease and prevent its return. Your job is to make certain that you follow these instructions:

1. **Carefully follow all oral self-care tips**. Do not allow anyone to use your toothbrush. Use only the softest toothbrush possible to gently but thoroughly clean your teeth. Allow your brush to dry between uses.
2. **Follow through with all your appointments**. Because you are no longer in severe pain does not mean the infection is gone. The underlying periodontal infection can recur if it is not completely treated.
3. **A warm salt water rinse** every hour is advised while the acute symptoms exist.
4. **Avoid using tobacco** products in any form.
5. **Balance your diet** with whole grains, green vegetables, proteins, and fruits. Avoid highly seasoned food and alcoholic beverages. We may prescribe a vitamin for you during this time as well.
6. **Get adequate rest**. The body will heal much faster when it has been adequately rested.
7. If you have been prescribed any rinse or medication, be sure to use it following the instructions carefully.

Necrotizing periodontal disease can be a serious medical condition that will need to be closely monitored. Because necrotizing periodontal disease can recur, it is essential that we have your full cooperation and understanding of the treatment before we start.

If you have any questions about necrotizing periodontal disease, please feel free to ask us.

Periodontal Disease

Periodontal disease is an infectious process classified according to how much damage has been done to the structures surrounding the teeth, namely the gingiva (gums) and bone. **It is an infection in your mouth.** It can happen anytime, around any teeth, affecting some or many of your teeth to varying degrees. There are genetic predisposing factors to periodontal disease, and our immune systems play a role in gum health, but it is usually related to how well you are able to keep your teeth clean through proper oral self-care. The better you clean your teeth to remove all the plaque bacteria, the less likely you will be to develop periodontal disease.

Progress of the Disease
The bacteria that cause this disease first cause the gum tissue to become inflamed and pull away from the teeth. As the problem becomes more serious, the bone that supports the teeth also becomes infected and begins to break down and dissolve. The teeth then become loose. Once the bone disappears, it is extremely hard, if not impossible, for new bone to be rebuilt. The damage is permanent and your teeth, the surrounding bone, and your general health will be compromised.

Periodontal disease is classified into several types. You will be given a separate handout with the appropriate description of the severity of your infection.

The mildest form of this infection will show up in red and swollen gum tissue that bleeds easily. There is seldom any pain involved at this stage. You may notice also that your breath becomes offensive and you feel the need to use mouthwash. Our sense of smell does become immune to the same odors, so we can lose our ability to detect our own offensive, diseased breath. As the disease progresses, the gum tissue becomes more red and swollen, more bleeding can be seen, and the teeth begin to become loose. This tooth mobility is a sign that there is a severe problem. There may still be no pain at this advanced stage. As more and more bone is lost and more teeth become involved in the infection, it becomes harder to treat. At this point, many times, the management of your problem will involve periodontal surgical procedures. If this is the case, you may be referred to a periodontist (gum specialist) for further treatment. Most of the time, periodontal disease starts and continues because of neglect. Brushing and flossing of teeth are not being done effectively on a daily basis. You may have been neglectful in getting your teeth checked and cleaned within the time frame intervals you need. Once we have diagnosed this disease, we will inform you of the problem and suggest treatment. If treatment is not completed, however, the disease will continue to progress. Unfortunately, the disease is quite invisible to most people until severe and possibly irreversible damage has occurred.

Solution
If it has been diagnosed in the early stages and has not progressed to bone loss, a proper cleaning (prophylaxis) will solve the problem. Scaling and root planing over multiple appointments may be needed for more advanced cases. In the most advanced cases, periodontal surgery and tooth loss are inevitable. You will receive an estimate of fees for the recommended treatment.

Periodontal disease is a condition that must be treated quickly. We believe that if the infection is aggressively treated in its early stages, conservative periodontal treatment may be possible and effective. Although we do not automatically rule out periodontal surgical intervention, we hope you can either avoid it or reduce the amount you will need.

Successful treatment of your periodontal problem will depend on several factors. But the most important of these is your ability to perform excellent oral self-care—brushing, flossing, and use of periodontal aids—on a routine, daily basis. Without this, periodontal treatment will fail, and the disease will return.

If you have any questions about periodontal disease, please feel free to ask us.

Periodontal Disease and Systemic Health

Research clearly shows that there is a strong correlation between oral (periodontal) infections and generalized (systemic) medical problems. There are over 300 different types of bacteria normally found in the human mouth, and the mouth is connected to the entire body.

A gum infection is similar to an infection that might occur elsewhere in your body. Bacteria are everywhere, including in our mouths. When the bacteria multiply past a critical number, problems begin. Why would the bacterial count change? Poor oral self-care, genetics, prescription medication, illness or systemic problems, and diminished salivary flow might contribute. When the body recognizes bacterial invaders, the immune system initiates a response to fight off the invader.

You might say, "My gums have always bled like this," and not seek treatment. Imagine seeing blood gushing from your eyes when you washed your face. You would seek immediate medical attention, perhaps even go to an emergency room!

Gum disease is an infection in your mouth, no different than an infection elsewhere in your body. The bacteria invade the soft tissues and the bone and get into the blood stream. In this way, they are then able to circulate throughout the entire body. Along with the bacteria are dead cells, metabolic by-products, toxins, food debris, and viruses.

Just as we know that smoking has an adverse affect on our health, science is examining a link between gum disease and many systemic conditions such as cardiovascular and respiratory disease, chronic obstructive pulmonary disease, premature birth and low birth weight, stroke, diabetes mellitus, and possibly rheumatoid arthritis. Although the scientific data have yet to confirm the links as diagnostic indicators, it is important for us to recognize the possible implications. The oral cavity is part of the human biology linked to all other body systems and is a portal of entry for a host of infective organisms. It only makes sense to keep it as clean as possible to reduce the risk of not only oral infection but possibly systemic inflammation as well.

Thorough oral self-care need not be difficult or time-consuming. The benefits are more than just sweet breath and a great looking smile. Spending just a few minutes a day caring for your teeth and gums and coming in for the professional hygiene visits at the intervals we advise can make the difference between whole body health and disease. After all, the jaw bones are connected to all our other bones!

Periodontal Treatment Recommendations: Initial Therapy

You have been diagnosed as having periodontal disease. This disease and infectious process is classified by its severity. The amount of destruction of the hard and soft supporting structures of the teeth is also indicated in the classification. The classification for your periodontal disease is:

Type I	**Gingival Diseases**
Type II	**Chronic Periodontitis**
Type III	**Aggressive Periodontitis**
Type IV	**Periodontitis as a Manifestation of Systemic Disease**
Type V	**Necrotizing Periodontal Disease**
Type VI	**Abscesses of the Periodontium**
Type VII	**Periodontitis Associated with Endodontic Lesions**
Type VIII	**Developmental or Acquired Deformities and Conditions**

The written explanation of your periodontal disease type has been given to you on a separate handout. You have also received a verbal explanation of your periodontal diagnosis.

Periodontal disease is an infection of the gingival (gum) tissue in your mouth. Treatment of the disease depends on the extent of the problem, the severity, and the length of time it has been present. The disease is site-specific and episodic in nature, as explained previously.

Successful treatment of your periodontal problem will depend on several factors. These factors include the position and alignment of your teeth, the loss of bone support for the teeth, the amount of plaque and calculus (tartar) present, existing restorations, broken teeth, decay, and the present state of inflammation of the periodontal tissues. Probably the most important factor in the successful treatment of your periodontal disease is your ability to perform proper oral maintenance procedures on a routine basis. These include brushing, flossing, and use of recommended periodontal cleaning aids, as instructed. This is of the utmost importance in the successful treatment of your periodontal disease and preservation of your teeth.

We recommend that for the treatment of your periodontal disease, you have the following procedures performed. We will take time to explain each procedure, including the time and fee involved, and to answer all of your questions.

If you have sustained severe and/or permanent damage to your periodontal tissue from this disease, it is possible that you may require periodontal surgery to correct any remaining periodontal problems. Final evaluation for this will be made following the initial periodontal therapy. At that time, if appropriate, we will refer you to a periodontal specialist. If you wish, all the procedures we have recommended, as well as the surgery itself, can be performed by the specialist.

The quoted fees are all inclusive and irrespective of the number of office visits and time it requires to complete the initial periodontal therapy. The number of visits needed is the probable minimum necessary.

Approximate number of office visits needed: _____

❑ **Prophylaxis**	$
❑ **Polishing**	$
❑ **Topical fluoride**	$
❑ **Scale and root plane by:**	
❑ **quadrant** ❑ **sextant** ❑ **half mouth** ❑ **full mouth** ❑ **tooth**	$
❑ **Local anesthesia needed**	$
❑ **Subgingival irrigation with a medicated solution**	$
❑ **Oral self-care instruction and evaluation**	$
❑ **Periodontal charting and reevaluation**	$
❑ **Other:** _____	$

Total initial periodontal therapy treatment fee: $

If you have any questions about periodontal treatment, please feel free to ask us.

Pocket Depth Measurement

When a dentist or physician is preparing a treatment agenda to heal a disease, test results are analyzed. Treatment decisions regarding a potential cure depend on information gathered. The more accurate the diagnostic information, the better the diagnosis and treatment. In the realm of periodontal disease, diagnosis is based in part on the collection and analysis of many numbers, specifically, measurements of the depth of the sulcus (crevice) of gum tissue that surrounds each tooth.

A periodontal charting generally consists of taking at least six measurements around every tooth. Areas of bleeding are also recorded. The evidence of bleeding is significant. Healthy gum tissue does not bleed when gently probed. There are certain factors, such as found in smokers that restrict bleeding, so lack of bleeding alone does not signify a healthy site.

These measurements (in millimeters) are one of the diagnostic tools (along with tissue color, position, and shape) a dentist and dental hygienist use to determine the severity of periodontal (gum) disease. Measurements generally range from 0 to 12 mm. Probing of the sulcus around the tooth often shows normal depths of 1 to 2 mm with greater depths in between the teeth where they touch as opposed to the direct cheek side or tongue side. The numbers will vary from position to position and tooth to tooth. They are rarely uniform throughout the entire mouth. The higher numbers indicate more severe soft and hard tissue involvement, and the greater the number of higher readings, the more likely surgical intervention is needed.

0 to 3 mm with **no bleeding:** Great numbers. No periodontal disease present.

1 to 3 mm **with bleeding:** Gingivitis (the mildest form of gum disease) present. Probably no bone loss. Usually treated with a good professional prophylaxis (cleaning) and improved oral self-care.

3 to 5 mm with **no bleeding:** May or may not have gum disease present. Smoking may be a factor in lack of bleeding. Since a patient cannot reliably clean deeper than 3 mm on a routine basis, there is high potential for gum disease to begin. Recommend professional recare visits 3 to 4 times a year.

3 to 5 mm **with bleeding:** Early to moderately advanced periodontal disease. Treatment is professional prophylaxis consisting of scaling and root planing and possibly systemic and/or site-specific antibiotics and other medications. Supporting bone may be involved. More frequent and extensive recare appointments are required. Some surgical intervention is possible.

5 to 7 mm **with bleeding:** Soft and hard tissue damage. Bone loss likely. Treatment will involve a more aggressive prophylaxis—scaling and root planing. Multiple appointments will be needed. Localized surgical intervention probable. Systemic and site-specific medications commonly used. Teeth may have started to become loose.

7 mm and above **with bleeding:** Advanced periodontal disease. Aggressive treatment required if teeth are to be saved. Surgery almost always required. Referral to periodontist is common. Systemic and site-specific medications commonly used.

In short, low numbers are good and high numbers are bad. The presence of deep periodontal pockets corresponds to more extensive gum disease and the need for more periodontal treatment.

Smoking and Adult Periodontitis

If you are a smoker, you are at a higher risk for not only lung and circulatory problems but oral disease as well. Smoking causes cell death and may be responsible for more than 50% of cases of adult periodontitis. It has been reported that more than 85% or all periodontal cases are present in people who smoke. And, more than 90% of gum infections that appear to be resistant to treatment (refractory gum disease) are found among smokers. Smokers are 2.6 to 6 times more likely to have periodontal disease. Former smokers are more likely to have periodontal disease. A person who smokes will not heal as well and does not respond as well to periodontal therapy as does a nonsmoker.

Thousands of chemicals are released during smoking, which causes a profound effect on the immune system that is responsible for helping us ward off infections. And since we now know that periodontal disease is an infection, it is easy to make the connection. Many smokers show few areas of bleeding during a periodontal charting because one of the effects of smoking is reduced circulation.

If you are reading this, you are most likely a smoker who has periodontal disease. Many smokers would like to stop this habit. Quitting is not as difficult as you may imagine. The thought of it is probably the most difficult aspect. There really are many aids today to help us to make that leap to a healthy decision about our dental and general well-being. Our office can be a great source for some suggestions to help you stop smoking. If you would like us to make suggestions for a healthier lifestyle, do not hesitate to ask!

Cosmetic Elective Periodontal Plastic Surgery: Tissue Recontouring

It is not uncommon for us to suggest to a patient who has absolutely no signs of periodontal (gum) disease to seriously consider having elective periodontal procedures performed. In these cases, the procedures are almost always needed to improve appearance. Sometimes they are suggested to promote future periodontal health or attend to a potential problem that might develop.

When you smile or talk, your teeth are framed by your lips and the visible gum tissue. People looking at you notice your teeth. People notice missing teeth, tooth alignment, gum color, discolored fillings, silver fillings, tooth color, and how much of your teeth actually show. If everything is integrated well and looks natural, people say you have a nice smile. If something does not look natural, it may be easy to define, such as crooked, stained, or yellow teeth; periodontal disease shown by red-colored gum tissue; or discolored fillings. Or it may be something not as readily discernable. Something does not look quite right.

That "something" may be related to the teeth and gum architecture. The position of the gums where they meet the teeth is esthetically important. If the teeth look too short, there may be more gum tissue covering them than is considered attractive. You may show too much gum tissue when you smile. There may be a difference in height of the gum of one tooth versus an adjacent tooth or its partner on the other side of the mouth. This could be caused by recession from brushing too hard; gum disease; poor or defective restorations, especially crowns; or just a problem with the way the tooth erupted into place. All of these things can detract from your appearance.

Several different simple periodontal procedures can correct most of these routine problems. Some involve removal of unwanted tissue; some involve grafting of tissue. Orthodontics might be helpful in some cases. The more extensive procedures will require referral to specialists.

In one common type of cosmetic periodontal plastic surgery, the gum tissue is reshaped and recontoured without the use of sutures (stitches). This procedure is done in the dental office. One tooth or several teeth may benefit from treatment. Postoperative discomfort is usually minimal. There may be transient sensitivity of the teeth if tissue is removed. The improvement generated by this type of procedure can be startling.

We will show you and describe in detail how you can benefit from cosmetic periodontal procedures. In many cases, the cosmetic periodontal surgery will complete the treatment you need. In some cases, it will be part of a larger treatment plan including crowns, veneers, or bonded restorations.

If you have any questions about cosmetic elective periodontal plastic surgery, please feel free to ask us.

Electrosurgery

Dental electrosurgery is a surgical procedure for the removal of periodontal or soft tissue. You may be more familiar with the scalpel and suture surgical procedure. Electrosurgery accomplishes the same thing, but in a different fashion. The choice is determined by your particular conditions and needs.

Electrosurgery is most often used to remove or recontour small amounts of gingival (gum) tissue, stop minor soft tissue bleeding (prior to impressions for crowns or placement of restorations), and/or expose sound tooth structure when:
- Insufficient clinical tooth structure remains to allow the proper retention of a crown.
- The sound tooth structure is beneath the gingival tissue.
- The gingival tissue is in poor position or contour.

Conventional surgery is needed when more extensive tissue removal, repositioning, or modification is required.

Electrosurgery is used in dentistry on a regular basis. A local anesthetic is given before the procedure is begun. A calibrated electric current is delivered to the site by a special handpiece and a selection of differently shaped tips. The different shapes are used to accomplish different things. The tip of the electrosurgery handpiece "draws" a line on the soft tissue and the soft tissue "falls off." There is usually very little postoperative bleeding associated with electrosurgical procedures.

There is generally very little postoperative pain associated with the electrosurgical procedure. Most patients say it feels like the burn from hot cheese on a pizza. Any nonprescription pain reliever is usually adequate for pain relief. Postoperative discomfort from conventional surgical crown lengthening is also usually minimal and the healing time is fast.

As with all soft tissue alterations in crown and bridge procedures, there may be an unavoidable delay before the final impression can be made. This is especially true when the crowns being prepared are easily visible when you speak or smile. While the soft tissue looks as if it is healed in a week or so, the tissue will continue to slowly change position and heal more fully for up to 8 weeks. At that time, the tooth may need to be slightly reshaped to compensate for the change before the impression is made. This is especially critical for upper front teeth. Obviously, the more tissue that is removed, the longer the healing time will be and the more likely final impression procedures will need to be postponed. If the procedure is done in a not critically cosmetic area, the impression will usually be made on the same day.

Sometimes the periodontal soft tissue changes that are needed are so extensive that they cannot be adequately accomplished by electrosurgery or a small conventional surgical procedure. If this is the case for you, you will be referred to a periodontist for the procedure. There will be an unavoidable delay in the final restoration while the tissue heals and matures. A wait of 4 to 12 weeks or longer is not unusual.

If you have any questions about electrosurgery, please feel free to ask us.

Flap Procedures

Periodontal flap procedures may be the most universal and commonly used of all periodontal surgical techniques. A *flap* is a section of gum tissue that has been freed from its underlying attachment in order to gain direct vision and access to the periodontal structures that are underneath. These periodontal structures are not normally accessible to the patient or dentist. The length and shape of the flap relate to the particular region of the surgery and the nature of the required treatment. An excellent analogy is that the procedure is like lifting the flap of an envelope to look at the contents, then closing the flap when done.

Indications

Flap procedures are indicated in cases of periodontal disease with active or nonresponsive pockets that are too deep to be treated successfully with scaling, root planing, or curettage. The flap may be raised to treat one tooth, a sextant (six teeth), or a quadrant (eight teeth). The advantage of the flap procedure is the shorter treatment time needed due to the improved access to the affected area. The root surfaces can be seen directly for better and more accurate cleaning. Pockets can be selectively reduced, or regeneration of lost tissues can be attempted. Many times the flap procedure is used strictly for correcting soft tissue defects. At other times, when the damage is more severe, the flap is used to gain access to the hard periodontal supporting structures for osseous (bone) surgery.

Procedures

Preoperative radiographs, clinical observation, and periodontal charting assist in planning which procedures are required during the flap procedure. However, none of these procedures give a direct view of the treatment site. Flap procedures are most often done by a periodontal specialist (a periodontist). While the periodontist may have a specific treatment plan for treating the diseased areas, when the flap is raised, the method for treating your particular problem may be modified. It may involve regenerative procedures. Bone grafting with natural or synthetic bone may be done. Guided tissue regeneration (GTR) may be attempted. These procedures may be done separately or in conjunction with one another. Other options include direct scaling and root planing of calculus (tartar) that might exist and the reshaping of a bone in a particularly difficult area.

The procedure involves the use of a local anesthetic so there is no pain during treatment. After the procedure is done, there is normally little postoperative discomfort. Prescription medication may be provided to deal with this. It is uncommon for surgical problems to arise after the flap is closed. Sutures will be used and a periodontal dressing (pack) may be placed for one week. After that time, the pack may be left off or reapplied, depending on your individual healing progress. Flaps normally heal quickly and well. Four to eight weeks after the procedure, the tissue appears normal. If indicated, further dentistry (fillings, crowns, etc.), can then be completed.

If you have any questions about periodontal flap procedures, please feel free to ask us.

Gingival Grafts

Periodontal (gum) surgery is most often associated with the removal of soft tissue. But there are times when it is necessary to use soft tissue to cover an area that has too little soft tissue remaining. Exposed roots may be due to improper brushing, periodontal disease, or genetic structure. Brushing too hard and/or with a hard toothbrush can cause the gingival tissue to disappear. The gingival margin (gumline) changes, and one or more millimeters of root structure can be exposed. Active periodontal disease can cause loss of this soft tissue too. In either case, this can lead to teeth that are very sensitive to temperature changes, root decay, or are quite unsightly. The disfigured soft tissue line can lead to a plaque trap, causing more disease and further problems.

Two methods of resolving these problems are free and attached gingival grafts. Both of these are periodontal surgical procedures. In both cases a local anesthetic will be used to numb the treatment site. In the case of an attached graft, gingival tissue is taken from a donor site and moved to the area where root coverage is required. The graft tissue is sutured into place, and a dressing is placed over the treated area. The dressing remains in place for several weeks and is then removed. An attached graft is not completely removed from the donor site. The donor site is adjacent to the site that needs root coverage. There is an incision made in the gum tissue, and the tissue is moved sideways, up, or down and sutured into place. Again, a protective dressing is placed to protect the area while healing occurs. Any anticipated postoperative discomfort is resolved with medication. Most discomfort will come from a free graft donor site.

A periodontist (gum specialist) usually performs these procedures, as well as other types of grafts and root coverage treatments. After the periodontist examines the areas needing treatment, you will have a better idea of what treatment will consist of, what the appearance may be, anticipated healing times, postoperative discomfort, and cost.

Most patients have heard that they should take better care of their teeth—brush and floss the teeth. Some patients brush too hard and in a back-and-forth motion; and some facial, bony structures and biting forces are such that root exposure happens, resulting in longer looking teeth. The grafting procedures mentioned here can restore the proper gingival marginal architecture, prevent root decay, reduce or eliminate thermal sensitivity, and make your smile look great again.

If you have any questions about gingival grafts, please feel free to ask us.

Gingivectomy and Gingivoplasty Procedures

There are two reasons for gingivectomy and gingivoplasty procedures to be performed. One is to correct a periodontal pathology or abnormality and the other is to reshape the gum tissue around a tooth or teeth so that a restoration, usually a crown, can be made.

A *gingivectomy* is the removal of a portion of the periodontal (gum) tissue. *Gingivoplasty* is a reshaping of the soft tissue. Although both obviously refer to some soft tissue removal, the gingivectomy involves more tissue reduction. In both cases, there is no alteration of the underlying bone support for the teeth. These procedures might be considered the simplest form of periodontal surgery.

The most frequent reason for a gingivectomy is that bleeding gum tissues still persist even after the teeth have been thoroughly cleaned and polished and oral self-care is excellent. There may be areas where it is impossible for the patient to clean effectively due to different situations. Therefore, the tissue never has a chance to heal and inflammation and infection remain. Removal of some soft tissue helps reposition the gums so the area can be properly cleaned on a regular basis. If the pocket is too deep, unwanted bacteria will colonize the area and cause periodontal infection to persist. Removing the extra soft tissue allows the patient better access for proper oral self-care at that location.

The tissue rarely grows back, unless other medical factors are present or oral self-care is neglected. These procedures can be done with either a laser or scalpel, depending on the extent of the therapy.

While time-consuming to perform, both of these procedures are technically simple to complete. Visibility and access to the surgical sites are usually very good, and results can be predicted with great reliability.

In brief, a local anesthetic is given, the specific soft tissue is removed, sutures (stitches) are placed, and a periodontal surgical dressing or medicated oral bandage may be used to cover the treated area. The dressing will be removed about 7 days later. Sometimes the dressing may be reapplied for another week. This depends on your healing progress. While the dressing is in place, it is helpful to rinse with an antibacterial mouthrinse and not eat on the side that is being treated. Hard, crunchy foods or chewing gum can displace the periodontal dressing, so beware.

If you are having this procedure done in order to make enough tooth structure available for a crown, final impression for the crown will be delayed for this 4- to 8-week healing period.

Postoperatively, there may be some discomfort. Antiinflammatory or pain relief medication may be prescribed for you.

Periodontal tissue is really thin, pink skin. New periodontal tissue will mature and will become stronger and will reach its final healed position around the tooth during the next 4 to 8 weeks.

If you have any questions about gingivectomy and gingivoplasty procedures, please feel free to ask us.

Gross Debridement

Gross debridement defines a large-scale removal of calculus (tartar) and debris from around the teeth and gums to permit adequate clinical evaluation of the periodontal tissues. In order for us to do a proper evaluation and examination of the soft gum tissues, the tissues must be easily visualized and measured. If the gums are inflamed (infected), swollen, bleed easily, or covered with calculus, plaque, and food debris, this cannot be accomplished.

A gross debridement is usually done by a registered dental hygienist. The hygienist will, in one or more appointments, clean off a great amount of the visible and easily accessible debris above the gumline. The tissue must be allowed some healing time before treatment can proceed. Often, there is a considerable amount of bleeding around the sites being cleaned. Even a minor amount of bleeding can obscure visibility. This initial debridement is always followed by scaling and root planing.

A hygienist or dental assistant will at some point spend time demonstrating the proper and most efficient manner of using a toothbrush and dental floss and any other tools to help to prevent further periodontal problems. You may be asked to demonstrate the brushing and flossing techniques you have been shown. We will review these particular techniques with you at future appointments to ensure that you are performing them effectively.

You may be given a prescription for an antimicrobial mouthrinse to use for a period of time after the gross debridement. It is often chlorhexidine gluconate. This rinse (not a bad breath rinse) will act on the undesirable bacteria and help the gum tissues to heal faster. You will only need to use the chlorhexidine gluconate rinse for a limited time. You must still brush and floss daily as instructed.

There is generally no need for local anesthetic for gross debridement. Most patients report that it is only slightly uncomfortable. The bleeding that will be present will stop quickly. In fact, most people say that their gums feel better right away after it is done—like an itch that has been scratched. There is rarely postoperative pain of any significance. Aspirin, Tylenol®, and any over-the-counter pain relievers are all strong enough to take care of any pain that might occur. Warm salt water rinses can help tissues to heal and feel better as well.

Once gross debridement is completed, the examination can proceed properly, and other potential treatment can be suggested. As long as the oral self-care we recommend is followed and your routine dental care intervals are adhered to, gross debridement need never be done again.

If you have any questions about gross debridement, please feel free to ask us.

Osseous Surgery

Indications

When periodontal (gum) disease progresses to a more advanced stage, it is common for the underlying supporting bone to become involved. First, the soft, periodontal tissue becomes infected and inflamed. When the inflammation increases, the bone reacts to the infection. Bone is destroyed, and it does not return. You will generally not feel the gums becoming infected or the bone disappearing. Unfortunately, it is painless. Generally, by the time pain is involved, the condition is quite serious.

Since periodontal disease is site-specific, the bone loss will not be uniform. Some teeth will show slight bone loss, some teeth will show more serious loss, and some teeth will exhibit no bone loss at all. The bone loss around a specific tooth or teeth may be regular or irregular in form. The bone loss may be vertical, horizontal, or both. If irregular, surgery to correct the bone loss will be needed. It is not possible at this time to reliably regenerate all lost bone. Once it is gone, it is gone. Research involving the possibility of periodontal bone regeneration has been underway for some time. But at this time, there are few ways to regrow periodontal supporting bone after it has dissolved from periodontal disease.

Treatment

Until fairly recently, the only method of correcting the irregular bone was to smooth off the high spots. The new bone height between teeth would be even at the level of the most severe bone loss. Although the problem was now corrected, other teeth might lose healthy bone in the leveling process. This could and would make those teeth less stable, an unavoidable and undesirable consequence. In some cases, the nature of the bone defect still dictates that this procedure be done.

A better approach is to augment or build up the irregular bone in locations where it has been lost. This is accomplished with the placement of natural or synthetic bone in a procedure known as *grafting*. Natural bone has been used for over 3 decades and there have been no reported immune system problems. There are also autografts that use your own bone. Allografts are synthetic or freeze-dried natural bone.

Preoperative radiographs, clinical examinations, and periodontal charting will give us an understanding of the type of osseous surgery that is necessary. However, the full extent of the problem may not be fully discovered until the area is exposed during surgery. Radiographs are a two-dimensional, black-and-white representation of a three-dimensional, full-color area. For this reason, treatment goals will remain the same, but the surgery method may be modified. Prognosis of the teeth needing surgery, options, and a best guess for treatment progress will be discussed prior to treatment.

To perform periodontal osseous surgery, a flap must be raised. (Please refer to the **Periodontal Flap Procedures** page.) A local anesthetic is used and postoperative discomfort is handled with medication. After this surgical procedure, sutures and a periodontal dressing are placed.

Osseous surgery may be the only treatment that will successfully help to retain your teeth after severe periodontal disease has been present for some time. Keeping your own natural teeth is generally better than having dentures.

If you have any questions about periodontal osseous surgery, please feel free to ask us.

Periodontal Surgery

Periodontal surgery is required for a variety of reasons. Any surgery would be initiated only after all signs of infection have been eliminated and you are involved in high-quality oral self-care. Periodontal surgery involves the contouring of the soft (gum) and hard (bone) tissues. The simplest type of periodontal surgery involves the reshaping and/or repositioning of the soft tissues only. The surgery may be required in order to eliminate or reduce problem pocket depths around one, several, or all teeth. The problem areas are usually places where you are having some difficulty keeping the area free of infection, plaque, and calculus.

It may also be necessary to reshape soft tissues to improve your appearance (cosmetic periodontal surgery) or to gain access for proper preparation and placement of any type of restorations. Different periodontal surgical procedures that do not involve the underlying bone can include correcting a frenum (muscle attachment) that is poorly positioned and grafting tissue to a new area where there is a deficient amount of periodontal tissue. These procedures may require some suturing of the gum tissue.

If you have experienced a more severe periodontal breakdown, your bone may have been affected by periodontal disease and may also require reshaping. This surgery is more extensive than soft tissue surgery. If your whole mouth has been affected, the surgery may be done in sections in separate appointments. Sutures and a periodontal dressing (intraoral bandage) are placed while healing occurs. A local anesthetic is used for these procedures. Postoperative discomfort will be alleviated with a prescription or over-the-counter medication.

Results

Once the healing has been completed, you will notice several things. Unless there was a graft placed or a frenum (muscle) cut, there will be soft tissue removed from around the teeth. This usually means that the teeth will look longer—because more of the teeth will be exposed. From an appearance standpoint, this is not usually welcomed, but it may be unavoidable. If you have experienced bone loss, the tissue may have to be repositioned in order to have the correct distance between the bone and gum. The soft tissue change may be slight or significant. Before the periodontal procedure, we will discuss with you the expected appearance of the teeth after surgery. We will also discuss with you whether there are other methods that can be used to improve the appearance of your teeth after the tissues have healed. If you are being referred to a periodontal specialist for these procedures, the expected results will be explained to you there as well.

After surgery, you may experience increased sensitivity to hot and cold stimulation—ice cream and cold or hot drinks, for example. The sensitivity may be slight or severe; it may be short-lived or last for months. There is no way to predict how you will respond. If the sensitivity is severe and lingering, there are several procedures that can be done to reduce or eliminate the problem.

Preventing Recurrence

The question most often asked by patients who require surgery to correct the damage caused by periodontal disease is whether the disease can come back after the surgery is finished. The answer is, simply and clearly, yes. If the same circumstances that caused the periodontal disease reoccur after surgery, you can develop the disease again. You have already shown a compromised resistance to periodontal disease. However, if you do your part with the brushing and flossing as we have instructed you and maintain your scheduled dental hygiene recare visits at the office, the odds in your favor increase greatly. You reduce the chance that you will redevelop periodontal disease. Your responsibility is to understand the nature of your periodontal problem and brush, floss, and use the recommended periodontal aids effectively.

If you have any questions about periodontal surgery, please feel free to ask us.

Prophylaxis

There is nothing more important to your dental health than maintaining a clean mouth. Prevention or absence of infection optimizes our general health. A clean mouth will be disease-, infection-, and trouble-free. A clean mouth will not be predisposed to developing either decay or periodontal (gum) disease. One of our very important functions in dentistry is to teach you how to properly maintain your teeth and gums, and to regularly remove anything that you are unable to remove yourself.

The theory and practice of preventive dentistry have undergone revolutionary changes in recent years. We now know that the preventive needs of every individual differ. The adage of "see your dentist regularly; get your teeth cleaned twice a year" has changed too.

Your Personal Plan

The recare and examination interval that we have recommended for you is designed for your unique situation. And it, too, can change. The interval between regular prophylaxis (cleaning) appointments that is established for you is a function of many things.
    These include:

- general health
- dexterity and hand/eye coordination
- age
- diet
- stress levels
- oral habits
- position and alignment of the teeth
- number, type, size, and location of restorations
- restorative materials used
- periodontal history
- location of bone and periodontal tissues

Simply stated, the more complex your dental situation and the more your tooth position and alignment deviate from the normal, the harder you will find it to keep your teeth clean and your gums healthy.

Recent studies have identified many of the microorganisms that cause gum disease and decay. They can be controlled with your help and with ours. These studies also show that a "cleaning" every 6 months may not be adequate for some patients. In order to prevent destructive oral disease, prophylaxis appointments in intervals of anywhere from 2 months to a year may be recommended. Periodontal (gum) disease can happen anywhere in your mouth at any time.

You don't have to let it happen to you! We are here to be your guide to good health.

If you have any questions about your oral care maintenance intervals, please feel free to ask us.

Ridge Augmentation

It is an unfortunate fact that teeth sometimes must be extracted. After an extraction (except for wisdom teeth), most people wisely choose to have the missing teeth replaced. When possible, the patients would like to have a replacement that is as close as possible to the original tooth in appearance. This usually means a fixed bridge, which will consist of crowns on both sides of the extraction site joined by the pontic, or replacement tooth.

Once a tooth is removed, the gum tissue and bone at the extraction site begin to change. First, the hole created by the missing tooth begins to fill in with new bone. Site changes occur rapidly for the first few months and then the changes slow down. The tissue shrinks at the extraction site. If there was significant periodontal disease, the shrinking will be quite noticeable. If there was a need for a surgical extraction, if the bone had to be removed or cut, or if there was trauma, there will be more shrinking of the tissue. If you were to run a finger along the gum from tooth to tooth, your finger would sink in at the extraction site. The architecture of the underlying bone has been altered, and since the gum follows the bone, the gum will change too.

In order to construct a bridge, the teeth on either side of the space are prepared (drilled) to allow the proper shape and thickness of metal and porcelain to be fabricated in a tooth shape. These are called *abutment teeth*. The missing tooth is replaced or "bridged" with a pontic. The pontic will abut or lay against the residual ridge area in the extraction space. You can imagine that if there is a great deal of tissue shrinkage, the pontic may need to be much longer than it should be and much different from its mirror image on the other side. When extensive tissue shrinkage has occurred, it is often impossible to get a pleasing esthetic result with a new bridge unless careful examination, diagnosis, planning, and a ridge augmentation procedure are performed.

Ridge augmentation involves building back shrunken tissue to its original height and width. The procedure is surgical and usually performed by a periodontist (gum specialist). The defective site is rebuilt through the use of free or attached grafts of the soft tissue, bone fill or pumping of the depressed area. Most often it will be done in two or three treatment appointments. The site is slightly overbuilt with tissue and allowed to heal for several weeks. Then a reshaping procedure will be completed to do the fine sculpting necessary to make a pontic appear as if it is growing out of the gum, not merely butting up and laid against it. Usually, we will do this fine sculpting procedure to maximize the appearance and function of the future bridge. Done properly, a new pontic shape will appear as if the tooth was never lost, but rather is again growing out of the gum (an ovate pontic form). The procedures are done in the office under local anesthetic and are well tolerated by patients. Postoperative discomfort is minimal and treated with simple pain relief medication.

Done correctly, ridge augmentation may take some time to complete. The original extraction site must be healed, the augmentation procedure and then the tissue reshaping procedure must be done separately, and allowed to heal before the final preparations and impression for the bridge can be made. Although it will take extra months of work, the result will be well worth the effort.

If you have any questions about ridge augmentation, please feel free to ask us.

Root Hemisections and Root Amputations

Indications

At times, a portion of a molar (or the bone surrounding part of it) is hopelessly damaged, but the other portion of it is still sound. Depending on the individual problem, it may be possible and desirable to retain the good part of the tooth and remove the damaged portion. Molars generally have two or three roots. One of the roots may be severely decayed, periodontally involved (with reduced gum and bone support), or split. Most commonly if a root is split, the tooth has already had endodontic therapy (a root canal). If the problem is decay, there may be no root canal on that tooth and it will need to have a root canal on the roots that will be retained.

Procedure

A *root amputation* is the removal of part or all of an individual root. A *root hemisection* is the dividing of the tooth through the middle to make two separate roots and two separate teeth out of what was once a single tooth with two joined roots. The hemisection procedure is most often performed on lower molars.

The procedure for either is similar. If the tooth did not have a root canal, this therapy will be completed on the root or roots that will remain. A periodontal flap is raised (please see the **Periodontal Flap Procedures** handout for more information). The area is viewed directly and the hopeless root section is removed or the tooth is divided. Usually, the removal of the root is not a difficult procedure.

The flap is then closed in the usual fashion and the area heals in a minimum of 6 to 8 weeks. When sufficiently healed, the remaining tooth is finally restored. Nearly 100% of the time, the tooth will need a cast restoration. For a root resection, in which the molar tooth has been divided into two premolar-sized portions, each root will receive a post and core, and then joined with splinted crowns. If necessary, other teeth may be crowned and added to the hemisected molar for additional support. In a tooth that has had a root amputated, a single crown may be placed, or it may be attached to another tooth for support. Your individual needs will dictate which is best for you.

The critical aspects for the success of these procedures are the diagnosis and execution of treatment. Posts and cores might be necessary. Often, the treated teeth must be splinted to adjacent teeth. The roots and cast crowns must be shaped just right to ensure that the remaining parts can be easily and thoroughly cleaned with a toothbrush and dental floss or other oral self-care tools.

In some cases, implant procedures have replaced root hemisection and amputation. However, your particular situation may indicate that either of these is best for you.

If you have any questions about root hemisections or root amputations, please feel free to ask us.

Scaling and Root Planing

The Procedure

Scaling is a periodontal dental procedure in which plaque and calculus are removed from the tooth both above (supragingival) and below (subgingival) the gum (gingiva). *Root planing* is a procedure in which diseased or altered portions of the root surface, the cementum, and dentin are removed and the resulting new surface is made smooth and clean. The more altered and damaged the root surface has been from calculus (tartar) accumulation, the more the need for root planing.

The purpose of scaling and root planing is to remove all debris from the teeth. Any item that can cause inflammation of the gum tissue must be eliminated. The root surface must be made as smooth as possible. Irregularities in the root surface can contribute to gum inflammation. Irregularities are sites for bacteria and plaque buildup. The bacteria and the toxins they produce in the plaque are held against the tooth by the calculus. In this way, plaque and calculus on the teeth have been positively linked to gum disease.

Depending on the severity of your particular periodontal problem, scaling and root planing may be the definitive treatment and no further procedures will be required. In many cases scaling and root planing are only a necessary part of the overall therapy. It is a demanding procedure. It requires much more time than the familiar adult prophylaxis (cleaning). It is usually done in multiple appointments, treating a quarter, half mouth, or your full mouth at each appointment. In this office we find that most patients are most comfortable if the area to be treated during the root planing procedure is anesthetized with a local anesthetic.

The scaling and root planing may have to be repeated in the future. It is customary to place the patient on a 3- to 4-month hygiene recare schedule. Scientific evidence clearly shows that for individuals who have demonstrated a predisposition to periodontal disease, an interval of 6 months is too long. We are familiar with your particular periodontal situation and will determine the appropriate interval for you. As your situation changes, there may be changes in the length of these intervals as well.

Other than the teeth being somewhat sensitive after the scaling and root planing procedure, there is little postoperative discomfort. The sensitivity will diminish with time. If you have been diagnosed as having severe periodontal infection, the sensitivity may remain for quite some time and further procedures may be needed to eliminate sensitivity. Although many procedures in dentistry can be considered elective, we consider scaling and root planing to be a necessity for your dental health.

Preventing Recurrence

Once scaling and root planing has been completed, it is most important for you to practice the brushing and flossing techniques in which you will be instructed. If we have recommended any additional periodontal aids, you must use them, too. Your cooperation is vital if the procedures are to be successful. To remain disease-free, you will need to remain constant in your oral self-care regimen.

If you have any questions about scaling and root planing, please feel free to ask us.

Scaling and Root Planing: Postprocedure Instructions

❏ The dental prophylaxis just completed has been preventive in nature due to your thorough oral self-care. That means that there was no gum disease evident. The prophylaxis was completed quickly and with the minimum of trauma to your teeth and soft tissues. In this event, you should have insignificant postoperative discomfort in your mouth. Congratulations on a job well done. Keep up the good work. We would rather assist you in preventing periodontal disease than in curing the problems periodontal disease can cause.

❏ A therapeutic prophylaxis has been completed. In this case, the gingival (gum) tissue showed signs of infection and inflammation and you may have had significant calculus (tartar) buildup. You may notice that your teeth feel different where the calculus was removed. The soft tissues may be sensitive or sore for approximately one day as they begin to heal. You may find that taking an over-the-counter pain reliever (aspirin, ibuprofen, etc.) will help during this 24-hour period. You may also rinse your mouth every few hours with warm salt water. Make sure that you brush and floss your teeth during this time period as you have been instructed. Be gentle, because the brushed areas may be sore, but be thorough! You do not want to have the periodontal infection begin again.

❏ When you have had scaling and root planing, or other more involved periodontal procedures, you can expect your gingival (gum) tissues to be quite sore. This is normal when the gum tissues have been infected and inflamed for some time. The more severely they have been affected, the more discomfort you can expect. This soreness should go away very quickly. You may rinse with warm salt water every few hours until the soreness is gone.

❏ You may also notice that the teeth have become sensitive to temperature changes after the scaling and root planing. This sensation frequently occurs when the surfaces of the roots of your teeth have been cleaned. Removal of the debris covering the roots and attached to the roots leaves the roots open to temperature stimulus. If the problem persists, please let us know.

❏ When you examine your gums closely in a mirror, you will also observe that the color, texture, and position of your periodontal tissues will undergo a change as the healing takes place. The swollen, reddened gum tissue will shrink, become more firm, and return to a healthy pink color. Watch for these welcome signs of improvement and be encouraged by the healing process.

❏ Please do not forget to brush, floss, and use other periodontal cleaning aids as you have been taught. It is important that you begin establishing proper oral self-care habits immediately. If you find that the recently treated areas are sensitive to the brushing and flossing, be gentle—**but be thorough!** With proper technique you cannot damage the teeth or gingival tissues.

❏ Brush after every meal with a fluoride-containing toothpaste. Rinse with a fluoride-containing mouthrinse once each day.

❏ Use the oral irrigator with the periodontal attachment as instructed. Fill the reservoir with:
    ❏ water   ❏ chlorhexidine gluconate 0.12%   ❏ other_____

❏ Use the periodontal cleaning aids as you have been shown.

❏ Please return in _____ weeks for a _____ minute appointment. During this time, your periodontal tissues will be evaluated for the expected improvement and effectiveness of your oral self-care and to determine the possible necessity of further periodontal treatment. This appointment will include reprobing the periodontal tissues.

❏ Because of your periodontal condition, we strongly recommend that you return for your next examination and preventive prophylaxis appointment in _____ months.

If you have any questions about these instructions, please feel free to ask us.

Scaling and Root Planing: Reevaluation

The goal of scaling and root planing is to remove all plaque, toxins, and calculus both above and below the gumline. After healing has occurred, the tissues will shrink, and a reevaluation of the condition of the gum and supporting structures will reveal any areas that may need re-treatment. Your oral self-care habits will be reevaluated at the same time and any revisions to our recommendations will be made. We will be polishing your teeth at this appointment. As you will recall, we did not polish your teeth during the root planing and scaling appointments. Although the polishing can, in theory, be done then, we believe that allowing tissues proper time to heal will allow us to make the best reevaluation of our treatment and oral self-care recommendations. That is why there is a time period of several weeks between the root planing and scaling appointment and this prophylaxis and evaluation. Once all tissues have responded and the goals of scaling and root planing are met, a recare interval will be established for you.

At the recare appointment, we will once again be evaluating your oral self-care to determine whether we need to recommend different procedures to keep your oral health at its best. We will reexamine your periodontal tissues for evidence of healing by remeasuring the probing depths around each tooth. Any areas of bleeding will be noted and treated; your teeth will then be polished and a topical fluoride treatment will be applied.

Topical fluoride provides a bacteriostatic action to the oral bacteria during treatment and for several hours afterward. It appears to be harder for the bacteria that cause gum disease to multiply and cause problems when topical fluoride is used.

If the goals of scaling and root planing have not been met, we will either re-treat those areas that have reinfected or refer you to a periodontist for specific periodontal surgery. The periodontal surgery will correct some of the hard (bone) and soft tissue defects that were caused by the periodontal infection.

At this time we may also consider using one or more of the newer nonsurgical therapies available for localized sites that have not healed as much as we would like. The site-specific therapy may be recommended for the first time or as a re-treatment. We will then monitor the results to determine whether a referral to a periodontist is appropriate.

A final word about how often you should have your teeth cleaned: modern dentistry considers a patient who has had gum disease to be always recovering, never completely "cured." If you do not take care of your teeth and gums, the problem can come back again. It is in the best interest of your oral health to have your teeth examined and cleaned at an interval of 3 to 4 months in most cases, not every 6 months as you have heard for years.

If you have any questions about the prophylaxis and reevaluation appointment, please feel free to ask us.

Soft Tissue Management

You have been diagnosed as having periodontal disease. Your specific periodontal problems may be slight and localized, slight and generalized, moderate, or severe. You may be a new patient or a patient who has been receiving treatment by us for some time. Treatment may be simple or quite complex and arduous. If you have been receiving continuous, regular hygiene care by us, there may have been a change (for the worse) in the condition of your periodontium (gums and supporting bone structure) or you may have had existing pockets that have not responded to conventional treatment. If you are a new patient, we are starting necessary treatment. Periodontal infection is site-specific and episodic: it can happen around teeth at any time.

Initial periodontal therapy, also known as *soft tissue management*, is an aggressive yet the most conservative method of treating periodontal (gum) disease. It is not periodontal surgery. It is done to attempt to minimize or eliminate the need for periodontal surgery. Initial periodontal therapy involves a thorough root planing of all infected areas. The root planing is designed to remove the toxins produced by the bacteria in plaque.

When initial periodontal therapy is coupled with an oral self-care regimen of brushing, flossing, and use of periodontal cleaning aids as instructed, the results can be dramatic! You have a great deal of the responsibility and can affect the outcome of treatment. Oral self-care instructions will need to be followed carefully; otherwise, what we do for you at our office can all too easily be undone at home.

You have been given other written information about procedures that will be performed, such as subgingival irrigation. Other procedures may be required, but we will discuss these with you before we do them.

What dentistry believes is true about periodontal disease this year is very different from what it considered fact several years ago. We now know that periodontal disease is not caused by one organism. It is caused by many different organisms that can be active and inactive during different periods of the disease process. We know you will not experience symptoms until bone destruction is advanced. This disease does not hurt until advanced stages. As research continues and dentistry learns new facts about the beginning and progression of periodontal disease, the treatment recommended and provided by the dentist and/or periodontist will change. You will particularly notice this if you have been treated for this disease in the past, either here or elsewhere. New discoveries, new treatments, and new medications will continue to change the way we treat this disease process. Some people may still think that correct procedure to maintain periodontal health is to get your teeth cleaned only twice a year. That hasn't been the case for 20 years. We now know that periodontal disease is an infection that affects about 95 of 100 adults. It can occur in bursts of activity and can cause profound bone loss.

We promote oral health for all of our patients. However, every patient is different. The treatment you need will differ from that of another. The fact is that our goal for you is to **prevent** both tooth decay and periodontal disease.

If you have any questions about initial periodontal therapy (soft tissue management), please feel free to ask us.

Splinting Teeth

In their normal state, teeth surrounded by healthy supporting structures exhibit very little mobility. *Mobility* can be defined in this case as movement of the teeth. Pushing on the teeth with dental instruments may cause the tooth to be deflected slightly from the "at rest" position, but this movement will be very, very slight.

Why Teeth May Need to Be Splinted

When the supporting bone is compromised and affected by periodontal disease, the teeth will show more mobility. If the tooth or teeth are subjected to trauma, they can be loosened in their sockets. Bruxing and grinding habits can also loosen teeth.

Teeth that are not too severely damaged by trauma will return to their former stability. Temporary splinting of the loosened teeth to each other or to other undamaged teeth may be required.

If the mobility is caused by clenching or grinding of the teeth, adjustment of the bite (occlusion) and the fabrication of a protective antigrinding/bruxing appliance may be indicated. In this case, no splinting of the teeth would be required.

The most common reason for splinting teeth is mobility caused by periodontal disease. The teeth show more movement as the bone support for the teeth diminishes. Multi-rooted teeth (molars) often show less mobility than single-rooted teeth with the same amount of bone loss. But the need for treatment is just as important. The more mobile the teeth, the more damage has been done, and the more splinting will be necessary.

The Splinting Procedure

The first step in elimination of tooth mobility is to begin to correct the periodontal problem. If the teeth are mobile, the periodontal problem is probably advanced and the corrective measures could be both involved and time-consuming. Splinting may be started immediately. It involves attaching the mobile and perhaps nonmobile teeth together with a wire, acrylic, or a combination of the two. Attaching the teeth together gives them all more strength. Splinting may be temporary or considered final, depending on your particular situation. Splinting has a limited life expectancy and must be repaired or replaced periodically. There is often a fee separate from the initial splinting fee associated with these procedures. You will be informed as to what your particular condition requires for short- and long-term therapy.

A more extensive form involves splinting the teeth together with cast and cemented restorations—crowns, bridges, bonded metal retainers, etc. This type of splinting will last much longer and is more expensive. The purpose is the same as that of external splinting—to attach the mobile teeth together so that they derive more strength and move less.

Teeth that are splinted will also require different and more involved brushing and flossing on your part. We will demonstrate these procedures for you.

Fees

Costs for splinting procedures vary greatly. It will depend on the number of teeth to be splinted, severity of the mobility, prognosis of the teeth, and the type of splinting selected.

If you have any questions about splinting teeth, please feel free to ask us.

Chlorhexidine Gluconate Oral Rinse 0.12%

Chlorhexidine gluconate oral rinse 0.12% provides long-term antimicrobial benefits. It is effective in reducing the redness, swelling, and bleeding of gum tissue that are present in gingivitis and periodontitis. This is not a cure for periodontal disease and should not be considered as a major treatment for this type of infection. Use of this rinse for up to 6 months does not appear to cause any significant changes in bacterial resistance or overgrowth of opportunistic bacteria or other organisms. It does not appear to cause any adverse changes in the normal microbial system that exists in the mouth.

The normal dosage is ½ fluid oz per use. (Use measuring cup provided or see markings inside cap.)

Use during Periodontal Therapy

If you are currently undergoing periodontal therapy, rinse as we have directed. Rinse twice a day, for 30 seconds each time, morning and evening after brushing and flossing. Do not eat, drink, or rinse with water for 30 minutes after rinsing. Continue this routine until all phases of your periodontal therapy are complete. If you are instructed to do so, you can also use this rinse in your oral irrigator (e.g., WaterPik).

Use during Crown and Bridge Procedures

If you are having a crown, inlay, onlay, or bridge procedure, please rinse with chlorhexidine gluconate 0.12% for 2 weeks before the tooth preparation appointment through 2 weeks after the final restoration is cemented or bonded into place. Dental research has shown that the use of this rinse will help to make gum tissue tight and healthy. The preparation and impression appointment will be easier and faster with less bleeding. The tissue also returns to normal faster after these procedures. For this use, rinse only once each day, before you go to bed.

Precautions

Use of this rinse can cause staining of the teeth, tongue, and some types of restorations. The stain can be easily removed by a professional cleaning. If you brush and floss your teeth thoroughly, this will be much less of a problem. Some patients may notice a slight change in taste sensations while using the rinse. This taste alteration will return to normal after the rinse is discontinued.

Do not use this product if you are pregnant (or are currently trying to conceive). This product has not been tested for use in children under age 18.

If you have any questions about the use of this rinse, please feel free to ask us.

Oral Rinse Protocol

The recommended standard of care for the treatment of moderate to severe periodontal disease is selective use of periodontal surgical procedures. These procedures may involve removal of bone and gum tissues or augmentation of bone and gum tissues. These techniques have shown a predictable level of success for many years. You have been diagnosed with periodontal disease and have been advised to have one of these standard periodontal treatments. For any of a variety of reasons (age, financial, health, emotional, time, etc.), you may have rejected this recommendation. Yet you wish to try to keep your teeth as long as possible. The following will describe a nonsurgical technique that is based on respected, long-term research. This is not a substitute for periodontal surgery. It is another modality we can use in the treatment of periodontal disease.

If you have decided that you wish to decline periodontal surgery at this time, we suggest the following maintenance routine in an effort to maintain the teeth that have periodontal disease. Results can vary from patient to patient. Understand also that you may have some teeth that have a questionable or hopeless prognosis. These teeth may eventually need to be removed. We will let you know which teeth can be left and which are better removed. Remember, if you have a periodontal infection, there is an infection in your body 24 hours each day. Your immune system is being called on to fight it 24 hours a day, every day. This is not good for your overall health.

Protocol

Initial:
- ❑ Scaling/root planing and subgingival irrigation where indicated.
- ❑ Adult prophylaxis.

Maintenance:
- ❑ Periodic professional treatment: every _____ months.
- ❑ Adult prophylaxis.
- ❑ Subgingival irrigation with four alternating oral rinses.

Oral self-care:
- ❑ Brush and floss daily as instructed.
- ❑ Use alternating prescribed oral rinses once daily.
- ❑ Every _____ months; after the adult prophylaxis at our dental office, we will advise you to switch to the next oral rinse in the regimen (the same that is used for the subgingival irrigation).
- ❑ If you have an intraoral irrigator (such as a WaterPik) and proper attachments, you can also use the oral rinse solution for daily subgingival irrigation.

The oral rinses prescribed will be chlorhexidine gluconate, phenol compounds with essential oils, chlorine dioxide, and stannous fluoride. We will advise you when to switch to the next solution based on the progress (or regress) of you disease.

If you have any questions about oral rinse protocol, please feel free to ask us.

Periostat: Systemic Submicrobial Dose of Doxycycline

You have been diagnosed with periodontal disease. Up until now, the treatment for periodontitis has included cleaning the area of debris (plaque, calculus, etc.), instructions in proper oral self-care, and when necessary, surgically correct the defects caused by the disease.

In the 1980s it was discovered that the antibiotic tetracycline used in daily small doses is useful in inhibiting the destructiveness of the enzymes that cause a breakdown of tissue that is a result of periodontal diseases.

Periostat is a doxycycline (20 mg, twice daily systemically) that is used to reduce the number of destructive enzymes. Side effects are minimal. It cannot be given to people who are allergic to tetracycline. It has been shown to improve the attachment of fibers to teeth and reduce pocket depth. It is not to be considered a cure for the disease. It is an adjunctive procedure to root planing and scaling. It is administered by taking it orally twice a day for at least 3 to 9 months. Please take this prescription as directed: do not skip a day. Research has shown that the use of this medication along with the treatment of scaling and root planing has a more positive effect than when just root planing and scaling are done alone.

This medication works more effectively in severely diseased teeth than in moderately diseased sites. The use of this medication as directed can reduce or eliminate the need for certain periodontal surgical procedures, or at least place a "hold" on the destructive process for a limited time until the corrective and definitive surgery can be accomplished.

Periostat is a new, nonsurgical or presurgical modality that helps in the long-term management of adult periodontal disease. You can benefit from this prescription if it is used in conjunction with root planing and scaling. It is not a "magic bullet" that will cure your periodontal disease forever: it does not replace your daily brushing and flossing, and you must take it twice a day.

If you have any questions about Periostat, please feel free to ask us.

Site-Specific Antibiotic Therapy

Oral bacteria are a major factor in periodontal (gum) disease. Gum disease is an infection around a tooth or teeth and often there are no symptoms. You may find out that you have gum disease when you have your teeth cleaned and a periodontal charting is performed.

For many years, physicians have been treating infections in other areas of our bodies with antibiotics. We now have the ability to treat individual infected areas in our mouths with a site-specific antibiotic. It does not have to be taken orally and then carried by the blood stream throughout our entire body. There are several types of medications that can be placed directly into the site of the infection. The material can be placed exactly where it is needed; therefore, only a very small amount of the drug needs to be administered.

A site-specific antibiotic is generally used where a 5 mm or deeper pocket is present or where other treatments may have been performed and were not successful in keeping the infection under control. It is a most conservative treatment and not a surgical procedure.

The Procedure
The first step is generally a thorough cleaning.

The selected antibiotic material is placed in the affected site. Multiple sites may be treated at the same time. You should not brush or floss the area where the material has been placed for a few days, as instructed. You may not notice an immediate improvement in the area. The healing process may take several months, during which the placement of the medication may need to be repeated. This is not unusual. During every dental hygiene recare appointment, we will evaluate your total periodontal condition.

These are several site-specific periodontal therapies that have evolved over time. While the dental insurance industry and the American Dental Association years ago agreed on an assigned procedure code for site-specific antibiotic therapy, it may not yet be a payable benefit with your particular dental insurance plan. Don't let possible insurance coverage (or lack thereof) dictate your recommended treatment.

We will select the most appropriate form of site-specific antibiotic therapy for your periodontal condition.

- ❑ Atridox—A doxycycline hyclate gel is placed into the diseased pocket, where it will dissolve in 7-10 days.
- ❑ Arrestin—A minocycline hyclate powder is placed into the diseased pocket, where it will dissolve in 7-10 days.
- ❑ PerioChip—A chlorhexidine gluconate gelatin disk is placed into the diseased pocket, where it will dissolve in 7-10 days.
- ❑ Other_____.

You should not brush or floss the area for _____ days. Avoid vigorous chewing in the treated area. You will need to return to our office in _____ days for evaluation of this site.

Until site-specific antibiotic therapy became available, a regular and thorough cleaning and excellent oral self-care were your only options for some areas of difficulty in your mouth. We can now offer a treatment option for difficult-to-treat areas.

The other option you have is no treatment of the problem or a referral to a periodontist for possible surgical correction. Site-specific treatment is a much more conservative approach than surgery. The site-specific treatment has the potential to reduce or eliminate surgical corrective procedures.

If you have any questions about site-specific antibiotic therapy, please feel free to ask us.

Illustration on CD-ROM

Subgingival Irrigation

Subgingival irrigation (flushing) of the periodontal tissues is a nonsurgical, additional treatment for periodontal (gum) disease.

In a healthy mouth, there is a crevice or ditch-like space around every tooth called a *sulcus*. We have an instrument called a *periodontal probe* to gently measure this sulcus space. The sulcus should measure between 1 and 3 millimeters, and no bleeding or pain should occur during probing. Gum tissue should be tightly attached to the bone surrounding each tooth. When the gum tissue is infected and periodontal disease is present, the tissues become red and swollen. When the sulcus is over 3 millimeters, it is difficult, if not impossible, to keep the bacteria levels under control with normal oral self-care.

Subgingival irrigation may aid in the removal of debris, bacteria, and toxins that cannot be routinely removed with normal oral self-care. A stream of fluid under slight pressure is delivered under the gum tissue to the appropriate site(s). The area is flushed out. The irrigation in the office is usually done with an antimicrobial that has a substantive effect: the molecules of the antimicrobial cling to your teeth and tissues and keep working for hours after the subgingival irrigation is completed. Water or other chemicals can also be used. If you are told that subgingival irrigation should be part of your daily oral self-care routine, you will be instructed in the proper solution to use.

If the subgingival irrigation is properly accomplished, you can remove a high percentage of problem bacteria and toxins out of the sulcus that cannot be reached with normal care efforts. The flushed and disturbed area should show a reduced level of bacteria. It may take some time for the bacteria and debris to build up to a level where they can again cause further or continued problems.

Subgingival irrigation is not a substitute for excellent oral self-care or for periodontal surgery, but it is another modality we can use in the treatment or prevention of periodontal disease. If you are in active initial periodontal therapy, the subgingival irrigation will be a part of your treatment. If you are in maintenance, it may be part of the routine treatment rendered when you come in for your recare appointment. If we recommend that you perform this procedure daily as part of your normal oral self-care, you will receive further instructions.

If you have any questions about subgingival irrigation, please feel free to ask us.

chapter 11

Prosthodontics

Content at a Glance: Prosthodontics

Have Missing Teeth Replaced
Details the adverse effects of not replacing missing teeth as soon as possible.

Implants, Crowns, and Bridges vs. Natural Teeth
While heavily suggesting that natural teeth are the best choice, this document describes the possibilities of natural looking restorations with crowns, bridges, and implant crowns.

Fixed Restorations
Crowns
Crowns: An Overview
Gives a general overview of procedures for and maintenance of fixed prosthetics.

Crown Design
Explains crown design and construction and insurance coverage possibilities. Includes a checklist for patient preferences and the fees involved.

Crowns and Bridges: Procedural Overview
Provides the patient with a general overview of the crown and bridge technique including impressions and temporaries.

Crown and Bridge Fees
Takes the confusion out of crown and bridge fees. Presents a checklist of items covered by the crown or bridge fee, as well as those procedures, which, though necessary, will require additional fees.

Crown and Bridge Preoperative Instructions
Reviews healthy habits to be followed prior to crown and bridge appointments.

Materials Options
Materials Options: An Overview
Advantages and disadvantages of the materials commonly used in crown and bridge restorations.

Cast Gold Restorations
Describes when and why these restorations are used.

Cast Gold and Ceramic Restorations
Reviews the advantages of cast gold and ceramic restorations.

Cast Porcelain Fused to Metal Restorations
Reviews the advantages of porcelain fused to metal restorations.

Full Porcelain/Full Ceramic Restorations
Reviews the advantages of full porcelain and full ceramic restorations.

Bridges
Bridges: An Overview
States the benefits of replacing missing teeth with bridges.

Full Ceramic and Porcelain Bridges
Describes the advantages of all-ceramic bridges.

Maryland Bridge (Bonded Resin Retainer)
A description of an alternative to a dual abutment bridge.

Ovate Pontic
Describes the benefits to esthetics of the ovate pontic form.

Partial Coverage Bonded Bridges
Explains the application of partial coverage bridges to preserve tooth structure.

Content at a Glance: Prosthodontics—cont'd

Implants

Implants: Options
Gives a general overview of implants, the procedure, success information, and alternatives.

Implant: Procedural Overview
Detailed explanation of the three phases in the dental implant procedure.

Procedures and Applications

Biologic Width
Defines biologic width and its importance in prosthetics.

Cementation: Postoperative Instructions
An explanation of what a patient can expect after cementation of his or her new restoration.

Crown Lengthening Procedures
An explanation of why sufficient tooth structure is needed and description of the procedure.

Extraction Site Defect
Details why this problem should be resolved prior to restoration with a bridge.

Ferrule
Describes a ferrule and its importance for restoration longevity.

Impressions
Describes impressions, their use, and procedures for taking impressions.

Posts
Gives a detailed description of post composition, use, and placement.

Posts, Core-Crown Buildups, and Crown Lengthening
Informs the patient of the use of posts and core-crown buildups, with brief information on electrosurgery.

Provisional Crowns
Reasons behind the use of provisional crowns are explored.

Provisional Crowns: Postoperative Instructions
Instructions for the patient to prolong the life and function of provisionals.

Study Models and Wax Ups
Explains the use of diagnostic study models and wax ups in the formation of treatment plans. This same document also appears in the "General Dentistry" section.

Removable Prosthodontics

Full Dentures
Explains how full dentures are custom-made and fit for individuals. Encourages patients to retain natural teeth where possible, characterizing full dentures as a last choice.

Immediate Dentures
Explains the role of immediate dentures in the tooth extraction and denture procedure.

Partial Dentures
Describes the appearance, fabrication, and function of a partial denture.

Have Missing Teeth Replaced

Most adults can expect to have 32 teeth. The four third molars, or "wisdom" teeth, are often extracted because they do not grow into the mouth well or there is not enough room for them to remain in proper alignment. It is very unusual to have wisdom teeth replaced. But the other 28 teeth are needed. Your mouth, jaw, and body developed together over millions of years. They are designed to operate together at peak efficiency. When you lose a tooth, the efficiency decreases and function suffers. When you lose a tooth, you lose some ability to chew food properly. This may mean that you either place more stress on the other teeth in order to chew all the food you eat, or you do not chew well enough and what is swallowed is not quite ready to be digested. This can lead to digestive difficulty. Or you might switch to a diet that consists of softer foods that do not have to be chewed as much. You might have to eliminate certain favorite foods because you cannot chew them thoroughly. For each missing tooth, you lose approximately 10% of your remaining ability to chew food.

Other problems also occur. The teeth adjacent to the space left by the missing tooth will eventually shift. If for example, a lower tooth is extracted, the opposing tooth in the upper jaw will grow slowly (or sometimes quickly) longer in a downward direction into the missing tooth space. This is called *extrusion* or *supereruption*. The teeth on either side of the missing tooth space will move and tilt off their proper vertical axis and drift into the missing tooth's space. This can make these teeth more prone to decay and gum disease because it is much harder to keep the teeth clean when they are not aligned properly. Root structure that is normally covered by gum and bone may become exposed. All this can happen if one tooth is lost. Other major problems can occur if multiple teeth are lost. There is a loss of the arch length, the distance from the back of the last tooth on one side of your mouth to the back of the last tooth on the other side of your mouth. With collapsed bite and loss of vertical dimension, the distance from your chin to the tip of your nose decreases, making your face shorter. Extrusion and movement of your maxillary (upper) alveolar bone until the gum tissue from the upper jaw can touch the teeth or gum tissue of the other jaw causes loss of facial tone and shape. The facial muscles of the cheeks and mouth sink into the edentulous (extraction) site. There can also be severe cosmetic problems when the extracted tooth's space is visible when you talk or smile. This is not a pretty sight to anyone. There is loss of self-image and self-esteem and a feeling that you are getting old. Once you start losing teeth, you can actually start to look old. Losing a tooth is pretty serious. The longer you wait after a tooth is extracted, the more difficult and expensive it can become to make the replacement you need. With very few exceptions, it is better to replace missing teeth as soon as possible. Evolution designed you to chew your food with 28 teeth.

We will discuss with you the type of replacement that would be best suited for you. You can choose to do nothing at all and leave the space or spaces, but as you can tell, this is not usually recommended. You can have a fixed replacement made that could be an implant, a conventional bridge (crowns/caps), a bonded resin bridge, or a combination of implants and bridges. You could also have a removable partial denture made. The advantages of the fixed replacements are that they are not designed to come out of your mouth at any time, they are the easiest to live with, feel more like the original teeth, and are perhaps more cosmetic than removable dentures. A removable partial denture is held in place by metal clasps that may be visible. It is bulkier and may interfere with your speech for a period of time. However, generally, dentures cost less than a fixed replacement.

Your chewing apparatus, jaws, and teeth were evolved to function in a particular fashion. The interaction is complex and marvelous. Loss of teeth degrades this function. Preserve your health. Replace missing teeth as soon as suggested.

If you have any questions about replacing missing teeth, please feel free to ask us.

Implants, Crowns, and Bridges vs. Natural Teeth

Nothing can replace the natural teeth you were born with for chewing and function. However, very few people go through life without having teeth filled, crowns (caps) placed, or bridges and implants used to replace missing teeth. Crowns, bridges, and implants are the best answer and closest to your natural teeth, but they are not the same as healthy, natural teeth.

Crowns

Crowns are used to reconstruct a single tooth broken down by dental decay. Crowns are made of ceramic, resin, porcelain, porcelain plus metal, or resin plus metal materials. They are bonded or cemented onto the prepared tooth and cannot easily be removed from the tooth once placed. If the tooth was in good alignment before the crown was prepared, the crown will be in good alignment. If the tooth was misaligned before the crown, sometimes the crown may be made to obtain a more ideal shape and position. It is cleaned and flossed just like a natural tooth and is most like real teeth.

Bridges

Bridges are crowns that are attached together, suspending the crown portion of a false tooth in or over the space left by the missing tooth. A bridge can be used to replace one or several teeth. Sometimes a bridge is used to splint loose teeth together in order to make the teeth more stable. Bridges are usually made of metal covered with either porcelain or resin. Some of the newer bridges are made of all resin or all ceramic materials. They are cemented or bonded onto the existing prepared teeth and are not easily removed once placed. The bridge teeth can be brushed the same as natural teeth, but since they are attached together, must be flossed differently by using a floss threader or other device.

The teeth are generally the same shape as natural teeth. However, if the existing teeth (abutments) that are used to anchor the bridge have moved from their original position because a tooth or teeth have been missing for years, the added tooth (pontic) may be longer or shorter than the tooth that it is replacing. With a bridge, the false tooth will most often butt up against the soft tissue ridge where the removed tooth was.

The shape of the tongue side of the false tooth varies. It is usually smaller on the tongue side and completely fills the space. Food will have more of a tendency to collect in this area, so you must be prepared to clean it. If the missing tooth has been gone a long time, the ridge may have shrunk considerably, and the pontic tooth will be longer than the teeth on either side. If this is the case, there are several periodontal procedures that can be done prior to the construction of the bridge. These procedures will build up the tissue to its former height. The more your mouth has changed from its normal state, the harder it is to make new teeth look and feel natural.

Implant Crowns

Implant crowns are used to replace single or multiple missing teeth. They are either cemented or screw-retained onto an implant fixture. The crowns are made of porcelain or resin and metal. But they have some significant differences from the natural teeth they replace. Teeth are supported by a root or roots that are irregular in shape. Implants are round. The cross-sectional of the implant will never match that of the tooth it is replacing. A multirooted tooth may be replaced by a single implant, so the manner in which an implant crown comes out of the soft tissue ridge will appear different from a natural tooth. There will be more space between the implant root and the adjacent teeth. Implant crowns are often cemented with temporary cement. This allows the dentist to easily take off the crown and evaluate how the implant is doing. Crowns on teeth are usually cemented with a final cement. Implant-supported crowns are wonderful, but not the same as natural teeth with crowns. Be prepared for some differences. Expect more maintenance on your part and in the dental office with crowns, bridges, and implants.

☛ *Smokers take note:* *There is a heightened risk of dental implant failure among smokers—as much as a 20% greater failure rate!*

If you have any questions about implants, crowns, and bridges vs. natural teeth, please feel free to ask us.

Crowns: An Overview

There are usually three reasons for the placement of crowns (caps) and bridges:

The first reason is that a tooth has been so badly damaged by decay or so heavily restored by fillings that it can only be saved with cast restoration.

The second reason is that a tooth has been treated endodontically (root canal treatment). These teeth are almost always restored with a cast restoration because they have lost a great deal of tooth structure from fracture, decay, or the drilling process. These teeth are prone to fracture under normal and light chewing forces.

The third reason a crown might need to be placed is that the tooth needs to be used as an abutment (anchor) for a bridge to replace missing teeth.

The procedure involves:

❑ Preparing (drilling) the tooth in an appropriate fashion for the type of crown chosen.
❑ Making impressions of the prepared tooth, opposing teeth, and the occlusal (bite) relationships.
❑ Selecting a shade for tooth-colored crowns.
❑ Fabricating a provisional restoration that will remain in place while the crown is being constructed.
❑ Cementing or bonding the completed crown into position. If the work to be done is extensive, there may also be several appointments needed for preliminary seating (try-in) of the crowns or castings.

Crowns are made from many different types of materials. We have prepared written information describing the advantages and disadvantages of each. If you have not seen this information, please ask for it. If you have any known sensitivity to metals, please let us know prior to treatment. If you would prefer that no metals be used in the construction of the crowns, please let us know. We will discuss your options prior to preparation of the tooth (or teeth).

It is important for the ultimate success of the crown(s) that you understand and can perform thorough plaque removal. You should immediately begin following the oral self-care instructions that you have been given. It will make the procedure more comfortable and efficient, and the resulting restorations will look better. Final impressions cannot be taken until the gum tissue is healthy. Your cooperation is appreciated and necessary.

Maintaining Your Fixed Prosthetics

As is true with your natural teeth and especially with teeth that have been restored with any dental material, you should avoid chewing on excessively hard or sticky foods after the crowns have been cemented. It is especially important not to bite down on hard foods with just one tooth. The porcelain material can fracture from the metal substructure under extreme forces. Anything you chew that could break a natural tooth could break a crown!

Be sure to brush and floss daily as instructed. We also advise using a fluoride mouthrinse as part of your daily routine. Please be sure to return for your regular examinations and prophylaxis (cleaning) appointments at the time intervals we suggest.

After observing these types of procedures for many years, we note that the gingiva (gums) can recede from the crown margins and the surrounding tooth structure may become visible. This recession usually takes place over a period of several years and may require restoration replacements or a periodontal plastic surgery procedure to correct it.

We expect that you will receive many years of service from the cast restoration.

If you have any questions about crowns and bridges, please feel free to ask us.

Crown Design

There are many different types of full coverage cast restorations (crowns) that can be used to restore a tooth or become part of a bridge. There are also certain essentials in the design that cannot be changed without risk of a compromise of the final restoration. The most common design is one in which there is a noble metal used for the substructure and a porcelain material is fused to the metal, hiding most but perhaps not all of the metal. Over time it is possible that more metal may be displayed if the tissue recedes from the area. This recession may be a result of the normal aging process or due to a dental pathology. At the interface of the crown and tooth, there is a 0.4-mm wide metal collar that encircles the tooth and marks the limits of the crown. There are other designs that use different metals, such as a higher gold content and different amounts of visible metal in the crown. More metal may be desirable if the patient has a bruxing (grinding) habit or if the crowns are being made for periodontal splinting reasons. Less metal display may be desired if there is a cosmetic compromise.

The more involved the construction of the cast restorations, the more each crown will cost. Some of the costs are fixed, as in the substitution of a metal margin with a porcelain margin. Some costs change, as in the price of gold, platinum, and other metals used in the substructure. The basic, least expensive crown will have some metal visible. It will contain noble metal, have a circular metal collar, and porcelain coverage of 85% of the crown. If you have an allergy to any type of metallic or ceramic material, you must let us know prior to crown fabrication. A metal allergy will affect the choice of metal.

The construction of the crown also involves a laboratory, which will perform the actual casting of the metal and porcelain application. There is also a difference between the level of expertise among the labs. The esthetic component of crowns relates directly to the level of ability of the laboratory technician and the dentist's artistic capabilities. Some laboratories specialize in esthetic crowns. Crowns that look and fit properly cost more because the best laboratories charge more for their work. We only use laboratories that have shown that they can consistently produce excellent dental crowns and bridges. Where your oral health is in question, we do not compromise.

Dental insurance coverage typically includes only the most basic type of crown. They do not pay for the esthetic component of crowns or any improvements over the base type of crown you have selected. This will naturally reduce their payment ratio for the procedure. The reimbursement to you will be approximately 40% to 50% for each crown. You may have been informed that it is 50% or more. This may not necessarily be an accurate statement: you need to know just what kind of crown your dental insurance covers.

Please consider the following options for your full coverage cast restorations. The options have already been explained to you verbally and/or in a written document. Keeping this information in mind, place a check mark next to the options you desire.

❑ Porcelain to semi-precious metal, full 360-degree metal collar, partial metal lingual,
   palatal surface (standard crown design) $
❑ Porcelain butt joint facial (cheek side) surface $
❑ Full precious metal (not semi-precious metal) $
❑ Minimal metal display on lingual (palatal) $
❑ Captek® type $
❑ Full cast porcelain or ceramic (no metal used, may be bonded into place) $
❑ Full occlusal (chewing surface) metal; porcelain on facial only $
❑ Other:_____ $

                                    Total $

If you have any questions about crown design or fees, please feel free to ask us.

Crowns and Bridges: Procedural Overview

TOOTH PREPARATION, IMPRESSION, AND PROVISIONAL RESTORATION

Appointment Expectations

Crown and bridge tooth preparation involves multiple appointments. The first appointment will include preparing the tooth (teeth), taking impressions, and making a provisional (temporary) restoration. This appointment will usually take the longest and be the most involved. In your case, you can expect to have an appointment that will be approximately _____ hour(s). The more teeth that we prepare for crowns, the longer the appointment will last.

Tooth Preparation

The preparation of the teeth consists of shaping and removing tooth structure. This tooth reduction allows the ideal thickness of metal, porcelain, or metal and porcelain. The amount of tooth reduction necessary depends on the material we have selected; different types of crowns require different designs. We will make sure that you are comfortable throughout the entire procedure by numbing the area as needed.

Sometimes, because of the position of the soft tissue (gums), it may be necessary to trim or shape the soft tissue around the teeth. If we find that, due to unforeseen circumstances, the tissue removal will be complicated, you may be referred to a periodontist (gum specialist) for this procedure. If the tissue does not need to be reshaped, we most often use a "retraction cord" that is fitted and placed around the tooth. This cord temporarily repositions the gum tissue away from the prepared portion of the tooth and makes it possible to get a better impression.

Taking Impressions

Once the teeth have been adequately prepared, the final impression is made. During this impression procedure, the prepared portions of the tooth must be clearly visible. The cleaner the prepared teeth are, the better the impression will be. To ensure accuracy we often take a second impression. This is a difficult and exacting task and some of the aspects of getting an acceptable impression are not in our control.

The impression material is mixed and placed into a special tray that conforms to the size of your mouth. Impression material is fairly soft when mixed, similar to cold molasses. Once placed in your mouth, the impression material will set in just a few minutes. Depending on the type of impression technique used, a separate model of the opposing teeth may also be made.

An impression of your bite (bite registration) will be used to be sure your final crown(s) will fit together with the opposite jaw, just as they did before.

Temporary or Provisional Restorations

After the impression is taken, the provisional (temporary) restoration(s) will be constructed. The temporary plastic/resin crown(s) replaces the prepared tooth structure and protects the tooth while the final crown is being fabricated. Provisional restorations are held in place with a temporary cement and will usually remain in your mouth for a minimum of 2 weeks—longer if the required treatment is complex.

Your New "Look"

At the initial appointment we will make a determination of the shade of porcelain (or resin) to be used in order to obtain the best esthetic results. You will, of course, participate in this process. Many times we will take photographs of your teeth to better match the shade. The impression, bite registration, and shade information are sent to a laboratory; and the crown(s) or bridge(s) is constructed according to our explicit work order. The returned restoration will be ready for cementation (if simple) or for a casting try-in (if more complicated).

Following the First Appointment

How will you feel after the appointment is completed? Most patients note their gingival (gum) tissue is sore for a day or two. The less modification or manipulation of the gingival tissues, the less sore you will be. Some patients notice tooth sensitivity, especially to cold, but that it goes away pretty quickly. Analgesics (pain relief medication) are not usually necessary. If we expect you to be more than normally uncomfortable, we will inform you at the end of the appointment.

If you have any questions about tooth preparation, impression, and provisional restoration for crowns or bridges, please feel free to ask us.

Crown and Bridge Fees

Although we make a great effort to explain specific treatment and related fees, we find that for cast restorations (crowns, bridges, inlays, onlays of metal and/or porcelain, also known as *caps*) there sometimes remains some confusion. Please carefully read the following so you understand what is included in the fees for each procedure and where other fees might apply.

Cast Restorations: Crowns and Bridges

The fee for cast restoration includes:

- ❑ The preliminary impressions and models
- ❑ Local anesthesia
- ❑ Preparation of the tooth (teeth)
- ❑ A provisional (temporary) restoration
- ❑ Bite registrations
- ❑ Models
- ❑ Final and withdrawal impressions of the prepared tooth and its opposing teeth
- ❑ Trial fittings
- ❑ Shade selection with photographs where indicated
- ❑ Trial cementation
- ❑ Adjustments
- ❑ Final cementation
- ❑ One year of follow-up and adjustments

The fee does **not** cover:

- ❑ Post and core buildup needed on a tooth previously treated by root canal
- ❑ Buildups to replace tooth structure where significant portions of the natural tooth are missing
- ❑ Periodontal (gum) surgery to expose adequate clinical tooth for crown retention
- ❑ Electrosurgery procedures to remove gum tissue where the decay of the tooth, fracture of the tooth, or previous tooth preparation has moved the sound tooth structure underneath the gum to the extent that the tooth cannot be properly prepared, visualized, or an impression made.

Unfortunately, the need for electrosurgery will often not be known until the tooth preparation begins. Usually we can complete this procedure in our office, but for more extensive cases, you will be referred to a specialist. If there is a potential that you will need a post, core, crown buildup, or soft tissue removal, we will inform you of the procedure and the associated cost before the preparation is begun (when possible). These procedures have separate dental insurance codes and are considered separate procedures and are not included in the fee for the crown or bridge.

If you have any questions about crown and bridge fees, please feel free to ask us.

Crown and Bridge Preoperative Instructions

Because you have decided to proceed with a fixed prosthetics procedure (crown, bridge, inlay, or onlay), we want to stress the importance of oral self-care. Any soft tissue infection, even if it appears to be minor, can cause difficulty with the preparation or final impression and cause a delay in treatment. If you brush and floss as we have instructed you, there will be no gum problems and the preparation and impression will be faster and easier for you and for us. Daily maintenance is necessary to ensure gum health. The better you take care of your teeth and laboratory-processed restorations, the longer they will usually last and the less trouble you will have in the future. Any problem that does develop will usually be small and easily corrected. We recommend that you continue to have your teeth checked by us at the interval we have established for you.

When the gums are irritated due to inadequate oral self-care, the tissue will become swollen and red and will bleed readily. When the gum tissue is swollen, the preparation margins of the tooth are not as easy to isolate and dry for the impression. The true contour of the tissue can become disfigured, making it virtually impossible to take a correct impression of the preparation. Impression materials do not work well in moisture. If the impression is not correct, the crown will not fit correctly. When tissue conditions become too difficult to work with, we may decide not to make the preparation or impression and will have to reschedule the appointment until the tissue improves.

It is important for you to practice thorough plaque removal, especially before we begin the preparation of the tooth. You will need to continue your excellent self-care while the temporary restoration is in place, through the impression and the final cementation of the restoration. Of course, we hope you can keep up these good habits forever!

As an extra measure of protection, we are prescribing an antimicrobial rinse, shown to help keep the soft tissues healthy and reduce potential bleeding problems. Please use the rinse _____ times a day, beginning 2 weeks before the tooth preparation appointment to 2 weeks after the final cementation.

Other Instructions: _____

_____

_____

If you have any questions about these preoperative instructions, please feel free to ask us.

Materials Options: An Overview

When a natural tooth undergoes extensive damage, it cannot be successfully restored for the long term with a "regular filling"—one placed by the dentist in a single office appointment. Materials constructed and processed in a laboratory are stronger and will last longer. All materials for cast restorations have advantages and disadvantages. The following is a summary of the materials that can be used.

Partial Coverage Restorations: Inlays and Onlays

Partial coverage restorations are indicated when there is sound remaining tooth structure that does not need to be included in the preparation. Advantages of an inlay or onlay include less drilling than for a full coverage crown. Because of esthetics and concern over potential allergic reactions to metal, dentistry is and has been moving away from any restorations that have metal in them.

❑ Gold Alloy—Gold has been used successfully in tooth restoration for many years with a long history of service. The yellow color might be visible when you speak or smile and for that reason is not considered an esthetic material. It is, however, useful for small to medium restorations and for those who brux or grind.

❑ Laboratory-Processed Resin—This is an excellent cosmetic choice because it can closely match natural tooth color. Laboratory-processed resins are wellsuited for small to medium restorations but not as successful in patients with a tooth grinding habit. The restorations have a tendency to break under extreme compressive forces. A mouthguard may be recommended for protection.

❑ Porcelain/Ceramic—Excellent for use in cosmetic dentistry, porcelain/ceramic restorations are used to restore small- to medium-sized cavities. The material is more wear-resistant than resin but can wear opposing enamel. It is not as successful for patients who brux or grind and has the potential to break under extreme biting forces. A mouthguard may be recommended for protection.

Full Coverage Restorations: Crowns and Bridges

Full coverage restorations are indicated when the entire remaining tooth structure needs protection or is vulnerable to fracture. A full coverage crown requires more preparation than an inlay or onlay.

❑ Full Cast Gold (High Noble)—Made of a gold alloy, full cast gold is the longest lasting of any of the laboratory-processed materials—20+ years. The alloy consists of gold, silver, palladium, and sometimes zinc, copper, and platinum. Although it is a very strong material, the yellow color makes it not as esthetically pleasing as other options.

❑ Full Cast Noble—Similar in properties and qualities to full cast gold, this material contains mostly palladium plus silver, gold, and other trace metals. Full cast noble material is more silver in color than a full noble metal.

❑ Porcelain Fused to Gold (High Noble or Noble Alloy)—This material is very esthetic and can last 10 to 20 years. The gold substructure is covered with porcelain, which can wear opposing teeth or fracture under forceful biting or grinding. The porcelain can be applied to just the surface of the crown facing on cheek. The result will not be as esthetic, but will last longer. A mouthguard may be recommended for protection.

❑ All Ceramic or Porcelain—This is the newest technology in laboratory-processed restorations and is considered very esthetic. No metal is used in the process, and therefore no metal will ever be visible. It is excellent for restoration of back teeth; expected service life is 10+ years. This type of restoration can be cemented or bonded in place. The same cautions exist as with any porcelain or ceramic material: it can wear opposing natural enamel, and a mouthguard may be recommended for protection from bruxing or grinding. Some processes in fabrication of the all ceramic or porcelain crown are actually controlled by a computer.

All the above take at least two appointments to finish. Tooth preparation, impressions, and temporary crown, bridge, or inlay/onlay will be done at the first appointment. Permanent cementation will take place during the second appointment. Because of the highly technical nature of the process and our exacting standards, we may need to take more than one impression. If we detect an irregularity with the returned laboratory restoration, we will take a new impression and redo the onlay or crown.

We will recommend the best material to meet your specific needs and answer any questions you have. Longevity of any of the restorations depends on the quality of the materials (and we only use the best), the technical skills in construction and placement (and we provide the best service possible), and what you do to and with the restorations once they are in your mouth. Clenching and grinding habits will significantly shorten the useful life of any restoration placed. What can break your natural tooth can break any restoration. Your oral self-care will affect the length of service of the restoration. You will need regular dental examinations and hygiene maintenance (cleaning) at intervals determined by your particular oral health requirements. A rule of thumb is that the more restorations you have in your mouth, the more care you (and they) will need. Any problem that begins can be discovered and corrected when it is small: with regular dental examinations, you can protect your investment.

Cast Gold Restorations

A cast gold restoration will give you the longest and most trouble-free service of any type of dental material available today. A full gold crown can be used when a tooth has undergone significant destruction. A much smaller and conservative type of restoration, called an *inlay*, is used when more enamel and original tooth structure exists. Cast gold restorations have been known to last for 25 to 40 years. A cast gold restoration is not likely to break. The gold casting is held in place by a dental cement (glue). It can even be bonded.

These gold restorations are especially recommended for patients who brux (grind) or clench their teeth. They are indicated for patients who want the most trouble-free, longest-lasting type of dental restoration. They are recommended when there is moderate to extensive tooth destruction. The gold castings are then used to cover the biting surfaces and weakened areas and to prevent fracture during normal chewing. Only cast restorations can do this. Silver fillings cannot strengthen teeth. Bonded tooth-colored fillings that are not laboratory fabricated do not strengthen teeth like cast gold. A laboratory is involved in the fabrication of the gold crown or inlay. Therefore there will be two visits needed for the restoration to be completed. A temporary plastic crown or inlay will remain in place on the tooth while the final restoration is being made. The appointments will be about 2 weeks apart.

Initially, the cast gold restorations are more expensive than silver fillings. Because cast restorations do not have to be redone as frequently as silver (if at all), you end up saving time and money in the long run. The longer the gold restorations are in place, the less you eventually spend getting the same tooth restored over and over. Another potential disadvantage of cast gold is the color. They are an obvious "wedding band" yellow. If you want restorations to be the same color as your teeth, cast gold is not for you. Depending on the type of restoration you require, the gold color may be able to be disguised or hidden when you smile, but when you open your mouth, the color may be visible. If this is objectionable to you, you should consider a tooth-colored inlay, onlay, or porcelain fused to metal crown. You may be able to have the esthetics you want: gold castings for back teeth that are not easily seen and tooth-colored restorations where they might be seen.

For patients who desire the longest-lasting, most trouble-free restoration and who understand the initial investment in time and money and don't find the display of yellow gold objectionable, this is the restoration of choice. We highly recommend this type of restoration.

If you have any questions about cast gold restorations, please feel free to ask us.

Cast Gold and Ceramic Restorations

Several types of partial coverage restorative materials are available today. Two that appear to be the strongest and have the longest life expectancy are gold and ceramic/porcelain materials. Although there are some significant differences between them in their design and fabrication, they are really quite similar in concept.

The major advantages of gold are proven reliability and long life expectancy. Gold restorations have been successfully used for many years in dentistry and can last 40 years or more. Gold is the longest-lasting restorative material that dentists have to work with today. Two disadvantages of the cast gold are high initial cost and a yellow color that looks nothing like a real tooth. Comparatively, a conventional filling costs less initially, though repeated replacement costs over the course of time will be more than the cast gold restoration. The yellow color of the gold can sometimes be masked so that it is not as visible or objectionable. The smaller the restoration and the further back in your mouth, the less the gold color will show. As with the porcelain/ceramic materials, gold can be used to replace an entire tooth (a full crown) or part of a tooth (partial coverage—inlay or onlay).

Two advantages of porcelain/ceramic restorations are a natural appearance and projected long-term wear. When completed, porcelain/ceramic restorations are bonded to the prepared tooth (unlike a cast gold restoration, which is most often only cemented) and like gold, take two visits to finish. Preparation of gold and porcelain/ceramic are similar. An impression is made of the preparation and a temporary restoration is placed on the first visit. The impression is sent to a lab for fabrication. Two weeks later, the final restoration is placed. Disadvantages of porcelain/ceramic restorations include high initial cost and high degree of technical expertise needed by the dentist and laboratory.

A gold restoration is especially recommended for patients who brux (grind) or clench their teeth. Gold is also indicated for patients who want the most trouble-free, longest-lasting type of dental restoration. They are also recommended when a moderate amount of tooth destruction is evident. Gold castings are then used to cover the biting surfaces and weakened areas of the teeth to prevent fracture during normal chewing. Only cast restorations can do this. Silver amalgam fillings cannot strengthen teeth in this way. Bonded tooth-colored restorations are also not laboratory fabricated and therefore do not offer additional strength.

Porcelain/ceramic restorations are not recommended for patients who grind or brux their teeth. When placed in these patients, the patients must expect to wear a protective anti-bruxism appliance to protect the restorations. These materials are recommended for patients who demand the strongest, best looking, most esthetic materials available today.

If you have any questions about cast gold or ceramic restorations, please feel free to ask us.

Cast Porcelain Fused to Metal Restorations

A porcelain fused to metal restoration can be used in the same areas as the cast gold restoration. Since the metal is covered with a layer of porcelain, it has a much more natural appearance than a gold casting and more closely resembles a natural tooth. It also has a fairly long life expectancy of 8 to 10 years and can last longer than 25 years. This is the most common crown fabricated by dentists in the United States. When made with a noble or semi-precious metal, it usually has a high content of gold, platinum, or palladium. With porcelain fused to metal crowns, the porcelain usually covers the metal or the biting, cheek side and part of the tongue side surfaces. There is often a narrow band of uncovered metal on the tongue side. Some preparations need to have a metal collar on the cheek side, near the gum. **If you think that you will find any display of metal objectionable, let us know before the tooth is prepared.** We will discuss your concerns and either modify the porcelain to metal crown preparation or change to an all-ceramic crown if possible.

An outside laboratory is involved in the construction of the porcelain to metal crowns, which adds to the cost and extends the treatment time. Crowns are held in place by a dental cement that permanently fixes the crown onto the tooth.

Some of the disadvantages of porcelain fused to metal crowns are similar to those of the cast gold crown. They are expensive. They require at least two appointments to complete. Porcelain fused to metal crowns, require more preparation of the tooth than is necessary for gold crowns. Because it is a restoration composed of several different materials (metal, porcelain, and opaque), there are potentially more problems. Cohesive fracture of the porcelain or a fracture of porcelain from the metal is possible. The crown in these instances may still be useful, but not as esthetic. Sometimes it can be repaired and sometimes it must be replaced. Because porcelain is hard, it may wear the enamel of the opposing teeth at a rate of approximately 100 microns (0.1 mm) per year. This may not sound like a lot of wear, but in the context of the mouth, it can be quite significant. Porcelain fused to metal crowns are not usually considered a conservative type of restoration, but in cases where there has been considerable destruction of the natural tooth structure, they are the restoration of choice. In the preparation (drilling) of the natural tooth, the nerve in the tooth may become damaged and endodontic therapy (root canal treatment) may be required. While unfortunate and unpredictable, this is not uncommon.

If recession of the gum tissue occurs around the crown, a dark metal line may appear or the root may become exposed. This does not necessarily mean that the crown has to be replaced. It may still function well but not be as esthetically pleasing in appearance. Correction by periodontal plastic surgery is possible.

The cast porcelain fused to metal restoration produces a more natural looking appearance than with a gold crown, although some of the metal substructure may be visible. This restoration can be successfully used to replace a great deal of missing tooth structure. They can last a long time with proper care.

If you have any allergies to metals, please let us know before the preparations are begun.

If you have any questions about cast porcelain fused to metal restorations, please feel free to ask us.

Full Porcelain/Full Ceramic Restorations

One of the most esthetic ways to restore teeth today is to use a full cast ceramic or porcelain crown. The construction of the crown is slightly different when using a ceramic or porcelain material. The decision of material to use will need to be left to our discretion.

This type of crown contains no metal, so it approximates the total appearance of an undamaged, natural tooth more closely than any other type of full, cast crown. With today's adhesive technology, these restorations are most often bonded into place with an enamel and dentin bonding agent. The crown fabricated from all porcelain or all ceramic is much more difficult to prepare and bond into place and is technically more sensitive and demanding. It usually will take slightly longer to complete. Laboratory costs are also higher. Consequently, this type of crown is more costly.

Since the biting or incising surfaces are covered with porcelain, similar to those of a porcelain to metal crown, the wear of the opposing teeth will be the same as that of a porcelain to metal crown. There are no other significant differences.

Although some of the ceramic crowns appear to be, as are porcelain veneers, they are well supported and very strong once they have been bonded onto the tooth. It is not advised that you chew ice cubes, nuts, or hard candies with these types of restorations or with your natural teeth. It is not recommended that these restorations be used in a patient with a bruxing or grinding habit unless the patient will faithfully wear a protective mouthguard or other appliance during times of bruxing.

These are beautiful restorations, possibly the most beautiful full coverage restorations available. These restorations are more complicated to accomplish, but the rewards are well worth the effort. You can expect them to last for a long time. They will last as long as or almost as long as porcelain fused to metal crowns. If you need a full coverage restoration, and esthetics is of maximum importance to you, porcelain and ceramic crowns should be considered.

If you have any questions about full porcelain and full ceramic crowns, please feel free to ask us.

Bridges: An Overview

Replacing missing front teeth can obviously improve the appearance of your smile. What most people don't think about is what happens when a missing back tooth is not replaced. Replacing a back tooth will help you regain your normal ability to chew food and digest it properly. Each time you lose a tooth, you lose about 10% of your ability to chew. When a tooth is lost, the other teeth surrounding the space tend to move into the empty space. This contributes to an increased opportunity for decay and gum disease to begin, along with bite problems and a potential for other dental problems. Missing teeth should always be replaced—the sooner, the better.

Fixed bridges are one of the possibilities that exist for the replacement of one or more missing teeth. Other alternatives are dental implants, Maryland (bonded) bridges, partial coverage bridges, and removable partial prosthodontics.

Advantages of the fixed bridge include proven reliability and longevity. Disadvantages include cost, increased difficulty in proper cleaning by the patient, and occasionally, the necessity of preparing a tooth for an abutment (bridge support), which might not have been previously filled or even damaged.

One or more teeth can be replaced by a fixed bridge. The design of the bridge is affected by, among other factors, the number, strength, and position of the remaining teeth and the patient's ability to properly clean the completed bridge. Generally speaking, the support for the bridge should be equal to or better than the root support of what the missing teeth had.

The teeth that are to be the supports for the bridge are prepared similar to the preparation of a single crown. The tooth is made smaller by about 1 to 2 millimeters, depending on the part of the tooth being drilled. An impression is made of the prepared teeth and sent to a lab. While the bridge is being made, the prepared teeth are protected by a well-designed temporary bridge. Once the final bridge has been put in with final cement, it is not easy to get it off again without permanently damaging the porcelain and metal.

Your oral self-care must include thorough plaque removal, especially around the bridge. We will show you how to properly clean it. It is important that you follow our recommended dental hygiene recare schedule. Frequent examinations are one way to protect your investment and to maintain optimal oral health.

If you have any questions about fixed bridges, please feel free to ask us.

Full Ceramic and Porcelain Bridges

For several years, dentistry has provided very strong single-unit all tooth-colored crowns. Problems with metal sensitivities and obtaining an excellent color match with porcelain fused to metal crowns were the driving forces in promoting research and development for metal-free crowns.

For several years, dentists have been able to place full ceramic/porcelain bridges to replace a missing front tooth. Biting on front teeth does not generate as much force as biting on back teeth. Recently, dental research has developed a very good metal substructure substitute for replacing missing back teeth. These full ceramic/porcelain bridges can be used in combinations of up to five missing and supporting teeth. The ceramic substructure is not quite as strong as metal, but it is clinically acceptable.

Advantages over metal/porcelain bridges include an excellent esthetic appearance, absolutely no metal display, and no considerations of possible metal allergy. Disadvantages include a slightly higher cost and higher technique sensitivity. As with metal supported bridges, the patient's oral habits, types of food eaten, and daily oral self-care will have a great effect on the longevity of the bridge. We feel confident enough of the full ceramic and porcelain bridges to offer this service to you.

A newer option for metal-free full ceramic/porcelain crowns and bridges is the LAVA system. This innovative system uses a zirconium oxide base, which provides greater strength than was previously possible in full ceramic/porcelain crowns and bridges. The LAVA system uses a conventional impression as with other crown and bridge procedures, but the manufacturing of the crown or bridge is accomplished in a computer-controlled milling unit. This technique requires less preparation of the tooth. The crowns and bridges produced by this system are four times stronger than the full ceramic/porcelain crowns and bridges and are highly fracture-resistant with excellent esthetic properties.

As with full ceramic/porcelain crowns and bridges, there are additional costs to produce these high-quality LAVA restorations. We will provide you with information regarding your oral conditions to help you select the strongest and longest-lasting material for your new restoration.

If you have any questions about full ceramic and porcelain bridges, please feel free to ask us.

Maryland Bridge (Bonded Resin Retainer)

The Maryland bridge, or bonded resin retainer, is an alternative to implants and conventional crowns to replace missing teeth. This type of replacement procedure can be considered when the space to be restored is next to teeth in good alignment that are not heavily restored with filling materials. Because this type of bridge is adhesively bonded to the enamel on the abutment teeth, having adequate enamel is important. A Maryland bridge is fixed into place and is not meant to be removed at night.

One advantage of this process over a conventional bridge is that a missing tooth can usually be replaced with a minimum amount of preparation (drilling) of the remaining teeth. It is not necessary to prepare the tooth to the same extreme degree as with full tooth coverage restorations (crowns or caps). This method is an extremely conservative procedure. It is also less expensive (about one quarter less) than a conventional bridge. Tissue health around the abutment teeth is usually excellent because little or no preparation of the tooth structure near the gingival (gum) tissues is needed. Unlike conventional full coverage restorations, teeth prepared for a Maryland bridge retainer will not need endodontic treatment (root canal therapy) at a later date.

If the patient has abusive eating or bruxing (grinding) habits, this type of restoration is contraindicated. Although we do consider it more of a restoration for posterior (back) teeth rather than anterior teeth, it does display metal more so than a conventional bridge. The biggest disadvantage of a Maryland bridge is that the expected life may not be as long as that of a conventional bridge made of full coverage crowns. This technique was only introduced in the early 1980s and therefore does not have the extensive successful history of full coverage bridges. While breaking of a Maryland bridge is not likely, debonding can occur, requiring a re-cementation. In some rare instances, it might have to be redone. In either case, you may be charged a fee for the procedure. A Maryland bridge is a fixed replacement for a missing tooth, but one that will need to be redone in the future. The success rate at 5 years of Maryland bridges in our practice is approximately 80%. However, this is a much better result than the national average, which shows a success rate of about 33% at 4 years. Maryland bridges are most appropriate for single-tooth replacement.

If dental implants are not an option for you for tooth replacement and you do not want to have the teeth on either side of the space to be radically prepared (cut down or drilled), then you should consider the Maryland bridge technique. For many patients, the advantages of less drilling of the teeth and the reduced cost make it a desirable alternative.

If you have any questions about the Maryland bridge technique, please feel free to ask us.

Ovate Pontic

When a tooth is lost through decay, trauma, or periodontal disease, the most common way to replace it today is with a fixed bridge. The most conventional bridge uses porcelain fused to metal in fabrication. Recent advances in reinforced resin and ceramic technology have resulted in metal-less bridges to replace missing teeth. No matter what materials are used, a dental bridge consists of anchor teeth (abutment teeth) on either side of the missing tooth space with a false tooth suspended between them. The false tooth (or pontic) is suspended over the space of the missing tooth. In many cases, this type of arrangement is sufficient to provide the restoration of form, function, and esthetics that are required, especially if this is a posterior (back) tooth. The gum tissue contacting side of the pontic is shaped to "sit on" or "lap" the soft tissue ridge, similar to a saddle thrown over the back of a horse. This type of pontic form is called a *ridge lap pontic*. A later alteration of this design is called a *modified ridge lap*. In this case the saddle is placed on the horse, but one side is picked up to the height of the horse's back so that it cannot touch the horse. The advantage of this design is that food has much less of a tendency to be trapped under the pontic and the patient could more easily clean beneath the false tooth. Until a few years ago, all pontics were constructed in this fashion.

A radically different, more cosmetic pontic design has recently been used with great success. It is called the *ovate (egg-shaped) pontic*. Unlike the ridge lap design where the pontic is butted up against the soft tissue, in the ovate pontic, a depression is created in the soft tissue ridge that mimics the shape of the natural root and crown. The false tooth is then made to appear as if it is growing out of the gum tissue, and not just resting on top of it. When done well, it is difficult to see which tooth is real and which tooth is a replacement. So why isn't this pontic form made all the time?

This ovate pontic takes more work and more time to accomplish, so it will cost more. The ovate pontic shape must be prepared into the bed of ridge soft tissue. This simple, minimally invasive surgical procedure uses electrosurgery or laser to create the egg-shaped depression in the tissue ridge. After this area is allowed to heal in the correct shape, guided by the form of the provisional (temporary) bridge, the impressions are taken for the construction of the final prosthesis. If a ridge is badly deformed by the extraction of the tooth or by ridge shrinkage, an additional surgical procedure (ridge augmentation) may be necessary to build out the ridge prior to shaping it for the ovate pontic. This will also add cost and time to the construction of the bridge. So while the shaping can be done in one appointment, two or even three procedures may be necessary.

The ovate pontic will give you maximum cosmetic improvement, look the most natural, and be the easiest to clean. If you have a high lip line, showing much of your teeth when you talk or smile, or demand the best esthetics available, then you need to consider the ovate pontic. After examining you, we will evaluate your tissue contour and smile line and determine what would be involved in creating the ovate pontic. This is the design we favor the most; it looks the best and is easiest to keep clean. Please understand that if the area has been missing a tooth for a long time, or if the area has shrunk from the normal position so that the normal architecture is destroyed, it will take a little more effort to create the ovate pontic.

If you have any questions about your particular needs, please feel free to ask us.

Partial Coverage Bonded Bridges

You may be familiar with the three common methods for replacing missing teeth—crowns and bridges (caps), dental implants, and removable partial dentures. The first two are permanently cemented onto the teeth and will, therefore, stay in the mouth at all times. The third option, a removable partial denture, must be taken out nightly. Bridges and implants work very well as anchors for replacing missing teeth. A disadvantage of implants is their cost and time to complete the crown or bridge fabrication. A disadvantage of a bridge is the amount of tooth that must be prepared (drilled away) to allow sufficient thickness of gold alloy and porcelain to be used. While this is acceptable with teeth that have large fillings, drilling away significant amounts of a tooth structure on a previously nonrestored tooth is not acceptable. Our treatment goal is to replace a missing tooth without removing the majority of natural tooth structure on the teeth adjacent to the missing tooth.

Recently, partial coverage bonded bridges have been used with great success. This new technique for partial coverage bridges requires a much smaller amount of tooth structure to be removed. If there is an existing restoration in the tooth, that filling will be removed, and the partial coverage bridge may be designed to include that preparation area. Currently, this is the most conservative type of bridge design available. An added advantage to a partial coverage bonded bridge is that the cost may be less than that for a conventional metal/porcelain bridge.

The appointment for the preparation and impressions for the bridge is similar to that for a conventional bridge. The partial coverage bridge is made from a laboratory-processed resin that is reinforced with a titanium bar. The bar is totally hidden within the resin material. The bridge will be bonded (not cemented) into place. The color match is usually excellent.

These types of bridges have been used successfully for years. The partial coverage retained bridge is a highly desirable option for replacing one missing tooth, especially a posterior (back) tooth if there are few or no fillings on either side of the missing tooth space.

Implants: Options

Twenty-five years ago, if someone described how missing teeth could be replaced with implants, it might have been called a miracle. Ten years ago, the use of dental implants to replace missing teeth might have been called astounding. Today, implant procedures are called routine. We would like you to have a basic understanding of what implants are, what can be expected from them, and what limitations they might have in your specific area of need.

A dental implant is a synthetic metallic root substitute that is placed or implanted in the jaw bone. It can be used to replace a single missing tooth, provide an abutment (anchor or retainer), replace several missing teeth, or provide added retention to a removable dental appliance such as a full denture. In fact, if you are missing all of your natural teeth, it is possible to have maxillary (upper) and mandibular (lower) fixed replacements. The replacements do not come out and you cannot remove them yourself.

Two separate events are needed when replacing a missing tooth with an implant. First is the surgical phase in which the implant is placed. In the second phase the replacement teeth are constructed and fixed into proper position.

The implant placement procedure involves making a small incision in the gum area where the implant is to placed, preparing a site in the underlying bone, inserting the implant into the prepared site, and closing the tissue over the implant with several sutures. This area is left undisturbed, usually for 4 to 6 months. More healing time may vary due to the density of your bone. The lower jaw is composed of bone that is more dense than that of the upper jaw. This healing time allows for the slow integration of the implant within your jaw. The implant is held in place by the bone.

After the healing and integration of the implant, the placement site is exposed by reopening the gum. A post will then be fastened to the implant by cement or with internal threads. The crown, bridge, or other type of replacement will be attached to this post. Some dentists prefer to do all phases of the implant procedure themselves, but many choose to perform either the surgical or prosthetic (the actual construction of the replacement device) only. If this is the case, you will be referred to a periodontist or oral surgeon who will perform the surgical portion of the implant placement.

Implants are very successful. Maxillary and mandibular implants are more than 90% successful. Lower implants have a somewhat higher success rate than upper implants. Occasionally, implants fail, but it is not common. Chances of an implant failure, many times, can be determined during or after the surgical phase before the replacement tooth or teeth are constructed.

☛ **Smokers take note:** *There is a heightened risk of dental implant failure among smokers—as much as a 20% greater failure rate!*

We will discuss with you the requirements and options for your particular situation. There are usually several possibilities for effectively replacing missing teeth. It is important to decide on the design of the implant-retained replacement prior to the actual implant surgical procedure. Position and alignment of the replacement teeth need to be carefully considered before determining the location of the implant.

If you have any questions about implants, please feel free to ask us.

Implants: Procedural Overview

Compared to a routine dental filling or crown (cap), replacement of a missing tooth or teeth with implants is a more complicated and lengthy process. It will take several phases. A periodontist or an oral surgeon will place the implant surgically. Then we will place the tooth or visible portion.

Phase One

In phase one of the treatment, the specialist evaluates the position, suitability, and strength of the bone that will surround the implant. This information will determine the length and width of the implants and how many implants will be necessary to replace the missing teeth. Impressions of all your teeth will be taken for study models in order to design the shape of the tooth or teeth to be implanted. A surgical guide will be made to indicate to the surgeon where the implants should be placed.

Phase Two

Phase two consists of the surgical procedures to place the implant in the bone. A local anesthetic is given, and the gum tissue is lifted to expose the implant site. The implant is placed into the bone and the gum is closed over it. You will not see the implant while integration with the bone takes place. The integration takes 4 to 6 months. After this time, the site is opened again and a healing collar will be threaded into the implant. This will guide the tissue into a shape that is needed for the future crown(s). The time that the healing collar needs to be in place will vary from person to person, but will be at least several weeks.

Phase Three

Phase three will begin once the tissue shape is sufficient. In this phase, specific attachments and components will be fitted to the implant. The implant components are similar in function to the wall or plaster anchors used to hang pictures on drywall. The healing collar is removed. Implant transfer copings, analogs, and other items are used to take an impression of the site. The healing collar is then put back on. The impressions and implant components are sent to the laboratory for fabrication of implant posts and temporary acrylic crowns.

When the temporary crown or bridge is returned from the laboratory, the healing collar is removed and the implant attachments are fastened to the implant. The temporary crowns are then seated and adjusted. They will be held in place by temporary cement or with screws, depending on your certain situation. We will explain the advantages and disadvantages of each in your particular case at the time you decide to have the implant.

Temporary crowns are placed because the bone that supports and surrounds the implant must be given the opportunity to be put into function gradually. Implant techniques dictate that the implants be slowly brought into biting function. This means you will be returning several times to have more acrylic added to the temporary crown. After the implant and temporary crown have been in biting function for a few months, the final crown(s) will be fabricated and cemented or screwed into place.

Maintaining All Your Teeth

To keep your implants and your natural teeth healthy and functional for the longest time possible, clean the implant and your other teeth daily, as instructed. You will also need to come in for dental hygiene recare appointments at a 3- to 4-month interval. You have invested time and money in these state-of-the-art tooth replacements. Maintaining them as instructed will give you the best chance of success.

We feel that the benefits of replacing teeth with implant-supported crowns and bridges far outweigh the inconvenience of the long start to finish time. This is especially true when the teeth on either side of the implant are sound, unfilled teeth that would not otherwise require dental treatment. Implants help you preserve your natural tooth structure.

If you have any questions about dental implants, please feel free to ask us.

Biologic Width

When a tooth is severely damaged by decay, trauma, or fracture, its restoration becomes more difficult. The restoration of choice in these instances is a laboratory-processed crown or partial coverage onlay. Usually, it is much better and less costly in the long run to save the tooth rather than extract it and consider an artificial replacement. If the damage extends below the gumline, to near or beyond the crest of the bone, preliminary treatment is required before the restoration can be successfully placed.

Biologic width is a term used by dentists to describe a 2.5-mm distance that must exist between the crest of the bone (closest to the biting surfaces of the tooth) and the end of any restoration. If this 2.5-mm distance is not kept, the soft tissue (gum tissue) will become chronically inflamed and the crown or onlay will be a failure. Insufficient biologic width must be corrected.

There are several possibilities for creating sufficient biologic width. What we recommend will depend on the severity of the damage, which tooth is affected, and the bone and gum architecture of the adjacent teeth.

For posterior (multi-rooted) teeth, the corrective therapy involves a periodontal surgical procedure. An incision is made in the gum tissue around the tooth. The tissue is reflected, and the fracture site, visualized. Then, the height of bone is reshaped so that it is not near the place where the restoration will end. Only enough bone is removed to establish the 2.5-mm biologic width. Obviously, there will be a limit as to how much bone can be reshaped. Most of the time, this can be determined before surgical entry. At times, this may not be known until the affected site is clearly visible. Radiographs do not always give the whole picture. After the surgery, there will be a 3- to 4-month wait so that the site can heal. After that time, the final restoration can be started.

For single-rooted teeth, surgery can be done. But rather than cutting away gum and bone, sometimes it is possible to orthodontically erupt the tooth so that the fracture site is moved away from the crest of the bone. This can be done in about 4 months. If the tooth is moved in this manner, the bone will slowly come along with the tooth. After the tooth has reached its final position, the bone will need to be trimmed to the proper relationship with the adjacent tooth. For some teeth, rapid eruption may be possible. When done in 3½ to 4 weeks, the bone will not move along with the erupting tooth so it may not have to be adjusted. When the orthodontics is done, the tooth must be stabilized in the new position for about 6 months before the final restoration can be begun. In some situations, a combination of both types of approaches will be used.

If you need to have a proper biologic width restored before restoration of a tooth, it can be established orthodontically or surgically or in combination. If this is not done, the final restoration will never be successful. What we will recommend to you depends on the nature of the break, which tooth is broken, and the position of the adjacent teeth, gingival tissues (gum), and bone.

If you have any questions about the need for adequate biologic width, please feel free to ask us.

Illustration on CD-ROM

Cementation: Postoperative Instructions

The dental laboratory has completed the fabrication on your following dental work:
- ❑ **crown(s)**
- ❑ **bridge(s)**
- ❑ **inlay(s)**
- ❑ **onlay(s)**

These restorations have been cemented with a:
- ❑ **glass ionomer**
- ❑ **zinc phosphate polycarboxylate cement**
- ❑ **bonded with a resin bonding cement**

Tooth Sensitivity

Occasionally, following the cementation or bonding process, there may be some transient (passing) sensitivity that can last from several days to several months. This is not unusual and may relate, in part, to the cementation/bonding procedure or the amount of tooth that was removed during the preparation for the restoration.

Sensitivity may also be related to the occlusion (bite). If your teeth have been anesthetized for the cementation/bonding procedure, it may be difficult for you to tell if your bite feels normal following the cementation/bonding of a new restoration. This occasionally results in a bite that is not correct. When the anesthetic wears off, you might notice that the bite does not feel correct. It will feel high and the new restoration will meet the opposing teeth too soon. This can cause the nerve in the tooth to become irritated and sensitive to hot or cold stimulation. Adjusting the occlusion will usually rectify this problem.

Occasionally, this sensitivity does not go away and may, in fact, get worse. This is not usually related to the cementation/bonding procedure but is a result of the extensive amount of original tooth destruction you experienced from decay. Although the tooth may appear to be fine while the provisional (temporary) restoration is in place, the nerve may in reality be slowly dying. In this situation, the restored tooth may eventually experience nerve death. The tooth will then need endodontic treatment.

Care of Your New Restoration

After the cementation or bonding, it is advisable to **not** use the tooth to chew food until normal sensation returns to the area (if the area was anesthetized). Cements set only partially while you are in the office and require at least 24 hours to achieve better physical properties. So do not stress the cemented or bonded teeth for 24 hours (i.e., no gum chewing, taffy, biting on nuts or bagels, etc.).

It is very important to your continuing oral health to brush and floss the teeth normally after this procedure. Please return to us for your normal preventive recare appointments at intervals of _____ months. Problems that may develop around the restorations (or any other teeth, for that matter) can then be found at an early stage and repaired easily. We will send you a notice when you are due for the appointment, but you should also indicate on your own calendar when it is time to return, and call the office if the notice is not received.

We also recommend daily use of a fluoride-containing mouthrinse. Follow the instructions on the label. Regular topical application of fluoride has been shown to reduce the incidence of some types of dental problems.

Expectations

You should receive many years of service from these restorations. We have used the best information, procedures, and materials available today in their fabrication. It is possible that they may require replacement if they fracture due to extreme force or trauma—the same as with natural teeth. Do not bite extremely hard objects with the teeth that have been cemented or bonded. The gingiva (gums) may also recede from the margins of the restoration, exposing metal or original tooth structure. It can take several years before it is noticed. Recession is usually a result of the normal aging process and does not indicate that the restoration is a failure. If a cosmetic problem results from the recession, however, you may want the restoration redone. Decay may also begin near the restoration. If the decay is caught at an early stage, it is not a major problem to fix.

If you have any questions about these instructions, please feel free to ask us.

Crown Lengthening Procedures

A crown lengthening procedure is necessary when there is insufficient tooth structure remaining clinically visible or accessible for proper retention of a cast restoration (a crown or onlay) or for routine restoration (filling). It is also necessary if the gum tissue has poor position or contour or for improving the cosmetic appearance of the teeth. It may also be required in order to make a successful impression for a cast restoration. The soft gingival tissues will be modified, repositioned, or reshaped so that a restoration can be placed. If the tooth has been severely decayed, crown lengthening may be necessary to more completely expose the decayed area and allow better preparation for the final filling.

Many times, this crown lengthening will be minimal and it can be done in our office. This may involve electrosurgery or a scalpel and suturing procedure. We will select the method based on your individual circumstances. If the modification is extensive, involving many teeth or the supporting bone, you may be referred to a periodontist (gum specialist) for evaluation and treatment. At times, after the crown lengthening is completed and the tissue is healed, the tooth may exhibit temporary sensitivity to thermal changes. With time, the sensitivity decreases. Also, we do not want the tissue that is removed to grow back. If it does grow back, which can happen, it may need to be removed again.

Restorations placed on sound tooth structure will last the longest possible time. One tooth or several teeth may be involved in the lengthening procedure. In many cases, it would be impossible to obtain a satisfactory result if the crown lengthening were not performed. Postoperative discomfort is usually minimal unless the crown lengthening has been extensive, as when the underlying bone must be recontoured. Over-the-counter pain relievers are usually very adequate. Healing time varies, depending on the extent of the procedure. Sometimes we will elect to finish the restoration or make the final impression at the time of the crown lengthening; other times we must wait for the site to heal. Healing time may be 4 to 6 weeks. This will be discussed with you when the crown lengthening procedure is suggested.

If a crown lengthening is recommended, you should have it done, or the final restoration may be compromised and the chance of obtaining a clinically successful restoration would be seriously reduced.

If you have any questions about the crown lengthening procedure, please feel free to ask us.

Extraction Site Defect

Teeth are removed for several reasons, including periodontal disease, extreme decay, and for orthodontic reasons. Once a tooth is removed, the shape of the ridge (i.e., the supporting bone and gum in which the tooth was situated and retained) changes. If there has been extensive bone loss, or if the tooth needed to be surgically removed (bone had to be cut away to gain access to the area), the change will be more dramatic. The ridge shrinks, collapses into itself, and over time decreases in width and height. As more time passes after the extraction, the more change occurs. This is an extraction site defect.

The extraction site defect presents a problem when the area is to be restored with a bridge or an implant. When the ridge architecture has significantly changed, the replacement tooth will have to deviate from the ideal shape. This could easily make the area more difficult to keep clean, difficult for the dentist to restore, and cosmetically quite unsightly. Perhaps the cosmetics may not matter to you when there is a back tooth being replaced—one that is not visible when you speak or smile. An extraction site defect in an area visible when you speak or smile will create a severe esthetic problem. The more the ridge has changed, the more the pontic will need to be either longer, wider, or fatter in order to fill up the extraction site. If you have a smile line that shows the tooth or gumline, the replacement tooth will be very obviously misshaped. It will never look right and will always be a cosmetic failure.

It is clear that for the replacement tooth to have a normal appearance, the extraction site must be rebuilt. The closer it can be made to the ideal, the better the replacement tooth will appear. The site (or *ridge* as it is called by dentists) will be restored through soft tissue or soft and hard tissue minor periodontal surgical procedures. If the ridge needs only a small amount of augmentation, only soft tissue procedures will be needed. If there is a large defect, the underlying supporting bone will have to be replaced as well. If the site is especially visible or needs an extensive amount of rebuilding, more than one augmentation procedure may be necessary. Our goal is to make the replacement tooth appear to be growing out of the extraction site, not merely lying against the soft tissue ridge.

If a dental implant is to be placed to act as an anchor for the replacement tooth, the extraction site must have enough bone thickness and height to properly surround the implant. These procedures almost always involve hard (bone) and soft tissue modification. We will let you know what is appropriate for you.

If you have any questions, please feel free to ask us.

Ferrule

If a tooth is going to receive a full coverage laboratory-processed restoration that will be successful for the long term, there are several variables that must be addressed. There must be no decay left on the prepared tooth. Its periodontal position (gum and bone) must be sound. The crown placed on the tooth must have an accurate fit, with the bite adjusted well and the margins of the crown/tooth interface sealed and adapted well. There must be sufficient tooth structure left to retain the crown and resist external forces that could dislodge the crown or fracture the underlying tooth.

While all these things are important, one of the most important factors in a successful long-term crown is that there is adequate tooth structure remaining around the circumference of the tooth so that the crown can resist lateral forces. These are forces that are not directed straight up and down (parallel to) the long axis of the tooth, but are rather tangential vector forces applied from the side (perpendicular to the long axis of the tooth).

You have a tooth that has been extensively damaged due to decay or fracture and there is very little of the tooth remaining above the gumline. In dentistry, a ferrule is an average 2-mm width of sound, undamaged, unrestored tooth that is available 360 degrees around the tooth for the crown to "grab." Even if posts (used on endodontically treated teeth) or pins and bonded core buildups are used to restore tooth structure under a crown, unless this adequate ferrule is present, the tooth can quite possibly be too weak to support a restoration and break under normal chewing forces. The longevity of the restoration is compromised.

If the necessary 2-mm ferrule is not available around the circumference of the tooth, one must be artificially created. There are two methods of developing a ferrule. If the tooth is broken off at the gumline or below, the tooth can be orthodontically erupted (a forced extrusion of the remaining tooth from the bone, considered a very controlled, slow, painless extraction) until enough tooth is available to use. This can be done in a matter of a month or so in most instances. The second method is to remove gum tissue (and/or bone) to expose the necessary 2 mm of tooth. This may be done by a laser or electrosurgery procedure or periodontal surgery. The procedure chosen will be a function of how much tooth needs to be exposed, where the tooth is, where the gumline is in respect to the adjacent teeth, and how far the fractured site is, at its deepest distance, from the underlying bone. There needs to be at least 2.5 mm of distance between the margin of the prepared tooth (and thus the final restoration) and the top of the bone. This space is called the *biologic width*. It is critical to have sufficient biologic width. If there is less space available and it is not created, the gum tissue will never heal properly.

After using radiographs, clinical inspection, and a periodontal measuring probe, we will determine which course of action is best. There may be extra time and expense in establishing the correct ferrule, but it is vital that this be done if the tooth is to be restored successfully for the long term.

If you have any questions about the procedure(s) needed to gain a clinically acceptable ferrule, please feel free to ask us.

Impressions

There are two types of impressions that we routinely take in this office. The first type is for the fabrication of study models and diagnostic casts. The second is for the construction of laboratory-processed crowns, bridges, and removable partial dentures.

Study Model or Preliminary Impressions

Study model impressions are the most common impressions made in a dental office. A sterilized metal tray or a disposable plastic tray is used for this procedure. The tray is fitted approximately to the dimensions of your upper or lower jaws and will cover your teeth and gum tissue. Once fitted, the tray is partially filled with a soft, viscous impression material. This material has the consistency of thick cookie dough batter. The filled impression tray is placed over your teeth and gently pressed into place. The material will take from 1 to 2 minutes to set. The impressions are absolutely painless and require no medication or special preparation. The material has a moderately pleasant taste.

From this impression, stone models will be made that are a very close duplicate of your teeth. These models allow us to analyze your teeth and properly design your dental treatment. We investigate the possibilities of orthodontics (braces), custom trays for whitening teeth, and replacement of missing or severely damaged teeth. We make custom trays for final impressions, guides for temporary crowns, mouthguards, splints, etc.

Final Impressions

This type of impression is for fabrication of crowns, bridges, or partial dentures. The impressions are made with a different material, one that is much more accurate in demonstrating the smallest details of the prepared area. Because of the increased need for precision, the impression is different. A custom-fabricated tray is often made from the model made in the preliminary impression. This material will be in place for 3 to 6 minutes. Often, a local anesthetic has been used to prepare the tooth so there should be no discomfort. It is not uncommon that a second or third impression might be taken to ensure the accurate fit of the finished restoration. If the impression is not right, the final restoration will be compromised.

Occlusal Registration

With both types of impressions, it is standard practice to take an occlusal (bite) registration during the appointment. This gives us the ability to relate the upper and lower jaw models. The impression may be placed on a tray or directly onto the biting surface of your teeth; you will then be instructed to bite down and hold your bite in place until the material sets. The bite registration impression sets very quickly.

If you have any questions about impressions, please feel free to ask us.

Posts

After a tooth has had its nerve tissue removed by endodontics (root canal treatment), often there is very little remaining tooth structure. Before a crown (cap), silver amalgam, or bonded resin restoration can be placed, a post may be positioned into the tooth to help give support and retention to the remaining tooth and restoration. The post can be a cast custom or a prefabricated post.

The prefabricated posts can be made of stainless steel, titanium, or a tooth-colored ceramic or reinforced resin. They are designed in various diameters and lengths. If you think you might be allergic to any metals, especially nickel, let us know before we select which post is to be used. A special drill is used to remove some of the root canal filling material (gutta percha) and shape the canal for the post. The length and diameter of the post correspond to the dimensions of the prepared canal space. Once the post has been fitted, it will either be cemented with a glass ionomer or other cement or bonded into place with a resin. The choice of the cementing medium is affected by the length and position of the tooth that will receive the post, the type of restoration to go over the post, and your past history of dental decay.

If a root canal has been filled with silver points instead of gutta percha, the silver points probably need to be removed and replaced; that is, the root canal will be redone with the gutta percha material. The cement that holds the silver points in place has a tendency to dissolve and the points will become loose. The new post and crown must be placed over a sound root canal filling in order to avoid future problems that could require removal of the newly placed post and crown.

The post will help the crown (or filling) resist some of the stresses that a tooth undergoes when you chew hard or sticky foods. It will reduce the possibility that the tooth will shear off at the gumline. It will serve to retain any filling, crown, or core buildup that is used to reconstruct the tooth. It is still possible that the tooth can shear off at the gumline, filling, or crown or come out even with the post in place. It is more likely to become dislodged if you eat very hard or sticky foods or bite into them the wrong way. The more remaining undamaged tooth structure, the less likely that this will happen. Crown lengthening may be needed before a post and crown are placed to allow more tooth structure to be used.

A cast post will entail more work on the part of the dentist. At least one extra visit will be needed. It does cost more than a prefabricated post. It is not used as routinely as a prefabricated post, but rather in special situations. It is cemented or bonded into place.

If you have any questions about posts, please feel free to ask us.

Posts, Core-Crown Buildups, and Crown Lengthening

Posts

After a tooth has had its nerve tissue removed by endodontics (root canal treatment), very often there is little remaining undamaged tooth structure. Before a restoration is placed, whether it is a crown (cap) or a silver or bonded filling, a post is placed into the tooth to help give support and retention to the remaining tooth and subsequent restoration. The post can be a cast custom-fitted post or a prefabricated post. The prefabricated post is made in various diameters, materials, and lengths. It may be metal or tooth colored. A special drill is used to remove part of the root canal filling material (gutta percha) and prepare and shape the canal for the post. Once the post has been fitted, it is either cemented into place with a glass ionomer material or bonded with a resin cement. Choice of cementing medium is affected by the length of the post, location of the tooth that the post is to be in, and past history of dental decay. If the existing root canal has been filled with silver points, they must be removed before the crown can be constructed. The cement that holds the silver points in the canals has been shown to dissolve quickly. The new crown must be placed over a sound root canal filling in order to avoid future endodontic problems that might require removal of the new crown.

The post will help the tooth resist some of the stresses that it undergoes when you chew hard or sticky foods. It will reduce the possibility that the tooth will shear off at the gumline. It will also serve to retain any filling, crown, or core buildup material that has been used in the tooth. It is still possible for the tooth to fracture, even with a post in place. It is also possible that the post may become dislodged if you eat especially hard or sticky foods and bite the wrong way. The more original tooth you have left, the less likely this is to happen.

Core-Crown Buildups

A core buildup or crown buildup is placed when there is insufficient tooth structure remaining to retain the future crown. It can be made out of silver amalgam, bonded resin, or glass ionomer. The choice of the material used relates to how much tooth is missing and how long the tooth must be in place without the final crown being cemented. Usually, if a post is placed, a buildup is also required. The more real or artificially reconstructed (core buildup) tooth structure there is available, the better the final crown will stay in place.

Crown Lengthening

Crown lengthening by electrosurgery or conventional surgery is a procedure that is performed to correct one of the following conditions:

    insufficient tooth clinically remaining to allow proper retention of a crown

    sound tooth structure that is beneath the gingival (gum) tissue

    gingival tissue that is in poor position or contour

Electrosurgery permits the repositioning, modification, or removal of soft tissue by employing a calibrated electric current. Conventional surgery is done with a scalpel and involves suturing. When there is insufficient tooth structure available for crown retention, the adequate tooth structure must be exposed, and the necessary gum tissue, removed. When the tooth cannot be kept isolated and dry during dental procedures, it becomes much harder, sometimes impossible, to get a satisfactory result. Saliva, blood, and water from your mouth affect dental material in an adverse fashion. Removing excess and unwanted tissue allows the tooth to be kept dry, thus increasing the possibility of a good result. Simply stated, when the dentist cannot see the work area, the results will probably not be satisfactory.

There is very little postoperative pain associated with the electrosurgery procedure. Most patients say that it feels like a burn from hot cheese on a pizza. A nonprescription pain reliever is usually adequate. Occasionally, the crown lengthening cannot be adequately completed with electrosurgery. Surgical crown lengthening will require sutures and delay in the final impression for the crown while the tissue heals. Four to eight weeks' healing time is usual. When either type of crown lengthening is not done, the chance of clinical success of the crown is seriously reduced.

All posts, core-crown buildups, and crown lengthening are grouped together on this page because it is very common that these procedures need to be done together. If a tooth needs a root canal treatment, it is usually fairly well broken down and difficult to restore. Each procedure may be called for on its own, or with one or both of the other procedures. If any of these procedures need to be done, there will be a fee charged separate from the crown fee.

If you have any questions about posts, core-crown buildups, and crown lengthening, please feel free to ask us.

Provisional Crowns

When a crown is being fabricated for you, the tooth or teeth treated will have an acrylic provisional (temporary) restoration that is retained by temporary cement. This is part of the treatment and does not warrant an additional fee. However, there are several instances when provisional crowns need to be made as a separate and intermediate procedure. Because of extra time and work involved, beyond that needed for a crown or bridge, there is a separate fee for the procedure.

One situation where a provisional crown warrants a separate fee involves a tooth or teeth that are severely decayed or broken, where the vitality of the nerve or the periodontal (gum) health is in question. It may be necessary to rebuild the tooth as soon as possible so that the health of the nerve inside the tooth, and the periodontal tissue surrounding the tooth, can be evaluated over time before proceeding with the final crown. When multiple teeth need this treatment, it is customary to place the provisional crowns on each at the same time. If each tooth is taken to completion individually before beginning the next tooth, there is too much opportunity for the remaining damaged teeth to deteriorate further, thereby complicating treatment and adding to the total cost. Provisional crowns may be in place for several months before further treatment is started on the tooth, after which time the tooth will need to have further preparation and a new provisional crown made.

When the nerve in the damaged tooth has a chance of dying, it is easier to save the tooth with root canal therapy if the final crown has not been placed. It often takes months for the health of the nerve to be determined. And, in fact, despite using a long-term provisional crown, the nerve may die years after the final crown is placed. When that happens, the access for the endodontic treatment is made through the crown. With respect to the periodontal tissues, if they are infected or in poor health, they must be healed before final impressions are made. Periodontal treatment coupled with a well-fitted provisional crown will promote proper healing. After the periodontal tissue is healthy, its position with respect to the crown margins will change, and the tooth will be re-prepared and a second provisional restoration will be made.

Another reason for long-term provisional crowns to be placed is to stabilize loose teeth and determine the necessary support for the final cast crowns. When a tooth involved in support for a bridge or splint has a questionable prognosis, it is a good idea to make a provisional bridge first and let the tooth (or teeth) function together for some time to see how well they respond. If the tooth turns out to be hopeless, it can be removed. If teeth are restored in quadrants at a time (three, four, five, or more), it may be necessary to do the opposing arch in long-term provisional crowns in order to establish the ideal occlusal (biting) relationships between the arches.

There are many and varied reasons why long-term provisional bridges might be needed. They might stay in place from months to years, especially in very complicated cases such as many teeth that are broken down and moderate to severe gum disease needing correction before the crowns are finally placed. In larger cases, financial limitations may dictate that treatment be phased over a longer time frame. Rather than let the teeth get worse during this time, long-term provisional crowns are made to hold things in place until the treatment can continue.

It is important that you understand why provisional crowns might be necessary for your dental health.

If you have any questions about long-term provisional crowns, please feel free to ask us.

Provisional Crowns: Postoperative Instructions

You have received a:
- ❏ plastic provisional restoration retained by provisional cement
- ❏ final restoration that has been trial cemented with a provisional cement

- The provisional cement requires about 45 minutes to set properly. Please avoid chewing food during this period of time.
- The provisional restorations or final restorations are now held in place with a temporary cement. This weak cement is used in order to facilitate removal of the restoration for further procedures. Do not chew anything sticky while the temporary cement is being used. These provisional restorations are meant to be in place for only a short period of time. The final cement that will be used is much stronger.
- The provisional restoration may not resemble the final restoration in size, color, texture, shape, or in any other way.
- Certain foods may stick to the provisional restoration material. This will not happen with the final gold or porcelain restorations.
- Provisional restorations are **not** strong. They may break or come off. If this happens, call our office and we will attend to them. If you are somewhere where you cannot contact a dentist and the provisional crown or bridge comes off, go to a pharmacy and purchase a tube of cream denture adhesive. Clean out the provisional restoration and replace it on your tooth or teeth with some of the adhesive placed in each crown that fits over a prepared tooth. This denture adhesive will hold the provisional restoration in place until you can return to our office for further treatment. **Do not leave the provisional restoration out of your mouth for an extended period of time!** The teeth surrounding the prepared teeth or the prepared teeth themselves could move and the final restoration may then not fit properly.
- If you have **a final restoration that is cemented for a short time with provisional cement,** please avoid sticky foods such as gum, etc. Chewing these types of food items could cause the provisional cement to fail; and the final bridge, crown, onlay, or inlay could loosen.
- Please brush and floss your teeth daily as you have been instructed. If you have a provisional restoration in place, when you use floss, begin as usual but when it is time to remove the floss, let go of the floss with one hand and pull it from between the teeth with the other hand. This will reduce the possibility of the floss "catching" the edge of the provisional restoration and pulling it off the tooth.
- It is possible that the prepared teeth, now covered by the provisional restoration, will be sensitive to hot, cold, or sweets. This is not uncommon. The provisional restorations may leak saliva or other fluids onto the newly prepared (drilled) tooth. This will not be the case with the final restoration.

Additional Instructions
- ❏ Rinse with chlorhexidine gluconate _____ times daily until one week after the final cementation.
- ❏ Rinse with warm salt water as instructed.
- ❏ Rinse with _____.
- ❏ Brush and floss as instructed after every meal.

If you have any questions about these instructions, please feel free to ask us.

Study Models and Wax Ups

Quite often, a patient will have dental problems that require a more detailed analysis in order to determine possible solutions. Teeth can be directly examined, but because of the limitations imposed by the tongue, lips, cheeks, and the small angle of sight from the front of the mouth, the ability to provide an appropriate treatment plan can be compromised. As more teeth are missing and more teeth shift from where they belong, especially in cases where the problem has been in existence for many years, more options for treatment become possible. This can be the case for extensive dental treatment or for only a few teeth that need restoration.

We will need to make study models (impressions) of the teeth, and we will also make a registration of how the teeth meet, in order to help plan treatment. We will be able to see things on the models that we cannot see clinically. We can also work with the models of your teeth between appointments. And that's a definite convenience for you! The models will show us many factors, especially in tooth movement, such as whether teeth have moved, how far they have moved, how they may have affected other teeth, as well as other considerations. If you are planning on fixed bridges or crowns or removable bridges (partials) to replace the missing teeth, the design must be exact from the moment treatment starts for the best result.

We use a diagnostic "wax up" to help us (and you) visualize possible changes to the shape and alignment of your teeth. The wax up shows teeth and gum tissue, usually in white plaster with white wax added. The original study models provide a three-dimensional look at the "before" condition of your teeth, and the wax up will give a three-dimensional "after" picture of what your teeth, replacements of missing teeth, etc. will look like when the treatment is completed. The wax up is often used where there are moderate to significant cosmetic changes to be considered. In conjunction with the wax up, it is possible to have the before picture converted to a digital image and then computer modified to show an "after" image. The digitized picture will have your lips, cheeks, gum tissue, and face visible and in proper color.

The wax up is valuable for you too. You will be able to judge the proposed changes and approve them. If you don't like them, it is relatively simple to have the wax up changed for a different look. Once the wax up is approved by both you and us, it will be used as the foundation for the anticipated treatment. The better a treatment is planned, the better the chance of a successful result.

There is an additional cost for either the study models or the diagnostic wax up. Fees for the study models are fixed. Fees for the diagnostic wax up depend on the number of teeth that are being modified. For an extensive "makeover" a fee of several hundred dollars is possible.

If you have any questions about the need for or use of diagnostic study models or a wax up, please feel free to ask us.

Full Dentures

Full dentures replace a full arch of missing teeth to restore chewing and facial appearance. A denture can be constructed to replace missing top teeth, missing bottom teeth, or both.

A denture is normally constructed of an acrylic (plastic) base, colored pink to look like the gum tissue it covers. The teeth are either plastic or porcelain. Choice of which type of material to use for the teeth will be based on our judgment and what the teeth in the opposing arch are. Porcelain goes against porcelain. Acrylic goes against acrylic or natural tooth.

If you already have a denture or dentures, construction of new dentures is relatively easy. Your mouth is familiar with the feel of the denture. Preliminary impressions are made from which more exact impression trays are designed and fabricated. These trays are used to make a final master impression, from which the denture will be made. The line of the teeth and thickness of the denture are established in wax and checked. Teeth are selected by color, form, and material. They are placed in the wax and tried in place in the mouth. When you approve the form, design, and setup of the teeth, the dental laboratory will complete the process in acrylic. Then they are returned to the office and delivered to you. They will be adjusted at that time. Expect to make several visits with us, as the dentures settle in and sore spots develop. Do not expect the new dentures to fit the same as your old ones. Dentures cannot be exactly duplicated. The feel will always be different. Not worse, just different.

If you have recently had one or a few teeth extracted, or are having a full denture made after wearing a removable partial denture, you will need more time to adjust to the new full denture. It can take 3 to 6 months for soft tissue to heal and reshape itself fully after an extraction. The more teeth removed, the more change there will be and the longer it will take to heal. Many times, a denture is made before this time period has elapsed. Expect to have more sore spots and more adjustments before the denture feels comfortable. You may also expect to have the denture relined after a few months to compensate for that tissue change. The reline fills in the space that develops under the denture by the extraction site. Partial dentures have some mechanical retention from clasps on teeth. Full dentures do not have this help and are more difficult to keep in place.

If you have a denture or dentures, make sure to remove them daily. Do not sleep with them in. Your gums need a chance to have unimpeded circulation of fresh blood. Dentures tend to restrict blood flow. Plaque can accumulate on your denture and on your gum tissue. Use a very soft toothbrush to gently brush your gums. Be sure to keep your dentures clean by brushing them daily with a denture brush and denture cleanser—and be sure to store them in water when they are not being worn.

If you have any questions about full dentures, please feel free to ask us.

Immediate Dentures

Immediate full or partial dentures are made when teeth are extracted on the same day that the finished dentures are inserted. Immediate dentures are different from regular dentures in that the final impressions are made before some or all of the teeth that are to be removed are extracted. Traditionally, fabricated dentures are constructed to replace an already existing full denture. There is no healing time necessary and the initial fit will be much better because the impressions will exactly reflect the soft tissues on which the denture base rests.

With immediate denture construction, there is an approximation of the fit of the denture base. Because the teeth are still in place when the denture is being constructed and tried in, the fit will not be as exact initially. It is more difficult to try in the immediate denture to check for fit and appearance when the teeth are still in place. This is especially true when the natural teeth that will be removed have drifted far out of their original position. Immediate dentures are made so that the patient will not be forced to be without teeth while the gum tissues heal and the remaining tissue ridges reach their final shape. This final healing can take 3 to 6 months after the teeth are removed.

The immediate denture will be inserted the same day the teeth are removed. Because of this, the patient will be numb and swollen from the local anesthetic, and not really able to tell much about the comfort of the denture base and the set of the denture teeth against the opposing jaw and teeth. Expect several appointments with us during the healing period as the swelling goes down and the denture base settles. Your bite will change and need to be readjusted. The more teeth removed at the time the immediate denture is delivered, the longer it will take to heal and the more sore spots you will have.

Sometimes we will advise removing some teeth as the denture is being made, leaving only a few front teeth in place. This will help make a more accurate fit of the immediate denture. Of course, every case is unique. Expect many sore spots and places where the tissue is rubbed raw. When this happens, take out the denture and see us immediately. If you continue to wear the denture without adjustment, the gum tissue will be badly damaged and it will take longer to heal. Although the general process of making an immediate denture is close to that of a traditional full denture, the immediate denture construction poses different and more significant problems.

After the tissue completely heals at the extraction site, the denture base will need an addition of more plastic. This is called a *reline*. The extra plastic will fill in the space between the denture base and the new position of the soft tissue. Originally, this space was estimated in the sites where the teeth had not yet been removed. Tissue shrinkage will continue for some time, but after about 6 months, it slows down enough that it is practical to do the reline. With either immediate dentures, or after some years of wearing dentures, the tissue may change enough that relines are again necessary. As you age and have no teeth, the bone in the jaws gets smaller. The plastic base of the denture does not change along with the jaw changes, so a periodic reline is necessary.

It is possible that after many years of missing teeth, the bone on which the denture sits becomes so small that it is difficult, if not impossible, for a denture to remain properly in place. Dental implants may help retain the denture. Some surgical procedures may help.

If you have any questions about immediate dentures, please feel free to ask us.

Partial Dentures

A partial denture is designed to replace one or several missing teeth. You may consider a removable partial denture to replace the missing teeth, if:

- you have missing teeth
- the remaining teeth cannot accept a fixed bridge
- there is not sufficient bone for implants
- finances are limited

Removable partial dentures have been made by dentists and worn by patients for many years. Partial dentures are composed of three different materials. A cast metal base with clasping arms holds a pink plastic gum tissue and plastic or porcelain teeth. The metal clasps are silver in color and, depending on the individual circumstances, may or may not be visible when you talk or smile. These clasps are absolutely necessary to hold the partial in place. Their location and design are dictated by the shape and position of your remaining teeth and which missing teeth will be replaced. We will show you where the clasps are to be located in your mouth. Most of the time, the amount of preparation (drilling) of your natural teeth needed to ensure successful clasp design is minimal. Often there is no need for a local anesthetic injection. This is unlike fixed bridgework, which always requires significant tooth reduction for proper design and fit.

If you find that the appearance of the clasps will be objectionable, then you might consider different possibilities. It is common to place crowns on the teeth that are clasped by the metal arms, and then place the clasps **inside** the crowns. This will give you a more natural appearance, but it will add to the ultimate cost of treatment. It involves significant preparation of the natural tooth and you might also want to rethink about fixed bridges or implants.

The base of the partial denture will rest lightly on your gum tissue. At some time in the future it is expected that you will need adjustments to the base. Usually this means an addition of more pink material to the denture base. Clasp arms will loosen and need to be tightened at various times. Weight loss or gain will also affect the fit of the base of the partial.

Although a partial is less expensive than a fixed bridge, which is metal and porcelain cemented into place, there are several possible drawbacks. It is much more bulky than a bridge and is more difficult to wear initially. You may have to adjust the way you speak to accommodate the extra bulk. After awhile, this will not be much of a problem. And depending on the position of the retaining clasps, they may be visible when you talk or smile.

Do not sleep with the partial dentures in place. The partial dentures absolutely must be removed during sleep time to be cleaned and give the clasped teeth a chance to rest. The gum tissue under the denture needs a chance to breathe and reestablish proper blood circulation. The partial denture can compress the tissue and reduce blood flow in the area. Plaque can accumulate on your denture and your gum tissue. Use a very soft toothbrush to gently brush your gums. Also brush your partial denture daily with a denture brush and denture cleanser. Always store your partial denture in water when you are not wearing it.

If you have any questions about removable partial dentures, please feel free to ask us.

chapter 12

Restorative Dentistry

Content at a Glance: Restorative Dentistry

Restorations

Each document describes the use, advantages, and disadvantages of the following restorations:

Amalgam Restorations
Amalgam and Bonded Resins: Postoperative Instructions
Bonded Resin Restorations: Tooth-Colored Fillings for Posterior Teeth
Microdentistry: Preventive Resin Restoration
Partial Coverage Restorations
Porcelain Inlays and Onlays
Resin Inlays and Onlays
The "Permanent" Filling

Corrective Procedures

Defective Restorations

Explains that restorations may degrade and/or fail over time and need to be repaired or replaced. Describes types of defects and the needed service.

Enamel Recontouring

Relates the use of enamel recontouring, particularly in relation to other possible procedures.

Sedative Restorations

The indications and procedures for the use of sedative restorations are discussed.

Safety and Warranty

Safety of Silver Amalgam and Base Metals

Reassures the patient that silver amalgam and base metals are not used in this practice. Includes reasons.

Warranty for Restorative Materials

Document states the office policy for replacement of restorations with stress on adherence to recare intervals.

Warranty for the Severely Compromised Tooth

This document states the limits of restoring the severely compromised tooth along with the factors that may limit the longevity of the treatment.

Amalgam Restorations

Silver amalgam restorations are the traditional silver filling materials. They have been used with success by all dentists for more than 150 years. Silver amalgam fillings were originally meant to be a low-cost substitute filling material for those patients who could not afford the standard-of-care gold restorations. They can be used to replace small or large amounts of tooth structure lost through decay or fracture. They are not technique sensitive. They are composed of silver, tin, mercury, copper, and other metals. Some of the newer silver amalgam materials are mercury-free. We have no long-term studies on how well these mercury-free amalgams will serve.

The silver amalgams available have a life expectancy of 14 years with a plus/minus deviation of 14 years. They can last a long time or need to be replaced within a year of when they were originally completed. As with resin restorations, the smaller the filling, the longer it can last. This is still the restorative material of choice for many dentists but that number is declining. Most restorations for back teeth, regardless of size, are silver amalgam. With the advent of the newer bonded resin materials, many posterior (back) teeth that previously would have been restored with amalgam are now being restored with the more conservative and more naturally appearing tooth colored resin and porcelain materials. Silver amalgam fillings can now also be bonded when there is little remaining tooth. This, of course, will add to the total fee charged for the restoration.

Disadvantages of the silver fillings are esthetics. It is impossible to have them look natural, and the appearance deteriorates as time goes by. If the surrounding enamel is thin, the gray/black color of the metal will show through. They can make the tooth turn dark. They add no strength to the tooth (unless bonded). They weaken the tooth because they have a higher expansion/contraction ratio than the surrounding tooth. These forces can, after time, cause the tooth to fracture. They are not considered a conservative restoration because they require more tooth prepared (drilled) than is actually necessary to be removed due to the decay. This extra drilling is strictly to allow the retention of the restoration. In some instances, it might be more cost-effective and better for the gingival (gum) health to place a cast restoration (crown or onlay). This would be the case when the silver filling would be large. When there are extensive amounts of tooth structure to be rebuilt/replaced, it is often quite difficult to establish the proper physiologic contour to the tooth. Remaining tooth structure may be more prone to fracture.

Advantages of the silver amalgam fillings are that they are quick and easy to place, relatively inexpensive, and have a proven record of success.

If finances are a major concern and cosmetics are not important, then this material is well suited for all types of restorations. If the cavity is small or on a previously undamaged portion of a tooth, a more conservative resin restoration would be a better choice.

If you have any questions about silver amalgam restorations, please feel free to ask us.

Amalgam and Bonded Resins: Postoperative Instructions

You have just had one or more teeth restored (filled) with either silver amalgam or resin (tooth-colored/bonded) materials, or prepared for an inlay/onlay or crown. How quickly you adjust to the new restoration depends on the size of the restoration and the closeness to the pulp (nerve). The larger the restoration, usually, the longer it will take you to become accustomed to it.

Chewing

If you have been given a local anesthetic, please do not chew in that area until full feeling returns. When you are "numb," you cannot feel if you are biting your cheek or lip. If you have had a **silver/metal** filling placed, it will require a minimum of 2 hours after you leave the office before you can chew on it. If you eat before the silver filling is adequately set, the filling may break and require replacement. If you have had a **resin** restoration placed, the resin sets immediately, and you can eat when the effect of the anesthetic is completely gone.

Occlusion

The occlusion (bite) of the new restoration has already been adjusted. If you have been anesthetized, you may not be able to notice if the bite feels normal. Wait until the anesthesia wears off and then, if the occlusion is not comfortable, call the office to have it adjusted. We do not believe in a bite "wearing in," regardless of the material used. If you have had multiple restorations placed, please give yourself time to become adjusted to them before you call the office. This may take one or two days. However, if the bite is off and it is not corrected, you could break the filling or the underlying tooth. We have checked your occlusion before you left our office but your tooth was still anesthetized, and you may not have been able to feel the bite well. It is often difficult to make the teeth meet as they usually meet under these circumstances. It is not uncommon for the new restoration to need a slight adjustment.

Size

The following restorations were: ❑ **normal in size and shape**: tooth #s _____
                                      ❑ **deep and/or wide**: tooth #s _____

When restorations are very large, it is possible that in the future the tooth may fracture and may need a cast restoration (crown or onlay) to be properly restored. If the restoration was deep, it is possible that the nerve may die and you will need endodontic therapy (root canal treatment). This may become evident tomorrow or 10 years from now. If a very large silver amalgam or bonded restoration breaks soon after it is placed, there is a strong chance that the filling material is being called upon to replace more tooth structure than it was designed to replace. In this situation the tooth will be better restored with a cast restoration.

Exposure

The nature of the design of the preparation for the restoration or the extent of the decay has caused the nerve to be **exposed** on tooth #s _____ or a **near exposure** on tooth #s _____. When the nerve was exposed, a medication was placed on the exposure site and there may be healing, but it is probable that endodontic treatment (root canal therapy) will be needed at some time in the future. If there was a near exposure, medication was also placed on the site, but there is a reduced possibility of future endodontic treatment. In either case, expect the tooth to be very sensitive to temperature changes, especially cold temperatures, for several weeks.

Sensitivity

Any time a tooth is prepared (drilled) for a filling, tooth structure is removed very quickly. The natural wear process that occurs in everyone's teeth proceeds much more slowly. The response of a vital, healthy nerve to this wear is to recede and deposit an insulation layer between the nerve and the surface of the tooth. Normally, the wear of the tooth proceeds at more or less the same pace as the nerve recedes and deposits insulation. When a tooth is drilled, tooth structure is removed much more quickly than the nerve can "defend" itself. One response of the nerve is to become sensitive to temperature changes. This will persist until the recession and insulation process can catch up to the rapid removal of the tooth structure caused by the drill. This sensitivity can last from several days to several months. Usually, the more drilling, the more and longer the sensitivity you will experience. Several other factors also contribute to postoperative temperature sensitivity, but choice of filling material—silver amalgam or bonded tooth-colored resin filling—is **not** a usual cause. When done correctly, white fillings are no more likely to be sensitive than silver fillings.

Oral Self-Care and Recare

You may (and please do!) brush and floss your teeth after the local anesthetic has worn off. There is no need to refrain from your normal, daily oral self-care routine. Continue with your oral hygiene maintenance appointments at the interval we have previously recommended. Problems that might develop around the restorations can be found at an early stage and easily repaired. If you wait too long, the entire restoration may have to be redone.

If you have any questions about these instructions, please feel free to ask us.

Bonded Resin Restorations: Tooth-Colored Fillings for Posterior Teeth

Tooth-colored restorations have been used in dentistry for a long time. Several variations of these materials have been used in front teeth for many years. The newest generation of tooth-colored filling materials (resins) is also used to restore cavities in back teeth. This is especially true when the restoration would be easily visible when you talk or smile. The use of silver amalgam filling materials in small- to medium-sized restorations is declining. These posterior (back) tooth-colored resins can be expected to last for several years. A reasonable estimate at this time is approximately 10 to 12 or more years. Longevity of the resin fillings (and silver fillings) is a function of the position and size of the filling, the care the patient gives it, and the foods the patient eats.

Resin restorations in back teeth require less drilling than for silver fillings. Because of the filling material itself and the insulating liners and bases used under these resins, there can be fluoride release and a subsequent inhibition of new cavity formation. They are excellent for small one-, two-, and three-surface restorations in premolars and molars. Advantages of the resin restorations include a natural appearance similar to that of your real tooth and the most conservative preparation of your tooth. The less the dentist must drill your tooth, the better off you are and the fewer dental problems you will develop in the future. They also restore a high percentage of the tooth's original strength. When a tooth is prepared (drilled), it becomes weaker. Restoring it with a bonded resin material will help make it strong again. They require only one appointment for completion.

Disadvantages include technique sensitivity, that is, they are harder to place than silver fillings. They also cost about 50% more than silver fillings. They can be used only rarely in patients who have a grinding or bruxing (clenching) habit. They cannot be easily used in areas where there is not a sufficient amount of original tooth structure. They require more time to finish.

Resin restorations are among the most conservative restorations in dentistry today. They require the least amount of drilling. The smaller any filling can be, the longer it will last. They are best for small to medium fillings. In areas where the display of metal from a silver filling would be unsightly, they are of great cosmetic importance.

If you have any questions about bonded resin restorations, please feel free to ask us.

Microdentistry: Preventive Resin Restoration

With the advent of adhesive dentistry (bonding), the concept of how a tooth should be prepared for a filling has changed. In the old days, if you were to have a silver filling (silver amalgam filling material was invented in the early 1800s), the tooth would have to be drilled beyond what was necessary to remove the decay. The extra drilling is needed for undercuts to be placed to mechanically retain the silver material. The extra tooth that was removed would make the tooth weaker. With adhesive dentistry, the ability of the dentist to bond (attach) composite resin materials to the tooth has changed this concept. Now, all the dentist needs to do is remove decay and then bond the resin into position. This means less drilling, and the tooth remains stronger. The reduced need for drilling of a tooth allows the dentist to perform microdentistry procedures. The technical expertise needed on the part of the dentist increases while removal of the tooth structure decreases. Innovative ways of removing decay are constantly being developed. With use of magnifying loupes, dyes that can selectively stain decay, and the new bonding materials, more of the tooth is preserved.

A preventive resin restoration is a combination of a microdentistry procedure and a conventional tooth sealant. In the old days, when a back tooth became decayed, the nondecayed grooves near the decayed portion were removed routinely to prevent further decay from starting. With a preventive resin, only the decay is removed. Bonding is placed to restore the area and a resin sealant is then bonded over the remainder of the tooth to prevent further decay. In this way, less drilling is needed and the tooth remains strong.

In preparing a tooth for a preventive resin, a traditional dental handpiece drill can be used to remove the decay, or the recently re-introduced air abrasion unit may be used. An air abrasion unit emits a stream of aluminum oxide or other smaller-particle sand-like material under high pressure. This is equivalent to sandblasting—but on a very small scale. The particles under high pressure quickly abrade away the decay, quietly and often with no need for a local anesthetic injection to numb the tooth. Another major advantage of abrasion dentistry is that the "sandblasting" does not cause cracks to form in the brittle tooth enamel. The traditional dental drill does cause cracks to radiate out from the preparation. These cracks have been implicated in an accelerated deterioration of the tooth and need for filling replacement. With abrasion dentistry this problem can be eliminated. Air abrasion cannot yet be used to prepare crowns and bridges or any type of cast and laboratory-fabricated restoration.

Because microdentistry procedures require a higher level of training and expertise, the fees are slightly higher than those for a silver filling. Bonded resin restorations have considerable advantages over silver filling materials. Their conservative nature and the fact that they protect the tooth, making it as strong as it can be, make them well worth the extra expense.

If you have any questions about microdentistry and preventive resin restoration, please feel free to ask us.

Partial Coverage Restorations

One of our primary goals in providing you with the optimal oral care is to preserve as much of your natural dentition as possible. Prevention of oral disease is the best way to accomplish this goal. Unfortunately, dental decay is the most common disease known to the human body. In the early stages the caries process can be reversed with the use of fluoride. If, however, the decay progresses to the point when a filling is required, the decay can be removed and the tooth restored very conservatively with tooth-colored, bonded direct restorations. Direct restoration means that it is begun and completed in the office in one appointment. Although tooth structure must be removed in this event, the amount removed is small and the strength of the tooth is not significantly compromised. This should be reason enough to go to the dentist to have your teeth examined and cleaned on a regular basis. Needs differ, but most adults should go two to four times each year.

If the tooth has a moderate to large amount of tooth structure to be replaced, a direct restoration will not be as successful. For these teeth, a laboratory or externally processed restoration is more appropriate. These are not the same as a crown (cap). A crown involves removing a maximum amount of tooth structure. The cast restoration is then fitted over the prepared tooth, as a thimble fits over a fingertip. No natural tooth can be seen. While full cast crowns do have a proven track record of success, a great amount of tooth structure is sacrificed.

Partial coverage restorations can be made of gold, resin, porcelain, or ceramic materials. The gold restorations are the least esthetic. The color is similar to that of a gold wedding ring. The other three materials are tooth-colored and provide a wonderful match to your natural tooth structure.

There are several advantages that you will realize with partial coverage restorations. They require that less tooth structure be removed than for a crown so they are small in size. This conservative preparation preserves much of the tooth adjacent to the gum tissue, providing a much better opportunity for excellent periodontal health. With the edges of the restoration above the gum, the restoration becomes easier to check for continued service. New decay is more easily seen and treated at an early stage. The chances of drilling of the tooth, the potential risk for future nerve damage, and a resulting root canal all decrease.

On the negative side, the partial coverage restorations are harder for the dentist to prepare and place. They are very technique sensitive and time-consuming. This contributes to a higher fee along with the necessary laboratory fees for processing the restoration. But the result is well worth the extra effort and cost. The maximum amount of sound, natural tooth is preserved. There is nothing a dentist can put in your mouth that is as good as an undrilled, undamaged tooth. The less the dentist must drill, the better off you will be, over both the short and long term. We will always suggest to you the most appropriate treatment and material based on your individual oral needs.

If you have any questions about partial coverage restorations, please feel free to ask us.

Porcelain Inlays and Onlays

One innovative way to restore a tooth that has been moderately to extensively destroyed by decay, previous drilling, or fracture is with a porcelain inlay or onlay. An inlay is a restoration in which a portion of the occlusal (biting) surface is restored. An onlay will restore more of the entire biting surface of the tooth. You might need an inlay alone, an onlay alone, or a combination inlay/onlay. This is considered a very conservative restoration.

The porcelain material produces an excellent esthetic result. The porcelain inlay or onlay is bonded to the tooth, making it very strong. It can be used with wonderful results in small, medium, and even large restorations lasting more than 12 years, relatively trouble-free.

An outside laboratory is involved in the construction of this type of restoration. During the 2- to 3-week processing time while the inlay or onlay is being made, the tooth will be protected by a temporary restoration. Porcelain inlays and onlays do have some disadvantages. They are more expensive to make and place and they take two appointments to complete. They must be adjusted and polished well or they can cause wear of the opposing enamel, exactly like a porcelain fused to metal crown.

Advantages include the excellent esthetics, high strength, predicted longevity, and conservative preparation. If the porcelain does chip, it can be repaired. However, you should not chew ice cubes, "jaw breakers," or other hard candy with these or any other type of restoration.

Anything that you put in your mouth that can break a real tooth can break this type of restorative material.

For patients who want a strong, long-lasting, conservative restoration that very closely matches a tooth, porcelain is possibly the best choice. All things considered, it is not as expensive as it might appear. Once it is finished, the tooth, if cared for properly, should not have to be drilled again for years. It does allow the conservation of most of the natural tooth. Remember, our goal is to preserve as much of your natural tooth structure as possible.

If you have any questions about porcelain inlays and onlays, please feel free to ask us.

Illustration on CD-ROM

Resin Inlays and Onlays

Resin inlays and onlays are very natural in appearance and are bonded into place. They are extremely conservative restorations. They require two appointments to complete and, just as with porcelain inlays or onlays, laboratory support is needed. The tooth will be protected with a temporary plastic inlay or onlay while the laboratory processes the final restoration.

Fabrication at the dental laboratory takes about 2 weeks. The wear of the resin is similar to that of enamel. So unlike porcelain, it will not wear the opposing natural tooth structure.

The resin material itself may be slightly weaker than porcelain. However, because porcelain is more brittle and more difficult to repair, the difference in strength is not significant. The resin is more forgiving and is more easily finished or repaired and the resin is easier to work on. Resin restorations, however, are not advised for patients who have a bruxing (grinding) or clenching habit unless a protective mouthguard is constructed.

We will select and recommend the proper restorative material based on your dental needs. Costs of each are comparable. Both types are excellent choices and are considered highly conservative in the amount of drilling needed.

An excellent way to restore a tooth with moderate to extensive decay is with an inlay or onlay.

If you have any questions about resin inlays or onlays, please feel free to ask us.

The "Permanent" Filling

One of the most frequent questions patients ask is, "Is this a permanent filling?" Without getting too involved in technical aspects of modern restorative materials, the answer is usually no. All filling materials have a life span of several to many years, depending on the restorative material used. As a rule of thumb for moderate to large restorations, the more it costs, the longer it will last.

Dental restorative materials constructed and processed in a dental laboratory will be stronger and harder and will last longer than silver amalgam (metal) fillings and office-placed composites (tooth-colored/bonded) filling materials. These laboratory-constructed materials include indirect restorations such as full cast crowns, inlays and onlays of porcelain, gold and gold alloys, ceramics, and resins. While the dentist will have certain preferences, you have the final decision over which material is to be used. To make the decision process easier, here is a brief summary of the advantages and disadvantages of materials commonly used in partial coverage restorations. Porcelain fused to gold alloy crowns are not included here as they are in a different category.

Cast Gold: The color of the cast gold is yellow, the same as a wedding ring. It can last 25 to 40 or more years—the longest of any dental material. Gold has a long history of success. Esthetics are poor to fair. The cost is high. However, the use of cast gold results in the fewest postoperative problems. It is excellent for medium to large tooth restoration. Two appointments are necessary to complete the restoration.

Technique Requirements: High

Laboratory-Processed Bonded Porcelains, Ceramics, and Resins: These materials produce excellent esthetics: they match the tooth color almost perfectly. The cost is moderate to high. With respect to longevity, it is probably not as long as cast gold, but should last for 12 or more years. Usually, less tooth preparation (drilling) is required than when using gold. These are relatively new dental procedures. They do not have the long-term history of success enjoyed by gold. These materials can break if overstressed. Resin is easier to repair than porcelain, is less expensive than porcelain and ceramic, and is an excellent choice for medium to large restorations. Two appointments are needed to complete these restorations.

Technique Requirements: High

Direct Resins: Direct resins also provide excellent esthetics. Minimal tooth preparation is involved. These are the best materials for small to medium tooth restorations. Direct resins are less costly than gold or porcelains. They are bonded to the tooth. Life expectancy of the material is 12 or more years, and this newer technology strengthens the tooth. Direct resins can be completed in one visit.

Technique Requirements: High

Silver Metal Amalgam: Silver amalgam was first used as a filling material in 1816. Proven longevity of 14 years, plus or minus 14 years. Silver amalgam does not strengthen the tooth. It is not conservative in tooth preparation. The esthetics are poor. It blackens, corrodes, and expands over time. It is the lowest in cost of all of the restorative materials.

Technique Requirements: Low

We will select and recommend the restorative materials best suited to meet your dental needs. Insurance coverage (or lack of it) will **never** dictate what dental treatment we feel you need and deserve. Our goal is to be able to provide for you the best and longest lasting restorations possible. We will be glad to discuss these options with you.

If you have any questions about "permanent" fillings, please feel free to ask us.

Defective Restorations

Nothing lasts forever. For dentistry, this is a real problem. **Every** restorative material—be it a filling, crown, bridge, cement, etc.— has a somewhat limited lifetime. We are now living much longer lives. Most dental materials were not designed to serve as long as we can now expect to live. Some materials may last many years, and others, considerably less. There is really no such thing as a permanent filling. As a general rule, the more expensive the restoration or dental material, the longer it will last. If you want a restoration that will last the longest time, you will probably need a laboratory-processed inlay, onlay, or crown. Direct filling materials (placed in one office visit) are not expected to last as long. The longevity of these restorations will depend on the type of material, the location of the tooth, and the size of the preparation in the tooth. There are also outside considerations such as the skills and knowledge of the dentist at the time, the kinds of food you eat, your oral self-care habits, and the structural abuse you place on your teeth. Habits such as clenching and grinding your teeth and chewing hard candies, ice, etc. will tend to quickly degrade the filling material, as well as your teeth, much faster.

Even the best-placed fillings get old. Crown cement dissolves, porcelain breaks, metals fatigue, resins degrade, and so on. Eventually, pieces of filling material or tooth can fracture or chip. A new cavity may start on an unfilled surface of the same tooth. The restoration needs replacement. Silver amalgam fillings (the black or gray fillings most of us have) can absorb moisture from saliva, expand, and cause the tooth to break. The filling expansion can cause both the filling and the margin between the tooth and filling to become rough. This can promote plaque retention and the start of new decay. When this happens, it is best to replace the restoration as soon as possible with a bonded resin, which will require less drilling. The better the material, the less drastic the thermocycling (hot coffee/cold ice cream and any temperature variations), and the less abusive your personal habits, the longer the restoration will last. If you have any of these restorative problems, you should have them corrected as soon as possible. Waiting can cause increased severity, and more extensive and expensive treatment may be required, or the problem may become impossible to fix.

Definitions

Fracture: Filling material that has broken in two or more pieces. Pieces may or may not be moving and are not often felt by the patient. The restoration must be replaced.

Leakage: Fluids penetrate between a filling and the tooth, causing decay. A patient usually notices this condition when the tooth becomes sensitive to fluids, sweets, or hot or cold. The restoration must be replaced.

Loose crown: The crown cementing medium may have failed. In the case of endodontic treatment, the post holding the crown may have broken or its cementing medium may have failed. It can be caused by an improper bite relationship, eating the wrong foods, or parafunctional mouth habits. Sometimes the restoration can be repaired and reused; otherwise, it must be totally redone.

Open contact: When two teeth that should touch don't, it is referred to as an *open contact*. It may be due to unwanted tooth movement after an extraction but is usually a result of an undercontoured filling. It can trap food and cause severe gum infection, bleeding, and bone loss around the affected teeth. The filling (or fillings) may need to be replaced.

Open margins: When a filling does not meet the tooth preparation, the result is an open margin. Basically, a crevice exists between the filling and the tooth. Plaque is easily trapped, predisposing the tooth to additional decay. This can be especially serious in crowns. Infrequently, an open margin can be repaired, but usually must be replaced.

Overcontour: When a filling or crown is shaped incorrectly, especially when it is too wide, it can cause bleeding gums and infection. The restoration must be reshaped or replaced.

Overhang: The most common type of restoration defect is an overhang. When the restorative material extends beyond the normal contour of the tooth beneath the gum, it causes a plaque trap. One common indication is the ripping or shredding of dental floss. An overhang causes gum infection (red gums that bleed easily). The excess material must be removed by polishing or replacing the restoration.

Recurrent decay: New tooth decay is seen around the tooth/filling margin or under the filling. You may or may not notice this condition. Usually, we notice it in a clinical exam or on a dental radiograph. Recurrent decay requires immediate replacement.

Stained resin: A stained composite resin is often a sign of degradation of the resin. Older resins are more prone to show staining. The stain indicates the resin matrix that holds the inorganic components together is old, overstressed, and no longer resisting moisture. We can then determine urgency of replacement. When it is a cosmetic problem, we will recommend that you have it restored sooner.

Undercontour: When a filling or crown is of an improper shape, especially deficient in width, it is undercontoured. This condition causes food impaction and gum infections. An undercontoured filling must be replaced.

If you have any questions about defective restorations, please feel free to ask us.

Enamel Recontouring

Most people want straight, beautifully aligned, white teeth. Unfortunately, most people are not naturally born that way. When teeth are in poor alignment, rotated, tilted, and/or crowded, one obvious way to correct the problem is by orthodontics (braces). However, there are situations where it may not be possible or desirable to use braces to straighten teeth. You might feel that you are too old (although this is rarely the case), the cost of the orthodontics may preclude their use, you may not want to wear braces, or perhaps there are only a few areas that need attention and full orthodontics are not indicated.

In certain select cases, the appearance of your top and bottom teeth can be slightly or dramatically improved by recontouring the enamel. The upper and lower incisors and canines can be routinely altered. Sometimes teeth further back in your mouth can also be cosmetically improved. Recontouring is useful when there is slight to moderate overlapping of the front teeth, uneven wear, or teeth that do not have their biting and incising edges in harmony, in effect, an uneven "picket fence" look. Enamel recontouring is a painless procedure and no local anesthetic is needed. The enamel that is overlapping or poorly shaped is removed, recontoured, and polished. Depending on your individual needs, one or several teeth may require some reshaping. Different amounts of enamel may be removed from different teeth. The teeth do not become prone to decay, are not made more sensitive to temperature changes, and are not made significantly weaker or damaged by the procedure.

Many times, recontouring is all that is necessary to significantly improve your appearance. Other times, when the poor alignment is more pronounced, it may be done in conjunction with a bonding procedure. The extent of your treatment will depend on your present conditions and on what you would like to see changed.

The procedure is not difficult for the patient and can often be done in only one appointment. The resulting change is immediate and permanent. It does take an artistic approach on the part of the dentist to determine what possibilities for change exist. We need to determine what enamel needs to be removed, where we must add material, and where orthodontics is the treatment of choice. The fees are reasonable and depend on the extent of the treatment.

If you have any questions about enamel recontouring, please feel free to ask us.

Sedative Restorations

Sedative restorations are placed for several different reasons. The most common reason is tooth pain. The pain may be constant, intermittent, or a reaction to sweets or a cold or hot stimulus. If the sensitivity is due to decay and it is very deep and close to the nerve, there is the possibility of exposure of the pulp (nerve) once all the decay is removed. If the cavity is especially deep, as much of the decay as possible will be removed, and a medicated, sedative filling will be placed in the tooth. This will serve to calm the nerve and give it a chance to heal. The sedative restoration, if done for this reason, should stay in your mouth for _____ weeks. Then the sedative restoration will be removed and the tooth will be examined to determine the need for further treatment. It may be able to be restored with a filling or cast restoration. However, if the decay was quite deep and the nerve does not heal, endodontic treatment (root canal therapy) will be required to alleviate pain and save the tooth.

If you have multiple large cavities and/or other serious dental problems, we may choose to first restore all the teeth with sedative restorations. This will quickly stabilize all the teeth so that they do not continue to deteriorate from the decay. Then the other, perhaps more serious dental problems can be addressed and treated. Once you are out of an emergency situation, we will have the time to thoroughly plan the best methods to restore your teeth.

A third use of a sedative restoration is as an aid in diagnosing sensitive teeth. You may have a problem with a single tooth, or perhaps you are unable to specifically pinpoint the exact tooth. If the tooth (or teeth) already has a restoration in it, we may need to remove the restoration and directly look at the prepared portions of the tooth. If we do not feel that it is appropriate to place a final restoration at that time, we will place a sedative restoration to allow the tooth to settle down enough to receive the final filling. In your case, we expect the sedative restoration to be in place for approximately _____ weeks. Occasionally, the tooth feels better as soon as the sedative restoration is placed. However, it will still be necessary to observe the tooth for a few weeks before placing a final restoration.

Infrequently, the placement of the sedative restoration offers no apparent relief. In this case other possibilities must be explored. Most often the tooth will require endodontic treatment. Other times, it just takes several days to get a positive result. If possible, give the sedative restoration time to work. But under no circumstances must you live in constant pain. Do not be afraid to call and ask to be seen if the sedative restoration does not appear to be effective.

If you have any questions about sedative restorations, please feel free to ask us.

Safety of Silver Amalgam and Base Metals

The practice of the art and science of dentistry has changed tremendously during the last 15 to 20 years. Nowhere is this more evident than in the variety of dental materials now available for tooth restoration. Composite resins (tooth-colored bonding plastics) permit us to restore teeth with less removal (drilling) of sound tooth structure. The composites look like natural tooth structure, are bonded to the tooth for a tight seal, last a long time, and add back strength to the prepared tooth. Silver amalgam (metal filling) materials don't look like natural teeth; they leak fluids at the tooth/metal interface; can crack teeth by volumetric and thermal expansion; require more removal of tooth structure than is required to eliminate decay; make the tooth weaker; and can last a long time but often seriously damage the tooth while in place. Silver fillings were invented around 1814 by the French as a temporary, inexpensive filling material to be used until the patient could afford a better-quality gold restoration. Back then, the dentists in the United States were so horrified by the use of the silver/mercury material that it was not allowed to be imported into the United States, or even taught in the dental schools, for many years.

Base metals have been used in dentistry as an inexpensive alternative to the noble and high noble metals. Noble and high noble metals contain precious metals such as gold, palladium, and platinum in varying percentages. Base metals are composed of metals that can have high allergenic, toxic, or even carcinogenic properties. Since 1976, we have never specified base metals be used in any laboratory-processed restoration. We have used casting metals that are of proven high quality. Because we are considerate of your overall medical health, we do not offer base metals as an option for any crown, bridge, or implant-supported casting.

We have made a decision in our practice to provide you with the best and most appropriate procedures and materials that dentistry has to offer. This does not necessarily mean the most expensive treatment. We want them to look good and be functional and comfortable too. We feel that silver amalgam materials will not help you meet this goal. We feel that routine use of new silver fillings and base metal has no place in dentistry today. We have elected to eliminate this material and procedure from our practice.

If You Have Dental Insurance

Insurance carriers routinely provide benefits for tooth-colored, bonded composite restorations for back teeth that reflect the fee for silver metal fillings. Contracts with the carrier almost always state that the benefit is for the least expensive service possible (alternative benefit clause). The insurance carrier is not telling you or the dentist what treatment you should have, only what their responsibility for payment is. The higher the premium, the more that is paid in benefits. The lower the premium, the lower the benefits. As a silly example, a very low cost dental insurance may pay 100% of the fee for a wooden denture. But that does not mean any dentist will carve you a set. If better materials are used based on the dentist's discretion, you are responsible for the difference.

In Conclusion

For your general health, we will not place cast base metals in your mouth. For the health and longevity of your teeth, we will not place new silver amalgam fillings in teeth with new decay or as a replacement for an existing restoration.

If you have any questions about silver amalgam and base metals, please feel free to ask us.

Warranty for Restorative Materials

You have just had restorative treatment (fillings) or fixed prosthetics (laboratory-processed crowns, bridges, inlays, or onlays) placed. In all cases we use the best available and most appropriate materials and techniques. The completed treatment should serve you well for several years. Like anything else, the dental materials have an effective life span and require routine, ongoing maintenance. There is nothing available in dentistry today that is as good as or better than your natural tooth. Like any piece of fine machinery or an automobile, the better care you can give it, and the less abuse it is subject to, the longer it will last.

Subject to a few conditions, the following is the warranty for the materials and treatment you have received. Four possibilities could invalidate this warranty. (1) If you have been diagnosed as a clencher or bruxer, and/or if you have been advised to have a protective mouthguard and you do not wear it or do not have it made. (2) **If you do not adhere to the ongoing professional dental hygiene interval (cleaning by the dental hygienist) that has been determined based on your current oral needs. We recommend that you have your teeth examined and a dental prophylaxis performed every _____ months.** (3) New decay that requires the restoration to be redone. (4) Trauma, accident, neglect, or treatment to the treated tooth or an adjacent tooth that involves the restored tooth.

Dentists have no control over what a patient places in his or her mouth—food or otherwise. Chewing ice cubes or frozen or hard candy, grinding, or clenching can age your natural teeth or any restorative material at **many** times its normal rate. Please do not suck on hard candy or mints; this can rapidly cause decay around recently placed restorations.

WARRANTY

For direct placement restorations (completed in a single office appointment): If the restoration needs to be redone within **two years** of initial placement, the restoration will be replaced at no additional fee to you.

For laboratory-processed restorations: If the lab-processed restoration needs to be redone within **two years** of initial placement, the crown, bridge, inlay, or onlay will be replaced at no additional fee to you. **From two to three years,** the patient is responsible for 40% of the cost of retreatment. **From three to four years,** the patient is responsible for 60% of the cost of retreatment. **From four to five years,** the patient is responsible for 80% of the cost of treatment. **At five years from initial placement,** the warranty is completed.

If you have any questions about the warranty, please ask us. With proper care, you should get years of service from your new restorations. Do the required daily oral brushing and flossing and have your teeth checked and cleaned at the suggested interval. Nothing (usually) lasts forever, but if you take care of your mouth as directed, the restorations will be in satisfactory service for quite some time.

This warranty covers the following:

Tooth#_____   **Restoration Type**_____   **Date**_____

Warranty for the Severely Compromised Tooth

Nature created teeth strong enough to withstand years of daily service in the mouth. However, teeth can change and weaken for a number of reasons, some of which are:

- Decay
- Drilling of the tooth to remove decay
- Silver metal fillings that expand and break teeth
- Broken (fractured) teeth that can only be restored with crowns (caps)
- Gum disease resulting in bone loss surrounding the teeth
- Endodontic treatment (root canal treatment)
- Clenching and grinding
- Tooth movement after extraction of adjacent or opposing teeth

A tooth that has experienced one or more of these conditions may end up in such bad shape that it becomes difficult to restore and to provide a good long-term prognosis.

Although a dentist can restore almost any badly damaged tooth, there are risks. The real question is not whether the restoration can be done but, rather, will the tooth undergoing the procedure be strong enough to last for an appreciable length of time?

We like to give a warranty for restorations we place. You have a tooth that is severely compromised. While we feel that the tooth can be restored to clinical function, we cannot give our usual guarantee for longevity. It all depends on the strength of the tooth, and when a tooth is badly broken down it is often difficult to assess. The restoration may be excellent but your natural tooth could still break. This can occur soon after the tooth is restored or after several years. Depending on the nature of the break, the tooth could again be repaired or it could be broken so badly that no other treatment would work and the tooth must be removed.

We think that saving teeth is very important. We additionally recognize that, at some point, saving a tooth becomes impractical because of the expense: $2500 to save a tooth for 5 years makes economic sense, but $2500 to save a tooth for 6 months is not a good investment. Based on your oral needs and our clinical judgment, we recommend that you have the tooth in question restored, subject to the limitations described. Please understand there are many factors out of our control that relate to the long-term success of this tooth and restoration. The tooth may just not be strong enough to last for a long time.

If you intend to save the tooth in question, please sign below, showing that you have read and understand the information in this document and that while the best efforts and materials will be used, the tooth itself may prove to be inadequate to properly support a long-term restoration.

Tooth#(s) that are severely compromised: _____

Signed: _____   Date: _____

chapter 13

Patient Education Packets

Building Educational Packets

The material in this section will help you assemble useful educational packets for your patients. These packets can be built on a number of dental topics using documents from this dental communications package. Use the cover pages in this section and add the pages from the list of suggested topics. You may find it beneficial to compile and customize your own packets.

Content at a Glance: Patient Education Packets

Welcome to our Practice: *Having the Smile You Want*

Pulling any number of topics into an attractive package for a new patient says a lot about your practice and how patients can expect to be treated. This packet covers a range of topics from a general welcome to office policies to encouraging them to have the dental care they deserve.

Pediatric Dentistry Educational Packet: *Children's Dentistry*

The documents suggested for this packet cover both prevention and frequently asked questions regarding the child patient. Additional documents may be equally appropriate to include and can easily be inserted.

Periodontics Educational Packet: *Diagnosis and Treatment of Beginning to Moderate Gum Disease*

This packet is designed for the patient who is not in an advanced phase of periodontal disease and who needs to understand the role of regular professional oral care and appropriate oral self-care habits.

Periodontics Educational Packet: *Diagnosis and Treatment of Advanced Gum Disease*

This educational packet helps the patient seeking periodontal therapy to more clearly understand the nature of his or her disease and the recommended treatment procedures. Additional documents may be equally appropriate to include and can easily be inserted.

Prosthodontics Educational Packet: *Considerations in Tooth Replacement*

This educational packet helps the patient who is replacing missing teeth understand the necessity of prosthetic dentistry and the many treatment options available today. Additional documents may be equally appropriate to include and can easily be inserted.

Prosthodontics Educational Packet: *Considerations in Advanced Tooth Replacement*

The documents suggested for this packet help inform the patient who is contemplating a crown procedure to more fully understand the process and appropriate material selection. Additional documents may be equally appropriate to include and can easily be inserted.

Restorative Dentistry Educational Packet: *Restoring Your Teeth*

This packet will help the patient seeking restorative dentistry to understand the rationale for material selection, postoperative care of new restorations, and issues surrounding warranty. Additional documents may be equally appropriate to include and can easily be inserted.

How to Build Your Own Educational Packets

Directions to assist you with creating packets customized to your practice needs.

Welcome to our Practice

HAVING THE SMILE YOU WANT

As we begin this relationship in health care, there are a few things we would like you to know about our philosophy of treatment and our office policies. This packet is designed to acquaint you with just a few of those points and will hopefully answer a question or two that you may already have.

Please feel free to call us at any time to ask questions or discuss treatment options. We feel that the more education you have about dentistry, the better your treatment outcomes will be.

We look forward to providing you with great oral health and a winning smile.

Pediatric Dentistry Educational Packet

CHILDREN'S DENTISTRY

Your oral health, and certainly the oral health of your children, is an important part of overall well-being. We have prepared the following materials to provide you with information on prevention of disease and a handy reference guide of when your child will lose those baby teeth.

Please read the following information carefully. If you have any questions regarding this material or have other dentally related questions, please feel free to call our office at any time.

Periodontics Educational Packet

DIAGNOSIS AND TREATMENT OF BEGINNING TO MODERATE GUM DISEASE

Please read the attached information carefully.

You have been diagnosed with the earliest stage of active periodontal disease—gingivitis. The following pages will help you to understand our treatment recommendations, why these procedures need to be done, your options, and the consequences and risks of action or inaction on your part.

This packet contains information that will help you understand:

- An effective method for brushing and flossing your teeth. We will demonstrate these skills to you.
- The process of periodontal disease. You will be able to more fully understand the exact type of disease you have.
- The theory of proposed nonsurgical treatment, what is accomplished, and how you will benefit from this therapy.
- The exact procedures that are necessary in treating this disease.
- Adjunct or additional oral self-care procedures that may be necessary to treat the disease and maintain periodontal health.

Please note that all of the information is regarding nonsurgical treatment. At this time your periodontal health is at a critical stage. If left untreated, the current condition, which is reversible, can lead to the next stage of disease, which is irreversible. Any treatment options that we feel are appropriate to your treatment will be discussed prior to beginning treatment.

At times, patients with dental insurance ask if these procedures are covered benefits or if they are cosmetic in nature and would not be covered. The recommended treatment for periodontal disease is not cosmetic and most plans do include it as a payable benefit. An exception may occur for procedures such as subgingival irrigation or the placement of a site-specific therapy. If you like, we can submit a pre-estimate to your insurance carrier to determine which benefits will be covered and to what degree. However, since the procedures must be done in the right sequence, this may cause a delay in treatment. More damage can occur to your supporting structures while we wait to hear from the insurance carrier. Additionally, whether or not the procedure is a covered benefit, it is part of our recommended periodontal therapy to treat your disease.

Please read the following information carefully. It has been written to clearly explain what you need to know about the disease process and the necessary steps to treat it.

Periodontics Educational Packet

DIAGNOSIS AND TREATMENT OF ADVANCED GUM DISEASE

Please read the attached information carefully.

You have been diagnosed with active periodontal disease and the following pages will help you understand our treatment recommendations, why these procedures need to be done, your options, and the consequences and risks of action or inaction on your part.

This packet contains information that will help you understand:

- An effective method for brushing and flossing your teeth. We will demonstrate these skills to you.
- The process of periodontal disease. You will be able to more fully understand the exact type of disease you have.
- The theory of proposed nonsurgical treatment, what is accomplished, and how you will benefit from this therapy.
- The exact procedures that are necessary in treating this disease.
- Adjunct or additional oral self-care procedures that may be necessary to treat the disease and maintain periodontal health.

Please note that all of the information is regarding nonsurgical treatment. It is possible that you may need surgical treatment to correct the problems caused by the periodontal disease after the nonsurgical treatment is completed. The better you can brush, floss, and use other cleaning aids as we instruct you, the better you will heal, and the less surgery will be indicated. So do the best job you can—daily! If you do need surgery as part of your therapy, we will provide you with additional information. Most often, we refer the periodontal surgical procedures to a specialist (periodontist). You are also welcome to have the nonsurgical portion of this treatment completed with a periodontist and not at this office. If this is something you would like to discuss, please let us know.

At times, patients with dental insurance ask if these procedures are covered benefits or if they are cosmetic in nature and would not be covered. The recommended treatment for periodontal disease is not cosmetic and most plans do include them as a payable benefit. An exception may occur for procedures such as subgingival irrigation or the placement of a site-specific therapy. If you like, we can submit a pre-estimate to your insurance carrier to determine which benefits will be covered and to what degree. However, since the procedures must be done in the right sequence, this may cause a delay in treatment. More damage can occur to your supporting structures while we wait to hear from the insurance carrier. Additionally, whether or not the procedure is a covered benefit, it is part of our recommended periodontal therapy to treat your disease.

Please read the following information carefully. It has been written to clearly explain what you need to know about the disease process and steps necessary to treat it.

Prosthodontics Educational Packet

CONSIDERATIONS IN TOOTH REPLACEMENT

Please read the attached information carefully.

In consideration of having missing teeth replaced, we find it helpful to provide you with important background information. The following pages will help you understand our treatment recommendations, why these procedures need to be done, your options, and the consequences and risks of action or inaction on your part.

This packet contains information that will help you understand:
- Why missing teeth should be replaced.
- The variety of treatment options available today.
- The exact procedures that are necessary in treating this condition.
- The many contemporary dental materials available.

At times, patients with dental insurance ask if these procedures are covered benefits or if they are cosmetic in nature and would not be covered. The recommended treatment for replacing a missing tooth is not cosmetic and most plans do include them as a payable benefit. An exception, however, may occur. If you like, we can submit a pre-estimate to your insurance carrier to determine which benefits will be covered and to what degree. However, since the procedures must be done in the right sequence, this may cause a delay in treatment. More damage can occur to your supporting structures while we wait to hear from the insurance carrier. Additionally, whether or not the procedure is a covered benefit, it is part of our recommended periodontal therapy for your disease.

Please read the following information carefully. If you have any questions regarding this material or have other dentally related questions, please feel free to call our office at any time.

Prosthodontics Educational Packet

CONSIDERATIONS IN ADVANCED TOOTH REPLACEMENT

Please read the attached information carefully.

In consideration of an extensive restorative procedure, such as a crown, we find it helpful to provide you with important background information. The following pages will help you understand our treatment recommendations, why these procedures need to be done, your options, and the consequences and risks of action or inaction on your part.

This packet contains information that will help you understand:
- Why a crown is the best restorative procedure for your condition.
- The variety of treatment options available today.
- The exact procedures that are necessary in treating this condition.
- The many contemporary dental materials available.

At times, patients with dental insurance ask if these procedures are covered benefits or if they are cosmetic in nature and would not be covered. The recommended treatment for replacing a missing tooth is not cosmetic and most plans do include them as a payable benefit. An exception, however, may occur. If you like, we can submit a pre-estimate to your insurance carrier to determine which benefits will be covered and to what degree. However, since the procedures must be done in the right sequence, this may cause a delay in treatment. More damage can occur to your supporting structures while we wait to hear from the insurance carrier. Additionally, whether or not the procedure is a covered benefit, it is part of our recommended periodontal therapy to treat your disease.

Please read the following information carefully. If you have any questions regarding this material or have other dentally related questions, please feel free to call our office at any time.

Illustration on CD-ROM

Restorative Dentistry Educational Packet

RESTORING YOUR TEETH

Please read the attached information carefully.

In consideration of any dental restorative treatment, we find it helpful to provide you with important background information. The following pages will help you understand our treatment recommendations, why these procedures need to be done, your options, and the consequences and risks of action or inaction on your part.

This packet contains information that will help you understand:
- Why a defective restoration should be replaced.
- The variety of treatment options available today, including issues of safety.
- Issues of wear and longevity pertaining to dental restorations.

At times, patients with dental insurance ask if these procedures are covered benefits or if they are cosmetic in nature and would not be covered. The recommended treatment for replacing a missing tooth is not cosmetic and most plans do include them as a payable benefit. An exception, however, may occur. If you like, we can submit a pre-estimate to your insurance carrier to determine which benefits will be covered and to what degree. However, since the procedures must be done in the right sequence, this may cause a delay in treatment. More damage can occur to your supporting structures while we wait to hear from the insurance carrier. Additionally, whether or not the procedure is a covered benefit, it is part of our recommended periodontal therapy to treat your disease.

Please read the following information carefully. If you have any questions regarding this material or have other dentally related questions, please feel free to call our office at any time.

How to Build Your Own Educational Packets

You can easily build your own packets on any topic that you commonly discuss with patients. We recommend that you begin almost any of the packets with the document on p. 147, *Before Treatment Begins*. You can then find the document that specifically addresses the problems you are discussing, then the solutions, followed by a description of the specific procedures. You can add financial information, which is available on many topics as a final document. Be sure to use the attractive packet covers provided on the CD-ROM.

The more you review the documents in this communication package, the more you will find uses during every phase of patient interactions.

Illustrations

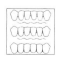

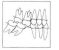

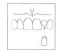

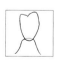

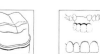

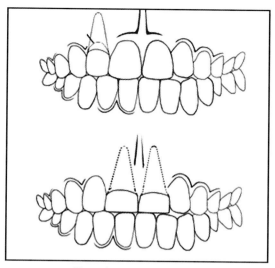

Altered passive eruption

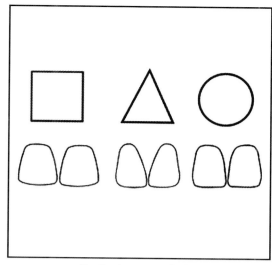

Tooth shape—anterior

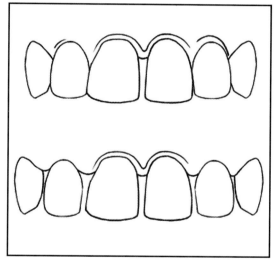

Diastemas

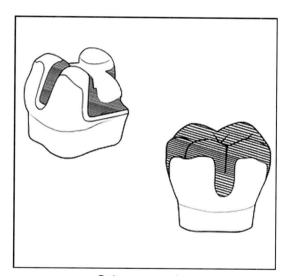

Onlay preparation

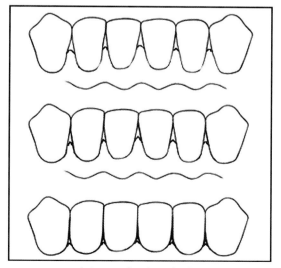

Interproximal contacts

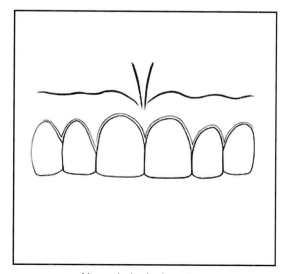

Normal gingival contour

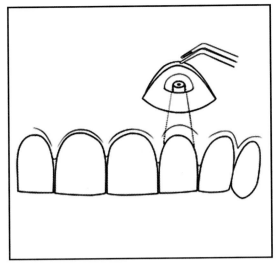

Apicoectomy

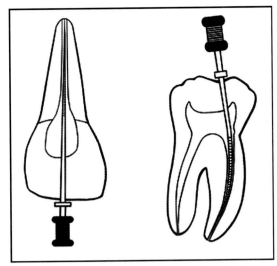

Endodontic therapy—anterior and posterior

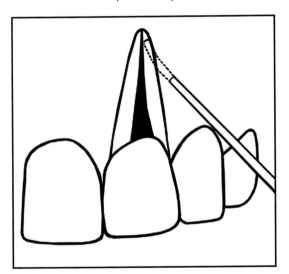

Fistulas tract

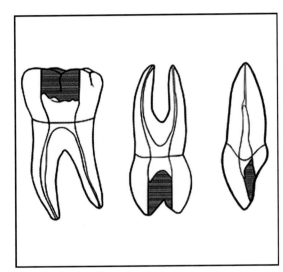

Endodontic access

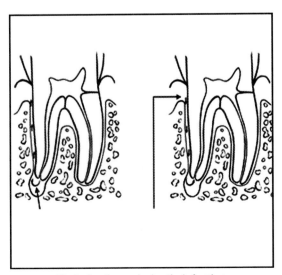

Endodontic-periodontic infection

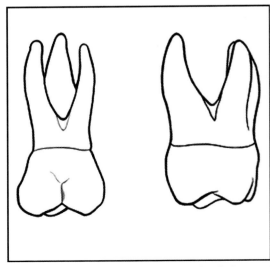

Maxillary molar—facial and proximal view

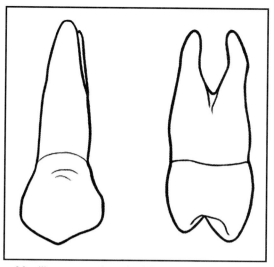

Maxillary premolar—facial and proximal view

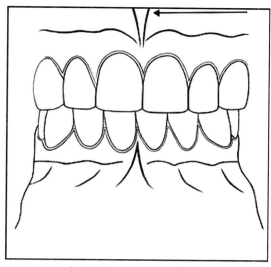

Labial frenum—maxillary

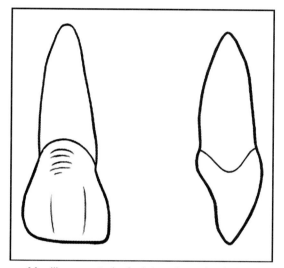

Maxillary central—facial and proximal view

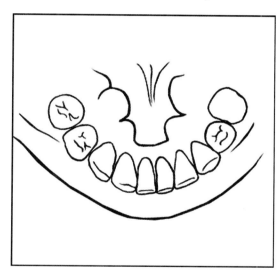

Mandibular tori

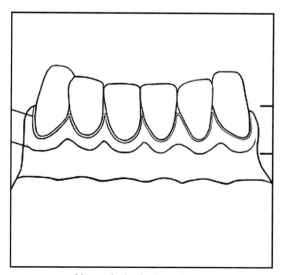

Normal gingival anatomy

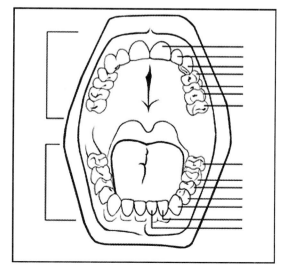

Full mouth view

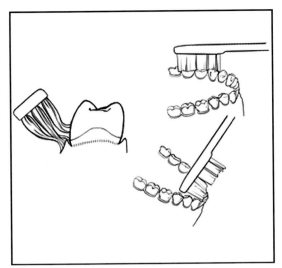

Toothbrush positioning

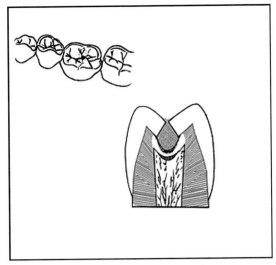

Dental caries—occlusal

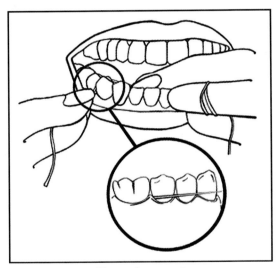

Floss placement

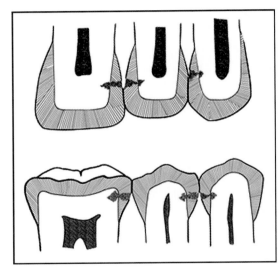

Dental caries—proximal

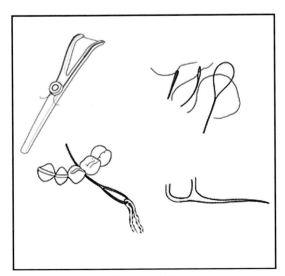

Flossing aids

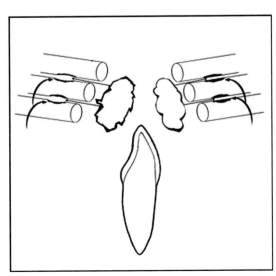

Demineralization and remineralization

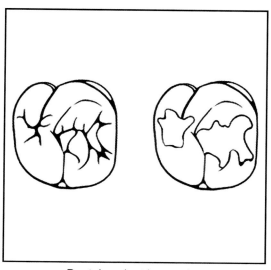

Dental sealant in a molar

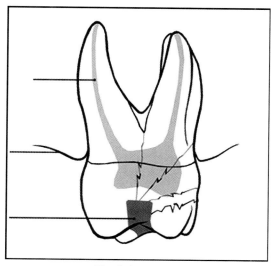

Tooth fractures

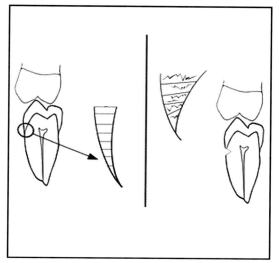

Abfraction

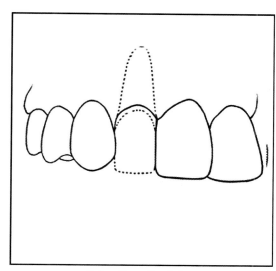

Extraction site defect

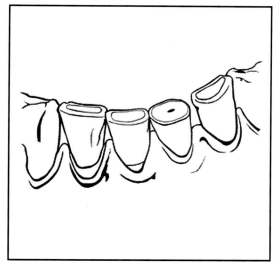

Attrition

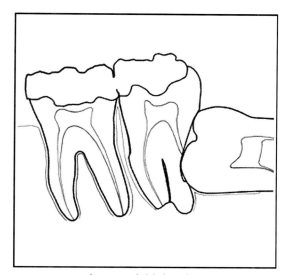

Impacted third molar

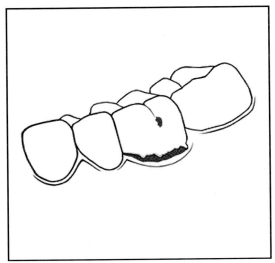

Dental caries—gingival margin and facial

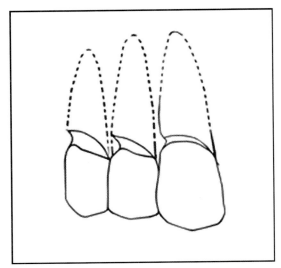

Toothbrush abrasion

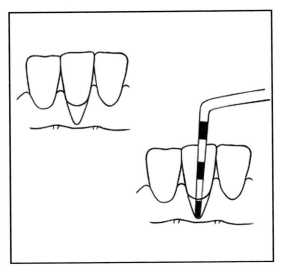

Recession

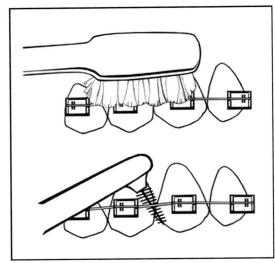

Oral care for orthodontic bands

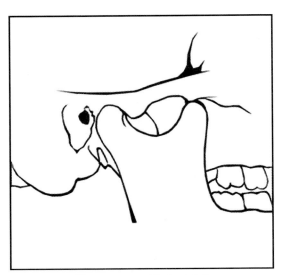

Temporomandibular joint

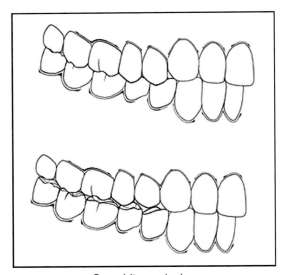

Crossbite occlusion

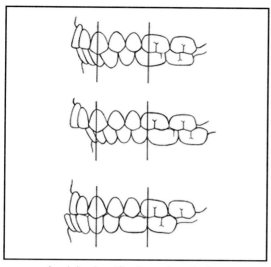

Angle's classification of occlusion

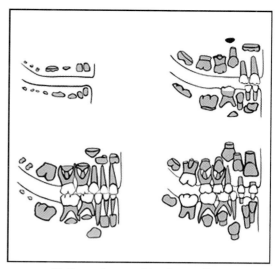

Pattern of normal tooth eruption

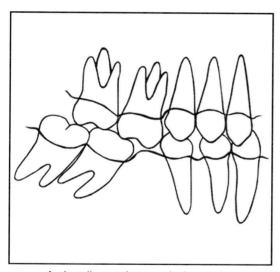

Arch collapse due to missing molar

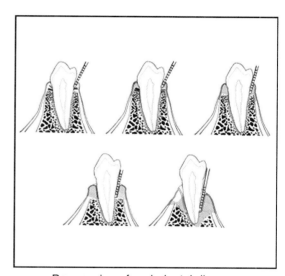

Progression of periodontal disease

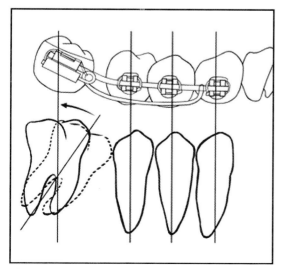

Orthodontic tooth movement—uprighting a tilted molar

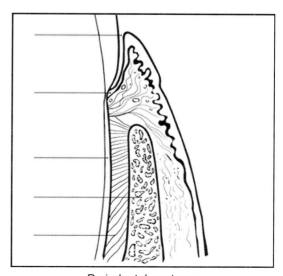

Periodontal anatomy

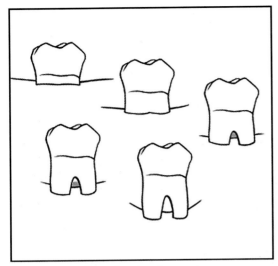

Furcation involvement

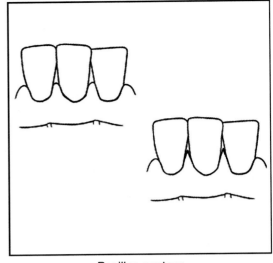

Papillae contour

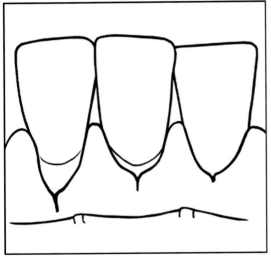

Gingival recession and clefting

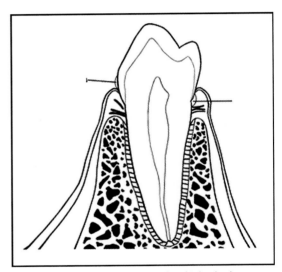

Calculus—supra- and subgingival

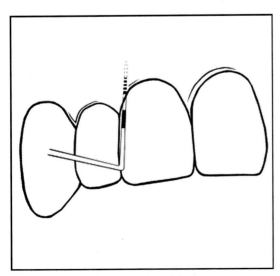

Periodontal probing

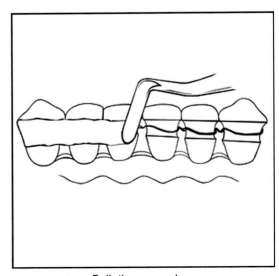

Splinting procedure

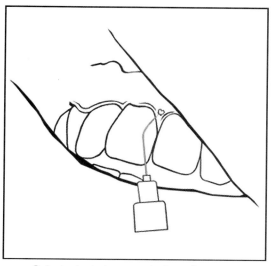

Subgingival placement of medicament

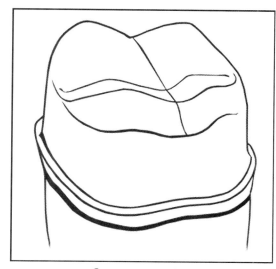

Crown preparation

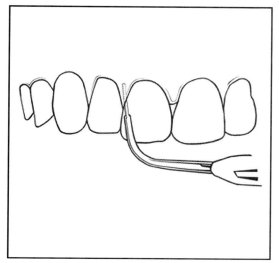

Subgingival irrigation

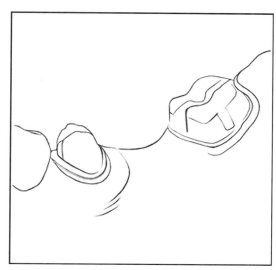

3-unit bridge preparation

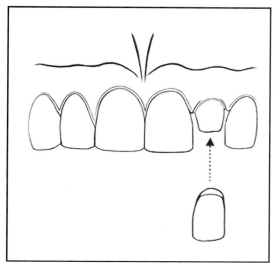

Single crown

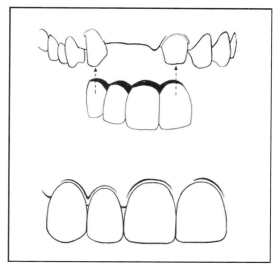

Anterior bridge preparation and seating

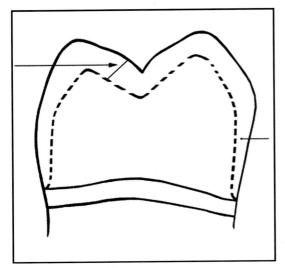

All metal crown

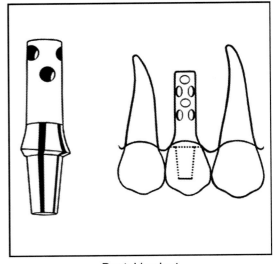

Dental implant

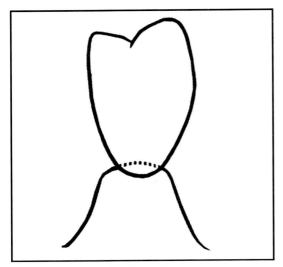

Ovate pontic

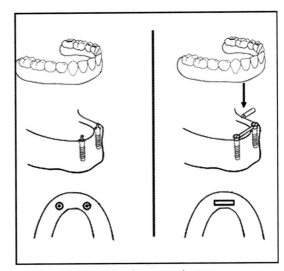

Dental implant overdenture

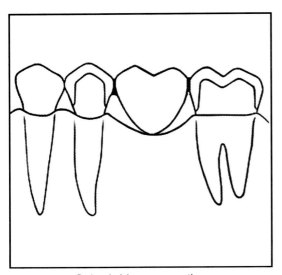

Onlay bridge preparation

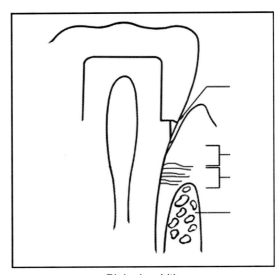

Biologic width

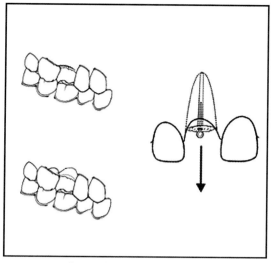

Crown lengthening option

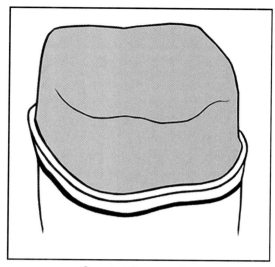

Core build-up—molar

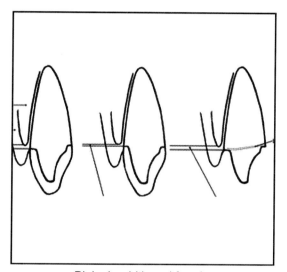

Biologic width and ferrule

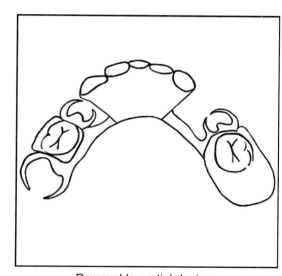

Removable partial denture

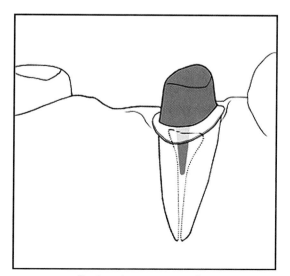

Post and core—premolar

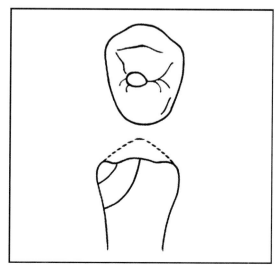

Tunnel preparation—hard tissue

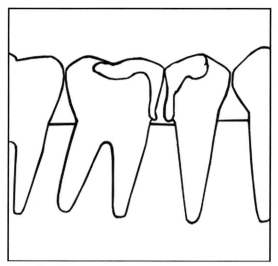

Poorly contoured amalgam restoration

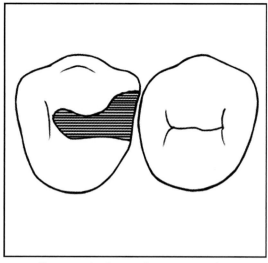

Open contact—amalgam restoration

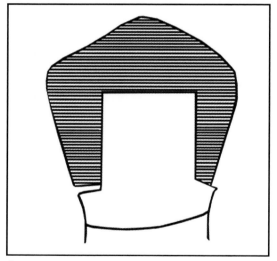

Open margin and underfinished margin on crown

Educational Packet Cover Art

This section contains seven pieces of artwork that can be used as attractive cover sheets for any educational packet you want to customize for a patient. The topics for which you can provide educational packets include the following:

Having the Smile you Want
Children's Dentistry
Diagnosis and Treatment of Beginning to Moderate Gum Disease
Diagnosis and Treatment of Advanced Gum Disease
Consideration in Tooth Replacement
Considerations in Advanced Tooth Replacement
Restoring your Teeth
The text that is included in the cover art can be customized to reflect your personal preferences.

Having the Smile you Want

As a new patient to our practice, we want you to know that you can expect the best in oral care. Our goal is to determine the dental treatment you both need and want, help you explore financial options, and provide your dental care in an efficient and courteous manner. Please review the information in this package prior to your first appointment. We will be glad to discuss any questions or concerns that you may have relative to your oral health before treatment begins.

This package includes the following materials:

Welcome to the Neighborhood
Welcome to Our Practice
Cancellation and No-Show Policy
Dental Emergencies
Dental Insurance Coverage
Dental Insurance – Points to Consider
Initial Oral Examination
Have the Dentistry You Need, Want, and Deserve
    for a Lifetime of Great Oral Health

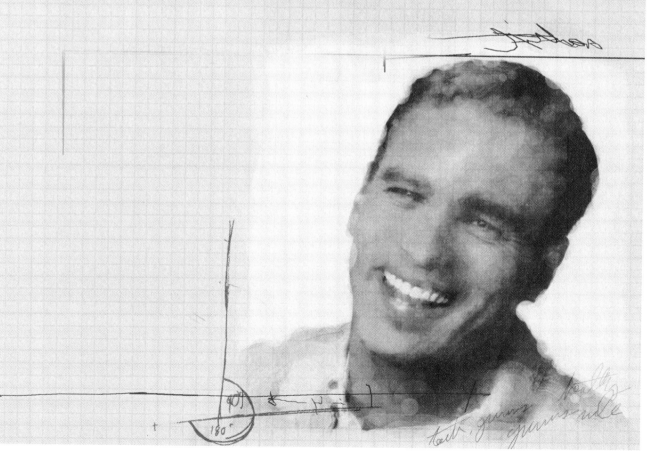

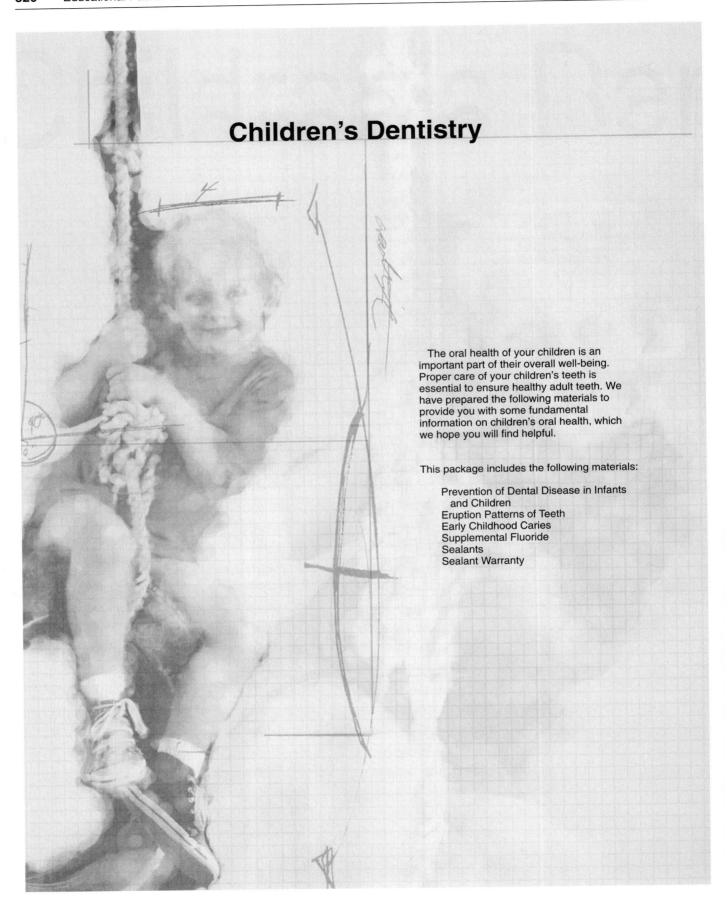

Children's Dentistry

The oral health of your children is an important part of their overall well-being. Proper care of your children's teeth is essential to ensure healthy adult teeth. We have prepared the following materials to provide you with some fundamental information on children's oral health, which we hope you will find helpful.

This package includes the following materials:

Prevention of Dental Disease in Infants
  and Children
Eruption Patterns of Teeth
Early Childhood Caries
Supplemental Fluoride
Sealants
Sealant Warranty

Diagnosis and Treatment of Beginning to Moderate Gum Disease

Periodontal disease is an infection that affects the gum tissues and bone around your teeth. You have been diagnosed with active periodontal disease that must be treated. The information in this package will help you understand our treatment recommendations and the part you will play in ensuring the success of that treatment.

Please review these information sheets prior to your appointment. We will be glad to discuss any questions or concerns that you may have before treatment begins.

This package includes the following materials:

Before Treatment Begins
Gingivitis
Early Signs of Periodontal Disease
How to Brush! How to Floss!
Prophylaxis
For a Lifetime of Great Oral Health

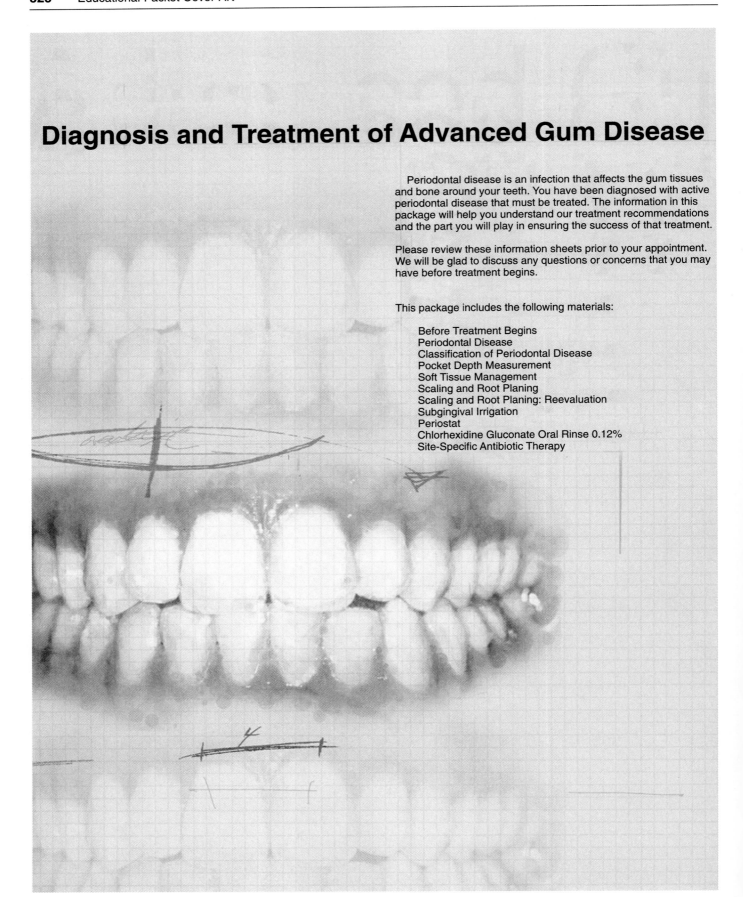

Diagnosis and Treatment of Advanced Gum Disease

Periodontal disease is an infection that affects the gum tissues and bone around your teeth. You have been diagnosed with active periodontal disease that must be treated. The information in this package will help you understand our treatment recommendations and the part you will play in ensuring the success of that treatment.

Please review these information sheets prior to your appointment. We will be glad to discuss any questions or concerns that you may have before treatment begins.

This package includes the following materials:

Before Treatment Begins
Periodontal Disease
Classification of Periodontal Disease
Pocket Depth Measurement
Soft Tissue Management
Scaling and Root Planing
Scaling and Root Planing: Reevaluation
Subgingival Irrigation
Periostat
Chlorhexidine Gluconate Oral Rinse 0.12%
Site-Specific Antibiotic Therapy

Considerations in Tooth Replacement

There are many options available to restore teeth to complete function. The decision to fill a tooth, to place a crown, or to replace missing teeth with a bridge or implant will be based on the conditions that are unique to your mouth. This package will provide information to help you understand our treatment recommendations and discusses the different options available.

Please review the information in this package prior to your appointment. We will be glad to discuss any questions or concerns that you may have before treatment begins.

This package includes the following materials:

Before Treatment Begins
Have Missing Teeth Replaced
Crowns and Bridges: Procedural Overview
Crown and Bridge Fees
Materials Options: An Overview
Cast Porcelain Fused to Metal Restorations
Bridges: An Overview
Full Ceramic and Porcelain Bridges

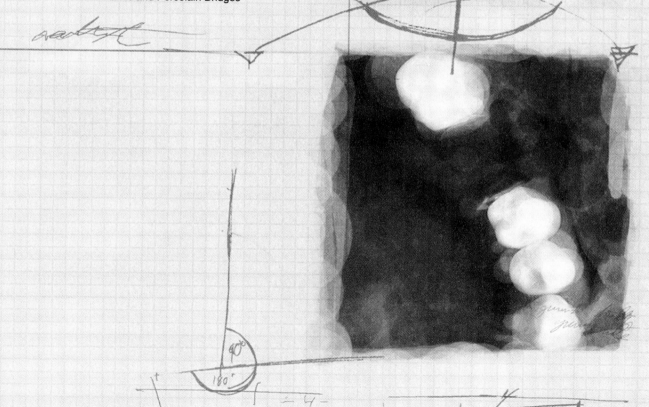

Considerations in Advanced Tooth Replacement

There are many options available to restore teeth to complete function. The decision to fill a tooth, to place a crown, or to replace missing teeth with a bridge or implant will be based on the conditions that are unique to your mouth. This package will provide information to help you understand our treatment recommendations and discusses the different options available.

Please review the information in this package prior to your appointment. We will be glad to discuss any questions or concerns that you may have before treatment begins.

This package includes the following materials:

Before Treatment Begins
Implants, Crowns, and Bridges vs. Natural Teeth
Crowns: An Overview
Crown and Bridge Fees
Crowns and Bridges: Procedural Overview
Materials Options: An Overview
Cast Gold Restorations
Cast Gold and Ceramic Restorations
Cast Porcelain Fused to Metal Restorations
Full Porcelain/Full Ceramic Restorations

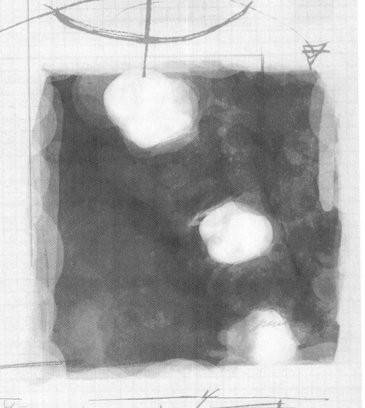

Restoring your Teeth

There are many options available to restore teeth to complete function. The decision to fill a tooth, to place a crown, or to replace missing teeth with a bridge or implant will be based on the conditions that are unique to your mouth. This package will provide information to help you understand our treatment recommendations and discusses the different options available.

Please review the information in this package prior to your appointment. We will be glad to discuss any questions or concerns that you may have before treatment begins.

This package includes the following materials:

Before Treatment Begins
Amalgam Restorations
Bonded Resin Restorations
Defective Restorations
Safety of Silver Amalgam and Base Metals
Warranty for Restorative Materials

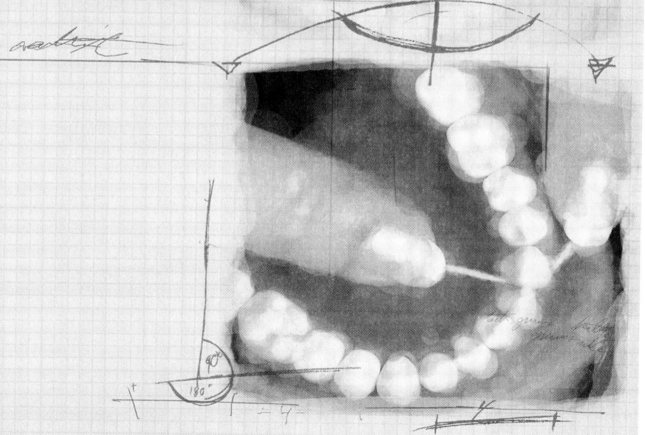

Index

Contenido

i

Contenido Detallado

primera parte

Comunicación con los Negocios/Ejecutivos

Revisión del Contenido:
Administración de la Práctica

Contacto con el Paciente

Formulario de Admisión del Paciente Nuevo
Use esto para asistir a la recepcionista al obtener la información necesaria cuando se fijan las citas de pacientes nuevos.

Matrícula del Paciente Nuevo
Información del paciente necesaria para procesar las reclamaciones de seguros.

Registro de la Visita Inicial del Paciente
Mantenga un historial de los aspectos consistentes con la Terapia Endodóntica: Largos Estimados bajo la Gráfica del Paciente de una visita inicial: necesidades del paciente, co-consultaciones y temas discutidos.

Lista de Verificación para la Discusión con el Paciente
Use esta lista para estar al día con la información escrita entregada a los pacientes para mejorar el diálogo.

Documentos para la Educación del Paciente
Esta lista de verificación asegura que los pacientes reciben la información que necesitan y duplicados.

Preferencias del Paciente
Encuesta de las expectativas y preocupaciones dentales del paciente.

Preferencias del Paciente: Niño
Encuesta de las expectativas y preocupaciones dentales de los padres acerca de su niño(a).

Preferencias del Paciente: Joven Adulto
Encuesta de las expectativas y preocupaciones dentales del paciente joven adulto.

Plan de Tratamiento
Use esto para seguir con atención la historia concisa del tratamiento planeado y las fechas de su conclusión. Útil para tratamientos que consisten de fases.

Formularios para la Gráfica Dental del Paciente

Terapia Endodóntica: Largos Estimados
Mantenga un historial sobre el largo de los canales del paciente durante de todas las sesiones de tratamiento endodóntico.

Terapia Endodóntica: Consentimiento Informado
La firma del paciente indica que entiende la terapia endodóntica, los honorarios envueltos y que se contestaron sus preguntas a su satisfacción.

Extracción: Consentimiento Informado
La firma del paciente indica que entiende la razón para la extracción dental, las posibles complicaciones y que se contestaron sus preguntas a su satisfacción.

Comunicaciones

Comunicaciones en la Oficina

Registro Diario de Información en la Gráfica Dental
Mantiene un historial para la oficina principal de las necesidades de citas y tratamiento de los pacientes, y el registro es usado como una lista de verificación de haber completado todos los papeles relacionados.

Directivos para el Tratamiento de la Higiene Dental
Una lista de verificación para asegurar una comunicación eficiente entre el dentista y el higienista.

Revisión del Contenido: Administración de la Práctica—continuación

Códigos de los Procedimientos Dentales
Una lista de códigos CDT-4 que se usará en la oficina para comunicar el tratamiento rendido en una hoja de trámite.

Hojas de Trámite
Use éstas para comunicar el tratamiento provisto y necesario para el paciente al personal de negocios.

Comunicaciones con el Laboratorio
Casos en Progreso en el Laboratorio
Para organizar, hacer citas y proveer un historial de los casos en el laboratorio.

Orden de Trabajo del Laboratorio
Lista de verificación para proveer al laboratorio con instrucciones completas para la construcción del caso.

Mercadear Su Práctica
Ayudas de Mercadeo
Ideas para ayudarle a planear su estrategia de mercadeo.

Guía para el Comunicado de Prensa
Se puede usar este comunicado de prensa tal como está o como una base para otros comunicados de prensa. Ofrece varias alternativas de anuncios.

Listas y Formularios de Teléfono
Llamadas Misceláneas por Completarse
Use estos para proveer al personal de negocios una lista de las necesidades de información de otras fuentes.

Pacientes Que Necesitan un Cambio de Cita
Una lista para mantener un historial de citas canceladas por pacientes o pacientes que no se presentaron a sus citas.

Cambios de Citas por Prioridad
Use esto para llenar vacantes en el horario y para mantener un historial de pacientes que quieren una cita más temprana o más conveniente cuando haya una vacante, aún con poco tiempo de anticipación.

Profesionales Solicitando Información del Paciente
Mantiene un historial de llamadas de dentistas, especialistas o médicos en cuanto al tratamiento del paciente.

HIPAA
Acto de la Portabilidad y de la Responsabilidad del Seguro Médico de 1996 (HIPAA)
El Acto de la Portabilidad y de la Responsabilidad del Seguro Médico de 1996 (HIPAA): qué es y qué cubre.

HIPAA—Contrato para los Asociados de Negocios
Lista de responsabilidades de los asociados de negocios con respecto a la información de salud protegida.

HIPAA—Registro del Entrenamiento del Personal
Lista para mantener un registro de los empleados que han recibido la política de la oficina respecto al Acto de la Portabilidad y de la Responsabilidad del Seguro Médico de 1996.

Formulario de Admisión del Paciente Nuevo

Fecha:_____   **Alerta de Salud:**_____

Paciente:_____   **Enviado por:**_____

Teléfono(s): Hogar:_____   **Trabajo:**_____   **Otro:**_____

Correo electrónico:_____

Razón para llamar:
❑ Dolor de diente o dolor, ¿por cuánto tiempo?_____
❑ Examen de paciente nuevo
❑ Hinchazón, ¿dónde?_____
❑ Empastadura perdida
❑ Problemas con la dentadura
❑ Diente roto
❑ Consulta

Comentarios (queja principal). Por favor escriba según como el paciente lo explicó:

_____

_____

Última cita dental o higiene dental:_____
Actitud: ❑ Agradable   ❑ Asustado   ❑ Otro
¿Se le ha dicho al paciente alguna vez que necesita **premedicación** antes de la cita dental?
❑ No ❑ Sí   ¿Por qué y qué medicación?_____
        Nombre y número de teléfono del médico:_____

¿Seguro dental?   ❑ Sí ❑ No
Si la respuesta es sí, diga al paciente: "Para que pueda recibir el reembolso máximo y más rápido de su seguro dental, debe traer su folleto de beneficios dentales y al menos un formulario de reclamación con su sección completamente llena y firmada. Por favor esté preparado para pagar por todo el diagnóstico y tratamiento de emergencia cuando venga. Si tratamiento futuro es necesario, será informado por el doctor. En este caso, se hará un estimado y usted puede hacer los arreglos financieros apropiados. ¿Usted tiene alguna pregunta?"

Diga al paciente el honorario anticipado por el examen oral inicial, examen de emergencia o radiografías si son necesarias. Diga al paciente que el honorario del examen incluye el examen inicial, diagnóstico, plan de tratamiento y consulta.

Diga al paciente: Las radiografías (rayos X) pueden ser requeridas para un diagnóstico exacto. El doctor determinará qué radiografías son necesarias cuando le examine.

Diga al paciente: Venga con 15 minutos de anticipación a la cita para llenar el formulario de historial de salud. Diga al paciente que si una cita debe ser cancelada, debe notificarlo al menos 24 horas antes de la cita, como cortesía a la oficina y a los otros pacientes.

Llamada tomada por:_____   **Fecha:**_____

Matrícula del Paciente Nuevo

Por favor complete este formulario. Si usted tiene seguro dental, no podemos someter una reclamación a menos que la información solicitada sea exacta. Si usted tiene cobertura de seguro dental doble, complete la información para el portador secundario. Gracias por su atención al detalle.

Nombre del Paciente: _____   Fecha de Nacimiento: _____

Número de Seguro Social del Paciente: _____
Dirección: _____
Ciudad: _____   Estado: _____ Código Postal: _____
Teléfono del hogar: ( ) _____   Teléfono del trabajo: ( ) _____
Correo electrónico: _____
Patrón del Paciente: _____

Información del Asegurado:
Nombre: _____   Fecha de Nacimiento: _____
Número de Seguro Social: _____   Patrón: _____
Dirección: _____
Ciudad: _____   Estado: _____ Código Postal: _____
Teléfono del hogar: ( ) _____   Teléfono del trabajo: ( ) _____

Información del Seguro:
Por favor seleccione el portador de seguro dental:
❏ Tradicional   ❏ Delta
❏ AETNA/Prudential PDO   ❏ CIGNA PPO   ❏ MetLife PPO   ❏ BC/BS PPO
Número de ID del Grupo: _____   Número de Teléfono de Reclamaciones: _____
Dirección para Someter Reclamaciones:
Calle: _____
Ciudad: _____   Estado: _____ Código Postal: _____

Información del Seguro Secundario:
Nombre _____   Fecha de Nacimiento: _____
Número de Seguro Social: _____   Patrón: _____
Calle: _____
Ciudad: _____   Estado: _____ Código Postal: _____
Teléfono del hogar: ( ) _____   Teléfono del trabajo: ( ) _____

Por favor seleccione el portador de seguro dental:
❏ Tradicional   ❏ Delta
❏ AETNA/Prudential PDO   ❏ CIGNA PPO   ❏ MetLife PPO   ❏ BC/BS PPO
Número de ID del Grupo: _____   Número de Teléfono de Reclamaciones: _____

Dirección para Someter Reclamaciones:
Calle: _____
Ciudad: _____   Estado: _____ Código Postal: _____

Registro de la Visita Inicial del Paciente

Paciente:_____ **Fecha:**_____

❑ Tiempo con el paciente:_____

Necesidades del Paciente *(escriba la fecha e iniciales cuando lo complete)*
❑ ___ ___ Necesidades del paciente ❑ Interproximal ❑ Examen de boca completa ❑ Plan de tratamiento ❑ Otro
❑ ___ ___ El paciente necesita recibir folletos en los tópicos:_____
❑ ___ ___ El paciente necesita ver visuales de los temas:_____
❑ ___ ___ El paciente necesita que nuestra oficina llame al dentista anterior para ❑ Radiografías ❑ Registrar información en
        la gráfica periodontal
        Nombre del Dentista:_____ Teléfono #:_____
        Fecha que se llamó:_____ Se habló con:_____
❑ Paciente informado acerca de la enfermedad periodontal:
        Tipo de caso: ❑ 1   ❑ 2   ❑ 3   ❑ 4   ❑ 5   ❑ 6   ❑ 7   ❑ 8
        ❑ Generalizado   ❑ Localizado—áreas específicas:_____
❑ Paciente aconsejado para tener el siguiente tratamiento:
        ❑ Alisado/Raspado radicular: ❑ Toda la boca   ❑ cuadrante_____   ❑ diente #_____
        ❑ Irrigación subgingival: ❑ Toda la boca   ❑ cuadrante_____   ❑ diente #_____
        ❑ Instrumento de higiene oral
        ❑ Re-evaluación/examen con sonda en _____ (fecha).
        ❑ Profilaxis de adulto
❑ Paciente aconsejado para estar en el intervalo de cuidado repetido de_____.
❑ Examen general para el plan de tratamiento

Paciente enviado al:
Endodontista
❑ Para evaluación del diente #_____
❑ Para tratamiento del diente #_____
❑ Endodontista:_____

Cirujano Oral
❑ Para la extracción del diente #_____
❑ Para evaluación de:_____ Área/diente_____
❑ Cirujano oral:_____

Ortodoncista
❑ Para evaluación:_____
❑ Para tratamiento:_____
❑ Ortodoncista:_____

Periodontista
❑ Para evaluación:_____ Área/diente_____
❑ Para tratamiento:_____ Área/diente_____
❑ Periodontista:_____

Discusiones con el Paciente
❑ Paciente informado de los riesgos, opciones, ventajas, desventajas del tratamiento.
❑ Se le ha dicho al paciente que el tratamiento periodontal se debe terminar antes de comenzar el tratamiento restaurativo.
❑ Se le ha dicho al paciente que el tratamiento puede cambiar si las condiciones orales cambian o no son como se esperaba
    del examen.
❑ Estimado del tiempo de tratamiento y honorarios discutidos con el paciente.
❑ El paciente necesita/pidió el tratamiento en fases.
❑ El paciente tiene objeciones al tratamiento: ❑ financieras ❑ tiempo ❑ emocionales
❑ El paciente no tiene ninguna otra pregunta.

Lista de Verificación para la Discusión con el Paciente

Paciente:_____   **Fecha:**_____

Información Dental a Dar al Paciente:

❑ **Visión general de la oficina**   ❑ Verbal   ❑ Escrita

                                         ❑ Bienvenido a Nuestra Práctica

❑ **Información dental general**   ❑ Verbal   ❑ Escrita

  ❑ Para una Vida con una Magnífica Salud Oral
  ❑ Examen Oral Inicial

❑ **Enfermedad periodontal**   ❑ Verbal   ❑ Escrita

  ❑ Enfermedad Periodontal
  ❑ Enfermedad Periodontal y Salud Sistemática

❑ **Cuidado repetido del mantenimiento de la higiene**   ❑ Verbal   ❑ Escrita

  ❑ Profilaxis

❑ **Odontología cosmética**   ❑ Verbal   ❑ Escrita

  ❑ Odontología Cosmética
  ❑ Opciones Caseras de Blanqueo
  ❑ Blanquear los Dientes: Visión General y Opciones
  ❑ Reemplazar Restauraciones Antiestéticas

❑ **Restauraciones**   ❑ Verbal   ❑ Escrita

  ❑ Restauraciones de Amalgama
  ❑ Restauraciones de Resina Adherida
  ❑ Coronas: Visión General
  ❑ Puentes: Visión General
  ❑ Implantes: Visión General

❑ **Prevención**   ❑ Verbal   ❑ Escrita

  ❑ Prevención de la Enfermedad Dental en Infantes y Niños
  ❑ Prevención del Deterioro
  ❑ Selladores
  ❑ Selladores y Fluoruro: Beneficios a Pacientes Adultos
  ❑ Fluoruro Suplementario
  ❑ Fluoruro Tópico

❑ **Necesidad de radiografías necesarias**   ❑ Verbal   ❑ Escrita

  ❑ Radiografías

Información de Negocio a Dar al Paciente

❑ **Información del pretratamiento**   ❑ Verbal   ❑ Escrita

  ❑ Cancelación y Política de No Presentarse
  ❑ Estimado de Honorarios
  ❑ Procedimiento de la Próxima Cita
  ❑ Objetivos del Tratamiento

❑ **Coordinación del seguro**   ❑ Verbal   ❑ Escrita

Acuerdos Financieros

  ❑ Cobertura del Seguro Dental
  ❑ Seguro Dental—Puntos a Considerar
  ❑ Estimado de Honorarios
  ❑ Arreglos Financieros
  ❑ Programa para Pagos

Documentos para la Educación del Paciente

Cuadros marcados indican la información que se dará al paciente. Por favor ponga la fecha y sus iniciales cuando se entrega la información al paciente.

Odontología Cosmética
Condiciones Congénitas

    Fecha   Inicial

- ❏ Erupción Pasiva Alterada: Tejido Suave — 450
- ❏ Erupción Pasiva Alterada: Tejido Duro — 451
- ❏ Dientes Que Faltan Congénitamente — 452
- ❏ Diastemas: Cerrar Espacios entre los Dientes — 453
- ❏ Fluorosis, Esmalte Veteado y Manchas Blancas — 454
- ❏ Incisivos Laterales Coniformes — 455

Procedimientos Cosméticos

- ❏ Restauraciones de Resina Adherida: Empastaduras del Color del Diente para los Dientes Posteriores — 456
- ❏ Odontología Cosmética — 457
- ❏ Recontorno del Tejido Cosméticamente — 458
- ❏ Recontorno del Esmalte — 459
- ❏ Laminados de Porcelana y Resina: Adhesión — 460
- ❏ Inlays y Onlays de Porcelana — 461
- ❏ Reemplazar Restauraciones Antiestéticas — 462
- ❏ La Sonrisa Perfecta — 463

Blanqueo
Información General

- ❏ Blanquear los Dientes: Visión General y Opciones — 464
- ❏ ¡Usted Puede Tener Dientes Más Blancos! — 465

Procedimientos Específicos

- ❏ Opciones Caseras para Blanquear los Dientes — 466
- ❏ Instrucciones para el Sistema Casero para Blanquear los Dientes con Cubetas — 467
- ❏ Técnica Potente de Blanqueo de Dientes en la Oficina sin Activación de Luz — 468
- ❏ Técnica Potente de Blanqueo de Dientes en la Oficina con Activación de Luz — 469
- ❏ Instrucciones Postoperatorias para el Blanqueo de Dientes en la Oficina — 470
- ❏ Opciones No Vitales para Blanquear los Dientes — 471
- ❏ Dientes Desteñidos por Tetraciclina: Opciones para la Mejoría Cosmética — 472

Endodoncia

- ❏ Apicectomía — 475
- ❏ Síndrome de Periodoncia-Endodoncia — 476
- ❏ Terapia Endodóntica: Una Visión General — 477
- ❏ Terapia Endodóntica: Procedimiento — 478
- ❏ Re-tratamiento de los Canales Radiculares — 479
- ❏ Hemisecciones y Amputaciones Radiculares — 480

Odontología en General
General

    Fecha   Inicial

- ❏ Antes de Comenzar el Tratamiento — 485
- ❏ Anatomía Dental y Oral — 486
- ❏ Obtenga la Odontología Que Usted Necesita, Quiere y Se Merece — 487
- ❏ Procedimientos de Control de Infecciones — 488
- ❏ Examen Oral Inicial — 489

- ❏ Medicamentos Recetados — 490
- ❏ Ejemplo de Folleto para el Paciente — 491-492
- ❏ Antibióticos Profilácticos para la Premedicación — 493-494
- ❏ Línea de la Sonrisa — 495
- ❏ Quedando Bien: Cómo Mantener Su Boca Saludable — 496
- ❏ Tratar a un Paciente Adulto — 497

Prevención

- ❏ Para una Vida con una Magnífica Salud Oral — 498
- ❏ ¡Cómo Cepillarse! ¡Cómo Limpiarse con Hilo Dental! — 499
- ❏ Alerta de Bebidas Chatarras — 500
- ❏ Prevención del Deterioro — 501
- ❏ Cuando las Radiografías Son Necesarias — 502
- ❏ Dar Marcha Atrás al Deterioro — 503
- ❏ Selladores y Fluoruro: Beneficio para los Pacientes Adultos — 504
- ❏ Fluoruro Tópico: En el Hogar y en la Oficina — 505

Problemas: Causas y Curas

- ❏ Abfracción: Un Nuevo Término Dental — 506
- ❏ Reflujo Ácido (Enfermedad de Reflujo Gastroesofágico) — 507
- ❏ Atrición y Abrasión — 508
- ❏ Mal Aliento — 509
- ❏ Síndrome de Diente Fraccionado — 510
- ❏ Síndrome de Diente Fraccionado: Instrucciones Postoperatorias — 511
- ❏ Deterioro de la Dentina — 512
- ❏ Displasia del Esmalte — 513
- ❏ Desgaste Excesivo — 514
- ❏ Extracción — 515
- ❏ Extracciones: Instrucciones Postoperatorias — 516
- ❏ Dolores de Cabeza: La Conexión Dental — 517
- ❏ Cómo Fomentar el Deterioro de los Dientes (Humor) — 518
- ❏ Dientes Impactados — 519
- ❏ Grietas Inducidas en el Esmalte por las Empastaduras de Metal — 520
- ❏ Sensibilidad al Metal — 521
- ❏ Protectores Oclusos (de Mordida) — 522
- ❏ Pericoronitis — 523
- ❏ Caries en la Superficie Radicular — 524
- ❏ Dientes Sensibles — 525
- ❏ Cuestionario de Disfunción de la Articulación Temporomandibular — 526
- ❏ Síndrome de Disfunción de la Articulación Temporomandibular — 527
- ❏ Abrasión por el Cepillo de Dientes: Evitando la Destrucción del Diente — 528
- ❏ Oclusión Traumática: Equilibración Oclusal o Ajuste de la Mordida — 529
- ❏ Muelas Cordales—Terceros Molares — 530
- ❏ Xerostomía: Síndrome de Sequedad en la Boca — 531

Siga

Documentos para la Educación del Paciente—continuación

Ortodoncia

		Fecha	Inicial
❑ Cuidado de los Frenillos	534		
❑ Dientes que Faltan Congénitamente	535		
❑ Ortodoncia Fija y Removible	536		
❑ Ortodoncia (Frenillos)	537		
❑ Enderezar los Molares Inclinados	538		

Odontología Pediátrica

		Fecha	Inicial
❑ La Primera Visita del Niño al Dentista	541		
❑ Caries Tempranas en la Infancia	542		
❑ Patrones de Erupción de los Dientes	543		
❑ Prevención de la Enfermedad Dental en Infantes y Niños	544		
❑ Selladores	545		
❑ Garantía del Sellador	546		
❑ Fluoruro Suplementario	547		
❑ Fluoruro Tópico: En el Hogar y en la Oficina Dental	548		

Periodoncia
Evaluación y Enfermedades

		Fecha	Inicial
❑ Clasificación de la Enfermedad Periodontal	552		
❑ Señales Tempranas de la Enfermedad Periodontal	553		
❑ Involucración de la Furcación	554		
❑ Hiperplasia Gingival	555		
❑ Gingivitis	556		
❑ Gingiva Adherida Insuficiente	557		
❑ Enfermedad Periodontal Necrótica	558		
❑ Enfermedad Periodontal	559		
❑ Enfermedad Periodontal y la Salud Sistémica	560		
❑ Recomendaciones para el Tratamiento Periodontal: Terapia Inicial	561		
❑ Medida de la Profundidad del Bolsillo	562		
❑ El Fumar y la Periodontitis del Adulto	563		

Opciones de Tratamiento

❑ Cirugía Plástica Periodontal Electiva Cosmética: Recontorno del Tejido	564		
❑ Electrocirugía	565		
❑ Procedimientos de Colgajo	566		
❑ Injertos Gingivales	567		
❑ Procedimientos de Gingivectomía y Gingivoplastia	568		
❑ Desbridamiento Completo	569		
❑ Cirugía Ósea	570		
❑ Cirugía Periodontal	571		
❑ Profilaxis	572		
❑ Aumento de Reborde	573		
❑ Hemisecciones y Amputaciones Radiculares	574		
❑ Raspado y Alisado Radicular	575		
❑ Raspado y Alisado Radicular: Instrucciones para después del Procedimiento	576		
❑ Raspado y Alisado Radicular: Reevaluación	577		
❑ Manejo del Tejido Suave	578		
❑ Colocar Férulas en los Dientes	579		

Agentes de Quimoterapia

❑ Enjuague Oral de Gluconato de Clorohexidina 0.12%	580		
❑ Protocolo de Enjuague Oral	581		
❑ Periostat: Dosis Submicrobiana Sistémica de Doxiciclina	582		
❑ Terapia Antibiótica Específica al Lugar	583		
❑ Irrigación Subgingival	584		

Prostodoncia

		Fecha	Inicial
❑ Reemplazo de Dientes Que Faltan	588		
❑ Implantes, Coronas y Puentes versus Dientes Naturales	589		

Restauraciones Fijas
Coronas

❑ Coronas: Una Visión General	590		
❑ Diseño de Coronas	591		
❑ Coronas y Puentes: Una Visión General del Procedimiento	592		
❑ Honorarios por Coronas y Puentes	593		
❑ Instrucciones Preoperatorias para Coronas y Puentes	594		

Opciones de Materiales

❑ Opciones de Materiales: Una Visión General	595		
❑ Restauraciones de Molde de Oro	596		
❑ Restauraciones de Molde de Oro y Cerámica	597		
❑ Restauraciones de Molde de Porcelana Unida a Metal	598		
❑ Restauraciones Completas de Porcelana/Cerámica	599		

Puentes

❑ Puentes: Una Visión General	600		
❑ Puentes Completos de Cerámica y Porcelana	601		
❑ Puente de Maryland (Retenedor de Resina Adherida)	602		
❑ Pontic Ovalado	603		
❑ Puentes Unidos de Cobertura Parcial	604		

Implantes

❑ Implantes: Opciones	605		
❑ Implantes: Una Visión General de los Procedimientos	606		

Procedimientos y Aplicaciones

❑ Ancho Biológico	607		
❑ Cementación: Instrucciones Postoperatorias	608		
❑ Procedimiento de Alargamiento de la Corona	609		
❑ Defecto en el Lugar de Extracción	610		
❑ Estructura Coronaria Remanente (Abrazadera)	611		
❑ Impresiones	612		
❑ Postes	613		
❑ Postes, Construcciones de Base-Corona y Alargamiento de la Corona	614		
❑ Provisionales/Coronas	615		
❑ Coronas Provisionales: Instrucciones Postoperatorias	616		
❑ Modelos de Estudio y Modelos de Cera	617		

Siga

Documentos para la Educación del Paciente—continuación

Prostodoncia Removible
❑ Dentaduras Completas   618 _____ _____
❑ Dentaduras Inmediatas   619 _____ _____
❑ Dentaduras Parciales   620 _____ _____

Odontología Restaurativa

	Fecha	Inicial

Restauraciones
❑ Restauraciones de Amalgama   623 _____ _____
❑ Amalgamas y Resinas Adheridas:
  Instrucciones Postoperatorias   624 _____ _____
❑ Restauraciones de Resina Adherida:
  Empastaduras del Color del Diente para los
  Dientes Posteriores   625 _____ _____
❑ Microodontología: Restauración Preventiva
  de la Resina   626 _____ _____
❑ Restauraciones de Cobertura Parcial 627 _____ _____
❑ Inlays y Onlays de Porcelana   628 _____ _____
❑ Inlays y Onlays de Resina   629 _____ _____
❑ La Empastadura "Permanente"   630 _____ _____

Procedimientos Correctivos
❑ Restauraciones Defectuosas   631 _____ _____
❑ Recontorno del Esmalte   632 _____ _____
❑ Restauraciones Sedativas   633 _____ _____

Seguridad y Garantía
❑ Seguridad de la Amalgama de Plata y de los
  Metales Comunes   634 _____ _____

❑ Garantía de los Materiales Restaurativos   635 _____ _____
❑ Garantía del Diente Severamente
  Comprometido   636 _____ _____

Instrucciones Pre- y Postoperatorias

	Fecha	Inicial

❑ Amalgamas y Resinas Adheridas:
  Instrucciones Postoperatorias   624 _____ _____
❑ Antes de Comenzar el Tratamiento   485 _____ _____
❑ Cementación: Instrucciones
  Postoperatorias   608 _____ _____
❑ Síndrome de Diente Fraccionado:
  Instrucciones Postoperatorias   511 _____ _____
❑ Instrucciones Preoperatorias para Coronas
  y Puentes   594 _____ _____
❑ Extracciones: Instrucciones Postoperatorias 516 _____ _____
❑ Técnica Potente de Blanqueo de Dientes en la
  Oficina con Activación de Luz   469 _____ _____
❑ Terapia Endodóntica: Consentimiento
  Informado   354 _____ _____
❑ Extracción: Consentimiento Informado 355 _____ _____
❑ Antibióticos Profilácticos para la
  Premedicación   493-494 _____ _____
❑ Coronas Provisionales:
  Instrucciones Postoperatorias   616 _____ _____
❑ Raspado y Alisado Radicular:
  Instrucciones para después del Procedimiento 576 _____ _____

Preferencias del Paciente

Paciente:_____   **Fecha:**_____

Brevemente, díganos cómo usted se siente acerca de sus dientes, su sonrisa y sus expectativas dentales.

1. ¿Cuáles son sus expectativas de esta oficina?_____
_____

2. ¿Le gustaría aprender cómo puede tener todos sus dientes por el resto de su vida?   ❑ sí   ❑ no

3. Si le están faltando ya algunos dientes, ¿le gustaría aprender cómo puede evitar el tener dentaduras completas?   ❑ sí   ❑ no

4. ¿Le gusta su sonrisa?   ❑ sí   ❑ no

5. Si la respuesta es NO, ¿qué no le gusta y qué cambios le gustaría ver?_____
_____

6. Si siente que sus dientes se han amarilleado, o no son lo suficientemente blancos, ¿le gustaría aprender sobre el blanqueo de diente?   ❑ sí   ❑ no

7. ¿Está usted interesado en una evaluación cosmética dental general?   ❑ sí   ❑ no

8. Si usted está contemplando un cambio cosmético dental, ¿cuál es el más importante para usted?
_____
_____

9. ¿Está usted enterado de cualquier cosa que pueda evitar que usted tenga un tratamiento dental básico o cosmético?   ❑ sí   ❑ no

10. ¿Todas sus pasadas experiencias en la oficina dental han sido positivas?   ❑ sí   ❑ no
Si la respuesta es NO, por favor explique:
_____
_____

11. ¿Hay algo en particular que quisiera que siempre hagamos para usted?   ❑ sí   ❑ no
Si la respuesta es SÍ, por favor explique:
_____
_____

12. ¿Hay algo en particular que nunca quisiera que hiciéramos?   ❑ sí   ❑ no
Si la respuesta es SÍ, por favor explique:
_____
_____

13. ¿Usted tiene algunas preocupaciones dentales no enumeradas aquí que quisiera traer a nuestra atención?   ❑ sí   ❑ no
Si la respuesta es SÍ, por favor explique:
_____
_____

¡Gracias por tomar tiempo para llenar este formulario!

Preferencias del Paciente: Niño

Paciente:_____   **Fecha:**_____

Brevemente díganos cómo usted se siente acerca de los dientes de su niño y sus expectativas dentales.

1. ¿Cuáles son sus expectativas de esta oficina para su niño?_____
_____

2. ¿Le gustaría aprender cómo su niño podría tener todos sus dientes por el resto de su vida?   ❑ sí   ❑ no

3. ¿Preferiría usted quedarse en el cuarto del tratamiento dental durante la visita de su niño?   ❑ sí   ❑ no

4. ¿Las experiencias de su niño en la oficina dental en el pasado han sido todas positivas?   ❑ sí   ❑ no
Si la respuesta es NO, por favor explique:_____
_____

5. ¿Hay algo en particular que le gustaría que siempre hagamos para su niño?   ❑ sí   ❑ no
Si la respuesta es SÍ, por favor explique:_____
_____

6. ¿Hay algo en particular que le gustaría que nunca hagamos para su niño?   ❑ sí   ❑ no
Si la respuesta es SÍ, por favor explique:_____
_____

7. ¿Usted tiene algunas preocupaciones dentales acerca de su niño no enumeradas aquí que quisiera traer a nuestra atención?   ❑ sí   ❑ no
Si la respuesta es SÍ, por favor explique:_____
_____

¡Gracias por tomar tiempo para llenar este formulario!

Preferencias del Paciente: Joven Adulto

Paciente:_____   **Fecha:**_____

Brevemente díganos cómo usted se siente acerca de sus dientes, su sonrisa y sus expectativas dentales.

1. ¿Cuáles son sus expectativas de esta oficina?_____
   _____
   _____

2. ¿Es importante para usted el prevenir el deterioro, la enfermedad de las encías y el tener
   un aliento fresco?   ❏ sí   ❏ no

3. ¿Sus experiencias en la oficina dental en el pasado han sido todas positivas?   ❏ sí   ❏ no
   Si la respuesta es NO, por favor explique:_____
   _____

4. ¿Hay algo en particular que le gustaría que siempre hagamos para usted?   ❏ sí   ❏ no
   Si la respuesta es SÍ, por favor explique:_____
   _____

5. ¿Hay algo en particular que le gustaría que nunca hagamos para usted?   ❏ sí   ❏ no
   Si la respuesta es SÍ, por favor explique:_____
   _____

6. ¿Usted tiene algunas preocupaciones dentales no enumeradas aquí que quisiera traer
   a nuestra atención?   ❏ sí   ❏ no
   Si la respuesta es SÍ, por favor explique:_____
   _____

7. ¿Usted piensa que sus dientes están lo suficientemente derechos?   ❏ sí   ❏ no

8. ¿Ha visto alguna vez a un ortodoncista?   ❏ sí   ❏ no

9. ¿Hay algo sobre su sonrisa que particularmente no le gusta?   ❏ sí   ❏ no
   Díganos sobre ello:_____
   _____

10. ¿Cuál es su deporte y equipo preferido, qué tipo de música le gusta, cuál es su grupo musical preferido y cuál es la mejor
    película que usted ha visto?
    Deporte_____
    Equipo de Deporte_____
    Música_____
    Grupo Musical_____
    Película_____

¡Gracias por tomar tiempo para llenar este formulario!

Plan de Tratamiento

Paciente:_____

Procedimiento	Comentario	Proveedor del Tratamiento	Fecha del Diagnóstico	Fecha Que Terminó	✓

Terapia Endodóntica: Largos Estimados

Paciente:_____   **Fecha:**_____

Diente #

Canal: *Largo Estimado*
Fecha: MB es ____ mm a ____ B ____ a ____   P ____ a ____
                                DB es ____ mm a ____ L ____ a ____   ML ____ a ____

Canal: *Largo de Trabajo/Localizador de Ápice*
Fecha: MB es ____ mm a ____ B ____ a ____   P ____ a ____
                                DB es ____ mm a ____ L ____ a ____   ML ____ a ____

Canal: *Largo de Radiografías*
Fecha: MB es ____ mm a ____ B ____ a ____   P ____ a ____
                                DB es ____ mm a ____ L ____ a ____   ML ____ a ____

Canal: *Largo Final—Ajustado*
Fecha: MB es ____ mm a ____ B ____ a ____   P ____ a ____
                                DB es ____ mm a ____ L ____ a ____   ML ____ a ____

MB = Mesiobucal   B = Bucal   P = Palatino
DB = Distobucal   L = Lingual   ML = Mesiolingual

Paciente:_____   **Fecha:**_____

Diente #
Canal: *Largo Estimado*
Fecha: MB es ____ mm a ____ B ____ a ____   P ____ a ____
                                DB es ____ mm a ____ L ____ a ____   ML ____ a ____

Canal: *Largo de Trabajo/Localizador de Ápice*
Fecha: MB es ____ mm a ____ B ____ a ____   P ____ a ____
                                DB es ____ mm a ____ L ____ a ____   ML ____ a ____

Canal: *Largo de Radiografías*
Fecha: MB es ____ mm a ____ B ____ a ____   P ____ a ____
                                DB es ____ mm a ____ L ____ a ____   ML ____ a ____

Canal: *Largo Final—Ajustado*
Fecha: MB es ____ mm a ____ B ____ a ____   P ____ a ____
                                DB es ____ mm a ____ L ____ a ____   ML ____ a ____

MB = Mesiobucal   B = Bucal   P = Palatino
DB = Distobucal   L = Lingual   ML = Mesiolingual

Terapia Endodóntica: Consentimiento Informado

Nombre del Paciente:_____   **Fecha:**_____

Entiendo que la terapia endodóntica (terapia del canal radicular) planificada para el diente # _____ es intentada cuando el tejido del nervio en el diente tiene tratamiento y se está haciendo en un diente vital como parte de un plan de tratamiento exhaustivo. La razón de la muerte del nervio puede ser deterioro, infección, trauma o como parte de los procedimientos restaurativos que requieren que un dentista prepare el diente para una restauración grande o una corona. Este procedimiento se ha explicado para mi satisfacción. También me han informado que ocasionalmente hay complicaciones durante o después del procedimiento del canal radicular.

Estoy enterado de las posibles complicaciones que incluyen: dolor, hinchazón, sensibilidad a la presión o a las fuerzas normales de morder. Puedo tener una reacción alérgica a los medicamentos o a los anestésicos usados. Entiendo que deben tomarse varias radiografías para ayudar a asegurar la instrumentación apropiada de el (los) canal(es) y el ajuste del material de empastadura en el canal radicular.

Entiendo que el tratamiento puede ser complicado, puede necesitar ser modificado o incluso descontinuado debido a las dificultades imprevistas incluyendo, pero no limitadas a: canales calcificados, perforación de la raíz o corona, canales inaccesibles o severamente torcidos, resorción interna o externa del diente, limas/instrumentos separados o rotos o fractura de la raíz o de la estructura de la corona. Algunas de estas complicaciones pueden requerir que sea enviado a un especialista endodóntico (endodontista) para evaluación o tratamiento adicional. Puede que necesite tener este procedimiento hecho enteramente por un endodontista.

Los procedimientos quirúrgicos del canal radicular pueden ser requeridos en el futuro debido a problemas continuos con el diente. La cirugía puede ser necesaria para quitar cualquier quiste(s) u otras infecciones relacionadas que se formen o que no curen correctamente.

La parte visible del diente y/o la raíz puede obscurecerse eventualmente. Esto podría causar un problema cosmético con el diente. El diente podría llegar a ser frágil y ser propenso a una fractura. Entiendo que está recomendado que este diente tenga una restauración con un molde de cobertura completa (corona u onlay). Las restauraciones con amalgama de plata no son apropiadas para los dientes tratados endodónticamente.

Me han explicado el tratamiento del canal radicular (o al guardián, si el paciente es un menor). En este momento no tengo ninguna otra pregunta. Entiendo que si preguntas se presentan durante el curso del tratamiento del canal radicular, puedo pedir más explicaciones al dentista que me está tratando. Entiendo que no hay garantía para este tratamiento endodóntico. Reconozco que el único otro tratamiento alternativo a la terapia endodóntica es extraer el diente. En este caso, puedo requerir un tratamiento dental aún más costoso.

Estoy de acuerdo con el tratamiento del canal radicular para el diente #_____ a ser realizado por el Dr._____ y con las radiografías, medicamentos o anestesia local que puedan ser utilizadas durante esta terapia. También entiendo que el tratamiento endodóntico puede requerir varias visitas a la oficina para completarse, dependiendo del número de canales que se tratarán, grado de dificultad, progreso de la curación y la resistencia de la infección radicular.

Me han dicho que los costos estimados son:
Tratamiento endodóntico para el diente #_____ $_____
Restauración final recomendada: $_____
   ❏ Molde del poste hecho a la medida
   ❏ Construcción del poste y la base del color del diente, en titanio o acero inoxidable
   ❏ Construcción de la base solamente
   ❏ Corona completa   ❏ Onlay en oro   ❏ Onlay en porcelana
   ❏ Otro:_____

_____   _____
Firma del Paciente o Guardián   Fecha

Extracción: Consentimiento Informado

Razones para recomendar la extracción de un diente:
- Enfermedad periodontal severa
- Daño irreparable al tejido del nervio dentro del diente
- Fracaso de la terapia endodóntica
- Fractura o deterioro severo de la superficie del diente
- Colocación incorrecta del diente o para propósitos ortodónticos

Me han informado la razón de la extracción del diente #_____ y me han explicado qué esperar durante este procedimiento. Entiendo que se requerirán radiografías dentales antes de la extracción, y posiblemente durante el procedimiento. Entiendo que requeriré un anestésico y que suturas pueden ser necesarias.

Me han dado y entiendo las instrucciones postoperatorias. También entiendo que me han dado una medicación antibiótica que debo tomarla hasta que la prescripción entera se acabe. Si me han recetado una medicación para el dolor, la tomaré solamente *si es necesaria*. Si la medicación para el dolor contiene un narcótico tal como codeína, podría ser peligroso operar maquinaria o conducir un vehículo de motor y podría causar daño a mí o a otros.

Espero sangrar por el área de la extracción por las primeras 24 horas.

Si prefiero puedo solicitar que la extracción sea hecha por un cirujano oral.

Algunas complicaciones de extracciones rutinarias incluyen (pero no se limitan a):
- Fractura de dientes o restauraciones adyacentes
- Dolor postoperatorio—leve, moderado o severo y durando de horas a días
- Hinchazón en y alrededor del área de la extracción
- Puntas o fragmentos de raíces separadas, fragmentos de hueso separados
- Daño temporal o permanente del nervio del área resultado del adormecimiento
- Curación incompleta resultando en dolor severo (alvéolo seco)
- Fractura del hueso circundante

Si usted tiene cualquier pregunta sobre la razón de la extracción, siéntase con libertad de preguntar.

He leído y entiendo la información presentada. No tengo otras preguntas sobre la extracción del diente #_____.

Doy mi permiso para extraer el diente.

_____   _____
Firma del Paciente o Guardián   Fecha

Registro Diario de Información en la Gráfica Dental

Fecha: _____

Proveedor del Tratamiento: _____

Nombre del Paciente	Cita Necesarias	Gráfica Dental Completada	Plan de Tratamiento Necesario	Higiene Necesaria	Carta para Paciente Nuevo	Verificar el Balance de la Cuenta	Pre-D Necesario	Seguro Completado	Seguro Enviado	Folletos Enviados

Directivos para el Tratamiento de la Higiene Dental

Paciente:_____   **Fecha:**_____

Por favor realice los siguientes servicios para el paciente. Cuando se terminen, por favor marque los servicios para revisión. Los números adyacentes al tratamiento son la secuencia de la cita y los servicios que se lograrán en esa visita.

Servicio Necesario	**Secuencia**	**Terminado**	
___	___	___	Radiografías: Interproximales
___	___	___	Radiografías: Series de boca completa
___	___	___	Radiografías: Otro_____
___	___	___	Instrucciones del cuidado oral de sí mismo
___	___	___	Divulgar
___	___	___	Divulgar, volver a examinar el cepillado y limpieza con hilo dental en cada cita de terapia. Haga que el paciente demuestre estas técnicas. Por favor ponga la fecha y anote en la gráfica periodontal del paciente cuando se logra.
___	___	___	Paciente aconsejado a comprar un irrigador oral. Por favor enseñe su uso con el accesorio periodontal.
___	___	___	Instrucción de la higiene oral de sí mismo incluye: ❑ cepillado de dientes ❑ limpieza con hilo dental ❑ cepillo Proxybrush ❑ enhebrador de hilo dental ❑ desbridamiento completo ❑ irrigador oral/accesorio periodontal
___	___	___	Reexaminar el proceso de la enfermedad periodontal
___	___	___	Registrar la información en la gráfica periodontal
___	___	___	Profilaxis de Adulto
___	___	___	Alisado/Raspado radicular de boca completa (1 visita)
___	___	___	Alisado/Raspado radicular de un cuadrante_____ visitas ❑ SD ❑ SI ❑ ID ❑ II ❑ con anestesia local
___	___	___	Alisado/Raspado radicular diente #_____
___	___	___	Irrigación subgingival, todos los bolsillos de 5mm o más. Áreas específicas.
___	___	___	Volver a sondear, reevaluar para terapia antimicrobiana local diente #_____
___	___	___	Colocar terapia antimicrobiana local: diente #_____
___	___	___	Colocar al paciente en un intervalo de cuidado repetido de_____ meses.
___	___	___	Cita para volver a sondear después de_____ semanas. Evaluar para terapia periodontal futura.
___	___	___	Reportar al Dr._____ los resultados de la terapia.
___	___	___	Después del tratamiento periodontal, haga que el paciente haga una cita de _____ minutos con el Dr._____ para evaluar y empezar otra odontología.
___	___	___	Otro:_____

Comentarios del higienista, recomendaciones u otras áreas que necesitan la evaluación del dentista.

_____

_____

Códigos de los procedimientos dentales (CDT-4 completo)

Diagnósticos/ Preventivos

0120 __ Examen oral periódico
0140 __ Examen oral limitado
0150 __ Examen oral exhaustivo
0160 __ Examen oral extensivo, detallado
0170 __ Re-evaluación limitada
0180 __ Evaluación exhaustiva periódica
0210 __ Rayos X, serie de boca completa
0220 __ Rayos X peri-apical, 1ra película
0230 __ Rayos X peri-apical, cada película adicional
0270 __ Rayos X interproximales, 1 película
0272 __ Rayos X interproximales, 2 películas
0274 __ Rayos X interproximales, 4 películas
0277 __ Rayos X interproximales verticales, 4 películas
0330 __ Panorámica
0460 __ Prueba de pulpa
0470 __ Moldes de diagnóstico
0471 __ Fotos diagnósticas
1110 __ Profilaxis - adulto
1120 __ Profilaxis - niño
1203 __ Fluoruro - niño
1204 __ Fluoruro - adulto
1330 __ Instrumento de Higiene Oral
1351 __ Selladores por diente
1510 __ Mantenedor de espacio unilateral
1515 __ Mantenedor de espacio bilateral
1550 __ Re-cementar el mantenedor de espacio

Restaurativos
Amalgamas

2140 __ Restauración de amalgama-1 superficie
2150 __ Restauración de amalgama-2 superficies
2160 __ Restauración de amalgama-3 superficies
2161 __ Restauración de amalgama-4+ superficies

Resina

2330 __ Restauración de resina-1 superficie, anterior
2331 __ Restauración de resina-2 superficies, anteriores
2332 __ Restauración de resina-3 superficies, anteriores

2335 __ Restauración de resina-4+ ángulo incisal
2390 __ Restauración de compuesto de resina de la corona, anterior
2391 __ Restauración de resina-1 superficie, posterior
2392 __ Restauración de resina-2 superficies, posteriores
2393 __ Restauración de resina-3 + superficies, posteriores
2394 __ Restauración de resina-4+ superficies, posteriores

Inlay

2510 __ Inlay metálico-1 superficie
2520 __ Inlay metálico-2 superficies
2530 __ Inlay metálico-3+ superficies
2610 __ Inlay de porcelana/cerámica-1 superficie
2620 __ Inlay de porcelana/cerámica-2 superficies
2630 __ Inlay de porcelana/cerámica-3+ superficies
2650 __ Inlay-compuesto/resina 1 superficie (procedimiento de laboratorio)
2651 __ Inlay-compuesto/resina 2 superficies (procedimiento de laboratorio)
2652 __ Inlay-compuesto/resina 3+ superficies (procedimiento de laboratorio)

Onlay

2543 __ Onlay-metálico-3 superficies
2544 __ Onlay-metálico-4+ superficies
2642 __ Onlay-porcelana/cerámica - 2 superficies
2643 __ Onlay- porcelana/cerámica - 3 superficies
2644 __ Onlay-porcelana-4+ superficies
2662 __ Onlay-compuesto/resina-2 superficies (procedimiento de laboratorio)
2663 __ Onlay-compuesto/resina-3 superficies (procedimiento de laboratorio)
2664 __ Onlay-compuesto/resina-4+ superficies (procedimiento de laboratorio)

Coronas - Individuales

2710 __ Resina de laboratorio
2740 __ Porcelana

2750 __ Porcelana con metal noble alto
2752 __ Porcelana con metal noble
2790 __ Molde de corona completa de metal noble alto
2792 __ Molde de corona completa de metal noble
2799 __ Provisional

Otros Restaurativos

2910 __ Re-cementar el inlay
2920 __ Re-cementar la corona
2930 __ Corona de acero inoxidable-diente primario
2931 __ Corona de acero inoxidable permanente
2932 __ Corona prefabridada de resina
2933 __ Corona de acero inoxidable con resina
2940 __ Empastadura sedativa
2950 __ Construcción de corona con pernos
2951 __ Retención de perno por diente
2952 __ Molde de poste y base
2954 __ Poste y base prefabricados
2955 __ Remoción de poste
2960 __ Laminado labial de resina/ en la oficina del dentista
2961 __ Laminado labial de resina/ laboratorio
2962 __ Laminado labial de porcelana /laboratorio
2970 __ Preformado provisional
2980 __ Reparación de la corona
2999 __ Restaurativo no especificado

Endodoncia

3110 __ Tapado directo de la pulpa
3220 __ Pulpotomía
3221 __ Desbridamiento de la pulpa
3230 __ Terapia primaria de pulpa anterior
3240 __ Terapia primaria de pulpa posterior
3310 __ Tratamiento de canal radicular anterior
3320 __ Tratamiento de canal radicular premolar
3330 __ Tratamiento de canal radicular molar
3346 __ Volver a tratar canal radicular de diente anterior
3347 __ Volver a tratar canal radicular premolar
3348 __ Volver a tratar canal radicular molar

3999 __ Endodontología no especificado

Periodontología

4210 __ Gingivectomía/ Gingivoplastia–cuadrante
4211 __ Gingivectomía/ Gingivoplastia–1-3 dientes
4249 __ Alargamiento de la corona
4260 __ Cirugía ósea-cuadrante
4261 __ Cirugía ósea—1-3 dientes
4320 __ Férula intracoronal
4321 __ Férula extracoronal
4341 __ Raspado y alisado radicular por cuadrante
4342 __ Raspado y alisado radicular-1-3 dientes
4355 __ Desbridamiento periodontal – boca completa
4381 __ Tratamiento de quimioterapia específico al lugar
4910 __ Mantenimiento periodontal
4920 __ Cambio de vendajes no citado
4999 __ Tratamiento periodontal no especificado

Prótesis Removibles

5110 __ Dentadura maxilar superior completa
5120 __ Dentadura mandibular completa
5130 __ Dentadura inmediata maxilar superior completa
5140 __ Dentadura inmediata mandibular inferior completa
5211 __ Dentadura maxilar superior parcial removible con base de resina con broches
5212 __ Dentadura mandibular parcial removible con base de resina con broches
5213 __ Dentadura maxilar superior parcial removible con armazón de metal moldeado
5214 __ Dentadura mandibular parcial removible con armazón de metal moldeado
5410 __ Ajustar dentadura maxilar superior completa
5411 __ Ajustar dentadura mandibular completa
5421 __ Ajustar dentadura maxilar superior parcial removible
5422 __ Ajustar dentadura mandibular parcial removible

Siga

Códigos de los procedimientos dentales (CDT-4 completo)—continuación

5510 __ Reparar base de la dentadura

5520 __ Reparar cada diente roto o que falta

5610 __ Reparar base de dentadura parcial removible

5620 __ Reparar armazón de la dentadura parcial removible

5630 __ Reparar/reemplazar broche roto

5640 __ Reemplazar cada diente roto

5650 __ Añadir diente a dentadura parcial removible

5660 __ Añadir un broche a dentadura parcial removible

5750 __ Revestir dentadura maxilar superior completa

5751 __ Revestir dentadura mandibular completa

5760 __ Revestir dentadura maxilar superior parcial removible

5761 __ Revestir dentadura mandibular parcial removible

5810 __ Dentadura maxilar superior completa interino

5811 __ Dentadura mandibular completa interina

5820 __ Dentadura maxilar superior parcial removible interina

5821 __ Dentadura mandibular parcial removible interina

5850 __ Acondicionamiento de tejido maxilar superior

5851 __ Acondicionamiento de tejido mandibular

Prótesis Fijas
Pontic (Puentes)

6210 __ Molde de metal noble alto

6212 __ Molde de metal noble

6240 __ Porcelana pegada a metal noble alto

6242 __ Porcelana pegada a metal noble

6253 __ Provisional

Anclajes

6545 __ Molde de metal pegado a resina

6720 __ Resina pegada a metal noble alto

6740 __ Porcelana/cerámica

6750 __ Porcelana pegada a metal noble alto

6752 __ Porcelana pegada a metal noble

6790 __ Molde de metal noble alto

6792 __ Molde de metal noble

6793 __ Provisional

Otras Prótesis Fijas

6930 __ Re-cementar puente

6970 __ Poste y base de molde

6972 __ Poste y base prefabricados

6973 __ Construcción de base

6975 __ Capas – cada diente

6999 __ Prótesis fija no especificada

Cirugía Oral

7111 __ Extracción de remanentes de dientes primarios

7140 __ Extracción rutinaria

7210 __ Extracción quirúrgica

7220 __ Extracción de tejido suave impactado

7230 __ Extracción de diente parcialmente impactado

7240 __ Extracción de diente completamente impactado

7250 __ Extracción quirúrgica de residuos de raíz

7285 __ Biopsia de tejido duro

7286 __ Biopsia de tejido suave

7287 __ Citología de cepillo

7510 __ Incisión y drenaje de un absceso

Servicios Suplementarios

9110 __ Tratamiento paliativo

9310 __ Consulta 2da opinión

9430 __ Visita en la oficina-observación

9440 __ Visita en la oficina-fuera de horas normales de trabajo

9450 __ Presentación del caso

9910 __ Medicamento de-sensibilizador

9940 __ Protector oclusal

9950 __ Montura oclusal analítica

9951 __ Ajuste de oclusión limitada

9952 __ Ajuste de oclusión completo

9970 __ Micro-abrasión del esmalte

9999 __ No especificado

Hojas de Trámite

Hoja de Trámite
Paciente:_____ Proveedor:_____

Tratamiento Terminado
    Diente # ___ Código del Procedimiento:_____
    Diente # ___ Código del Procedimiento:_____
    Diente # ___ Código del Procedimiento:_____

Servicios de Higiene
    ❏ Profilaxis 01110
    ❏ Fluoruro 00120
    ❏ Selladores Diente #_____
    ❏ Alisado Radicular 04341 SI II SD ID

Predeterminación
    Diente #_____ Código del Procedimiento:_____
    Alisado/Raspado Radicular 04341
    Otro_____

Comentarios:_____

Hoja de Trámite
Paciente:_____ Proveedor:_____

Tratamiento Terminado
    Diente # ___ Código del Procedimiento:_____
    Diente # ___ Código del Procedimiento:_____
    Diente # ___ Código del Procedimiento:_____

Servicios de Higiene
    ❏ Profilaxis 01110
    ❏ Fluoruro 00120
    ❏ Selladores Diente #_____
    ❏ Alisado Radicular 04341 SI II SD ID

Predeterminación
    Diente #_____ Código del Procedimiento:_____
    Alisado/Raspado Radicular 04341
    Otro_____

Comentarios:_____

Hoja de Trámite
Paciente:_____ Proveedor:_____

Tratamiento Terminado
    Diente # ___ Código del Procedimiento:_____
    Diente # ___ Código del Procedimiento:_____
    Diente # ___ Código del Procedimiento:_____

Servicios de Higiene
    ❏ Profilaxis 01110
    ❏ Fluoruro 00120
    ❏ Selladores Diente #_____
    ❏ Alisado Radicular 04341 SI II SD ID

Predeterminación
    Diente #_____ Código del Procedimiento:_____
    Alisado/Raspado Radicular 04341
    Otro_____

Comentarios:_____

Hoja de Trámite
Paciente:_____ Proveedor:_____

Tratamiento Terminado
    Diente # ___ Código del Procedimiento:_____
    Diente # ___ Código del Procedimiento:_____
    Diente # ___ Código del Procedimiento:_____

Servicios de Higiene
    ❏ Profilaxis 01110
    ❏ Fluoruro 00120
    ❏ Selladores Diente #_____
    ❏ Alisado Radicular 04341 SI II SD ID

Predeterminación
    Diente #_____ Código del Procedimiento:_____
    Alisado/Raspado Radicular 04341
    Otro_____

Comentarios:_____

Casos en Progreso en el Laboratorio

Hoja de Seguimiento

Paciente	Laboratorio	Caso	Para	Fecha de Envío	Fecha de Regreso	De vuelta

Orden de Trabajo del Laboratorio

Fecha:_____   Fecha de Regreso:_____

Paciente:_____   Edad:_____   Sexo:_____

Por Favor Llame sobre el Caso   sí   no   **Desinfectado**   sí   no

Tipo de Restauración:

- ❏ Unidad Sola
- ❏ Puente
- ❏ Molde Completo
- ❏ Porcelana
- ❏ Procera
- ❏ Empress I

- ❏ Empress II
- ❏ Targis/Vectris
- ❏ Cristobal Plus
- ❏ LAVA Completo en Cerámica
- ❏ Porcelana/Noble
- ❏ Porcelana/Noble Alto

- ❏ Inlay
- ❏ Onlay
- ❏ Implante
- ❏ Implante Soportado
- ❏ Temporal Procesado en el Laboratorio

- ❏ Carga Progresiva Provisional
- ❏ Con Férula
- ❏ Modelo de Cera para Diagnóstico
- ❏ Otro

Diente #:_____

Línea Final: 360 bisel   270 bisel   Chaflán Bucal   Chaflán Completo

Diseño de Corona: Collar de Metal Completo Mínimo (.4mm máximo)   Juntura Bucal de Cabo a Cabo de Porcelana
Margen de Porcelana Completo   Diseño Modificado que Toca el Reborde

Adjunto:

- ❏ Impresión Final del Arco Completo
- ❏ Impresión del Cuadrante
- ❏ Registro Oclusal
- ❏ Impresión de la Separación
- ❏ Arco Completo Contrario
- ❏ Modelos de Estudio S I

- ❏ Moldes
- ❏ Cubeta de Mordida Triple, Impresión Contraria y Final
- ❏ Tabla de Transferencia del Arco de la Cara
- ❏ Cubeta de Mordida Triple y Contraria

Fotografías incluidas: sí   no
Sombra:_____

- ❏ Por favor vierta las impresiones
- ❏ Montura
- ❏ Devuelva terminado, listo para sellar o ligar
- ❏ Devuelva para tratar el molde e impresión de la separación
- ❏ Aplique la porcelana y regrese la porcelana bizcochada

- ❏ Regresar para zanjar

- ❏ Matriz/Matrices de zanja

- ❏ Aplique la porcelana y devuelva terminado

Instrucciones Especiales:

_____

_____

_____

Dr._____   Licencia #_____

Ayudas de Mercadeo

Esta colección no está diseñada para ser un paquete completo de mercadeo, pero le proveerá con muchos documentos que le ayudarán con su estrategia de mercadeo.

Comunicados de Prensa
La prensa puede ser su amiga; empiece por establecer amistad con alguien en la prensa. Consiga a una persona de contacto en el periódico que sirve el área donde viven sus pacientes. Siempre que usted agregue personal nuevo, equipo, técnicas, etc., envíe un comunicado de prensa a su contacto. Revise la **Guía para el Comunicado de Prensa (p. 364)** en este capítulo para ayudarlo con esto. Muchos periódicos tienen columnas disponibles para las historias de interés humano sobre éxito y oportunidades en la comunidad.

Coloque un anuncio simple en el periódico que anuncie un acontecimiento especial tal como una casa abierta o un día de "Conozca los Especialistas".

Considere patrocinar los acontecimientos de la comunidad que destacan negocios del área; su nombre y/o anuncio aparecerán en la publicidad de antes del acontecimiento o en el programa. Cuando usted es un participante del acontecimiento, esté seguro de tener folletos disponibles en temas "calientes" por ejemplo **Odontología Cosmética (p. 457), Blanquear los Dientes: Visión General y Opciones (p. 464), Señales Tempranas de la Enfermedad Periodontal (p. 553)** y **Para una Vida con una Magnífica Salud Oral (p. 498).**

Tablón de Anuncios de Educación Continua
Mantener un tablón de anuncios en su oficina les deja saber a sus pacientes acerca de conferencias, entrenamiento y otra educación continua en la cual usted y su personal participan. Exhiba los diplomas, los certificados y las cartas de recomendación también. Los pacientes son deseosos de cosechar los beneficios de la investigación y tecnología.

Pacientes Nuevos
La carta de **Bienvenido al Vecindario (p. 379)** debe ser enviada a todos los recién llegados junto con un imán con su nombre en él. Contacte el Welcome Wagon (grupo de bienvenida) de su comunidad, la Cámara de Comercio o la Asociación de Comerciantes, si ellos no proporcionan servicios a los recién llegados, probablemente pueden referirle a alguien que lo hace. Ofrezca información de salud gratis, sin obligación e invite a posibles pacientes a visitar la práctica para demostrar que usted se interesa por su comunidad y por las necesidades de los pacientes.

También, hay varias cartas excelentes en **Cartas y Formularios para el Paciente (Sección 3)** que serán muy útiles para los que acepten su oferta y quisieran más información sobre su práctica. Vea **Documentos para la Educación del Paciente (pp. 346-348)** para una lista de otros documentos para los posibles pacientes que puedan estar interesados en la lectura.

El Paciente Bien Informado
El ímpetu principal de esta publicación es la educación del paciente. No hay mejor herramienta de mercadeo que pacientes felices que dicen a todos sus amigos y conocidos sobre su dentista que toma tiempo para explicar todo lo que ellos necesitan saber para tomar una decisión informada. Mientras mayor es el conocimiento de los pacientes, mayor será su aceptación al tratamiento. Incluya la palabra escrita para ayudarles a mantener las cosas rectas.

Guardando Seguimiento
Mucho de la **Administración de la Práctica (Sección 1)** es dedicado a formularios para ayudar con el seguimiento de las citas y tratamiento del paciente. Estos formularios son inestimables para una suave transición del cuarto de tratamiento a la oficina. Considere **Casos en Progreso en el Laboratorio (p. 361), Documentos para la Educación del Paciente (pp. 346-348), Plan de Tratamiento (p. 352)** y los formularios bajo **Listas y Formularios de Teléfono (pp. 365-368).**

Gracias por Enviar Pacientes Nuevos
Anime el envío de pacientes nuevos recompensando a los pacientes que envían a otros a usted. Cartas como **Gracias por Enviar Pacientes Nuevos (p. 378)** contienen un certificado de regalo. Para un primer paciente nuevo, considere un certificado para una pizza. Con un segundo paciente nuevo puede ganar una comida en un restaurante agradable. El tercero puede ofrecer flores. Use su imaginación.

Finanzas
Manejadas correctamente, sus prácticas financieras pueden hacerle un héroe para sus pacientes. Los pacientes pueden ver claramente la necesidad para el tratamiento y desean tener el mejor, pero éste debe poderse pagar. Para ayudar a los paciente con las consideraciones financieras de la odontología:

1. Esté siempre tan alfrente como sea posible en divulgar todos los costos de cada opción de tratamiento por escrito. **Plan de Tratamiento (p. 352), Estimado de Honorarios (pp. 390-391)** son buenos formularios para usar.
2. Vea siempre que los pacientes estén al tanto de cuáles son sus opciones de pago por escrito. Use **Arreglos Financieros (p. 392),** para esto.
3. Provea un formulario de Verdades al Prestar, sin importar si tiene intenciones de cobrar interés.
4. Asegúrese que sus pacientes tienen una copia firmada de los arreglos financieros que han hecho con usted. Vea información de **Arreglos Financieros (p. 392), Preautorización de Pago (p. 393)** y **Programa para Pagos (p. 394).**
5. Asegúrese que sus pacientes entiendan cómo las aseguradoras dentales llegan a la cantidad del reembolso. Aquí serán útiles **Cobertura del Seguro Dental (p. 385), Seguro Dental: Puntos a Considerar (p. 386)** y **Determinación de Beneficios de Seguro (p. 387).**
6. Cuando envíe la carta para **Narrativos del Seguro (Sección 2),** envíe una copia al paciente también. Esto informa al paciente de su intento por obtener el reembolso apropiado para él o ella.
7. Asegúrese que sus arreglos financieros y formularios de consentimiento cumplan con las regulaciones locales y estatales.

Guía para el Comunicado de Prensa

Dr. (su nombre) se complace en anunciar (elija uno de abajo)

- la adición de (nombre) a nuestro personal. (Nombre) es un/una (nombre de la profesión), que estará (escriba los deberes generales). (Dé una biografía de algunas oraciones y mencione una o dos ventajas que este nombramiento da a sus pacientes.)
- la integración de (nombre del nuevo equipo o técnica) a nuestra práctica. Este/Esta nuevo/a (equipo o técnica) nos permitirá ofrecerle (nombre varias ventajas que esta nueva adición proporcionara a los pacientes).
- que (nombre), (nombre su profesión) ha terminado recientemente (entrenamiento, certificación, etc.) en (nombre del tema). (Nombre varias ventajas que este entrenamiento ofrece al paciente: puede incluir un nuevo servicio, más oportunidades para un servicio popular existente o un servicio más avanzado.)
- la integración de *Complete Dental Communication for Patients and Professionals,* un sistema educativo, en su práctica. Este software comprensivo da al Dr. _____ la capacidad para informar a todos los pacientes, detalladamente y por escrito, para su revisión casera, acerca de las necesidades dentales del tratamiento y las ventajas y desventajas de las opciones disponibles antes del tratamiento. También educará al paciente sobre diversos servicios dentales que el Dr. _____ puede proporcionar.

Llamadas Misceláneas por Completarse

Persona a Llamar	Teléfono	Información Necesaria	Llamar para el Dr.	Hecho

Pacientes Que Necesitan un Cambio de Cita

Paciente	Teléfono # (etiquéta: hogar, trabajo, etc.)	Tratamiento	Con Quién	Hora Deseada	Resultado de la Llamada	Fecha	Iniciales

- Mantenga este formulario a la mano; cerca del teléfono.
- Coloque el nombre del paciente y la información en la lista, un paciente por línea.
- Contacte cuando los espacios deseados ocurran en el programa.
- Registre los resultados de contacto (viene a la cita, etc.), fecha que llamó y las iniciales de la persona que llamó.
- Lleve la lista a la atención del doctor semanalmente, para revisión.

Cambios de Citas por Prioridad

Paciente	Tratamiento	Teléfono # (etiquéta: hogar, trabajo, etc.)	Hora Deseada	Resultado	Fecha	Iniciales

■ Mantenga este formulario a la mano; cerca del teléfono.

■ Coloque el nombre del paciente y la información en la lista, un paciente por línea.

■ Contacte cuando los espacios deseados ocurran en el programa.

■ Registre los resultados de contacto (viene a la cita, etc.), fecha que llamó y las iniciales de la persona que llamó.

■ Lleve la lista a la atención del doctor semanalmente, para revisión.

■ Después de tratar de contactar tres veces, si no se ha programado una cita, traiga a la atención del doctor.

Profesionales Solicitando Información del Paciente

Fecha/Hora	Paciente	Dentista, Médico que envío	Dentista, Médico Teléfono #	Tema

■ Cuando pacientes, otros dentistas o médicos llaman con relación al tratamiento del paciente, por favor registre el nombre del paciente y la información para lo que llamó en este diario.

■ **Esté seguro de anotar los detalles de la llamada en la gráfica dental del paciente también.** Inicié ambos este diario y la gráfica dental del paciente.

■ Si el mensaje es largo, la parte apropiada de este diario puede ser duplicada para la gráfica dental del paciente.

■ El dentista a cargo del tratamiento debe revisar este diario **diariamente**.

Acto de la Portabilidad y de la Responsabilidad del Seguro Médico de 1996 (HIPAA siglas en inglés)

¿Qué Es HIPAA?

El Acto de la Portabilidad y de la Responsabilidad del Seguro Médico de 1996 (HIPAA siglas en inglés) fue firmado como ley por el ex-presidente Bill Clinton el 21 de agosto de 1996. Las regulaciones finales fueron publicadas el 17 de agosto del 2000, para ser establecidas para el 16 de octubre del 2002. El HIPAA exige que las transacciones de toda la información del cuidado de salud de los pacientes sea formateada en un estilo electrónico estandarizado. En adición a proteger la privacidad y seguridad de la información del paciente, el HIPAA incluye legislación acerca de la formación de cuentas de ahorros médicos, la autorización de un programa para el control del fraude y abuso, el transporte fácil de la cobertura del seguro de salud y la simplificación de los términos y condiciones administrativos.

¿Qué Cubre HIPAA?

HIPAA abarca tres áreas primarias, y sus requisitos de privacidad se pueden separar en tres tipos: estándares de privacidad, derechos de los pacientes y requisitos administrativos.

1. **Estándares de Privacidad.** La preocupación principal de HIPAA es el uso cuidadoso y la divulgación de la información de salud protegida (PHI siglas en inglés), la cual generalmente es información de salud controlada electrónicamente, la cual es capaz de ser distinguida individualmente. La información de salud protegida también se refiere a la comunicación verbal, aunque la Regla de Privacidad de HIPAA no intenta dificultar la comunicación verbal necesaria. El Departamento de Salud y de Servicios Humanos de los Estados Unidos (USDHHS siglas en inglés) no requiere cambios de reestructuración, como por ejemplo a prueba de ruidos, cambios arquitectónicos y así sucesivamente, pero alguna precaución es necesaria cuando se intercambia información de salud por medio de la conversación.

   El Reconocimiento del Recibo del Aviso de las Prácticas de Privacidad, el cual permite que la información del paciente se utilice o se divulgue para tratamiento, pago u operaciones del cuidado de salud (TPO), se debe procurar de cada paciente. Una autorización detallada y sensible al tiempo puede también ser publicada, la cuál permite que el dentista divulgue la información en circunstancias especiales además de TPOs. Un *consentimiento escrito* también es una opción. Los dentistas pueden divulgar información de salud protegida *sin* reconocimiento, consentimiento o autorización en situaciones muy especiales, por ejemplo, abuso de niños percibido, supervisión de salud pública, investigación de fraude o aplicación de ley con permiso válido (por ejemplo, una orden judicial). Cuando se divulga información de salud protegida, el dentista debe tratar de divulgar sólo la información *mínima necesaria,* para ayudar a proteger la información del paciente tanto como sea posible.

   Es importante que los profesionales dentales se mantengan fieles a los estándares de HIPAA porque los proveedores de cuidado de salud (como también las oficinas de compensación del cuidado de la salud y los seguros médicos) quienes transmiten información de salud formateada *electrónicamente* a través de un servicio de facturación exterior o mercancía son consideradas *entidades cubiertas.* Las entidades cubiertas pueden enfrentarse con penalidades civiles y criminales serias por violación de la legislación de HIPAA. Fracaso en el cumplimiento de los requisitos de privacidad de HIPAA puede resultar en penalidades civiles de hasta $100 por infracción con un máximo anual de $25,000 por fracaso repetido de cumplir con el mismo requisito. Penalidades criminales resultando del manejo ilegal de la información de salud privada pueden extenderse desde $50,000 y/o 1 año de cárcel hasta $250,000 y/o 10 años de cárcel.

2. **Los Derechos de los Pacientes.** HIPAA permite a los pacientes, representantes autorizados y padres de menores, como también a los menores, a hacerse más consientes de la privacidad de la información de salud a la cual ellos tienen derecho. Estos derechos incluyen, pero no están limitados a, el derecho a ver y copiar su información de salud, el derecho a cuestionar violaciones a las políticas y regulaciones y el derecho a requerir formas alternas de comunicación con su dentista. Si alguna información de salud es publicada por alguna otra razón que no sea TPO, el paciente tiene derecho a un informe de la transacción. Por tanto, es importante para los dentistas el mantener registros fieles de dicha información y proveerla cuando sea necesario.

   La Regla de Privacidad de HIPAA determina que los padres de un menor tienen acceso a la información de salud del niño. Este privilegio puede ser anulado, por ejemplo, en casos que se sospecha de abuso del menor o el padre accede a un término de confidencialidad entre el dentista y el menor. Los derechos del padre a tener acceso a información de salud protegida también pueden ser restringida en situaciones donde una entidad legal, como una corte, interviene y cuando una ley no requiere el consentimiento del padre. Para una lista completa de los derechos del paciente provistos por HIPAA, esté seguro de adquirir una copia de la ley y entenderla bien.

Siga

Acto de la Portabilidad y de la Responsabilidad del Seguro Médico de 1996 (HIPAA siglas en inglés)—continuación

3. **Requisitos Administrativos.** El obedecer la legislación de HIPAA puede parecer como una faena, pero no necesita ser así. Es recomendable que se vuelva apropiadamente familiarizado con la ley, organice los requisitos en tareas simples, comience a obedecer temprano y documente su progreso en la obediencia. Un primer paso importante es evaluar la información actual y las prácticas de su oficina.

Los dentistas necesitarán escribir una *política de privacidad* para su oficina, un documento para los pacientes detallando las prácticas de la oficina en lo relacionado a información de salud protegida. El *HIPAA Privacy Kit* de la Asociación Dental Americana (ADA) incluye formularios que usted (el dentista) puede usar para preparar a su gusto su política de privacidad. Es útil el tratar de entender el papel de la información de cuidado de salud para sus pacientes y las maneras en la cual ellos tratan con la información mientras están visitando su oficina. Entrene a su equipo de trabajo, esté seguro que ellos están familiarizados con los términos de HIPAA y con su política de privacidad de la oficina y los formularios relacionados. El HIPAA requiere que usted designe un *oficial de privacidad,* una persona en su oficina que será responsable por aplicar nuevas políticas en la oficina, manejar reclamaciones y hacer las elecciones envolviendo los requisitos mínimos necesarios. Otra persona con el papel de *persona de contacto* procesará las reclamaciones.

Un *Aviso de las Prácticas Privadas*—un documento detallando los derechos del paciente y las obligaciones de la oficina dental en relación con información de salud protegida—también debe ser redactado. Además, cualquier papel de un tercer grupo con acceso a la información de salud protegida debe estar claramente documentado. Este tercer grupo es conocido como un asociado de negocios (BA siglas en inglés) y es definido como cualquier entidad quien, en nombre del dentista, toma parte en cualquier actividad que envuelve la exposición de la información de salud protegida. El *HIPAA Privacy Kit* provee una copia de "Los Términos del Contrato de los Asociados de Negocios" del USDHHS, el cual provee un plan concreto para interacciones de los asociados de negocios.

La fecha principal de obediencia con la privacidad HIPAA, incluyendo el entrenamiento del equipo de trabajo, fue el 14 de abril del 2003, aunque muchas entidades cubiertas quienes sometieron una petición y un plan de obediencia para el 15 de octubre del 2002, fueron concedidas a tener extensiones de un año. Es recomendable que los dentistas preparen sus oficinas con anticipación de todos los plazos, lo cual incluye preparar las políticas de privacidad y formularios, contratos de los asociados de negocios y las sesiones de entrenamiento de los empleados.

Para Más Información sobre HIPAA

Para una discusión extensa de todos estos términos y requisitos, una lista completa de las políticas y procedimientos de HIPAA, y una colección completa de los formularios de privacidad de HIPAA, contacte la Asociación Dental Americana (ADA) para un *HIPAA Privacy Kit*. El sitio Web de ADA es www.ada.org/goto/hipaa. Otros lugares Web que pueden contener información útil acerca de HIPAA son:

■ Oficina de Derechos Civiles del USDHHS (USDHHS Office of Civil Rights): www.hhs.gov/ocr/hipaa
■ Grupo de Trabajo en Intercambio de los Datos Electrónicos (Work Group on Electronic Data Interchange): www.wedi.org/SNIP
■ Salud de Phoenix (Phoenix Health): www.hipaadvisory.com
■ Oficina de USDHHS de la Secretaria Auxiliar para la Planificación y la Evaluación (USDHHS Office of the Assistant Secretary for Planning and Evaluation): http://aspe.os.dhhs.gov/admnsimp/

BIBLIOGRAFÍA

1. *HIPAA Privacy Kit*
2. http://www.ada.org/prof/prac/issues/topics/hipaa/index.html

HIPAA–Contrato para los Asociados de Negocios

El Acto de la Portabilidad y de la Responsabilidad del Seguro Médico (HIPAA siglas en inglés) requiere un contrato firmado entre el empleado individual designado como el Oficial de Privacidad y el dentista.

Este contrato entre la oficina del Dr.————————————————— (la *entidad*) y ————————————————— (el *asociado de negocio*) divulga las condiciones para asegurar el cumplimiento satisfactorio con la Regla de Privacidad del HIPAA.

Durante el periodo de este contrato los asociados de negocios deben cumplir con las siguientes responsabilidades con respecto a la información de salud protegida:

Un asociado de negocio debe limitar las peticiones de información de salud protegida a nombre de la entidad cubierta a lo que sea razonablemente necesario para lograr el propósito previsto; a la entidad cubierta le es permitido confiar razonablemente en tales peticiones del asociado de negocio de otra entidad cubierta como el mínimo necesario.

El hacer la información disponible, incluyendo la información retenida por un asociado de negocio, cuando sea necesaria para determinar la conformidad por la entidad cubierta.

Satisfacer los derechos de un individuo de tener acceso y de enmendar su información de salud protegida contenida en un sistema de registro, incluyendo información retenida por un asociado de negocio, si es apropiada, y recibir una explicación de la divulgación por un asociado de negocio.

Mitigar, en una medida practica, cualquier efecto prejudicial que es conocido a la entidad cubierta de un uso o una divulgación inadmisible por sus asociados de negocios de información de salud protegida.

Los asociados de negocios no pueden usar la información de salud protegida para sus propias utilidades. Esto incluye, pero no está limitado a, vender información de salud protegida a terceros grupos para las actividades de mercadeo de los terceros grupos, sin autorización.

Se requiere que la entidad cubierta asegure, en cualquier manera razonable considerada eficaz por la entidad cubierta, la cooperación apropiada por sus asociados de negocio para cumplir con estos requisitos.

Si la entidad cubierta descubre material en violación del contrato por el asociado de negocio, tomará medidas razonables para remediar la violación o terminar el contrato con el asociado de negocio. Si la terminación no es factible, la entidad cubierta reportará el problema a la Oficina para los Derechos Civiles del Departamento de Salud y Servicios Humanos.

HIPAA–Registro del Entrenamiento del Personal

El Acto de la Portabilidad y de la Responsabilidad del Seguro Médico (HIPAA) requiere que todos los empleados estén entrenados en la política de HIPAA en la oficina dental.

Certifico por este medio que los siguientes empleados de la oficina dental abajo nombrados han recibido la política de la oficina con respecto a la Regla de Privacidad del Acto de la Portabilidad y de la Responsabilidad del Seguro Médico.

Oficial de Privacidad _____ Fecha _____

Oficina Dental de   Nombre_____

                        Dirección_____

                        Cuidad_____ Estado_____

Entiendo la Política de Privacidad de la oficina y los procedimientos necesarios para proteger la privacidad de la información de salud de los pacientes y accesaré solamente la información que es necesaria para realizar mis deberes.

Nombre   Fecha

_____

_____

_____

_____

_____

_____

_____

_____

_____

_____

_____

_____

_____

_____

_____

_____

Cartas y Formularios para el Paciente

Revisión del Contenido: Cartas y Formularios para el Paciente

Bienvenido/Gracias
Evaluación de Nuestros Servicios
Permita que los pacientes conozcan que a usted le importa lo que ellos piensan y evite un malentendido por parte de todos. Excelente para mantener una alta calidad en el cuidado y en la tan importante primera impresión. Información sólida para mejorar el tratamiento.

Un Placer Conocerle
Cemente buenas relaciones con pacientes con esta carta de seguimiento dirigida a un paciente que usted ha conocido por primera vez. Ésta es más efectiva cuando se escribe a mano.

Gracias por Enviar Pacientes Nuevos
Una nota de agradecimiento dirigida a un paciente por haber enviado a un paciente nuevo a su práctica. Incluye una oración indicando que usted ha incluido un regalito como muestra de su apreciación. Es más efectiva cuando se escribe a mano.

Bienvenido al Vecindario
Preséntese a personas recién mudadas al vecindario y de le una impresión positiva y un incentivo para pasar por su oficina y visitarle.

Bienvenido a Nuestra Práctica
Preséntese a pacientes nuevos y ayúdeles a entender las políticas de su oficina en cuanto a citas, arreglos financieros y formularios del seguro. Asegúreles que siempre pueden esperar recibir explicaciones completas y un cuidado de alta calidad. También se puede enviar a pacientes nuevos que han hecho una cita.

Política de la Oficina
Política de Cancelación y de No Presentarse a una Cita
Una manera diplomática para informar a los pacientes de las responsabilidades suyas y de ellos en cuanto a las citas. Incluye información para emergencias, y también los cargos por cancelación/no presentarse.

Emergencias Dentales
Evite daño o dolor adicional al preparar a sus pacientes para que puedan manejar las emergencias dentales.

Cómo el Acto de la Portabilidad y de la Responsabilidad del Seguro Médico (HIPAA siglas en inglés) Afectará Su Próxima Visita Dental
Examina los tipos de divulgaciones de información de salud permitidas bajo HIPAA.

Seguro
Cobertura del Seguro Dental
Explique a los pacientes cómo trabaja el seguro dental, su responsabilidad financiera y cómo conseguir que se someta una reclamación.

Seguro Dental: Puntos a Considerar
¡Todas las coberturas de seguros no fueron creadas iguales! Un punto frecuentemente perdido por muchos pacientes. Esto da una visión general en lenguaje sencillo de muchos conceptos de beneficios dentales.

Determinación de Beneficios del Seguro
Informe al paciente que se ha recibido la pre-determinación, que ahora se pueden hacer los arreglos de pago y comenzar el tratamiento. Advierte de las posibles limitaciones de tiempo.

Petición de Información
Expida los problemas del formulario de reclamación del seguro con esta carta al paciente, pidiéndole que provea la información que falta o que contacte a la oficina en cuanto a su formulario de reclamación del seguro.

Financiero
Consentimiento de Pago
Un formulario de autorización con criterios de selección para los métodos actuales de pago con que ha acordado el paciente.

Revisión del Contenido: Cartas y Formularios para el Paciente—continuación

Estimado de Honorarios
Una visión general informativa para fomentar que el paciente entienda las recomendaciones de tratamiento y los honorarios correspondientes. Está dividido según las especialidades de tratamiento, con espacios separados para las responsabilidades financieras del seguro y del paciente. Da a los pacientes la información que necesitan para hacer sus arreglos financieros.

Estimado de Honorarios (Formulario Breve)
Un formulario diseñado para usarse en la comunicación con el paciente en cuanto al tratamiento planeado.

Arreglos Financieros
Explicación de seguros, posibles opciones de pago, garantías de honorarios y procedimientos de no haber pagado. Da a los pacientes la información que necesitan para escoger los arreglos financieros apropiados.

Preautorización de Pago
Preautorización de una tarjeta de crédito para que la oficina pueda tomar el pago directamente de la cuenta de la tarjeta a base de un plan de pago de una vez, semanal o mensual. Se puede usar con los formularios de arreglos financieros.

Programa para Pagos
Provee un programa de pagos actual con fechas. Espacio para los procedimientos que este programa cubre, la cuota total y la firma del paciente.

Tratamiento
Rechazo del Tratamiento
Declaración para la firma del paciente, en rechazo del tratamiento particular que usted ha recomendado.

Evaluación Cosmética Dental
Un formulario diseñado para captar toda la información cosmética dental específica al paciente antes de determinar el tratamiento apropiado.

Servicios de Higiene Dental: Visita de Profilaxis Dental
Este formulario de verificación permite que el paciente conozca lo que se ha hecho en la visita para profilaxis.

Visión General del Examen/Consulta
Una lista de verificación general de condiciones encontradas y el tratamiento propuesto y las co-consultaciones.

Actualización del Historial Médico
Da al paciente una oportunidad fácil para que pongan al día su historial médico en cada cita. Asegura que usted tenga la información más reciente y también un historial de las revisiones.

Procedimiento para la Próxima Cita
Da un perfil del próximo procedimiento al paciente, los servicios que se completarán y el tiempo aproximado requerido.

Petición para la Educación del Paciente
Para los futuros pacientes, este formulario está diseñado como un anexo para "Bienvenido al Vecindario" en esta sección.

Metas del Tratamiento
Resume la filosofía del tratamiento y envuelve al paciente en el proceso de la determinación del tratamiento.

Evaluación de Nuestros Servicios

¡Gracias por escogernos como su equipo dental! Nos esforzamos para proveerle con el mejor cuidado oral posible al ofrecerle lo más adelantado de la tecnología y filosofía dental y valoramos su opinión. Apreciaríamos que tome tiempo para evaluar nuestros servicios. Se usará la información que usted provee para identificar nuestros puntos fuertes y también las áreas donde podemos hacer que su experiencia sea aun mejor. Siéntase libre de comentar en el espacio provisto abajo.

Por favor circule 1 para Excelente, 2 para Bueno, 3 para Termino Medio, 4 para Regular y 5 para Pobre.

- ¿Fue comprehensivo el examen?   1   2   3   4   5
- ¿Este examen fue el examen más minucioso que usted ha tenido?   1   2   3   4   5
- ¿Cómo se pudo haber mejorado el examen?_____
  _____
- ¿Las explicaciones que usted recibió fueron claras?   1   2   3   4   5
- ¿El doctor explicó la diferencia entre el tratamiento requerido y el
  tratamiento electivo?   1   2   3   4   5
- ¿Usted entendió cuál tratamiento dental necesita?   1   2   3   4   5
- ¿El doctor usó medios auxiliares visuales adecuados para ayudar a explicar los
  problemas dentales y el tratamiento?   1   2   3   4   5
- ¿El doctor le dio información por escrita adecuada para cada problema dental
  y su solución?   1   2   3   4   5
- ¿El doctor le explicó los riesgos, las opciones para el tratamiento, las ventajas y
  desventajas del tratamiento, las consecuencias del tratamiento y del no-tratamiento
  para sus problemas dentales?   1   2   3   4   5
- ¿El doctor o recepcionista explicó claramente la política financiera de la oficina?
  (Usted paga cuando le proveemos el tratamiento a menos que haya hecho otro
  arreglo previamente.)   1   2   3   4   5
- ¿Usted se sentiría cómodo al sugerirle a un pariente o amigo que venga aquí para
  sus necesidades dentales?   1   2   3   4   5

Conteste las siguientes preguntas si usted tiene necesidades dentales extensivas.

- Si sugerimos que hiciera una co-consulta con un dentista especialista,
  ¿usted entendió por qué?   1   2   3   4   5
- Si sugerimos que hiciera una co-consulta con un especialista,
  ¿usted entendió cuándo debía ver el especialista?   1   2   3   4   5
- Si sugerimos que hiciera una co-consulta con un especialista,
  ¿usted entendió cuándo tendría un tratamiento por nuestra oficina?   1   2   3   4   5
- ¿El doctor le explicó que se puede hacer su tratamiento en fases a través de un
  período de tiempo?   1   2   3   4   5

Apreciamos cualquier persona que usted le sugiera que venga aquí y le trataremos con el mismo respeto, preocupación y atención profesional que le hemos tratado a usted.

Comentarios:_____
_____
_____

Gracias por haber tomado tiempo para contestar estas preguntas.

Un Placer Conocerle

¡PARA UN MAYOR IMPACTO, ESCRIBA ESTA NOTA A MANO!

(Fecha)

Estimado (Nombre del paciente),

Fue un placer conocerle hoy. Si usted tiene cualquier pregunta sobre cualquier tratamiento dental del cual hablamos, favor de sentirse libre para contactarme. Como mencioné durante nuestro diálogo, estoy incluyendo con esta nota información relacionada al(a la) (tema hablado). Estoy seguro que usted la encontrará interesante e informativa.

(Reitere cualquier información específica del examen que señale las partes de los folletos que serán de mayor interés al paciente.)

(Mencione, si es posible, cualquier conversación personal que pudieron haber tenido: ej. el equipo en el cual están los hijos de ambos, una sugerencia útil para su juego de golf, etc.)

Si tiene algunos amigos o parientes que comparten su visión de querer una salud oral excelente y que están buscando un dentista, usted puede sugerirle con confianza que vengan aquí. Espero verle de nuevo.

Sinceramente,

Gracias por Enviar Pacientes Nuevos

¡ESTA CARTA ES MÁS EFECTIVA CUANDO SE ESCRIBE A MANO!

(Fecha)

Estimado (nombre del paciente),

Muchísimas gracias por su recomendación tan amable de que _____ viniera a nuestra oficina. Uno de los mejores cumplidos que un paciente puede hacerle a un proveedor de cuidado de salud es sugerirle a sus amigos y familia le visiten. Valoramos mucho su confianza en nosotros. Uno de nuestros pacientes nuevos nos ha visitado a causa de su envío. Usted puede estar seguro que le daremos el mismo cuidado que le incitó a sugerirle que nos visitara.

Favor de aceptar la muestra adjunta de nuestra apreciación. Esperamos que la disfrute.

Gracias de nuevo.

Sinceramente,

Bienvenido al Vecindario

(EDITE EL TEXTO EN BASTARDILLA SEGÚN SU SITUACIÓN.)

Estimado Vecino,

Bienvenido a (nombre de la comunidad). Hemos estado en esta área desde el (año) y encontramos que es un lugar magnífico para vivir y criar a una familia—cualidades que estamos seguros que le motivaron a tomar su decisión final.

Una de las decisiones más difíciles al establecerse en un nuevo lugar es encontrar un excelente cuidado de salud para su familia. Nos gustaría ayudarle a encontrar su nuevo dentista. Permítanos presentarnos.

Adjuntos están los sucesos principales profesionales que destacan al Dr. Stephen Candio y Beth Stolar Candio, BS, RDH, MA. Proveemos un cuidado dental consistente y excepcional para todas las edades. A través de nuestra orientación de prevención, nos esforzamos en ayudarle a mantener su dentición natural. Nuestra meta es que usted tenga dientes funcionales, cómodos, de buena apariencia y sin dolor ahora y cuando usted tenga 95 años de edad. Nuestra área de pericia principal es la odontología estética adhesiva (la unión y las empastaduras conservadoras). Por muchos años llevamos a cabo investigaciones clínicas en esta área. Incluso hemos trabajado con un manufacturero para desarrollar muchos de los materiales dentales que se usan hoy en la odontología. En nuestra oficina tenemos dos especialistas dentales: un ortodoncista (frenillos) y un periodontista (limitado al tratamiento de enfermedades de las encías y el hueso oral). Si usted siente que necesita una consulta en cualquiera de estas áreas, ellos se complacerán en proveerle una evaluación.

Para su beneficio y salud, no usamos níquel ni metales inferiores en ninguna restauración que colocamos. No usamos materiales de empastadura directa (amalgama de plata). Nuestras restauraciones (inlay, onlay o corona completa) procesadas en el laboratorio están compuestas de cerámica, porcelana, resinas procesadas o aleación de alto contenido de oro. Si se necesita una subestructura de metal para coronas o puentes, solamente se usa una aleación de la más alta calidad de oro o metal precioso.

Adjunto, usted encontrará una lista de información útil que le puede ayudar a contestar las preguntas dentales que pueda tener. Para los niños menores en el hogar, tenemos información que describe cómo se puede ayudar a los niños a mantener dientes sin deterioro; cuándo los niños deben visitar al dentista; en qué edad generalmente salen los dientes de leche y los dientes permanentes; las dosis de fluoruro sistémico *(Sparta no tiene el fluoruro en el agua potable);* y los selladores protectores (se colocan rápidamente y son capas plásticas sin dolor que se colocan en la superficie de la mordida para evitar el deterioro). Independientemente de si usted selecciona a nuestra oficina para su cuidado dental, nos gustaría ofrecerle esta información gratis sobre éste y otros temas dentales que incluyen: el blanqueo casero, coronas, canales radiculares, implantes dentales y muchos más. Favor de referir al formulario adjunto y marque lo que le gustaría recibir. Entonces devuélvalo por correo con su nombre y dirección, tráigalo a la oficina o llámenos para dejarnos saber cuál información le interesa tener.

Cuando usted esté listo, estaremos contentos en ayudarle a mantener sus dientes en un estado saludable y hermoso para toda su vida. Tenemos una oficina dental única y apreciaríamos la oportunidad de proveerle un cuidado dental excepcional a usted y a su familia.

Sinceramente,

Bienvenido a Nuestra Práctica

Estamos muy contentos de que usted haya seleccionado a nuestra oficina para su cuidado dental. Nuestras metas serán el determinar cuál tratamiento dental usted necesita y ofrecerlo en la manera más eficiente con excelencia clínica y cortesía. Le enseñaremos cómo combinar una evaluación dental profesional con regularidad con el cuidado casero diario rutinario y apropiado para mantener una salud oral óptima para sí mismo para toda la vida. Queremos que usted tenga dientes cómodos, sin dolor, de buena apariencia y funcionales cuando usted tenga 95 años de edad.

(En este espacio, entre una biografía breve destacando los grados/certificaciones y otras actividades relacionadas a la ontología del dentista, la higienista y/u otro personal dental principal en esta oficina.)

Las horas de oficina son por cita. Cuando sea apropiado, preferimos fijar citas más largas y completar tanto tratamiento dental a la vez como sea posible. Esto permite la eficiencia máxima e interrumpe su horario diario lo menos posible.

Nuestra oficina ofrece arreglos financieros simples para evitar posibles malentendidos. A menos que se haya hecho otro arreglo previo, se espera el pago completo en el momento que se provee el tratamiento. Si usted tiene un seguro dental, para su protección, le enviaremos un pre-estimado del tratamiento dental a su portador de seguros. Cuando devuelvan el pre-estimado (6 a 8 semanas), indicarán su porción del pago. Le pedimos que pague esta porción en el momento que comience el tratamiento. Si el tratamiento es extensivo o tomará varios meses para completarse, se pueden hacer pagos parciales en las citas durante este período de tiempo. Para su conveniencia, se acepta VISA y MasterCard. Para procedimientos más complicados, se puede arreglar un préstamo sin interés (máximo 12 meses).

Usted puede esperar recibir el mejor cuidado dental que podemos proveer. La tecnología dental ha hecho avances notables. Usted podrá no estar consciente de algunos de los avances en el diagnóstico y tratamiento y cómo le pueden beneficiar. Si no ha visitado a un dentista recientemente o ha estado bajo el cuidado de alguien que no ha adoptado estas técnicas, notará una diferencia en el primer momento que entre a nuestra oficina.

Una vez que usted ha explicado sus preocupaciones dentales y se ha completado un examen dental minucioso y las radiografías necesarias, se desarrollará un plan de tratamiento. Explicaciones escritas y en video están disponibles y se le ofrecerán. Se presentarán las ventajas y desventajas del tratamiento, los riesgos del tratamiento o el no-tratamiento y las opciones y costos del tratamiento. Se contestará cualquier pregunta que usted tenga antes que el tratamiento comience.

Estamos comprometidos en proveer una cita inicial para cada paciente durante la cual se pueden atender las preocupaciones y deseos dentales del paciente. Respetamos el tiempo del paciente. No fijamos citas de más de un paciente a la vez. A menos que surja una emergencia dental no esperada, aseguramos que se vean a los pacientes en la hora señalada para su cita. Queremos que cada paciente se sienta cómodo, con un tiempo de cita adecuado para atender sus preocupaciones dentales. Favor de permitirse el tiempo adecuado para viajar a nuestra oficina.

Adjunto usted encontrará un formulario para el historial médico y dental que usted puede completar antes de su primera visita. Favor de traerlo consigo. Gracias por la oportunidad de proveerle el cuidado dental.

(En este espacio, entre los nombres del dentista, higienista y los otros mencionados arriba y pida que cada uno firme por encima de su nombre.)

Política de Cancelación y de No Presentarse a una Cita

Las horas de oficina son por cita y sí valoramos su tiempo. Esta oficina es una oficina dental de práctica privada y no una "clínica" dental. El tiempo de la cita está reservado sólo para usted. Cuando es apropiado, preferimos fijar citas más largas para completar tanto del tratamiento dental necesario como sea posible durante una sola cita. Creemos que este tipo de horario causará una interrupción mínima a su horario diario y será más eficiente para terminar su cuidado dental. Cuando usted hace una cita, favor de asegurarse que la podrá cumplir. Las citas por la mañana son las mejores para los procedimientos más complejos.

Emergencias y problemas de paciente no previstos pueden surgir, y causar cambios en el horario. Las emergencias son inesperadas y parecen llegar en las horas menos convenientes. Si usted tiene una emergencia dental que necesita atención inmediata, siempre ofrecemos atenderle inmediatamente. Esperamos que otros pacientes que pueden resultar un poco incomodados por esto puedan comprender que es una situación de emergencia. En algún momento ellos podrían necesitar la misma cortesía.

Diferente a muchas oficinas, esta oficina no le llama para confirmar su cita. Favor de apuntar cualquier cita dental que le hemos fijado en un lugar que le ayudará a recordarla fácilmente. Si usted no puede llegar a la cita, favor de notificar a la oficina. Para las citas antes de las 4 p.m. de lunes a viernes habrá un honorario de $25 por cada 30 minutos del tiempo citado si no se cumple o si hay una cancelación con menos de 24 horas de anticipación. Para las citas después de las 4 p.m. de lunes a viernes o los sábados el honorario es $50 por cada 30 minutos del tiempo citado si no se cumple o si hay una cancelación sin la notificación de 24 horas de anticipación.

Si nuestro personal puede conseguir que otro paciente venga a la hora de su cita, no habrá un honorario por la cita no cumplida.

Si usted tiene cualquier pregunta sobre nuestra política de cancelación y de no presentarse a una cita, favor de sentirse libre de preguntarnos.

Emergencias Dentales

El cuidado dental regular ayuda a prevenir las emergencias dentales inconvenientes. Sin embargo, las emergencias dentales pueden ocurrir y sí ocurren. Aquí hay una lista de las emergencias dentales más comunes y de lo que usted puede hacer hasta que pueda llegar a nuestra oficina. Una buena regla general: si le duele, NO espere para hacer una cita. Estaremos contentos de atenderle lo antes posible.

Dolor de Muela/Dientes Sensibles

Varios problemas diferentes pueden causar un dolor de muela o un diente sensible. A veces es señal de que un nervio se está muriendo dentro del diente. Una medicación sin receta puede aliviar el dolor temporalmente. Contáctenos para una cita tan pronto se de cuenta del problema. Un dolor leve, si no se trata, puede progresar a una hinchazón facial u oral y un dolor severo. Comúnmente, se puede eliminar el dolor de muela con el tratamiento endodóntico (terapia de la raíz radicular).

Un diente sensible puede ser el resultado de una raíz expuesta, una empastadura defectuosa o con filtración, deterioro, un problema relacionado a la mordida o un nervio que se está muriendo. Venga donde nosotros tan pronto como sea posible para una evaluación.

Diente Roto

Los dientes con empastaduras grandes pueden romperse o fracturarse con mucha facilidad. Llámenos tan pronto como sea posible para tener una evaluación y restauración del diente. Si el diente roto no se trata, puede desarrollar problemas más serios. Los dientes rotos pueden o no ser sensibles a los cambios del aire y temperatura. La sensibilidad y el dolor no son necesariamente una indicación de cuán dañado está el diente.

Diente Que Se Cae por Golpe

Coloque el diente en agua o dentro de un paño o toalla húmedo. **No trate de fregar o lavar el diente.** Traiga al diente y al paciente a nosotros inmediatamente. Mientras más rápido se pueda reposicionar el diente, mejor es la probabilidad de que se pueda salvar. **El tiempo es crucial.**

Objeto Atascado entre los Dientes

Use el hilo dental para remover el objeto. **No use objetos afilados o puntiagudos para sacar el objeto de entre los dientes.** Si el objeto no sale fácilmente, venga a donde nosotros para ayuda.

Caída de Corona/Puente Final o Provisional

Venga donde nosotros lo antes posible para que se recemente la corona. Si esto no es posible, usted puede usar un adhesivo para dentadura (FIXODENT®, por ejemplo) que se puede comprar sin receta. Coloque una cantidad pequeña en la corona y vuelva a ponerla en su lugar. No use fuerza para ponerla. No debe ser difícil de poner. Cuando usted no puede poner la corona en su lugar correctamente, guárdela y tráigala consigo a la cita. Nosotros haremos la cementación. La razón por la que se salió puede hacer imposible el que el dentista recemente la corona vieja. Se tomará esta decisión durante su examen.

Dentadura Completa o Parcial Rota

Traiga la dentadura completa o parcial aquí para que se repare. **No trate de pegar el plástico usted mismo. No use CRAZY GLUE® ni otros materiales similares.**

Problemas Ortodónticos

Si el aparato está suelto, lleve al paciente al ortondoncista. Si se ha expuesto un alambre afilado, cúbralo con un pedazo de cera, goma de mascar, una bolita de algodón—cualquier cosa para que el lado puntiagudo no hinque en los tejidos suaves.

Encías Hinchadas

Las encías hinchadas son señal de una infección. La infección puede ser resultado de un nervio que se está muriendo o un problema periodontal (de las encías). Enjuague su boca con agua salada tibia. Venga a donde nosotros lo antes posible. La hinchazón puede estar o acompañada por dolor. De cualquier modo, necesita atención inmediata.

(En este espacio, entre el nombre del dentista, dirección y número de teléfono.)

Cómo el Acto de la Portabilidad y de la Responsabilidad del Seguro Médico (HIPAA siglas en inglés) Afectará Su Próxima Visita Dental

El Departamento de Salud y de Servicios Humanos de los Estados Unidos ha publicado recientemente estándares nacionales para la información de salud privada. El Acto de la Portabilidad y de la Responsabilidad del Seguro Médico, una ley federal obligatoria conocida como HIPAA, es designada para:

- proveer protección para la privacidad de cierta información de salud identificable (llamada información de salud protegida—PHI siglas en inglés),
- asegurar la cobertura de seguro de salud cuando se cambian patrones y
- proveer estándares para facilitar transferencias electrónicas relacionadas a la información de salud.

Mientras la privacidad de la información de salud protegida personal se mantiene confidencial, ciertos aspectos de esta ley permitirán la divulgación de la información de salud protegida para facilitar las actividades de salud pública. Las siguientes tablas examinan los tipos de divulgación de información de salud permitida bajo HIPAA.

La información de salud protegida puede ser divulgada con su autorización en las siguientes categorías.
Usted puede pedir una limitación o restricción en la divulgación de esta información: Usted tiene el derecho a: • pedir una restricción o limitar alguna de las divulgaciones antedichas para usarse para tratamiento, pagos u operaciones de la oficina. • inspeccionar y copiar información que pueda ser usada para hacer decisiones acerca de su cuidado. • pedir una corrección de esta información si usted siente que es incorrecta o incompleta. • un informe de las divulgaciones que hemos hecho que no están relacionadas a tratamiento, pago u operaciones de esta oficina. Esta petición debe ser dirigida por escrito al gerente de esta oficina, y usted será informado de las especificaciones que son requeridas por esta petición.
Tratamiento—La información de salud protegida será usada para proveer el cuidado de salud apropiado ya sea por esta oficina u otros proveedores de cuidado de salud, laboratorios de diagnóstico o fabricación.
Pagos—La información de salud protegida será usada para facilitar el pago por el tratamiento rendido. Su plan de salud pide esta información para poder facturar, recaudar los pagos o para obtener aprobación antes del tratamiento.
Operaciones del Cuidado de Salud—Para asegurar que todos los pacientes reciban cuidado oportuno y de calidad, la información de salud protegida será usada para facilitar las operaciones diarias de nuestra práctica. Esto incluye, pero no esta limitado a: • estudios clínicos/investigación para mejorar nuestra práctica • recordatorios de cita por llamadas telefónicas o por correo • hojas para apuntarse usadas para notificarnos de su llegada • programas de citas fijadas • información con relación a sus opciones de tratamiento o beneficios y servicios relacionados • comunicaciones con familia o amigos que están involucrados en su cuidado o pago por su cuidado

La información de salud protegida puede ser divulgada sin su autorización en las siguientes categorías.		
Según los Requisitos de Ley	**Procedimientos Judiciales y Administrativos**	**Vigilancia** La información de salud protegida puede ser divulgada a una agencia de vigilancia de la salud según lo autorizado por ley para auditorias, investigaciones, inspecciones y dar licencias.
Salud Pública	**Pleitos y Conflictos**	**Compensación del Trabajador** La información de salud protegida puede ser divulgada para compensación del trabajador o programas similares que proveen beneficios para las lesiones o enfermedades relacionadas al trabajo.

Siga

Cómo el Acto de la Portabilidad y de la Responsabilidad del Seguro Médico (HIPAA siglas en inglés) Afectará Su Próxima Visita Dental—continuación

Riesgos de la Salud Pública	Aplicación de la Ley	Militares y Veteranos
Investigación de Salud La divulgación de la información de salud protegida esta permitida cuando sea requerido por las leyes federales, estatales, tribal o locales.	**Pesquisidor y Examinadores Médicos** La divulgación de la información de salud protegida a oficiales ocurrirá en respuesta a una orden de la corte, citación, petición de descubrimiento o citación judicial: para identificar a un fugitivo sospechoso, testigo o persona desaparecida; acerca de una víctima del crimen si no es posible obtener permiso de la persona; para identificar una persona difunta, determinar la causa de muerte, acerca de una muerte que se cree que pueda ser el resultado de conducta criminal: conducta criminal ocurriendo en la práctica; en situaciones de emergencia.	**Actividades de Seguridad e Inteligencia Nacional**
Abuso, Negligencia o Violencia Domestica La información de salud protegida puede ser divulgada para prevenir una amenaza a su salud y seguridad o la salud y seguridad de otros.	**Donaciones de Órgano, Ojo o Tejido** La divulgación de la información de salud protegida puede ser realizada a bancos de órganos como sea necesario para facilitar la donación y transplante de órgano o tejido.	**Servicios de Protección para el Presidente y Otros** La información de salud protegida puede ser divulgada según lo autorizado por ley cuando es pedida por autoridades de comandos militares, oficiales federales para seguridad nacional y protección del presidente y otros líderes del estado.

Cobertura del Seguro Dental

Responsabilidad de Pago

Su patrón, la gerencia o la unión ha comprado una cobertura de seguro dental de una selección de planes ofrecidos por una compañía o agente de seguros. Cada compañía de seguros ofrece muchos planes diferentes. El tipo de beneficios que están cubiertos se relaciona a la cantidad de dinero gastado en el paquete de beneficios. Generalmente, mientras más dinero se gasta en un plan, más servicios están cubiertos. La mayoría de los seguros dentales cubren sólo 50% a 80% del costo del tratamiento. Generalmente los servicios mayores (coronas, puentes, etc.) que son los procedimientos dentales más costosos usualmente sólo están cubiertos un 50%. Por ejemplo, algunos paquetes de beneficios dentales no cubrirán los honorarios por las coronas de porcelana (material del color del diente) que no son visibles cuando usted habla o sonríe; sólo pagan por una corona de metal. Bajo este tipo de plan usted tiene que pagar el costo completo de la porcelana para estos dientes. Según las compañías de seguros, las empastaduras colocadas en los dientes frontales tienen tanto un uso funcional como un componente cosmético. Ellos pagarán por la parte funcional pero no la cantidad completa por las restauraciones cosméticas.

Los honorarios cargados por el tratamiento dental reflejan las muchas partes diferentes de un procedimiento particular o los procedimientos particulares. El tratamiento para sus necesidades particulares puede o no caer dentro de los límites fijados por su plan dental particular. Muchos procedimientos dentales pueden no estar listados en el programa de procedimientos/pagos de su seguro. Si su procedimiento dental cae dentro de esta categoría, usted puede no recibir ningún reembolso del seguro por este procedimiento. **Al final usted tiene la responsabilidad de pagar el honorario completo por un tratamiento dental aceptado, no importa la cobertura de su seguro.**

Selección de Opciones de Tratamiento

Nuestra meta a través de sus fases de examen, diagnóstico y tratamiento es proveerle con la mejor salud oral posible. No permitimos que la compañía de seguro nos diga cómo le debemos tratar. Le recomendamos los tratamientos que creemos que usted necesita y le hablaremos sobre los planes alternos. Si o no el tratamiento recomendado es un beneficio dental cubierto está entre usted y su patrón y el portador de seguro.

Sometimiento de una Reclamación

Estamos contentos de ayudarle a recibir los beneficios máximos que le permita su cobertura dental. Para someter su reclamación al seguro, necesitaremos un formulario del seguro con su parte completada y firmada. Tratamos con las compañías de seguros diariamente; por esto tenemos mucha experiencia en el sometimiento de reclamaciones a los portadores de seguros. Tenemos mucho cuidado en someter las reclamaciones apropiadamente la primera vez. Hay tres cosas que **no podemos** hacer: 1) Alterar la fecha del tratamiento; 2) Someter una reclamación por más del honorario verdadero; 3) Someter una reclamación por procedimientos que no se hayan realizado. Como no es poco común que los portadores de seguros cometan errores, preferimos presentar las reclamaciones nosotros mismos, y después de verificar el pago apropiado. Los portadores de seguros pueden responder a las peticiones para el pago de un tratamiento preautorizado en tan poco tiempo como una semana o tan largo como 45 días. Favor de ser paciente; no tenemos control sobre el correo ni sobre la velocidad con la cual el portador de seguro procesa su reclamación.

Nuestra oficina no puede negociar con su compañía de seguro sobre el reembolso de los gastos dentales. Sólo su comprador del plan (su patrón) puede negociar una cobertura mejor. Si a usted le gustaría una cobertura mejor o mayor, necesitará hablar con el comprador de su plan sobre las características que quiere en su plan dental.

Si usted tiene cualquier pregunta sobre su cobertura del seguro dental, favor de sentirse libre de preguntarnos.

Seguro Dental: Puntos a Considerar

Lo siguiente es una sinopsis en un lenguaje sencillo de la mayoría de los contratos de seguro dental. Favor de leerlo con cuidado, y tal vez guardarlo para referencia en el futuro.

✓ Los beneficios del seguro dental no trabajan igual como los del seguro médico. Casi *siempre hay un co-pago* por parte del paciente para *casi todos* los procedimientos.

✓ Hay "deducibles" en todos los planes. En el pasado nunca se sacaron estos deducibles del tratamiento preventivo ("limpiezas"). Recientemente muchos portadores han comenzado a sacar los deducibles del tratamiento preventivo.

✓ Las compañías de seguros típicamente no proveen seminarios o libros de instrucciones sobre la mejor manera de obtener los reembolsos más altos de beneficios para el paciente.

✓ No importa los beneficios del seguro dental existentes, el paciente siempre tiene la responsabilidad legal por el costo completo del tratamiento dental.

✓ La medida de cobertura dental depende solamente en el plan de seguro dental comprado por el patrón. Mientras más alta la prima pagada por el patrón, mayores son los beneficios del seguro dental.

✓ Aun si hay una predeterminación por escrito de los beneficios devueltos por el portador de seguro, es posible que después de proveer el tratamiento, no hay beneficios pagables del seguro.

✓ Nosotros (la oficina dental) no tenemos absolutamente ningún poder o influencia para tratar con el portador de seguro. Sólo el empleado o el comprador del contrato tiene el poder. Cualquier queja sobre beneficios, pago o cobertura se debe dirigir a Recursos Humanos o al dueño de la compañía.

✓ Las letras *UCR* (siglas en inglés) en los comprobantes de seguro significan el honorario *Usual, Habitual y Razonable.* La cantidad de dinero que usted ve como UCR no tiene ninguna base en la realidad. Es una cantidad arbitraria determinada solamente por el plan seleccionado y la prima de seguro pagada por el empleado. No hay ninguna relación al honorario verdadero de la oficina dental. Mientras mejor el plan (es decir, mayor la prima pagada), más alto será el UCR.

✓ Un portador particular de seguros puede tener una docena de honorarios diferentes por el mismo procedimiento, la misma oficina y el mismo dentista.

✓ No se ha establecido una cobertura y programa de pago universal. El hecho que existe un código de seguro que describe un servicio dental no garantiza que éste será un beneficio pagado bajo su póliza. Hay muchos procedimientos dentales que son necesarios, y muchos de ellos son preventivos, pero no son beneficios cubiertos.

✓ Los beneficios financieros no se pueden ahorrar y llevar al próximo año.

✓ Sus beneficios dentales casi siempre tienen un nivel máximo de contribución anual. Esta cantidad es lo MÁS que su portador de seguro está obligado a pagar por un año (por calendario o de otra manera) por contrato. Cuando esta cantidad es alcanzada, no habrán más beneficios dentales pagables hasta al próximo año de beneficios. Si usted comenzó algún tratamiento dental antes de que el máximo fuera alcanzado, el portador no tiene obligaciones de pago más allá del máximo anual.

Determinación de Beneficios del Seguro

(Fecha)

Estimado (nombre del paciente),

Hemos recibido la predeterminación de beneficios terminada por su portador de seguro. Puede que usted también haya recibido una copia de este formulario de la predeterminación de beneficios.

Cuando usted esté listo para comenzar el tratamiento, favor de llamar a nuestra oficina para revisar los detalles del plan de tratamiento y hacer los arreglos financieros apropiados. Favor de notar que su plan puede tener una limitación que requiere que el tratamiento comience dentro de un período fijo de tiempo. Cuando el tratamiento no comienza dentro del período fijo de tiempo, su portador de seguro puede cancelar el estado de predeterminación.

Sinceramente,

Petición de Información

Fecha:

Estimado (Paciente):

Para procesar y someter su formulario de reclamación del seguro para el tratamiento suministrado el (fecha), necesitaremos la siguiente información (vea la lista abajo). Para su conveniencia, se ha incluido un sobre para regresarlo predirigido y con sello.

❑ Favor de completar todo el formulario incluido.
❑ Favor de completar la porción del paciente en el formulario incluido.
❑ Favor de firmar el formulario incluido en todos los sitios marcados con X.
❑ Favor de contactarnos sobre su formulario de reclamación.

Gracias por adelantadas por su atención inmediata a este asunto.

Sinceramente,

Consentimiento de Pago

Paciente:_____   **Fecha:**_____

Cuenta Núm:

Accedo a autorizar que se realicen los servicios dentales indicados (listados en el formulario del Estimado de Honorarios). Entiendo que en cualquier momento puedo terminar o posponer el tratamiento propuesto. Me han informado de las alternativas de tratamiento que están relacionadas a mis condiciones orales, sus respectivas ventajas y desventajas, los riesgos sustanciales y las consecuencias del tratamiento limitado, retrasado o el no-tratamiento. Me han informado de los costos del tratamiento dental y del tratamiento dental alterno. Me han informado de los arreglos financieros disponibles para mí. Se han contestado todas las preguntas a mi satisfacción y he leído y entiendo las directivas y advertencias.

Se hará el pago completo en cada cita para el tratamiento dental completado en esa cita. Pagaré con
❏ MasterCard   ❏ VISA   ❏ Dinero en efectivo   ❏ Cheque personal en cada cita.

Se harán los pagos por $_____ por mes por _____ meses.
El pago se vence a no más tardar que el día _____ del mes.

Los cheques con fecha posterior o la autorización de tarjeta de crédito por el balance de $_____ se pagará el _____ y el balance restante de $_____ se pagará el _____ .

Librito de cupones: Los pagos se recibirán para el día _____ del mes por _____ meses.
Los pagos mensuales serán de $_____ .

El estimado de honorarios por los servicios dentales se garantiza por 90 días. Si el tratamiento no se comienza dentro de 90 días de la fecha estimada, el costo del tratamiento dental puede variar. Una vez que se haya comenzado el tratamiento dental, se pueden requerir cambios en el plan de tratamiento anticipado dependiendo de las condiciones orales que se encuentren. Me informarán si esto ocurre y me darán la opción de continuar con el tratamiento, cambiar el tratamiento o cancelar el tratamiento.

Si mi balance se vence y no se paga por 60 días o más, la oficina se reserva el derecho de interrumpir o descontinuar el tratamiento dental y/o enviar mi cuenta a un abogado para el cobro. En el caso que se envíe mi cuenta para el cobro, seré responsable por todos los costos y honorarios, incluyendo los honorarios razonables de abogado incurridos. Si el pago no se hace dentro de 30 días, se cargará una tasa de 1.5% por mes a mi cuenta. Las normas dentales estatales y las opciones legales del estándar de cuidado requieren que me den opciones de tratamiento, una lista de procedimientos, honorarios totales por los procedimientos y arreglos financieros indicados. Esto es para la protección mutua de tanto el paciente como del dentista.

Coordinador Financiero:

_____   _____
Firma del Coordinador Financiero   Fecha

_____   _____
Firma del Paciente o Guardián   Fecha

Estimado de Honorarios

Paciente:_____   Fecha:_____

Seguro
Primario   Secundario
Máximo anual   Máximo anual
Deducible anual   Deducible anual

Diente	Tratamiento	Co-Consulta#	Honorario	Pago del Seguro*	Su Co-Pago*

Co-consulta#—Este tratamiento dental no es proveído por esta oficina dental. Le enviaremos a un especialista para evaluación y tratamiento. Ellos le informarán del tratamiento exacto propuesto, cuánto tiempo tomará, el costo envuelto y contestarán cualquier pregunta que usted pueda tener. *El honorario por este tratamiento no está incluido en el total de este plan de tratamiento.*

*Esto es *sólo un estimado* del pago de su seguro. La cobertura de seguro para los procedimientos dentales varía tremendamente entre los diferentes portadores y planes con el mismo portador o patrón. El verdadero pago del seguro puede ser diferente a lo que aparece aquí. Usted será responsable por el balance del honorario que aparece en la lista.

Este plan de tratamiento está diseñado con varias metas: la prevención de la enfermedad dental, cambios mínimos a la estructura saludable del diente y del tejido de las encías y la restauración de los dientes con materiales que durarán más tiempo y con los menos problemas futuros. Queremos que usted tenga dientes que son funcionales, una boca sin dolor y una sonrisa atractiva para toda su vida.

Estimado de Honorarios

(FORMULARIO BREVE)

Nombre del Paciente:_____   **Fecha:**_____

Lo siguiente es una lista del tratamiento dental propuesto y un estimado de honorarios por ese tratamiento.

Periodontal:

Honorario Total: $ Pago Estimado del Seguro: $ Pago del paciente: $

Restaurativo:

Honorario Total: $ Pago Estimado del Seguro: $ Pago del paciente: $

Endodóntico:

Honorario Total: $ Pago Estimado del Seguro: $ Pago del paciente: $

Prostéticas Fijas:

Honorario Total: $ Pago Estimado del Seguro: $ Pago del paciente: $

Prostéticas Removibles:

Honorario Total: $ Pago Estimado del Seguro: $ Pago del paciente: $

Cosmético:

Honorario Total: $ Pago Estimado del Seguro: $ Pago del paciente: $

Arreglos Financieros

Nuestra meta al discutir los arreglos financieros relacionados a sus necesidades dentales incluyen:
- informarle de las alternativas de tratamiento
- las respectivas ventajas y desventajas
- las consecuencias y/o riesgos del tratamiento limitado retrasado y/o el no-tratamiento

Discutiremos los costos del tratamiento dental y del tratamiento alterno. Con mucho gusto contestaremos sus preguntas hasta que usted esté completamente satisfecho.

Seguro Dental

Estamos contentos de ayudarle recibir sus beneficios máximos del seguro dental. El seguro dental es un contrato entre su patrón, quien selecciona sus límites de cobertura, y la compañía de seguros. Usted (el abonado) recibirá los beneficios dentales como se definan dentro de este plan. Los pagos del seguro recibidos por esta oficina se acreditarán a su cuenta o se reembolsarán a usted en caso de un sobrepago. No podemos garantizar pagos del portador de seguros en los estimados de reembolso de seguros generados en nuestra oficina. Usted es responsable por todos los honorarios (cargos) dentales que su compañía de seguros no ha pagado, no importa la razón, dentro de un período de 60 días del comienzo del tratamiento. Se espera que usted pague la cantidad total adeudada.

Nuestra oficina aceptará la asignación de los beneficios del seguro dental directamente a nuestra oficina. Favor de traer su librito de beneficios del plan dental a nuestra oficina para permitir que nuestro personal haga un estimado razonable de los beneficios que la compañía de seguro le pagará por un procedimiento dental dado. Para un estado exacto de beneficios se puede enviar a la compañía de seguro un formulario de predeterminación de beneficios. Este proceso requiere que se use un formulario del seguro dental con su parte completada para peticionar una predeterminación de beneficios de su portador de seguro. El portador de seguro regresará el formulario con una declaración de las responsabilidades de pago por parte de ellos su co-pago. Usted podrá necesitar traer un formulario del seguro completado para **cada** cita en la cual se comience un tratamiento **nuevo**.

Opciones de pago

Además de aceptar pagos directamente de su portador de seguro, se deben hacer arreglos financieros por su co-pago. El co-pago es la diferencia entre los costos de tratamiento y el pago del seguro. Ofrecemos un descuento de cortesía de 5% por el pago completo antes de comenzar el tratamiento. Nuestro coordinador financiero puede explicarle los arreglos de pago mensual tales como cheques con fechas posteriores, autorización de tarjetas de crédito y libritos de cupones.

Procedimientos de Garantías y de No-pagar

Las reglas estatales nos obligan a estar seguros que usted entienda sus necesidades de tratamiento dental, el tratamiento y las opciones apropiadas, los honorarios envueltos y los arreglos financieros. Esto es para la protección mutua tanto para el paciente como para el dentista.

Los honorarios estimados por los servicios dentales se garantizan por 90 días. Si el tratamiento no se comienza dentro de 90 días de la fecha estimada, el costo del tratamiento dental puede variar. Una vez se haya comenzado el tratamiento dental, se puede requerir cambios en el plan de tratamiento anticipado dependiendo en las condiciones orales que se encuentran. Se le informará si esto ocurre y se le dará la opción de continuar con el tratamiento, cambiar el tratamiento o cancelar el tratamiento.

Si su balance se vence y no se paga por 60 días o más, nuestra oficina se reserva el derecho de interrumpir o descontinuar el tratamiento dental y/o enviar su cuenta a un abogado para el cobro. En el caso que se envíe su cuenta para cobro, usted será responsable por todos los costos y honorarios, incluyendo los honorarios razonables de abogado incurridos. Si el pago no se hace dentro de 30 días, se cargará una tasa de 1.5% por mes a su cuenta.

Preautorización de Pago

Yo, (nombre del pagador), autorizo (nombre de la oficina dental) a mantener un archivo de mi firma y a cargar mi

❑ VISA   ❑ MasterCard   ❑ Otro _____

con el balance de los cargos no pagados por el seguro dental inmediatamente después de recibir el co-pago del seguro dental o el balance de los cargos no pagados dentro de 30 días de terminar el tratamiento dental y de no exceder $_____ por
   ❑ esta cita solamente
   ❑ todas las citas de este año.

Para los cargos que recurren por el tratamiento en progreso o el tratamiento completado de $_____ cada
   ❑ semana
   ❑ mes desde el (fecha) hasta el (fecha). Asigno los beneficios del seguro dental al proveedor arriba mencionado.

Entiendo que este formulario es válido por 1 año desde la fecha que aparece abajo a menos que cancele por escrito la autorización del proveedor.

Nombre del Paciente:
Nombre del Titular de la Tarjeta:
Dirección del Titular de la Tarjeta:
Ciudad, Estado y Código Postal:
de Cuenta de la Tarjeta de Crédito: Fecha de Expiración:

_____   _____

Firma del Titular de la Tarjeta   Fecha

Programa para Pagos

Paciente:_____

Arreglos de Pago

Entiendo el tratamiento dental recomendado listado abajo o adjunto. Se han explicado a mi satisfacción las ventajas/desventajas de los procedimientos y los procedimientos alternos, los riesgos y las consecuencias de la acción o de la falta de acción. Autorizo al dentista o a sus auxiliares a hacer el tratamiento listado. Estoy consciente de que puedo posponer o terminar el tratamiento en cualquier momento. Se puede terminar el tratamiento por la falta de pago por los servicios hechos. He leído el plan de pago cuidadosamente y he seleccionado una de las opciones de pago.

Si tengo un seguro dental, la oficina dental **estimará** el costo por mí parte. Cuando llegue el pago del seguro, seré responsable inmediatamente por lo que no está cubierto. Si la cobertura del seguro reembolsa a la oficina por más de lo que se estimó, tendré el derecho a un crédito o un reembolso, según la mí elección. Si decido pagar por adelantado la cantidad estimada entera antes de comenzar el tratamiento, por cualquier cantidad sobre $100, se descontará un 5% de esta cantidad. Entiendo que aceptan dinero en efectivo, cheques personales y tarjetas de crédito como métodos de pago.

❏ El pago completo en cada cita para el tratamiento terminado en ese día.

Fecha:_____ Cita 1 $_____	Fecha:_____ Cita 5 $_____
Fecha:_____ Cita 2 $_____	Fecha:_____ Cita 6 $_____
Fecha:_____ Cita 3 $_____	Fecha:_____ Cita 7 $_____
Fecha:_____ Cita 4 $_____	Fecha:_____ Cita 8 $_____

❏ Pago mensual de $ _____ por _____ meses.
  Pago inicial de $_____.
  Me enviarán un cupón para el pago mensual.

❏ Dejaré cheques con fechas posteriores para depositarse el día _____ de cada mes.
❏ Daré la autorización previa para el pago por tarjeta de crédito: ❏ VISA   ❏ MasterCard
  Se cargará $_____ a mi tarjeta de crédito el día _____ de cada mes hasta que los honorarios estén totalmente pagados.
  Tarjeta #_____ Fecha de Expiración:_____

Autorizo el pago directo a (nombre de la oficina dental) de mis beneficios dentales. Entiendo que sólo yo soy responsable por todos los costos del tratamiento dental. Autorizo al dentista y al personal dental a hacer todos los procedimientos diagnósticos, preventivos y terapéuticos necesarios para el cuidado dental. Permito al dentista que entregue cualquier información médica o dental a otros practicantes de salud o portadores de seguros. Se puede fotocopiar mi firma o usar la frase "firma archivada" para ayudar a conseguir los beneficios debidos del seguro.

Plan de Tratamiento

Diente # _____ Procedimiento: _____ Honorario: $_____

Esto es sólo un estimado. Las condiciones que se presenten cuando verdaderamente se traten los dientes pueden requerir un cambio en los honorarios. El tratamiento podría ser más o menos extensivo que lo que se determinó originalmente. Entiendo que la oficina dental ha hecho todos los esfuerzos para estimar todas las necesidades de procedimientos dentales con la mayor precisión posible. Si ocurre un cambio, me informarán inmediatamente y el tratamiento no procederá sin mi aprobación.

Honorario total por el tratamiento listado: $_____

_____   _____
Firma del Paciente/Guardián   Fecha

Rechazo del Tratamiento

Nombre del Paciente: _____   **Fecha:** _____

El (nombre del dentista) me recomendó el siguiente tratamiento dental el (fecha).

Se revelaron las ventajas y desventajas del tratamiento, los riesgos del tratamiento y del no-tratamiento, las opciones y los honorarios. Se contestaron todas mis preguntas a mi satisfacción. Entiendo que en el futuro, un cambio en mi salud oral puede hacer que sea imposible que se haga el tratamiento hoy sugerido o puede causar que haya un problema que sea más costoso de reparar. En este momento, rechazo que se haga el siguiente tratamiento para mí o para mi hijo(a) _____ .

Periodontal:

Preventivo:

Restaurativo:

Endodóntico:

Prostéticas:

Cirugía Oral:

_____   _____
Firma del Paciente/Guardián   Fecha

Evaluación Cosmética Dental

Pupilas: ❑ Horizontal   ❑ Izquierda Alta   ❑ Derecha Alta

Nariz: ❑ Centralizada   ❑ Izquierda   ❑ Derecha

Labios en reposo: ❑ Igual de largo izquierdo y derecho   ❑ Izquierdo más largo   ❑ Derecho más largo
❑ Horizontal   ❑ Izquierdo Alto   ❑ Derecho Alto

Línea del medio dental centralizada: ❑ Debajo de la nariz   ❑ Debajo del labio
❑ En la cara   ❑ Sobre los dientes de la línea del medio # 24 y 25

Simetría/reflejo de espejo izquierdo y derecho:

	8/9		7/10		6/11	
Largo	❑ dln	❑ no	❑ dln	❑ no	❑ dln	❑ no
Ancho	❑ dln	❑ no	❑ dln	❑ no	❑ dln	❑ no
Vertical	❑ dln	❑ no	❑ dln	❑ no	❑ dln	❑ no

(dln = dentro de los límites normales)

Comentarios: _____

Línea de sonrisa: ❑ Baja   ❑ Media   ❑ Alta   ❑ Alta Extendida
❑ Balanceada   ❑ Izquierda Alta   ❑ Derecha Alta

Extensión de sonrisa: ❑ Normal   ❑ Forzada/Artificial

Arquitectura Gingival en Forma de Concha: ❑ A nivel "Clásica"   ❑ Irregular #6 #7 #8 #9 #10 #11

Reflejo de Espejo de Forma de Concha:

	8/9		7/10		6/11	
	❑ sí	❑ no	❑ sí	❑ no	❑ sí	❑ no

Apuntes: _____

Análisis de Forma de Concha: _____

Evidencia de erupción–generada por el desgaste anormal:

	#7		#8		#9		#10	
	❑ sí	❑ no	❑ sí	❑ no	❑ sí	❑ no	❑ sí	❑ no

❑ **Consulta Ortodóntica**
❑ **Consulta Periodontal**

Dimensión Relativa de los Incisores:

	#6	#7	#8	#9	#10	#11
Largo	____	____	____	____	____	____
Ancho	____	____	____	____	____	____

Problemas con las Dimensiones Relativas de los Incisivos: _____

Sugerencias para el Mejoramiento: _____

Evaluación Cosmética Dental—continuación

Número de dientes visibles al ancho máximo de la sonrisa: _____ Maxilar _____ Mandibular

Línea incisa: ❏ Horizontal "Normal"   ❏ Sube izquierda–derecha   ❏ Sube derecha–izquierda

Línea gingival anterior/posterior: ❏ Normal   ❏ Alterada (describa) _____

❏ **Sobremordida** _____ mm   ❏ **Superposición** _____ mm   ❏ **Rotaciones,** diente #s _____

❏ **Dientes apiñados,** diente #s _____

❏ **Cemento visible,** diente #s _____

❏ **Dientes agrietados,** diente #s _____

❏ **Abrasiones de cepillo de dientes visibles,** diente #s_____

Atrición: Maxilar, diente #s _____   Categoría: 1   2   3   4
            Mandibular, diente #s _____   Categoría: 1   2   3   4

Desgaste de cerradura y llave en:
❏ Directo   ❏ Saliente   ❏ Lateral Derecho   ❏ Lateral Izquierdo   ❏ Oblicuo Derecho   ❏ Oblicuo Izquierdo

Bordes incisos manchados, diente #s _____

Color de dientes   ❏ Uniforme   ❏ Variable   Matiz dominante _____

Estriaciones   ❏ Ninguna   ❏ Presente, diente #s _____

Manchas blancas   ❏ Ninguna   ❏ Presente, diente #s _____

Restauraciones desteñidas, diente #s _____

Amalgamas visibles, diente #s _____

¿Diastema aceptable para el paciente?   ❏ sí   ❏ no

Comentarios _____

_____

Sugerencias para la mejoría _____

_____

Servicios de Higiene Dental:
Visita de Profilaxis Dental

Nombre del Paciente: _____

Su visita de profilaxis dental el _____ incluyó los siguientes servicios:

- ❏ Una revisión de historia médica y dental
- ❏ Un examen oral para el cáncer y evaluación del tejido suave
- ❏ Una evaluación de cuidado oral de sí mismo, incluyendo
  - a. uso correcto del hilo dental
  - b. técnica de cepillar los dientes
  - c. técnica del enhebrador de hilo dental
  - d. tabletas/solución de tintura
  - e. evaluación de los hábitos de cuidado oral diario de sí mismo
  - f. recomendación de producto para el cuidado oral de sí mismo
  - g. otro_____
- ❏ Radiografías intraorales
  - ❏ series de cuidado repetido　　❏ series completa　　❏ áreas seleccionadas
- ❏ Evaluación periodontal, incluyendo:
  - a. medida de las profundidades sulculares (examen periodontal con sonda)
  - b. movilidad del diente
  - c. involucración de furcación
  - d. retiro del tejido gingival (encías)
  - e. puntos sangrantes
  - f. depósitos de cálculo
- ❏ Caries dentales (cavidades) evaluación, incluyendo:
  - a. restauraciones defectuosas
  - b. dientes fracturados
  - c. deterioro
  - d. erosiones y abrasiones
  - e. desgaste
- ❏ Eliminación ultrasónica del cálculo (sarro)
- ❏ Alisado radicular
- ❏ Irrigación subgingival de los bolsillos periodontales con una solución medicada
- ❏ Profilaxis y pulido
- ❏ Aplicación de fluoruro tópico
- ❏ Aplicación de sellador en los dientes números_____.
- ❏ Fotografías/video intraoral
- ❏ Impresiones para modelos diagnósticos de estudio y registro oclusal para modelo de relación de mordida.
- ❏ Blanqueo vital/no-vital de dientes, dientes números_____.
- ❏ Aplicación de un agente desensibilizante en la superficie de la raíz, dientes números_____.
- ❏ Aplicación de medicamentos subgingivales específicos al lugar, dientes números_____.

Comentarios del higienista:

_____

_____

_____

_____

Visión General del Examen/Consulta

Nombre del Paciente:_____   **Fecha:**_____

Basado en el examen oral comprehensivo o una consulta, se observan las siguientes áreas de patología o preocupación dental. Favor de recordar que esto **no** es un plan de tratamiento específico. Es un bosquejo general de lo que se ha encontrado, el tratamiento propuesto y la secuencia del tratamiento. Lo seguirá un plan detallado de tratamiento con una lista de los servicios y honorarios específicos. Algunos dientes podrán tener más de un problema diagnosticado; sin embargo, un procedimiento dental puede ser todo lo que se necesita para corregir la condición.

Áreas de Patología o Preocupación Dental

Categoría de enfermedad periodontal:

Cantidad de Dientes	SD	SI	ID	II	
_____	____	____	____	____	❑ Dientes sueltos o incurables
_____	____	____	____	____	❑ Dientes rotos
_____	____	____	____	____	❑ Dientes frontales deteriorados
_____	____	____	____	____	❑ Dientes traseros deteriorados
_____	____	____	____	____	❑ Dientes que requieren tratamiento endodóntico (canal radicular)
_____	____	____	____	____	❑ Restauraciones defectuosas en los dientes frontales
_____	____	____	____	____	❑ Restauraciones defectuosas en los dientes traseros
_____	____	____	____	____	❑ Dientes que faltan que se reemplazarán
_____	____	____	____	____	❑ Dientes mal alineados
_____	____	____	____	____	❑ Coronas para dientes frontales
_____	____	____	____	____	❑ Coronas/onlays para dientes traseros
_____	____	____	____	____	❑ Abrasiones causadas por el cepillo de dientes
_____	____	____	____	____	❑ Atrición
_____	____	____	____	____	❑ Blanqueo cosmético de dientes
_____	____	____	____	____	❑ Unión cosmética (porcelana)
_____	____	____	____	____	❑ Unión cosmética (resina)
_____	____	____	____	____	❑ Reemplazo de empastaduras desteñidas
_____	____	____	____	____	❑ Reemplazo de empastaduras de metal
_____	____	____	____	____	❑ Cirugía plástica cosmética

Visión General de la Secuencia del Tratamiento

_____ Tratamiento Periodontal   Oficina:_____   Enviado a un especialista:_____

_____ Endodoncia   Oficina:_____   Enviado a un especialista:_____

_____ Cirugía Oral   Oficina:_____   Enviado a un especialista:_____

_____ Ortodoncia   Oficina:_____   Enviado a un especialista:_____

_____ Operatorio (empastaduras)

_____ Cosmética

_____ Prostético (coronas, inlays, onlays)

_____ Reemplazar dientes que faltan

_____ Otro:_____

Actualización del Historial Médico

Nombre del Paciente: _____

¿Hay algún cambio en su historial médico desde su última cita dental?   ❏ Sí   ❏ No
   Si la respuesta es sí, por favor explique: _____

¿Está usted tomando *algún* medicamento?   Este seguro de incluir cualquier medicamento SIN RECETA que esté tomando.
❏ Sí   ❏ No   Si la respuesta es sí, por favor enumere los medicamentos: _____

_____   _____
Firma del Paciente o Guardián   Fecha

¿Hay algún cambio en su historial médico desde su última cita dental?   ❏ Sí   ❏ No
   Si la respuesta es sí, por favor explique: _____

¿Está usted tomando *algún* medicamento?   Este seguro de incluir cualquier medicamento SIN RECETA que esté tomando.
❏ Sí   ❏ No   Si la respuesta es sí, por favor enumere los medicamentos: _____

_____   _____
Firma del Paciente o Guardián   Fecha

¿Hay algún cambio en su historial médico desde su última cita dental?   ❏ Sí   ❏ No
   Si la respuesta es sí, por favor explique: _____

¿Está usted tomando *algún* medicamento?   Este seguro de incluir cualquier medicamento SIN RECETA que esté tomando.
❏ Sí   ❏ No   Si la respuesta es sí, por favor enumere los medicamentos: _____

_____   _____
Firma del Paciente o Guardián   Fecha

¿Hay algún cambio en su historial médico desde su última cita dental?   ❏ Sí   ❏ No
   Si la respuesta es sí, por favor explique: _____

¿Está usted tomando *algún* medicamento?   Este seguro de incluir cualquier medicamento SIN RECETA que esté tomando.
❏ Sí   ❏ No   Si la respuesta es sí, por favor enumere los medicamentos: _____

_____   _____
Firma del Paciente o Guardián   Fecha

¿Hay algún cambio en su historial médico desde su última cita dental?   ❏ Sí   ❏ No
   Si la respuesta es sí, por favor explique: _____

¿Está usted tomando *algún* medicamento?   Este seguro de incluir cualquier medicamento SIN RECETA que esté tomando.
❏ Sí   ❏ No   Si la respuesta es sí, por favor enumere los medicamentos: _____

_____   _____
Firma del Paciente o Guardián   Fecha

Procedimiento para la Próxima Cita

En su próxima cita, se harán los siguientes procedimientos. Si le han dicho que usted necesita tomar un antibiótico profiláctico 1 hora antes de su cita, favor de recordarse de tomarlo. Se ha fijado la cita por _____ minutos. Es posible que en la próxima cita surgirá una situación que causará una modificación del tratamiento anticipado. Si esto ocurre, se le informará inmediatamente.

Periodontal
———— Raspado y alisado radicular
        Cuadrante ❏ SD   ❏ ID   ❏ SI   ❏ II   Puede requerir anestesia local.
———— Cirugía periodontal

Restaurativo
———— Restauraciones del color de diente, adheridas
        ❏ Dientes frontales
        ❏ Dientes traseros
———— Poste
———— Base
———— Alargamiento de corona
———— Preparación para ———— inlay ———— onlay de corona
———— Impresión para un ———— inlay ———— onlay de corona
———— Preparación para un puente _____
———— Impresión para un puente
———— Molde preliminar de prueba
———— Cementación provisional
———— Cementación final

Endodoncia
———— Comenzar canal radicular, diente #————
———— Continuar canal radicular, diente #————
———— Finalizar canal radicular, diente #————

Cirugía oral
———— Extracción
———— Otro

Prostéticas removibles
———— Impresiones preliminares, registros, transferencia de arco facial
———— Impresiones finales
———— Armazón preliminar de prueba
———— Estructura de cera preliminar de prueba
———— Entrega de dentadura completa o parcial

Si usted tiene cualquier pregunta sobre algún procedimiento u honorario, favor de hacerla antes de hacer su próxima cita.

Petición para la Educación del Paciente

Favor de marcar lo que le gustaría recibir. Entonces puede enviarnos el formulario por correo con su nombre y dirección, dejarlo en la oficina o llamarnos para dejarnos saber la información le gustaría que le enviemos.

Su Nombre: _____

Dirección: _____

_____

Ciudad, Estado, Código Postal _____

Metas del Tratamiento

Nuestra meta al recomendar el mejor tratamiento para cumplir con sus necesidades dentales específicas es ayudarle a tener la mejor salud oral posible. Nuestra recomendación para el plan de tratamiento se basará en los muchos años que tenemos de práctica e investigación clínica de tiempo completo. Cuando sea apropiado, también sugerimos opciones de tratamiento de las cuales usted puede hacer una selección. Le explicaremos todas las opciones con las ventajas y desventajas de cada opción. A base de esta información y del conocimiento de su propia situación personal (tales como el tiempo que usted tiene disponible para el tratamiento y las consideraciones financieras) y con nuestros años de práctica dental exitosa, podemos trabajar juntos para escoger el mejor plan para usted.

Diseñamos los planes de tratamiento con varias metas: la prevención de la enfermedad dental, un cambio mínimo a la estructura saludable de los dientes y del tejido de las encías y la restauración con materiales que sean los más duraderos y que tengan los menos problemas futuros. Al final, queremos que usted tenga dientes que sean funcionales, una boca sin dolor y una sonrisa atractiva cuando tenga 95 años de edad.

La cobertura de seguros para los procedimientos dentales varía tremendamente entre los muchos portadores diferentes de seguro, tal como pueden ser diferentes los planes con el mismo portador o patrón. Las variaciones pueden afectar las cantidades deducibles, los co-pagos del paciente y la cobertura de procedimientos. En ningún momento permitiremos que ninguna cobertura de seguro dental dicte su tratamiento. No importa si usted tiene o no algún tipo de seguro dental, nuestras recomendaciones serán las mismas.

Aunque le ayudaremos con el sometimiento del seguro para el tratamiento que usted haya terminado, usted es responsable por el pago no cubierto dentro de 60 días (por cualquier razón) por su portador de seguro. Se le pueden arreglar planes de pago para el tratamiento dental extensivo. Raramente el tratamiento dental para las mejorías cosméticas sea un beneficio dental cubierto, no importa el plan de seguro que usted tenga. Algunos de los métodos innovadores nuevos de restaurar dientes, reemplazar dientes que faltan (implantes dentales) o regenerar tejido de hueso o de las encías podrán ser costos no cubiertos. Esto no es porque sean procedimientos experimentales sino porque su patrón todavía no ha comprado una cobertura para ellos.

Si usted tiene cualquier pregunta sobre su tratamiento y su cobertura de seguro, favor de sentirse libre de preguntarnos en cualquier momento.

Narrativas del Seguro

Revisión del Contenido: Narrativas del Seguro

Evite que los procedimientos más frecuentemente malentendidos se atasquen en el proceso de negación/apelación ofreciendo la información de apoyo y los códigos apropiados desde el comienzo. Estas narrativas permiten que el consejero de la compañía de seguros entienda cómo y dónde varios procedimientos caben dentro del plan de beneficios. Todas las cartas tienen espacio para su membrete en la parte superior de la carta. Las cartas adicionales en esta sección pueden ayudar a resolver otros problemas comunes de seguros.

Estas cartas sirven dos propósitos:
1. Aumentar al máximo el reembolso del seguro al paciente.
2. Demostrar al paciente, a través de la copia para el paciente, que usted está tratando al máximo que pueda en obtener el reembolso apropiado para él.

Es posible que éstos puedan generar un mejor pago por un procedimiento, y de seguro ayudarán a cementar una relación más fuerte entre el paciente y el dentista.

Narrativa de Información del Procedimiento
Los documentos están organizados en tres áreas de temas dentales: Endodoncia; Preventivos/Periodoncia y la Odontología de Restauraciones.

Resolución de Problemas
Códigos de Beneficios Cambiados
Pide una revisión de los códigos que un portador de seguro ha alterado, para restituirlos como un servicio pagable.

Queja al Comisario de Seguro
Cuando la compañía de seguro no responde, se demora por mucho tiempo o sigue pidiendo información ya entregada, una ayuda externa puede obtener que las cosas se muevan de nuevo. Esta carta es fácil de individualizar según sus necesidades específicas.

Información Narrativa
Provee un formulario para la narrativa de un procedimiento específico.

Predeterminación de Beneficios
Formulario para pedir una predeterminación de beneficios, con espacio para comentarios narrativos específicos.

Respuesta a un Pedido de Radiográfico
Una respuesta a un portador de seguro cuando se han pedido unas radiografías que no añadirán nada a la determinación de la enfermedad y por ende tampoco al tratamiento apropiado.

Petición para una Recodificación del Seguro
Esta carta pide la reconsideración de una reclamación para un puente fijo cuando no es un beneficio del seguro.

Apicectomía

Paciente: **Portador de Seguro:**
Número de Seguro Social del Paciente: **Número de Grupo:**
Paciente ❏ **es**   ❏ **no es**   **el abonado**   **Patrón:**
                                                       Abonado:

Re: Números del código de ADA:
  ❏ D3410 Apicectomía de Diente Anterior, diente #
  ❏ D3421 Apicectomía de Primera Raíz Bicúspide, diente #
  ❏ D3425 Apicectomía de Primera Raíz Molar, diente #
  ❏ D3426 Apicectomía de Cada Raíz Adicional, diente #
  ❏ D3426 Apicectomía de Cada Raíz Adicional, diente #
  ❏ D3430 Empastadura Retrógrada, diente #   , primera raíz
  ❏ D3430 Empastadura Retrógrada, diente #   , raíz adicional
  ❏ D3430 Empastadura Retrógrada, diente #   , raíz adicional
  ❏ D3450 Amputación Radicular, primer diente #   , primera raíz
  ❏ D3450 Amputación Radicular, primer diente #   , raíz adicional

Fecha:

Estimado Consejero Dental:

La siguiente narrativa dará información adicional sobre el tratamiento suministrado al paciente el ____. Debido a la patología periapical residual después del tratamiento endodóntico, se hicieron los procedimientos indicados arriba. Se confirmó el diagnóstico por medio de:
  ❏ Dolor crónico
  ❏ Fístula
  ❏ Sensibilidad a palpación/percusión
  ❏ Evidencia radiográfica de patología periapical
  ❏ Síndrome endodóntico/periodontico
  ❏ Canales calcificados o severamente dilacerados, imposible de arreglar sin cirugía
  ❏ Aparato separado en el canal, imposible de remover sin cirugía
  ❏ Imposibilidad de remover el material de empastadura endodóntica existente
  ❏ Otro:

❏ Radiografía adjunta.

Todas las citas postoperatorias habituales se incluyeron en el honorario.

Si tiene cualquier pregunta, favor de sentirse libre de contactar esta oficina. Favor de aplicar los beneficios contractuales apropiados a los procedimientos listados en el formulario del seguro. Si los procedimientos listados no son procedimientos cubiertos y códigos de pago de su compañía de seguro, favor de recodificarlos y aplicar los beneficios alternos como se ha indicado.

Gracias.

Sinceramente,

copia/(paciente)

Blanqueo No Vital de Dientes

Paciente: **Portador de Seguro:**
Número de Seguro Social del Paciente: **Número de Grupo:**
Paciente ❑ **es** ❑ **no es** **el abonado** **Patrón:**
 Abonado:

Re: Números del código de ADA:
 ❑ D3999 Blanqueo no vital, diente tratado endodónticamente
 ❑ D9974 Blanqueo interno–por diente

Fecha:

Estimado Consejero Dental:

La siguiente narrativa dará información adicional sobre el tratamiento suministrado al paciente. El diente #_____, se había tratado endondónticamente
 ❑ el_____,
 ❑ aproximadamente _____ años atrás; desconocida la fecha de terminación.

El diente se ha desteñido significativamente a causa de la dentición natural. Se llevó a cabo una secuencia de blanqueo no vital en este diente. Esto consistió en remover el material de obturación gutapercha coronal y poner un sellador de ionómero de vidrio sobre la apertura del canal.

❑ Para hacer el blanqueo se usó una solución de blanqueo oxidante (peróxido de hidrógeno, 35%) y una aplicación de energía de luz/calor para activar los químicos de blanqueo.

❑ Para hacer el blanqueo se usó una solución oxidante en un procedimiento en la oficina que duró _____ minutos. La aplicación del blanqueador se repitió en _____ citas separadas en las siguientes fechas: (Entre las fechas aquí).

❑ Para hacer el blanqueo se usó una mezcla de perborato de sodio y Superoxol o agua mezclada para obtener una consistencia de pasta, seguido por una restauración provisional para asegurar la preparación del acceso. Es posible que sea necesario repetir este procedimiento varias veces antes de obtener el cambio de color adecuado.

❑ El honorario por la preparación inicial y la preparación del ionómero de vidrio /restauración adherida/ restauración es $

❑ El honorario por cada aplicación de blanqueo es $

❑ El honorario total por el blanqueo, sin la restauración final es $

Comentarios:

Favor de aplicar los beneficios contractuales apropiados a los procedimientos listados en el formulario del seguro. Si los procedimientos listados no son procedimientos cubiertos y códigos de pago de su compañía de seguro, favor de recodificarlos y aplicar los beneficios alternos como se ha indicado, para cumplir con su responsabilidad contractual con el comprador del contrato.

Si usted tiene cualquier pregunta, favor de sentirse libre de contactar esta oficina. Gracias.

Sinceramente,

copia/(paciente)

Retratamiento de Endodoncia

Paciente:
Número de Seguro Social del Paciente:
Paciente ❑ es ❑ no es el abonado

Portador de Seguro:
Número de Grupo:
Patrón:
Abonado:

Re: Números del código de ADA:
❑ D3346 Re-tratamiento Endodóntico, Diente Anterior
❑ D3347 Re-tatamiento Endodóntico, Diente Bicúspide
❑ D3348 Re-tratamiento Endodóntico, Diente Molar

Fecha:

Estimado Consejero Dental:

La siguiente narrativa le dará información adicional sobre el tratamiento suministrado al paciente el _____. El diente # _____ requirió un retratamiento de la endodoncia realizada previamente. La endodoncia previa se concluyó hace aproximadamente _____ años. La razón para el re-tratamiento es:

❑ Reinfección apical, notable por el drenaje de tracto fistuloso.
❑ Reinfección apical, área periapical radiolúcida radiográfica.
❑ Reinfección apical, designada por presión/hinchazón/dolor.
❑ Reinfección apical asociada con el síndrome endodóntico/periodontico.
❑ Relleno/condensación del canal endodóntico clínicamente inaceptable. No hay evidencia radiográfica de la curación apical.
❑ Puntos sueltos de plata en los canales, corrimiento de cemento de punto de plata.
❑ Este diente exhibió una obstrucción mecánica o natural que requirió más tiempo para arreglar.

El retratamiento requirió mayor destreza técnica y más tiempo de retratamiento para remover el material de empastadura endodóntico y arreglar el(los) canal(es). Es más difícil remover un sellador/cemento endodóntico endurecido y los materiales de obturación que tratar cualquier canal inicialmente.

Comentarios:

Favor de aplicar los beneficios contractuales apropiados a los procedimientos listados en el formulario del seguro. Si los procedimientos listados no son procedimientos cubiertos y códigos de pago de su compañía de seguro, favor de recodificarlos y aplicar los beneficios alternos como se ha indicado.

Si usted tiene cualquier pregunta, favor de sentirse libre de contactar esta oficina. Gracias.

Sinceramente,

copia/(paciente)

Bruxismo: Aparato de Arco Completo

Paciente:
Número de Seguro Social del Paciente:
Paciente ❑ **es**   ❑ **no es**   **el abonado**

Portador de Seguro:
Número de Grupo:
Patrón:
Abonado:

Re: Número del código de ADA:
D9940 Aparato Protector Oclusal

Fecha:

Estimado Consejero Dental:

Ésta es una petición para una predeterminación de responsabilidades de cobertura.

Este paciente se ha diagnosticado como un paciente que sufre los efectos del bruxismo y/o rechinar. Clínicamente el paciente exhibe evidencia clara de una dentición gastada anormalmente. El desgaste es claramente patológico y mayor de lo esperado para un paciente de esta edad. Los síntomas del síndrome de disfunción temporomandibular (DTM) ❑ están   ❑ no están presentes.

El tratamiento consistirá de modelos de estudio completos del arco superior e inferior para el análisis oclusal, seguido por la fabricación en el laboratorio de un aparato rígido del maxilar completo para el bruxismo. No es un plano llano sino uno que se ha ajustado con abolladuras para todos los puntos de las cúspides y los bordes de los incisivos. Donde sea posible, hay disclusión guiada exclusivamente para los caninos para las excursiones laterales izquierdas y derechas. En los movimientos protuberantes hay disclusión posterior. Se hará un ajuste final con el paciente en una posición sentada y supina.

Los honorarios por este procedimiento incluyen lo siguiente: modelos de estudio, análisis oclusal, fabricación del aparato para el bruxismo, ajuste final antes de la entrega, entrega, citas de seguimiento y reajustes como sean necesarios.

Si el paciente sigue bien las instrucciones, el pronóstico es bueno. La velocidad del desgaste de la dentición natural debe disminuir a los niveles fisiológicos normales. Si el bruxismo/rechinar sigue en la presencia del aparato, se espera que habrá que hacer un aparato nuevo en el futuro.

Si usted tiene cualquier pregunta sobre el diagnóstico o el tratamiento de este paciente con respecto a este procedimiento, favor de contactar esta oficina. Gracias.

Sinceramente,

copia/(paciente)

Bruxismo: Sistema de Suprimir Tensión

Paciente: **Portador de Seguro:**
Número de Seguro Social del Paciente: **Número de Grupo:**
Paciente ❏ es ❏ no es el abonado   **Patrón:**
                                                       Abonado:

Re: Número del código de ADA:
D9940 Aparato Protector Oclusal

Fecha:

Estimado Consejero Dental:

Ésta es una petición para una predeterminación de responsabilidades de cobertura.

Este paciente se ha diagnosticado como un paciente que sufre los efectos del bruxismo y/o rechinar. Clínicamente el paciente exhibe evidencia clara de una dentición gastada anormalmente. El desgaste es claramente patológico y mayor de lo esperado para un paciente de esta edad. Los síntomas del síndrome de disfunción temporomandibular (DTM) ❏ están ❏ no están presentes.

El tratamiento consistirá de la fabricación de un aparato intraoral con un sistema de suprimir tensión. Se fabricará este aparato de diseño particular en la oficina dental.

Los honorarios por este procedimiento incluyen lo siguiente: análisis oclusal, fabricación del aparato para el bruxismo, entrega, citas de seguimiento y reajustes como sean necesarios.

Si el paciente sigue bien las instrucciones, el pronóstico es bueno. La velocidad del desgaste de la dentición natural debe disminuir a los niveles fisiológicos normales. Si el bruxismo/rechinar sigue en la presencia del aparato, se espera que habrá que hacer un aparato nuevo en el futuro.

Si usted tiene cualquier pregunta sobre el diagnóstico o el tratamiento de este paciente con respecto a este procedimiento, favor de contactar a esta oficina. Gracias.

Sinceramente,

copia/(paciente)

Desensibilización: Dentición Completa

Paciente:
Número de Seguro Social del Paciente:
Paciente ❑ **es** ❑ **no es   el abonado**

Portador de Seguro:
Número de Grupo:
Patrón:
Abonado:

Fecha:

Estimado Consejero Dental:

❑ Se trató este paciente adulto con la aplicación en la oficina de fluoruro desensibilizante medicado (D9910) después de unos procedimientos de profilaxis de adulto (D1110). Esto se hizo con iontoforesis, aplicación con cubeta o una combinación de las dos modalidades. Se ha demostrado en numerosos estudios que estos procedimientos clínicos reducen y posiblemente eliminan el dolor producido por los cambios termales en los lugares afectados. El procedimiento se hizo para reducir la sensibilidad moderada a severa del diente, probablemente causada por la migración de los tejidos gingivales relacionada a la edad, el cuidado de sí mismo abusivo mecánica/inadvertidamente o la reposición quirúrgica de los tejidos gingivales marginales.

Si usted tiene cualquier pregunta en cuanto a los servicios suministrados, favor de sentirse libre de contactar esta oficina. Gracias.

Sinceramente,

copia/(paciente)

Desensibilización: Específica al Lugar

Paciente: **Portador de Seguro:**
Número de Seguro Social del Paciente: **Número de Grupo:**
Paciente ❑ **es**   ❑ **no es**   **el abonado**   **Patrón:**
                                                       Abonado:

Re: Números del código de ADA:
 ❑ D9910 Aplicación de Medicamento Desensibilizador
 ❑ D9911 Aplicación de Resina Desensibilizadora para la superficie cervical y/o de la raíz, por diente

Fecha:

Estimado Consejero Dental:

El paciente ha experimentado una sensibilidad extrema de la dentina del diente #s _____. Esta sensibilidad al calor y al frío se manifiesta cuando el paciente come o bebe cualquier cosa que está encima o debajo de la temperatura normal de la cavidad oral.

Se aisló y se trató cada diente individualmente con:
 ❑ Esmalte/agente para unir dentina y/o resina restaurativa
 ❑ Fluoruro
 ❑ Iontoforesis
 ❑ Solución desensibilizadora

Después de la aplicación del material desensibilizador en _____, se redujo o se eliminó la incomodidad causada por el cambio termal. Espero que se retenga el material por varios meses. Si la sensibilidad regresa, se reaplicará el material.

Si este procedimiento es un beneficio cubierto, favor de remitir la compensación apropiada. Si el procedimiento no está codificado correctamente para sus propósitos de informe, favor de recodificarlo según los detalles provistos en esta narrativa y solicitar el beneficio dental apropiado.

Si usted tiene cualquier pregunta, favor de sentirse libre de contactar esta oficina. Gracias.

Sinceramente,

copia/(paciente)

Cita de Higiene Dental

Paciente:
Número de Seguro Social del Paciente:
Paciente ❏ **es** ❏ **no es** **el abonado**

Portador de Seguro:
Número de Grupo:
Patrón:
Abonado:

Fecha:

Estimado Consejero Dental:

La siguiente narrativa dará información adicional sobre el tratamiento suministrado al paciente nombrado arriba en esta fecha.

❏ D1330 Instrucción para el Cuidado Oral de Sí Mismo

El honorario de $_____ es un honorario de una sola vez, cargado al momento de la primera cita solamente. Toda lo demás de la instrucción para el cuidado de sí mismo no tendrá un honorario separado.

Este paciente está recibiendo un tratamiento terapéutico periodontal para una enfermedad periodontal diagnosticada de tipo _____. **No** es una Profilaxis Periodontal Preventiva, ADA 01110. El honorario por la instrucción de cuidado oral de sí mismo incluye: Demostración e instrucción del cepillado de los dientes apropiado, uso del hilo dental, los medios auxiliares de limpieza periodontal, el descubrimiento de la placa, el uso de los enjuagues apropiados, la instrucción en el uso de la irrigación subgingival cuando sea requerida y presentaciones en video.

El paciente ha demostrado su entendimiento y puede hacer estas funciones con éxito.

El paciente recibirá una repetición de estas instrucciones de cuidado oral de sí mismo durante cada una de las _____ citas anticipadas en esta secuencia de tratamiento. El tiempo total pasado en la instrucción de cuidado de sí mismo será aproximadamente _____ minutos.

❏ D1110 Profilaxis de Adulto.
Se ha cargado a este paciente un honorario adicional de $ _____ por la profilaxis de adulto. Aunque se ha hecho un diagnóstico de gingivitis, se ha fijado un horario de ❏ tiempo adicional ❏ citas adicionales. La duración del tiempo adicional necesario: _____ minutos por cita. El número necesario de citas adicionales: _____.
La razón por el honorario adicional es:
❏ La duración de tiempo desde la última cita de profilaxis. La última cita de profilaxis del paciente se concluyó el_____.
❏ Acumulaciones excesivas de cálculo que requirieron tiempo adicional para removerse.
❏ La presencia de desteñimiento excesivo que requirió tiempo adicional para removerse.
❏ El paciente presentó un problema de manejo y por eso requirió más tiempo para el tratamiento y/o la instrucción de cuidado oral de sí mismo.

Favor de aplicar los beneficios contractuales apropiados a los procedimientos listados en el formulario del seguro. Si los procedimientos listados no son procedimientos cubiertos y códigos de pago de su compañía de seguro, favor de recodificarlos y aplicar los beneficios alternos como se ha indicado, para cumplir con su responsabilidad contractual con el comprador del contrato.

Si usted tiene cualquier pregunta, favor de sentirse libre de contactar esta oficina. Gracias.

Sinceramente,

copia/(paciente)

Diagnóstico Periodontal

Paciente:　　　　　　　　　　　　　　　　　　　　**Portador de Seguro:**
Número de Seguro Social del Paciente:　　　　　**Número de Grupo:**
Paciente ❏ **es** ❏ **no es** **el abonado**　　　　　**Patrón:**
　　　　　　　　　　　　　　　　　　　　　　　　　　Abonado:

Fecha:

Estimado Consejero Dental:

Esta carta provee información suplementaria para ayudarle en su revisión de esta reclamación para los beneficios dentales.

Las siguientes definiciones son de la Academia Americana de Periodontología (American Academy of Periodontology) para los tipos de casos usados para la identificación del diagnóstico.

　　I. Enfermedades Gingivales: Una inflamación o lesión de la gingiva caracterizada por los cambios de color, la forma gingival, la posición, la apariencia de superficie y la presencia de sangrado y/o exudado.

　II. Periodontitis Crónica: Una inflamación del periodonto asociada con la placa y el cálculo. La velocidad de la progresión está afectada por los factores locales, sistémicos o ambientales. Además se puede clasificar como localizada o generalizada.

　III. Periodontitis Agresiva: Velocidad rápida de la progresión de la enfermedad periodontal en un individuo quien aparte de eso es saludable, en la ausencia de grandes acumulaciones de placa y/o cálculo. Además se puede clasificar como localizada o generalizada.

　IV. Periodontitis como una Manifestación de Enfermedad Sistémica: Periodontitis asociada con las enfermedades hematológicas o genéticas.

　V. Enfermedades Periodontales Necróticas: Papilar y gingiva marginal ulcerada y necrótica. Además puede clasificarse como gingivitis necrótica ulcerativa o periodontitis necrótica ulcerativa.

　VI. Abscesos del Periodonto: Una infección purulenta del tejido periodontal localizada.

VII. Periodontitis Asociada con Lesiones Endodónticas: Bolsillo periodontal profundo localizado que se extiende hacia el ápice del diente después del necrosis de la pulpa.

VIII. Deformidades y Condiciones de Desarrollo o Adquiridas: Enfermedad gingival o periodontitis iniciada por factores localizados relacionados a un diente. Estos factores modifican o predisponen a la acumulación de placa o la prevención de medidas efectivas de cuidado oral de sí mismo.

El tratamiento en este momento consistió de una evaluación periodontal, registrar información en la gráfica periodontal, raspado, alisado radicular, irrigación medicada de bolsillos periodontales, pulido, instrucción del cuidado oral de sí mismo y reevaluación de la condición periodontal. El tratamiento requirió _____ citas.

Adjunto, favor de encontrar　❏ radiografías　　❏ formulario de reclamación　　❏ gráfica periodontal　　❏ otro:

Sinceramente,

copia/(paciente)

Pronóstico Periodontal

Paciente:
Número de Seguro Social del Paciente:
Paciente ❑ **es** ❑ **no es** **el abonado**

Portador de Seguro:
Número de Grupo:
Patrón:
Abonado:

Re: Pronóstico del tratamiento relacionado a lo periodontal

Fecha:

Estimado Consejero Dental:

En este momento, el pronóstico para las áreas envueltas en el tratamiento para la corrección de la patología periodontal se clasifica como

❑ I Enfermedad Gingival
❑ II Periodontitis Crónica
❑ III Periodontitis Agresiva
❑ IV Periodontitis como una Manifestación de Enfermedad Sistémica
❑ V Enfermedad Periodontal Necrótica
❑ VI Abscesos del Periodonto
❑ VII Periodontitis Asociada con Lesiones Endodónticas
❑ VIII Deformidades Desarrolladas o Adquiridas

La condición, sin las excepciones explicadas, es generalmente:

❑ excelentes   ❑ buenas   ❑ regulares   ❑ reservados   ❑ pobres   ❑ incurables

Comentarios:

Favor de observar que el pronóstico para este caso puede cambiar en cualquier momento. Algunos de los factores que afectan el pronóstico son los resultados del tratamiento, la curación, la motivación del paciente, la rutina diaria de cuidado por sí mismo, la salud sistémica del paciente y el intervalo de cuidado y mantenimiento preventivo (D4910).

Hasta esta fecha, la terapia periodontal activa:

❑ no ha comenzado   ❑ ha comenzado   ❑ fue completada

El tratamiento futuro (si la fase activa del tratamiento fue completada) envuelve los procedimientos de mantenimiento periodontal (código D4910) en un intervalo de mes(es), el registro y evaluación de _____ información en la gráfica periodontal en cada cita y la instrucción continuada del cuidado oral de sí mismo.

Si usted tiene cualquier pregunta sobre cualquier aspecto de este caso, favor de sentirse libre de contactar esta oficina.

Sinceramente,

copia/(paciente)

Raspado/Alisado Radicular

Paciente: **Portador de Seguro:**
Número de Seguro Social del Paciente: **Número de Grupo:**
Paciente ❏ **es** ❏ **no es** **el abonado**   **Patrón:**
                                                                  Abonado:

Re: Números del código de ADA:
    ❏ D4341 Raspado y Alisado Radicular por Cuadrante
    ❏ D4342 Raspado y Alisado Radicular, 1–3 dientes por Cuadrante

Fecha:

Estimado Consejero Dental:

La siguiente narrativa dará información adicional sobre el tratamiento suministrado al paciente en esta fecha. Se hizo un raspado y alisado radicular para este paciente para su(s) cuadrante(s) ❏ SD ❏ SI ❏ ID ❏ II. A estos cuadrantes les quedaron por lo menos cinco dientes naturales. Las razones para terminar dos cuadrantes completos de raspado y alisado radicular en una cita eran:

    ❏ El paciente viene a la oficina desde una larga distancia y las restricciones de tiempo en cuanto al empleo del paciente o su situación familiar eran evidentes. Era más fácil que el paciente se quedara para varias citas largas para el tratamiento en vez de venir para muchas citas más breves. No se disminuyó el tiempo actual de tratamiento.

    ❏ La cita de hoy era una cita doble, de 2 horas de duración. Esto es precisamente la misma cantidad total de tiempo que se pasaría para el procedimiento del código 4341 si se terminaran dos cuadrantes en dos fechas diferentes de tratamiento. El paciente no debe sufrir una pérdida financiera de beneficios dentales contratados porque se terminaron con los cuadrantes ❏ SD ❏ SI ❏ ID ❏ II en el mismo día.

Incluidos y adjuntos, favor de encontrar la gráfica periodontal y el diagnóstico inicial, y una copia de los servicios exactos y completos del tratamiento provisto, por cuadrante.

Favor de aplicar los beneficios contractuales apropiados a los procedimientos listados en el formulario del seguro. Con la información que he proporcionado, esperaría un pago completo de beneficios para los procedimientos completados hasta ahora bajo el código 4341. Si esto no se hace y los beneficios del paciente son menos del máximo permitido, pido que el consejero dental hable conmigo personalmente para explicarlo.

Si usted tiene cualquier pregunta, favor de sentirse libre de contactar a esta oficina. Gracias.

Sinceramente,

copia/(paciente)

Terapia Específica al Lugar

Paciente:
Número de Seguro Social del Paciente:
Paciente ❏ **es** ❏ **no es** **el abonado**

Portador de Seguro:
Número de Grupo:
Patrón:
Abonado:

Re: Número del código de ADA:

D4381　　Entrega localizada de agentes de quimioterapia por medio de un vehículo de liberación controlado en el tejido reticular enfermo, por diente, por informe.

Fecha:

Estimado Consejero Dental:

Los dientes #s: ＿＿＿＿ se han tratado con:

❏ Arestin®　　　❏ Atridox®
❏ Periochip®　　❏ Otro ＿＿＿＿

Esta terapia incluye el costo del material, la ubicación del material en el bolsillo enfermo, la instrucción de cuidado oral de sí mismo, remoción del material (si es necesario) y las citas necesarias de seguimiento para evaluar los resultados del tratamiento.

El raspado y alisado radicular del área tratada se concluyeron previamente como un procedimiento de terapia primaria. Se colocó este material porque el lugar no respondió a la terapia convencional. Este paciente tiene una historia de terapia periodontal previa.

El material mencionado arriba se colocó en el bolsillo periodontal enfermo debido a las siguientes profundidades registradas.

Diente # ＿＿＿＿ MB　B　DB　　　Diente # ＿＿＿＿ MB　B　DB
　　　　　　　ML　L　DL　　　　　　　　　　　　ML　L　DL

Adjunto, favor de encontrar:
❏ La gráfica periodontal
❏ Las radiografías

Favor de observar que, a causa del lugar del área tratada, es posible que la pérdida existente de hueso y/o la profundidad probable del bolsillo no sea evidente y que sólo se pueda detectar clínicamente.

Si usted no está familiarizado con el material o la técnica o si tiene preguntas en cuanto al tratamiento suministrado a este paciente, favor de contactar esta oficina.

Sinceramente,

copia/(paciente)

Férula

Paciente: **Portador de Seguro:**
Número de Seguro Social del Paciente: **Número de Grupo:**
Paciente ❏ es ❏ no es el abonado   **Patrón:**
                                                        Abonado:

Re: Números del código de ADA:
   ❏ D4320 Férula Provisional, Intracoronal
   ❏ D4321 Férula Provisional, Extracoronal

Fecha:

Estimado Consejero Dental:

La siguiente narrativa dará información adicional sobre el tratamiento suministrado al paciente el⎯⎯⎯.

❏ Se requiere el colocar férulas a los dientes **antes del tratamiento periodontal** debido a la movilidad del diente.

❏ Se requiere el colocar férulas a los dientes **después del tratamiento periodontal** debido a la movilidad del diente para ayudar en la curación de los tejidos periodontales suaves y duros.

Adjunto, favor de encontrar: ❏ Radiografía preoperatoria   ❏ Fotografía postoperatoria

Favor de aplicar los beneficios contractuales apropiados a los procedimientos listados en el formulario del seguro. Si los procedimientos listados no son procedimientos cubiertos y códigos de pago de su compañía de seguro, favor de recodificarlos y aplicar los beneficios alternos como se ha indicado.

Si usted tiene cualquier pregunta, favor de sentirse libre de contactar esta oficina. Gracias.

Sinceramente,

copia/(paciente)

Irrigación Subgingival

Paciente:
Número de Seguro Social del Paciente:
Paciente ❏ **es** ❏ **no es**   **el abonado**

Portador de Seguro:
Número de Grupo:
Patrón:
Abonado:

Re: Números del código de ADA:
   ❏ D9630 Otros Medicamentos y/o Medicinas
   ❏ D4999 No Especificado, por Informe

Fecha:

Estimado Consejero Dental:

El paciente   ❏ se ha sometido   ❏ se someterá a una medicación subgingival con el(los) siguiente(s) medicamento(s): Gluconato clorohexidina 0.12%, fluoruro de sodio 2.0%, peróxido de hidrógeno 1.7%, cloruro de zinc 1.0%. Se hizo este procedimiento para el diente #_____; o el(los) cuadrante(s)   ❏ SD   ❏ SI   ❏ ID   ❏ II. El propósito de la irrigación subgingival es entregar la solución medicada al área para mantener y remover las bacterias patogénicas. Se ha probado que la peor placa es la placa no ligada que reside en el bolsillo periodontal patológico. Este tipo de placa es más virulenta que la placa ligada supragingival, y el remover la placa subgingival por medio de la irrigación beneficiará a la salud periodontal del paciente. También se ha probado, en numerosos estudios, que la irrigación subgingival reduce o elimina el sangrado y otras señales de infección/inflamación periodontal de áreas de profundidad sulcular aumentada.

Los procedimientos de irrigación subgingival que se completarán se harán por:
   ❏ diente #s:_____
   ❏ cuadrante (definido como cinco dientes o más por cuadrante) número y localización del cuadrante:
   ❏ arco

Si la irrigación subgingival o la aplicación de una solución medicada es un beneficio cubierto para el o la paciente bajo el contrato de beneficios dentales, favor de asegurar la codificación de tratamiento apropiada para el procedimiento según su programa de los códigos de pago.

Si usted tiene cualquier pregunta, favor de contactarme personalmente. Gracias.

Sinceramente,

copia/(paciente)

Tratamiento de Fluoruro Tópico en la Presencia de Caries Activas

Paciente:
Número de Seguro Social del Paciente:
Paciente ❏ **es**   ❏ **no es**   **el abonado**

Portador de Seguro:
Número de Grupo:
Patrón:
Abonado:

Fecha:

Estimado Consejero Dental:

❏ Se trató este paciente adulto con un fluoruro tópico (código D9630 Otros Medicamentos y Medicinas por Informe) con una entrega por cubeta intraoral. La razón para la aplicación del fluoruro fue el descubrimiento de lesiones cariosas activas que se tratarán o una historia pasada reciente de lesiones cariosas activas. La aplicación del fluoruro tópico tiene la intención de retrasar la progresión del proceso de caries y/o reducir la severidad e incidencia de esta enfermedad.

Si usted tiene cualquier pregunta en cuanto a los servicios suministrados, favor de sentirse libre de contactar a esta oficina.

Sinceramente,

copia/(paciente)

Alargamiento de Corona

Paciente: **Portador de Seguro:**
Número de Seguro Social del Paciente: **Número de Grupo:**
Paciente ❑ **es**   ❑ **no es**   **el abonado**   **Patrón:**
                                                                 Abonado:

Re: Números del código de ADA:
   ❑ D4249 Alargamiento de la corona, por informe
   ❑ D4211 Gingivectomía

Fecha:

Estimado Consejero Dental:

Un procedimiento de alargamiento de corona   ❑ se llevó   ❑ se llevará a cabo en el diente #s_____
La razón por el alargamiento de la corona es:
   ❑ Extirpación del tejido hiperplásico y/o redundante.
   ❑ Extirpación del tejido edematoso.
   ❑ Exposición de la estructura subgingival deteriorada profunda o extensiva, extirpación del tejido saludable.
   ❑ Exposición del margen profundo o extensivo de la restauración subgingival existente, extirpación del tejido saludable.
   ❑ Exposición del lugar de la fractura del margen, extirpación del tejido saludable.
   ❑ Para obtener el largo clínico correcto para una retención adecuada de la corona, extirpación del tejido saludable. La(s) corona(s) clínica(s) era(n) demasiado corta(s) para la retención adecuada del/de los molde(s) de restauración.
   ❑ Una restauración colocada directamente.
   ❑ Una restauración de molde procesada en el laboratorio.
   ❑ Otro:_____

El procedimiento de alargamiento de la corona **no** es parte de los servicios usuales y habituales para el procedimiento dental restaurativo o prostético. El alargamiento de la corona es un procedimiento clínico completamente separado, que se usa solamente cuando existe una altura inadecuada de la corona. En ningún momento se considera que el alargamiento de la corona es parte del procedimiento dental restaurativo o prostético.

Si usted tiene cualquier pregunta, favor de contactar a esta oficina.

Sinceramente,

copia/(paciente)

Inlay/Onlay: Metálico

Paciente: **Portador de Seguro:**
Número de Seguro Social del Paciente: **Número de Grupo:**
Paciente ❑ **es** ❑ **no es** **el abonado**   **Patrón:**
                                                           Abonado:

Re: Números del código de ADA:
- ❑ D2510 Inlay Metálico (1 superficie)
- ❑ D2520 Inlay Metálico (2 superficies)
- ❑ D2530 Inlay Metálico (3 superficies o más)
- ❑ D2542 Onlay Metálico (2 superficies)
- ❑ D2543 Onlay Metálico (3 superficies)
- ❑ D2544 Onlay Metálico (4 superficies)

Fecha:

Estimado Consejero Dental:

Ésta es una petición para   ❑ el pago   ❑ la predeterminación para el diente #_____ de la restauración indicada arriba. El examen clínico del diente indica que una restauración colocada directamente estaría contraindicada a causa de:
- ❑ Cúspides socavadas
- ❑ Grosor inadecuado de la dentina para sostener el esmalte
- ❑ Extensión del daño/de la estructura preparada del diente
- ❑ La preparación estaba a 2/3 partes o más de la distancia de las laderas de las cúspides desde la ranura oclusal primaria.

Según los libros de texto de la operatoria científica dental, el inlay/onlay y el colocar coronas a las cúspides son obligatorios para proteger la estructura cuspídea subyacente débil para que no se fracture y para remover el margen oclusal cuando está sujeto a la tensión fuerte.

Una restauración colocada directamente, sea de amalgama o de resina adherida, no sería aceptable clínicamente ni sería el estándar de cuidado. A causa de la naturaleza no sostenida del diente sin la restauración de cobertura oclusal procesada en el laboratorio, se espera que las porciones debilitadas del diente se fracturarían bajo la carga oclusal normal. El abonado podría tener una cláusula de "materiales o restauraciones alternos" en el contrato de beneficios. Esto no se debe usar como una justificación para cambiar los beneficios o los códigos usados en el formulario del seguro que se ha sometido. Aunque el grado de preparación necesario podría no ser evidente en la radiografía sometida, es observable clínicamente.

Si usted tiene cualquier pregunta en cuanto a esta restauración, favor de contactar esta oficina. Gracias.

Sinceramente,

copia/(paciente)

Inlay/Onlay: Porcelana

Paciente:
Número de Seguro Social del Paciente:
Paciente ❏ **es** ❏ **no es** **el abonado**

Portador de Seguro:
Número de Grupo:
Patrón:
Abonado:

Re: Números del código de ADA:
- ❏ D2610 Inlay Porcelana/Cerámica (1 superficie)
- ❏ D2620 Inlay Porcelana/Cerámica (2 superficies)
- ❏ D2630 Inlay Porcelana/Cerámica (3 superficies o más)
- ❏ D2642 Onlay Porcelana/Cerámica (2 superficies)
- ❏ D2643 Onlay Porcelana/Cerámica (3 superficies)
- ❏ D2644 Onlay Porcelana/Cerámica (4 superficies o más)

Fecha:

Estimado Consejero Dental:

Ésta es una petición para   ❏ el pago   ❏ la predeterminación para el diente #_____ de la restauración indicada arriba.
El examen clínico del diente indica que una restauración colocada directamente estaría contraindicada a causa de:
- ❏ Cúspides socavadas
- ❏ Grosor inadecuado de la dentina para sostener el esmalte
- ❏ Extensión del daño/de la estructura preparada del diente
- ❏ La preparación estaba a 2/3 partes o más de la distancia de las laderas de las cúspides desde la ranura oclusal primaria.

Según los libros de texto de la operatoria científica dental, el inlay/onlay y el colocar coronas a las cúspides son obligatorios para proteger la estructura cuspídea subyacente débil para que no se fracture y para remover el margen oclusal cuando está sujeto a la tensión fuerte.

Una restauración colocada directamente, sea de amalgama o de resina adherida, no sería aceptable clínicamente ni sería el estándar de cuidado. A causa de la naturaleza no sostenida del diente sin la restauración de cobertura oclusal procesada en el laboratorio, se espera que las porciones debilitadas del diente se fracturarían bajo la carga oclusal normal. El abonado podría tener una cláusula de "materiales o restauraciones alternos" en el contrato de beneficios. Esto no se debe usar como una justificación para cambiar los beneficios o los códigos usados en el formulario del seguro que se ha sometido. Aunque el grado de preparación necesario podría no ser evidente en la radiografía sometida, es observable clínicamente.

Si usted tiene cualquier pregunta en cuanto a esta restauración, favor de contactar esta oficina. Gracias.

Sinceramente,

copia/(paciente)

Inlay/Onlay: Resina

Paciente: **Portador de Seguro:**
Número de Seguro Social del Paciente: **Número de Grupo:**
Paciente ❑ **es**   ❑ **no es**   **el abonado**   **Patrón:**
                                                                 Abonado:

Re: Números del código de ADA:
   ❑ D2650 Inlay de Resina (1 superficie)   ❑ D2662 Onlay de Resina (2 superficies)
   ❑ D2651 Inlay de Resina (2 superficies)   ❑ D2663 Onlay de Resina (3 superficies)
   ❑ D2652 Inlay de Resina (3 superficies o más)   ❑ D2664 Onlay de Resina (4 superficies o más)

Fecha:

Estimado Consejero Dental:

Estimado Consejero Dental:

Ésta es una petición para ❑ el pago ❑ la predeterminación para el diente #_____ de la restauración indicada arriba. El examen clínico del diente indica que una restauración colocada directamente estaría contraindicada a causa de:
   ❑ Cúspides socavadas
   ❑ Grosor inadecuado de la dentina para sostener el esmalte
   ❑ Extensión del daño/de la estructura preparada del diente
   ❑ La preparación estaba a 2/3 partes o más de la distancia de las laderas de las cúspides desde la ranura oclusal primaria.

Según los libros de texto de la operatoria científica dental, el inlay/onlay y el colocar coronas a las cúspides son obligatorios para proteger la estructura cuspídea subyacente débil para que no se fracture y para remover el margen oclusal cuando está sujeto a la tensión fuerte.

Una restauración colocada directamente, sea de amalgama o de resina adherida, no sería aceptable clínicamente ni sería el estándar de cuidado. A causa de la naturaleza no sostenida del diente sin la restauración de cobertura oclusal procesada en el laboratorio, se espera que las porciones debilitadas del diente se fracturarían bajo la carga oclusal normal. El abonado podría tener una cláusula de "materiales o restauraciones alternos" en el contrato de beneficios. Esto no se debe usar como una justificación para cambiar los beneficios o los códigos usados en el formulario del seguro que se ha sometido. Aunque el grado de preparación necesario podría no ser evidente en la radiografía sometida, es observable clínicamente.

Si usted tiene cualquier pregunta en cuanto a esta restauración, favor de contactar esta oficina. Gracias.

Sinceramente,

copia/(paciente)

Selladores

PARA EL ADMINISTRADOR DEL PLAN DE SEGURO MÉDICO EN EL LUGAR DE EMPLEO

Paciente:
Número de Seguro Social del Paciente:
Paciente ❏ **es** ❏ **no es** **el abonado**

Portador de Seguro:
Número de Grupo:
Patrón:
Abonado:

Re: Número del código de ADA:
❏ D1351 Selladores

Fecha:

Estimado Administrador del Plan de Seguro Médico:

Ha llegado a mi atención que su plan de beneficios dentales no incluye un pago para la aplicación de "selladores" (código de ADA D1351). Recientemente he colocado selladores en los dientes permanentes de uno de los niños de su abonado y no hubo un pago al abonado.

Sugeriría que su plan necesita una revisión en esta área. No se ha mantenido al día con las prácticas preventivas aceptadas y disponibles desde la última parte de la década del 1960. Ustedes están haciendo un daño tanto a sus abonados como a su compañía al no incluir los selladores dentales como un beneficio pagable. Los selladores son un tratamiento preventivo económico—son muchos menos costosos que la necesidad de colocar restauraciones, las cuales realmente se evitan con los selladores. Su plan sí paga para los procedimientos más costosos que se necesitan cuando surgen problemas.

El hecho que no se incluyen los selladores como un beneficio pagable indica que ustedes pueden no estar conscientes de lo que son y de lo que hacen. A pesar de las aplicaciones sistémicas y tópicas de fluoruro a los dientes, y a pesar del cuidado adecuado de sí mismo, las superficies oclusales (de mordida) de los dientes son las primeras áreas que se deterioran. Estas superficies se caracterizan por hoyos y aberturas que son más pequeñas que el diámetro de una cerda del cepillo de dientes. No se pueden limpiar fácilmente. Las bacterias colonizan los fondos de los hoyos y aberturas y comienzan el proceso de deterioro. Hay poco o nada que un paciente puede hacer en su casa para evitar que estas lesiones comiencen. El sellador es una capa plástica no invasiva, rápida de colocar y sin dolor que llena los hoyos y aberturas y así evita la colonización de bacterias y la deterioración subsiguiente. De hecho, los estudios han demostrado claramente que el deterioro activo en estas áreas se puede sellar efectivamente y evitar que cause más daño. La única otra alternativa a los selladores es una empastadura. El diente se taladra, se daña permanentemente y se condena a más taladrar y más empastaduras cuando el paciente avanza en edad. Estas empastaduras pueden ser costosas. Se puede necesitar terapia endodóntica y restauraciones de cobertura completa. Éstos pueden costar 25 veces más que el sellador. Los selladores son seguros y efectivos.

Los selladores pueden quedarse en los dientes por años. Una retención de 5 años no es poco común. Yo personalmente he puesto selladores que todavía funcionan después de casi 20 años de servicio. Ustedes no cubren los selladores que cuestan \$_____, pero sí cubren las restauraciones de molde que cuestan \$_____. También tienen que pagar para que se rehagan los moldes cada 5 años.

Los selladores están endosados por la Asociación Dental Americana, el Instituto Nacional para la Salud Dental y (en 1984 y 1994) por el Cirujano General. Si ustedes se preocupan por el control de los costos del cuidado de la salud para sus abonados, les aconsejo fuertemente que de inmediato hagan que los selladores sean un beneficio pagable en su plan dental. Sus abonados y ustedes se beneficiarán de esto. Consideren que esta acción es una práctica firme de negocio, una que tiene una relación de costo/beneficio maravillosa.

Sinceramente,

copia/(paciente)

Laminados: Indirectos

Paciente: **Portador de Seguro:**
Número de Seguro Social del Paciente: **Número de Grupo:**
Paciente ❑ **es**   ❑ **no es**   **el abonado**   **Patrón:**
                                                                     Abonado:

Re: Números del código de ADA:
   ❑ D2961 Laminados de Resina
   ❑ D2962 Laminados de Porcelana

Fecha:

Estimado Consejero Dental:

La siguiente narrativa dará información adicional sobre el tratamiento suministrado al paciente el_____.

❑ Debido a la naturaleza extensiva de la fractura/del deterioro del borde de diente incisivo #_____, una restauración de resina adherida directamente no sería clínicamente efectiva.

❑ Como han ocurrido fracasos repetidos de la resina fabricada en la oficina y colocada directamente, sólo se indica clínicamente para este diente una restauración procesada en el laboratorio.

Favor de aplicar los beneficios contractuales apropiados a los procedimientos listados en el formulario del seguro sometido. Si los procedimientos listados no son procedimientos cubiertos y códigos de pago de su compañía de seguro, favor de recodificarlos y aplicar los beneficios alternos como se ha indicado, para cumplir con su responsabilidad contractual con el comprador del contrato.

Si usted tiene cualquier pregunta, favor de sentirse libre de contactar a la oficina. Gracias.

Sinceramente,

copia/(paciente)

Laminados: Colocados para Corregir el Desteñimiento

Paciente:
Número de Seguro Social del Paciente:
Paciente ❑ **es**   ❑ **no es**   **el abonado**

Portador de Seguro:
Número de Grupo:
Patrón:
Abonado:

Re: Números del código de ADA:
- ❑ D2960 Laminados de Resina, Directos
- ❑ D2961 Laminados de Resina, Indirectos
- ❑ D2962 Laminados de Porcelana

Fecha:

Estimado Consejero Dental:

El paciente anticipa la colocación de _____ laminados, del tipo indicado arriba en los dientes #_____. Estos dientes muestran evidencia de desteñimiento por la tetraciclina ❑ moderado ❑ severo.

Los dientes parecen ser de color   ❑ azul   ❑ gris   ❑ morado   ❑ marrón y   ❑ están o   ❑ no están rayados.

La condición es extremamente desfigurante, y le causa al paciente una gran angustia mental. El paciente ha manifestado problemas en la interacción con otros en las actividades normales diarias sociales y relacionadas al trabajo. El paciente tiene una imagen baja de sí mismo y la autoestima baja a causa del color no usual y no deseable de los dientes.

La documentación del médico que recetó el medicamento de tetraciclina   ❑ está adjunta   ❑ no está disponible. Las fotografías diagnósticas también están disponibles si se piden.

Favor de informar a esta oficina si las coronas de porcelana/metálicas o laminados de cobertura completa son un beneficio cubierto para este paciente. Puede referirse al formulario completado de predeterminación adjunto para los detalles de los honorarios que se cobrarán.

Gracias por su atención inmediata a este asunto.

Sinceramente,

copia/(paciente)

Códigos de Beneficios Cambiados

Paciente: **Portador de Seguro:**
Número de Seguro Social del Paciente: **Número de Grupo:**
Paciente ❑ **es** ❑ **no es**   **el abonado**   **Patrón:**
                                                      Abonado:

Fecha:

Estimado Coordinador de Beneficios:

Ha llegado a nuestra atención que usted ha cambiado arbitrariamente un código de procedimiento sometido para el tratamiento para este paciente particular a un código de procedimiento que no refleja la terapia necesaria para este paciente. Usted ha hecho la determinación a base de las radiografías que este procedimiento se podría hacer de una manera más simple/diferente.

La pregunta del tratamiento apropiado sólo puede ser determinada por el dentista que trata al paciente en el momento del diagnóstico y de la planificación del tratamiento. A menos que su consejero dental examine al paciente usted no debería dictar ni sugerir posibilidades de tratamiento diferentes a lo que haya sugerido el dentista que trata al paciente.

Si no se reembolsa al paciente apropiadamente según la definición del contrato recomendaré al paciente y asegurado que:

■ El asegurado/paciente contacte a la Junta Estatal de Odontología con respecto a la manipulación de los códigos de tratamiento por su compañía de seguros y la conducta de su consejero dental.

■ El asegurado contacte al Comisario Estatal de Seguros con respecto a este asunto particular y presente una queja formal en contra de su compañía de seguros.

■ El asegurado contacte a su abogado y busque una compensación directa de la compañía de seguros o del individuo responsable de alterar el documento legal del formulario sometido de reclamación de seguro dental como se ha presentado.

Sinceramente,

copia/(paciente)

Queja al Comisario de Seguro

Al: Comisario de Seguro, Estado de _____

Re: Retraso en procesar el seguro dental
    ❏ Pre-determinación
    ❏ Petición para el pago

Fecha:

Estimado Comisario de Seguro:

Se ha presentado un formulario de reclamación de seguro dental a: (nombre de la compañía de seguro)

Localizado: (dirección de la compañía de seguros)

Se ha enviado toda la información necesaria para procesar la reclamación ❏ una ❏ dos ❏ tres veces.

❏ La compañía de seguro ha solicitado que se vuelva a someter información ya ha sido proporcionada.

❏ La compañía de seguro ha atrasado los trámites de esta reclamación arbitrariamente, con un marco de tiempo desmesurado.

❏ Quiero presentar una queja formal en contra de la compañía de seguro.

❏ Favor de referir a la información adjunta en cuanto a esta reclamación.

Gracias por su atención a este asunto.

Sinceramente,

copia/(paciente)

Información Narrativa

Paciente: **Portador de Seguro:**
Número de Seguro Social del Paciente: **Número de Grupo:**
Paciente ❑ es ❑ no es   el abonado   **Patrón:**
                                                             Abonado:

Re:

Fecha:

Estimado Consejero,

La siguiente narrativa dará información adicional sobre el tratamiento rendido al paciente el _____.

(Escriba la narrativa aquí.)

Favor de aplicar los beneficios contractuales apropiados a los procedimientos listados en el formulario del seguro. Si los procedimientos listados no son procedimientos cubiertos y códigos de pago de su compañía de seguro, favor de recodificarlos y aplicar los beneficios alternos como se ha indicado, para cumplir con su responsabilidad contractual con el comprador del contrato.

Si usted tiene cualquier pregunta, favor de sentirse libre de contactar esta oficina. Gracias.

Sinceramente,

copia/(paciente)

Predeterminación de Beneficios

Paciente:
Número de Seguro Social del Paciente:
Paciente ❑ **es** ❑ **no es**   **el abonado**

Portador de Seguro:
Número de Grupo:
Patrón:
Abonado:

Fecha:

Estimado Consejero Dental:

No se están colocando las restauraciones de molde por razones cosméticas, para restaurar/alterar la dimensión vertical o para servir de férulas periodontales.

❑ Unidad singular   ❑ Dientes de anclaje   ❑ Pontic

Diente maxilar que falta #s: _____
Diente mandibular que falta #s: _____

Código de ADA	Diente #s	Fecha de Colocación Inicial	Fecha de Colocación Anterior (Restauración anterior)

Unidad singular
Anclaje
Pontic

Fechas de extirpación de dientes reemplazados con pontic:

Razón para el reemplazo de restauraciones de molde existentes:
   ❑ Márgenes abiertos
   ❑ Restauraciones defectuosas, diente #s: _____
   ❑ Deterioro en el diente #s: _____
   ❑ Fracturas/grietas no visibles en el plano radiográfico
   ❑ Dientes restaurados previamente con materiales grandes colocados directamente que no se pueden restaurar adecuadamente sin restauraciones de molde
   ❑ Cúspides o bordes de incisivos socavados, diente #s: _____
   ❑ Dientes previamente tratados endodónticamente, diente #s: _____
      Fecha de tratamiento endodóntico: _____

Comentarios:

Documentos Adjuntos: ❑ Radiografías preoperatorias o impresos termales   ❑ Formulario del seguro
❑ Fotografías

Un retraso en tramitar esta reclamación de predeterminación podría perjudicar la salud oral del paciente. Podría requerir procedimientos dentales adicionales más costosos o la pérdida de dientes. El paciente y yo le agradecemos su atención inmediata a este asunto. Si tiene cualquier pregunta, favor de contactar a esta oficina.

Sinceramente,

copia/(paciente)

Respuesta a un Pedido Radiográfico

A: Revisión de Reclamaciones Dentales

Fecha:_____

Re:_____ Petición para Radiografías Dentales

_____ Pre-estimado de Radiografías

Paciente: **Portador de Seguro:**
Número de Seguro Social del Paciente: **Número de Grupo:**
Paciente ❏ es   ❏ no es   el abonado   **Patrón:**
                                                                      Abonado:

Diente #_____

Código de ADA_____

Numerosas patologías (tejido suave y duro) o problemas dentales no se prestan al diagnóstico radiográfico. Los problemas dentales de dientes y de tejido suave que rutinariamente no se pueden diagnosticar de las radiografías incluyen (pero no se limitan a):

- abfracción, atrición
- abrasión causada por el cepillo de dientes
- erosiones químicas (reflujo gástrico, etc.)
- lesiones cariosas oclusales desde incipientes hasta tamaño mediano
- deterioro facial y lingual clase V
- restauraciones fracturadas
- salientes faciales y linguales
- ancho bucolingual de restauraciones
- cúspides no sostenidas
- síndrome de diente fraccionado
- cúspides fracturadas y que faltan (especialmente si hay una restauración grande de metal existente)
- grietas en el esmalte y en la dentina que salen de una restauración de amalgama que ha absorbido agua y expandido
- superficies ásperas
- estructura de diente restante inadecuada para una estructura coronaria remanente clínicamente aceptable
- dientes sensibles (calor, frío, dulces)
- restauraciones con filtraciones, restauraciones con márgenes clínicamente inaceptables
- recesión de tejidos gingivales
- tejidos gingivales hiperplásicos o edematosos
- sangrado cuando se examina con sonda
- pérdida de hueso facial o lingual y profundidades aumentadas de bolsillos
- oclusión traumática
- movilidad de dientes
- pulpitis irreversible
- dientes con una reacción adversa a la presión o la palpación
- gingivitis
- cálculo facial o lingual
- exudado de surco
- deterioro recurrente debajo de las coronas y en una orientación mesial o distal con respecto a las restauraciones de metal y el plano de la fuente del rayos X y el aparato que capta la imagen

El diagnóstico requiere un examen físico. Un diagnóstico correcto y exacto de un problema dental no necesariamente requiere radiografías dentales. No se debe hacer un diagnóstico basado solamente en las radiografías o en una conversación con el paciente. En muchas de las anomalías mencionadas arriba, se puede hacer el diagnóstico sólo con un examen clínico. El uso de radiografías dentales puede ser contraindicado, innecesario, y de hecho, puede exponer al paciente a la radiación ionizante no-diagnóstica dañina que, al juicio clínico profesional del dentista que trata al paciente, no tiene ningún potencial de cambiar o modificar el diagnóstico. Se ha informado al paciente de la naturaleza del problema y éste entiende que las radiografías preoperatorias no añadirían nada al diagnóstico ni cambiarían el plan de tratamiento propuesto.

Las radiografías preoperatorias para el tratamiento dental propuesto podrían no demostrar o no pueden demostrar la naturaleza ni la extensión del problema. Si hay cualquier pregunta, favor de pedir al consejero dental que me llame.

Gracias.

Número de Teléfono_____

Sinceramente,

copia/(paciente)

Petición para una Recodificación de Seguro

Paciente:
Número de Seguro Social del Paciente:
Paciente ❏ **es** ❏ **no es** **el abonado**

Portador de Seguro:
Número de Grupo:
Patrón:
Abonado:

Fecha:

Estimado Consejero Dental:

Adjunto favor de encontrar ❏ un estimado de pretratamiento o ❏ una petición de pago. Si el formulario de reclamación que hemos sometido indica un puente de molde de porcelana a oro/metal noble y la póliza del asegurado no permite el pago ni para el puente ni para el pontic, favor de revisar la reclamación y recodificar para pago por dientes designados como dientes de anclaje, código de ADA #D6750; restauraciones de molde de unidad singular, código de ADA #D6250.

Si un puente fijo no es un beneficio pagable para este abonado, favor de referir a la siguiente documentación de apoyo. Razón para una cobertura completa de dientes de anclaje si un puente fijo no es un beneficio pagable (favor de referir a las radiografías):

- ❏ Restauraciones defectuosas grandes existentes que no se pueden restaurar con materiales colocados directamente, diente #s: _____
- ❏ Cúspides o bordes de incisivos no sostenidos, diente #s: _____
- ❏ Diente fracturado #s: _____
- ❏ Deterioro, diente #s: _____
- ❏ Líneas de fractura, fracturas no visibles en el plano de la radiografía, diente #s: _____
- ❏ Diente previamente tratado endodónticamente, diente #s: _____
- ❏ Dientes de anclaje se restauraron previamente con restauraciones de molde de cobertura completa que se están reemplazando a causa del deterioro recurrente.

Además, si un puente fijo no es un beneficio pagable para el asegurado, favor de recodificar, evaluar y aplicar los beneficios para una dentadura parcial removible para reemplazar el diente o los dientes que faltan.

Comentarios:

Si usted tiene cualquier pregunta, favor de contactar a esta oficina. Gracias por su atención inmediata a este asunto.

Sinceramente,

copia/(paciente)

Cartas y Formularios de Co-consultación

Revisión del Contenido:
Cartas y Formularios de Co-consultación

Estas cartas de co-consultación hacen que las co-consultaciones de pacientes sean precisas y sin complicaciones. Dan al especialista la información dental y comercial necesaria para mantener el tratamiento dentro del horario planeado. Están completas con las peticiones de evaluación/tratamiento necesarias y un anexo de cuadros de verificación.

Cartas de Co-consultación/Consulta
Solicitud de Consulta Médica
El tratamiento dental puede afectar o estar afectado por otros aspectos de una condición médica del paciente. Informe a los otros proveedores de cuidado de salud del paciente el tratamiento dental exacto que usted propone y anímelos a que contesten prontamente con las recomendaciones pertinentes.

Envío de un Paciente a un Especialista Dental
Use para informar a su paciente de lo que él o ella necesita específicamente para contactar al especialista requerido, el tratamiento que usted propone y cuándo debe él o ella buscar este tratamiento.

Co-consultaciones con Especialistas
Los documentos de Co-consultación y Consulta para Tratamiento Dental Especial resumen tanto los servicios pedidos como el seguimiento para después del tratamiento.

> **Co-consultación para Endodoncia**
> **Co-consultación para Cirugía Oral**
> **Co-consultación para Ortodoncia**
> **Co-consultación Periodontal**

Peticiones
Petición de Radiografías e Historiales
Pida las radiografías y los historiales dentales del otro proveedor de cuidado de salud.

Envío de Documentos Pedidos por el Paciente
Carta explicativa para los historiales de un paciente enviados a otra oficina a petición del paciente.

Solicitud de Consulta Médica

(Nombre y
Dirección del Médico que se consultará)

(Fecha)

Estimado Doctor:

Nuestro paciente mutuo, (Nombre del paciente), ha sido examinado y necesita el siguiente tratamiento dental:

❑ Cirugía oral (extracción(es))

_____

❑ Restauraciones

_____

❑ Tratamiento Endodóntico

_____

❑ Tratamiento Periodóntico (limpieza/raspado/profilaxis)

_____

❑ Tratamiento Periodóntico (tratamiento quirúrgico)

_____

❑ Prótesis fija (trabajo de puente)

_____

❑ Dentaduras completas o parciales

_____

❑ Otro:

_____

Favor de informarme de cualquier recomendación especial que usted tenga en cuanto a este tratamiento propuesto, especialment
de las premedicaciones necesitadas por el paciente antes del tratamiento dental y/o las contraindicaciones al tratamiento dental.
Si usted requiere que se posponga el tratamiento dental, favor de dejarme saber cuándo usted cree que se puede resumir.

Si usted tiene cualquier pregunta, favor de contactarme. En este momento el paciente no está citado para ningún tratamiento dental
y sólo se le citará para más tratamiento después de recibir su respuesta.

Favor de contestar en la parte inferior de esta carta y regresarla a mi oficina. Tanto el paciente como yo le agradeceremos por su
atención inmediata a este asunto.

Sinceramente,

Envío de un Paciente a un Especialista Dental

Paciente:_____   **Fecha:**_____

Le estamos enviando al siguiente especialista para una evaluación y/o tratamiento. Los detalles que queremos que el especialista evalúe están anotados. Cuando usted llame a la oficina del especialista para una cita, favor de leerle estas instrucciones.

Antes de su cita, hablaremos con el especialista y/o enviaremos una carta con un resumen de los aspectos técnicos de sus necesidades dentales.

Una vez que el especialista haya concluido el examen, le informarán del tratamiento exacto que ellos proponen, cuánto tiempo durará el tratamiento, el costo envuelto, hablarán con usted sobre los detalles postoperatorios y contestarán cualquier pregunta que usted tenga.

Antes de regresar a nuestra oficina para más tratamiento, favor de ver al especialista para:
❑ Evaluación solamente
❑ Evaluación y tratamiento

En cualquier momento durante el tratamiento en nuestra oficina, favor de ver al especialista para:
❑ Evaluación solamente
❑ Evaluación y tratamiento

Tan pronto como sea posible, favor de ver al especialista para:
❑ Evaluación solamente
❑ Evaluación y tratamiento

❑ **Endodontista** (canal radicular):

❑ **Periodontista** (encías, implantes):

❑ **Cirujano Oral** (extracciones, implantes):

❑ **Ortodoncista** (frenillos):

Co-consultación para Endodoncia

Paciente:_____   **Fecha:**_____

Enviado a :_____   **Enviado por:**_____

Estimado Doctor:

❏ Le hemos enviado al paciente nombrado arriba el (fecha).
❏ Entregamos su número de teléfono al paciente y le instruimos que le llamara para una cita.
❏ Al paciente le gustaría que usted le llame para fijar una cita.   Teléfono del hogar:_____
                                                                      Teléfono del trabajo:_____

Favor de   ❏ Evaluar   ❏ Tratar   ❏ Retratamiento   ❏ Apicoectomía

Diente #s:_____

Restauración final propuesta:

Otro:_____
_____

❏ Favor de enviar al paciente de vuelta a donde nosotros cuando haya concluido el tratamiento.
❏ Favor de llamar nuestra oficina si el paciente no le ha contactado para el: (fecha)
❏ Favor de llamarme para hablar de este caso después de su examen y antes de comenzar su tratamiento.
❏ Favor de enviar un informe por escrito en cuanto a su(s):
    ❏ diagnóstico inicial
    ❏ plan de tratamiento
    ❏ recomendaciones finales

❏ Al momento el paciente está citado en esta oficina el (fecha) para:_____
❏ Se le ha dicho al paciente que no debe hacer otra cita en esta oficina hasta que le haya visto a usted.

Comentarios:_____
_____

Adjunto: ❏ Posteroanterior ❏ Interproximal   Fecha:_____

Sinceramente,

Copia/archivo del paciente

Co-consultación para Cirugía Oral

Paciente:_____   **Fecha:**_____

Enviado a :_____   **Enviado por:**_____

Estimado Doctor:

❑ Le hemos enviado al paciente nombrado arriba el (fecha).
❑ Entregamos su número de teléfono al paciente y le instruimos que le llamara para una cita.
❑ Al paciente le gustaría que usted le llame para fijar una cita.   Teléfono del hogar:_____
                                                                       Teléfono del trabajo:_____

Favor de   Evaluar   Tratar

❑   ❑   Extracción, diente #_____
❑   ❑   Biopsia de_____, diente #_____
❑   ❑   Frenectomía, diente #_____
❑   ❑   Reducción de tuberosidad   ❑ I   ❑ D
❑   ❑   Apicoectomía, diente #_____
❑   ❑   Implante, diente #_____
❑   ❑   Otro: _____

Restauración final propuesta:

Comentarios: _____
_____

❑ Favor de enviar al paciente de vuelta a nosotros cuando haya concluido el tratamiento.
❑ Favor de llamarme para hablar de este caso después de su examen y antes de comenzar su tratamiento.
❑ Favor de enviar un informe por escrito en cuanto a su(s):
   ❑ diagnóstico inicial
   ❑ plan de tratamiento
   ❑ recomendaciones finales
❑ Favor de tomar una radiografía panorámica y enviar una copia a nuestra oficina.
❑ Al momento el paciente está citado en esta oficina el (fecha) para:_____
❑ Se le ha dicho al paciente que no debe hacer otra cita en esta oficina hasta usted haya
   completado su.   ❑ Examen   ❑ Tratamiento

Adjunto: ❑ Posteroanterior (Fecha)   ❑ Interproximal (Fecha)   ❑ Radiografías (Fecha)

Consideraciones especiales: _____
_____

Sinceramente,

Copia/(archivo del paciente)

Co-consultación para Ortodoncia

Paciente:_____   **Fecha:**_____

Padre/Guardián:_____

Enviado a:_____   **Enviado por:**_____

Estimado Doctor:

❑ Le hemos enviado al paciente nombrado arriba el (fecha).
❑ Entregamos su número de teléfono al paciente y le instruimos que le llamara para una cita.
❑ Al paciente le gustaría que usted le llame para fijar una cita.   Teléfono del hogar:_____
                                                                                              Teléfono del trabajo:_____

Favor de   ❑ Evaluar   ❑ Tratar para las siguientes condiciones:

Evaluación completa de ortodoncia:

Enderezar:_____
Intruir:_____
Extruir:_____
Otro:_____

Se ha completado toda la odontología operatoria para el paciente y se le ha aconsejado de tener intervalos de 3-meses de cuidado continuo de higiene mientras esté bajo el tratamiento activo. Se le ha asesorado de usar un tratamiento de fluoruro tópico diario mientras esté bajo el tratamiento activo.

❑ Favor de llamarme si el paciente no le ha contactado para el: (fecha)
❑ Favor de llamarme para hablar de este caso después de su examen y antes de comenzar su tratamiento.
❑ Favor de enviar un informe por escrito en cuanto a su(s):
   ❑ diagnóstico inicial
   ❑ plan de tratamiento
   ❑ recomendaciones finales
Al momento el paciente está citado en esta oficina el (fecha) para_____.

Agradecemos el cuidado que usted y su personal toman en reforzar la higiene oral de sí mismo correcta diaria y el intervalo de higiene de 3-meses de cuidado repetido.

Se le ha dicho al paciente que no debe hacer otra cita en esta oficina hasta verle a usted.

Comentarios: _____

_____

Sinceramente,

Copia/(archivo del paciente)

Co-consultación Periodontal

Paciente:_____   **Fecha:**_____

Enviado a :_____   **Enviado por:**_____

Estimado Doctor:

❑ Le hemos enviado al paciente nombrado arriba el (fecha).
❑ Entregamos su número de teléfono al paciente y le instruimos que le llamara para una cita.
❑ Al paciente le interesa que usted le llame para fijar una cita.

Teléfono del hogar:_____
Teléfono del trabajo:_____

Favor de   ❑ Evaluar   ❑ Tratar para las siguientes condiciones:

❑ Clasificaciones de enfermedad periodontal:
  Cuadrante   ❑ SD   ❑ ID   ❑ SI   ❑ II
  Sextante   ❑ SD   ❑ ID   ❑ SI   ❑ II
  Diente #: _____
❑ Evaluación de implante, diente #:_____
  Restauración final propuesta:_____
❑ Alargamiento de corona, diente #:_____
❑ Furcación, diente #:_____
❑ Otro:_____

Al momento, el paciente ha recibido y completado los siguientes servicios periodontales:

	Fecha
❑ Raspado y alisado radicular	_____
❑ Irrigación subgingival	_____
❑ Instrucción de higiene oral de sí mismo	_____
❑ Pulido	_____
❑ Terapia específica al lugar #:	_____ con (producto) _____

❑ Favor de enviar un informe por escrito en cuanto a su(s):
  ❑ diagnóstico inicial
  ❑ plan de tratamiento
  ❑ recomendaciones finales
❑ Al momento el paciente está citado en esta oficina el (fecha) para:_____
❑ Se le ha dicho al paciente que no debe hacer otra cita en esta oficina hasta que usted haya completado su
  ❑ Examen ❑ Tratamiento.
❑ Favor de citar al paciente para citas alternas de mantenimiento de higiene entre las oficinas.
  Intervalo:_____
❑ Favor de llamarme para hablar de este caso después de su examen y antes de comenzar su tratamiento.

❑ Favor de informarme por escrito si el paciente acepta o rechaza las recomendaciones de tratamiento. Si acepta el tratamiento, favor de enviar informes actualizados de progreso, la fecha anticipada de terminación y las recomendaciones de restauración. Favor de aconsejarme del pronóstico para los dientes a corto y largo plazo y de los intervalos recomendados para los intervalos de mantenimiento profesional de higiene.

Adjunto: ❑ Gráfica periodontal (Fecha)   ❑ Radiografías   ❑ Posteroanterior   ❑ Interproximal   ❑ Serie de boca completa (Fecha)

Sinceramente,

Copia/(archivo del paciente)

Petición de Radiografías e Historiales

(Nombre del doctor que tiene los historiales)
(Dirección del doctor que tiene los historiales)
(Ciudad, estado, código postal del doctor que tiene los historiales)

(Fecha)

Estimado Doctor:

A petición de (nombre del paciente o guardián), favor de remitir las radiografías e historiales más recientes para (nombre del paciente). Favor de enviar los materiales solicitados a:

    (Nombre de la oficina a donde se deben enviar los historiales)
    (Dirección de la oficina a donde se deben enviar los historiales)
    (Ciudad, estado, código postal a donde se deben enviar los historiales)

Gracias por su ayuda en este asunto.

Sinceramente,

Copia/(archivo del paciente)

Envío de Documentos Pedidos por el Paciente

(Nombre de la oficina a donde se deben enviar los historiales)
(Dirección de la oficina a donde se deben enviar los historiales)
(Ciudad, estado, código postal a donde se deben enviar los historiales)

(Fecha)

Estimado Doctor:

Adjunto, favor de encontrar los historiales dentales y las radiografías más recientes de (nombre del paciente). Nuestros registros indican que la última vez que se vio a este paciente en nuestra oficina fue el (fecha). Se están remitiendo estos historiales a su oficina según la petición del paciente.

Sinceramente,

Copia/(archivo del paciente)

Educación para el Paciente

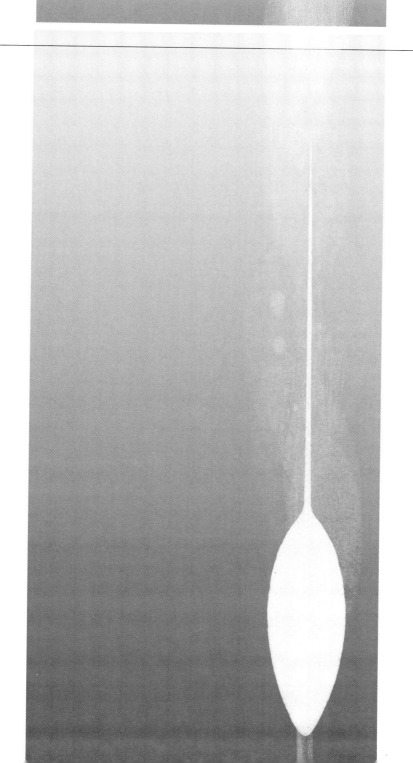

Odontología Cosmética

Revisión del Contenido: Odontología Cosmética

Condiciones Congénitas

Erupción Pasiva Alterada: Tejido Suave
Define la erupción pasiva alterada en lo referente a la apariencia y explica las opciones de tratamiento con el tejido suave. Describe como la proporción de diente y encía y líneas de los labios afectan la apariencia.

Erupción Pasiva Alterada: Tejido Duro
Define la erupción pasiva alterada en lo referente a la apariencia y explica las opciones de tratamiento con el tejido duro. Describe como la proporción de diente y encía y líneas de los labios afectan la apariencia.

Dientes que Faltan Congénitamente
Alerta al paciente de los problemas asociados con dientes que faltan congénitamente y el tratamiento que necesita.

Diastemas: Cerrar Espacios entre los Dientes
Define cómo y por qué los diastemas pueden ocurrir. Ofrece una visión general de los posibles tratamientos.

Fluorosis, Esmalte Veteado y Manchas Blancas
Describe fluorosis, esmalte veteado y manchas blancas y las opciones de tratamiento disponibles.

Incisivos Laterales Coniformes
Describe los incisivos laterales coniformes y las opciones disponibles de tratamiento dependiendo del grado de malformación y de la edad del paciente.

Procedimientos Cosméticos

Restauraciones de Resina Adherida: Empastaduras del Color del Diente para los Dientes Posteriores
Explica el uso, las ventajas y desventajas de las restauraciones de resina adherida para dientes posteriores. Asume que estas restauraciones estarán en lugar de las restauraciones de amalgama de plata.

Odontología Cosmética
Da una visión general y enumera muchas de las posibilidades y procedimientos disponibles en la odontología cosmética.

Recontorno del Tejido Cosméticamente
Aconseja cómo la cirugía periodontal puede mejorar la apariencia de los dientes y la arquitectura de la encía. Incluye opciones de tratamiento.

Recontorno del Esmalte
Relaciona el uso de recontorno del esmalte, particularmente con relación a otros posibles procedimientos.

Laminados de Porcelana y Resina: Adhesión
Una visión general de laminados: indicaciones, ventajas y desventajas de cada tipo.

Inlays y Onlays de Porcelana
Explica cuándo los inlays y onlays de porcelana son usados. También da ventajas, desventajas y la sincronización del tratamiento.

Reemplazar Restauraciones Antiestéticas
Señala las condiciones que harían el reemplazo de restauraciones más viejas deseable, incluso cuando las restauraciones siguen siendo funcionales, con precauciones en esperar demasiado tiempo.

La Sonrisa Perfecta
Da al paciente la perspicacia en el papel que juega la encía en la sonrisa perfecta.

Blanqueo

Información General

Blanquear los Dientes: Visión General y Opciones
Consideraciones importantes del blanqueo de los dientes y las opciones de tratamiento disponibles son repasadas.

¡Usted Puede Tener Dientes Más Blancos!
Información introductoria sobre los métodos caseros y de oficina del blanqueo de los dientes.

Siga

Revisión del Contenido: Odontología Cosmética—continuación

Procedimientos Específicos

Opciones Caseras para Blanquear los Dientes

Comparación de cubetas hechas a la medida, tiras blanqueadoras y geles aplicados con brocha para aplicación del blanqueador por el paciente.

Instrucciones para el Sistema Casero para Blanquear los Dientes con Cubetas

Información, direcciones específicas y honorarios para un protector bucal para la casa para blanqueo de dientes.

Técnica Potente de Blanqueo de Dientes en la Oficina sin Activación de Luz

Detalles de la técnica potente de blanqueo sin activación de luz son explicados.

Técnica Potente de Blanqueo de Dientes en la Oficina con Activación de Luz

Detalles de la técnica potente de blanqueo con activación de luz son explicados.

Instrucciones Postoperatorias para el Blanqueo de Dientes en la Oficina

Instrucciones postoperatorias para la técnica potente de blanqueo en la oficina.

Opciones No Vitales para Blanquear los Dientes

Discute las técnicas del blanqueo y blanqueo potente: indicaciones, procedimientos y resultados a esperar, a corto y largo plazo.

Dientes Desteñidos por Tetraciclina: Opciones para la Mejoría Cosmética

Descripción de dientes desteñidos por tetraciclina y las posibilidades para mejoría cosmética.

Erupción Pasiva Alterada: Tejido Suave

Asuntos Estéticos

Las sonrisas atractivas se determinan por la cantidad de estructura del diente visible cuando usted sonríe. Los dientes están compuestos de dos partes básicas—la porción de la raíz (debajo del borde la encía) y la corona (por encima del borde de la encía).

Esa proporción es aproximadamente 1.6:1, largo a ancho. Es decir, los dientes deben parecer más largos que anchos, o a una razón de largo (1.6:1) a ancho (1). Los dientes que no tienen esta proporción aproximada parecen menos atractivo en nuestra cultura.

Erupción Pasiva Alterada

Los dientes que parecen cortos y "regordetes" realmente pueden estar cubiertos con tejido de la encía. La proporción correcta de altura a anchura está presente, pero el borde de la encía descansa demasiado lejos en la corona del diente para que sea atractiva. Esta condición se llama *erupción pasiva alterada*. Aunque la causa exacta de la erupción pasiva alterada no se conoce, sí vemos esta condición en los primeros años de la adolescencia. La buena noticia es que se puede tratar a través de un procedimiento quirúrgico menor. Se pueden remover pequeñas cantidades del tejido de la encía con un láser o con un aparato elector-quirúrgico; muchas veces, no se requiere sutura ni cuidado postoperatorio extensivo.

Líneas del Labio

Un factor que complica la erupción pasiva alterada puede ser una línea del labio alta o una que expone más de los dientes y la encía cuando el paciente sonríe. Una línea del labio baja efectivamente "escondería" el tejido de la encía que cubre la corona. Mientras más alta la línea del labio, menos atractiva la sonrisa.

Líneas de Sonrisa

Ocasionalmente, puede ser necesario una ligera reformación de los bordes de la mordida para ayudar a formar una sonrisa atractiva. El rediseño más extensivo de la sonrisa puede incluir la verdadera fabricación de laminados finos que cubran la parte exterior y que se colocan sobre los dientes frontales reformados y se cementan en su lugar o puede incluir una corona de porcelana como el mejor tratamiento.

Usted puede tener la sonrisa sensacional que usted quiere y se merece. Después de un examen comprehensivo, recomendaremos el mejor plan de tratamiento para ayudarle a alcanzar esa meta.

Si usted tiene cualquier pregunta sobre la erupción pasiva alterada, favor de sentirse libre de preguntarnos.

Erupción Pasiva Alterada: Tejido Duro

Los dientes están compuestos de dos partes visibles básicas—la porción de la raíz y la porción de la corona (cubierta de esmalte). En este caso, el término corona no se refiere al tipo de reemplazo de diente fabricado por un laboratorio. Mejor dicho, es parte del diente que normalmente se ve cuando usted habla.

La filosofía estética dental actual, demostrado por las personas que tienen dientes y sonrisas hermosos, demuestra que debe haber una cierta cantidad de diente cubierto de esmalte visible para tener una sonrisa atractiva. Esa proporción es aproximadamente 1.6:1, largo a ancho. Los dientes que son más cortos se ven progresivamente menos atractivos. Parecen cortos y regordetes. Si de verdad están gastados a causa de un problema de apretar o rechinar, esto es un tipo de problema diferente. Sin embargo puede ser que los dientes mismos no sean demasiados cortos. Puede ser que no hay suficiente corona del diente para verse. El restante que se debe ver está cubierto con tejido de encía o encía y hueso. Esto se conoce como erupción pasiva alterada. No está enteramente claro por qué esto ocurre. Puede ser obvio tan temprano como a la edad de los 14 años. Los dientes pueden tener un color agradable y ser muy rectos, pero todavía falta algo porque son demasiados pequeños y se ve demasiado de la encía cuando usted sonríe.

Esto puede ser un problema cosmético severo cuando se junta con el tipo de línea del labio que enmarca los dientes. Una línea del labio baja probablemente esconderá casi todo o toda de la parte de la encía que cubre el diente, de modo que hay menos necesidad de corregir el defecto. Una línea del labio mediana o alta, especialmente una línea el labio alta, mostrará todo el diente y la encía. Mientras más alta la línea del labio, menos atractiva la sonrisa. La situación puede ser tan severa que el paciente entrenará sus músculos para mantener el labio superior rígido o cubrir la boca con una mano cuando está sonriendo. De esta manera, los dientes cortos o la expansión grande del tejido de la encía se esconderá de la vista. Esto puede causar problemas psicológicos significativos.

La solución puede ser fácil o complicada, dependiendo de la naturaleza exacta del problema. Si sólo hay que remover una cantidad pequeña del tejido de la encía de un solo diente, o de varios dientes, y hay una línea del labio mediana, entonces el tejido se remueve fácilmente con un láser o con un aparato de cortar electro-quirúrgico. No se necesitan ni los bisturíes ni los puntos en los casos pequeños. Cuando hay que remover más de la encía y exponer más del diente, puede ser necesario reformar algún hueso subyacente. Dos meses después de la eliminación del hueso, se elimina el tejido suave que se mencionó anteriormente. La primera cirugía tiene que sanarse con suficiente tiempo para que el tejido pueda llegar a su posición final antes de completar la segunda. Recuerde que usted está examinando unas diferencias desde varios milímetros a una fracción de un milímetro que causará que el caso sea un éxito o un fracaso. Un procedimiento de dos pasos es mejor que un procedimiento de un solo paso.

Se pueden reformar los bordes de la mordida (esmalte y/o dentina) de uno o más dientes si hay una necesidad no sólo de alargar los dientes sino también de hacerlos parecer más altos en la línea de la sonrisa. Esto es para los dientes superiores, por supuesto. Si hay que reformar gran parte del diente para alcanzar el efecto deseado, es posible que se exponga la raíz o la dentina, lo que hará que el diente sea sensitivo. Será necesario cubrir esos dientes con laminados de porcelana o con coronas para alcanzar la estética apropiada. Aun si se reforma sólo una pequeña cantidad del diente, los laminados o coronas pueden ser recomendables para conseguir la apariencia exacta que usted quiere. Hablaremos con usted sobre esto antes que usted comience el tratamiento. Es importante que usted conozca lo que se está haciendo, cuánto tiempo tomará para completarse y cómo usted se verá cuando se termine.

Nosotros haremos los laminados o coronas y reformaremos los dientes. Determinaremos lo que se puede hacer. Podríamos también hacer la reformación del tejido suave. Esto es lo más común. Para los procedimientos que envuelven la reformación de hueso, le podríamos enviar donde un periodontista (un especialista en encías). Como haremos el tratamiento restaurativo, sabemos exactamente dónde debe estar el tejido suave. Somos especialistas en lo cosmético. Estableceremos la posición final del borde de la encía. En los casos extremos, se corregirá el problema con una combinación de los procedimientos arriba mencionados y la cirugía ortognática para reposicionar la mandíbula y los dientes. Esto lo hace un cirujano oral. Con un examen comprehensivo, le podemos decir lo que es apropiado para usted. Usted no tiene que vivir con una sonrisa no atractiva porque tiene dientes que parecen ser cortos debido a la apariencia de tener demasiado tejido de encía. Estos problemas se pueden corregir. Permítanos saber lo que no le gusta de su sonrisa o sus dientes. Probablemente la sonrisa que usted tiene ahora se puede convertir en una que le gustaría exhibir.

Si usted tiene cualquier pregunta sobre la erupción pasiva alterada, favor de favor de sentirse libre de preguntarnos.

Dientes que Faltan Congénitamente

Algunos de nosotros tendremos 32 dientes desarrollados durante nuestra vida. Esto se ha considerado como un conjunto normal de dientes. Sin embargo, muchas veces no desarrollamos un juego completo de 32 dientes. Es bastante común que las personas les falte uno o más de los terceros molares (los cordales). Y como los tamaños de la mandíbula del ser humano moderno ha disminuido, no es raro que no haya espacio en la boca para la posición correcta de los terceros molares y hay que extraerlos.

No tan común, pero tampoco raro, es una condición en la cual algunos de los dientes frontales nunca se desarrollan. Cuando los dientes permanentes no se desarrollan, se consideran que faltan congénitamente. El término para esta condición se llama dientes *que faltan congénitamente*. Cuando esto ocurre, frecuentemente envuelve uno o dos de los incisivos superiores laterales, que son los dientes más pequeños en cualquier lado de los dos dientes frontales superiores. Con menos frecuencia no se desarrollan los colmillos (caninos) o premolares.

El problema que resulta de los dientes que faltan congénitamente envuelve el espacio donde el diente (los dientes) debía(n) estar. Los dientes más cercanos al espacio se mueven a posiciones diferentes para llenar la apertura, muchas veces el resultado es una sonrisa apiñada—¡cuando de hecho faltan algunos dientes!

Los problemas que resultan de los dientes permanentes que faltan se pueden reducir o eliminar con detección temprana y un plan de tratamiento futuro. El tratamiento común envuelve la ortodoncia para mover los dientes permanentes a una posición mejor o mantener los dientes permanentes en su lugar correcto. Como tratamos los incisivos laterales que faltan tan a menudo, la rutina de tratamiento está bien establecida. Se alcanza la mejor estética, la apariencia más natural, al dejar los incisivos centrales permanentes y caninos contiguos en sus lugares habituales.

Cuando faltan los incisivos laterales, es probable que recomendaremos que se muevan los colmillos (caninos) a sus posiciones. Esto mantendrá al hueso del espacio del diente que falta en su nivel correcto. Entonces recomendaremos que se regresen los colmillos a sus posiciones correctas. Esto puede sonar como tratamiento adicional, pero es necesario para mantener al hueso en la altura adecuada para tratamientos de reemplazo de dientes en el futuro.

La secuencia de tratamiento es la ortodoncia tan temprano como sea necesario para mantener el espacio. Mientras más lejos se han movido los dientes de la posición original, más tratamiento será necesario. Entonces mientras crecen el niño y su boca, se hace un reemplazo removible. Se usa este aparato hasta que los dientes estén listos para recibir el implante o el puente, más o menos después de la edad de 18 años cuando las estructuras dentales y de la boca estén más maduras.

Cuando faltan los dientes permanentes en la parte más atrás de la boca, es común que se retengan los dientes de leche en estos espacios. A veces los dientes de leche pueden durar por años pero no tienen la estructura de la raíz para quedarse estables durante toda la vida. Como los dientes de leche retenidos son apropiados para una boca pequeña, no tienen el tamaño, la forma o la función de un diente permanente. Cuando se pierden, se pueden reemplazar con implantes o un puente. Su propia situación particular determinará el desarrollo del tratamiento.

Si usted tiene cualquier pregunta sobre los dientes que faltan congénitamente, favor de sentirse libre de preguntarnos.

Diastemas: Cerrar Espacios entre los Dientes

Causa

Una diastema es un espacio entre dientes, es decir, dientes contiguos que no se tocan. Hay varias razones porque pueden existir espacios entre los dientes. Las dos más comunes son una discrepancia del largo del arco (los dientes son demasiados estrechos para el arco que les sostiene) o porque hay dientes que faltan congénitamente. Entonces los dientes restantes o se mueven o meramente no tocan el próximo diente disponible. Los espacios entre los dientes pueden ser de sólo una fracción de milímetro de ancho o tan anchos que se puede fácilmente pasar una pajilla entre los dientes. Los dientes que faltan pueden causar, y frecuentemente causan, un problema cosmético. En la cultura actual del mundo occidental, se considera que los espacios o aperturas no son deseables ni atractivos.

Opciones de Tratamiento

Hay varias opciones disponibles para tratar un diastema. La mayoría de estas opciones trabajan bien, no importa si los espacios son grandes o pequeños ni si hay varios espacios o sólo un espacio entre dos dientes.

Se puede usar la ortodoncia para mover los dientes a una alineación más agradable. Se podría hacer esto con un retenedor de bandas fijas y alambres. Los alineadores ortodónticos transparentes Invisalign son frecuentemente usados para cerrar estos espacios. La ventaja es que las restauraciones complejas generalmente son innecesarias y usted no tiene que preocuparse si la restauración se agrietará o se romperá después de los años de servicio. La desventaja de usar la ortodoncia para cerrar un diastema es el tiempo necesario para mover los dientes, que puede variar desde algunos meses hasta 18 meses.

La otra opción es de restaurar los dientes con una adhesión. La adhesión se puede hacer con resina o con porcelana. La resina será menos costosa y trabajará bien para cerrar los diastemas pequeños. La porcelana requiere una visita adicional, es más costosa y es más apropiada para casos más grandes donde hay que hacer una modificación mayor de la apariencia. Esto incluiría el cambio del color de los dientes, del largo de varios dientes o de la alineación de varios dientes. Como regla general para los espacios pequeños, una resina adherida trabajará bien; para los espacios más grandes hay que considerar la ortodoncia y la porcelana. Se puede hacer que tanto la porcelana como la resina sean del mismo color de sus dientes existentes.

Hay que examinar y evaluar cada situación individualmente antes del tratamiento. Frecuentemente, requerimos que se hagan impresiones de modelo de estudio para que podamos tomar las medidas del largo y ancho del diente y de la cantidad de separación entre los dientes. Usando este método, podemos mostrarle cómo usted se podría ver a través del uso de un modelo de cera diagnóstico que muestra la forma nueva de los dientes.

Un punto importante para recordar es si usted también quiere una sonrisa que sea más blanca, debemos terminar el proceso de blanqueo antes del proceso de adhesión. Los dientes se pueden blanquear pero no los materiales dentales tales como las porcelanas y las resinas. Se hacen las restauraciones para que sean del mismo color de sus dientes en el momento de colocarse, por lo tanto el blanqueo tiene que hacerse primero.

Después

Después de mover los dientes ortodónticamente o de reformarlos con porcelana o resina, ¡su apariencia cambiará! No sólo eso, sino que también sentirá que sus dientes son diferentes. Sus labios tendrán un sostén diferente. El aire se desviará de sus dientes de una manera diferente. Dependiendo de la cantidad del cambio, usted podrá hacer ajustes leves a su manera de hablar. La buena noticia es que todos los ajustes toman sólo algunas horas hasta algunos días. Muy rápidamente, las adiciones y los cambios se sentirán naturales y usted no notará que se hicieron, ¡con la excepción de que las personas le felicitarán de cuán afortunado es usted de haber nacido con dientes tan hermosos!

Si usted tiene cualquier pregunta sobre el cierre de diastemas, favor de sentirse libre de preguntarnos.

Fluorosis, Esmalte Veteado y Manchas Blancas

Fluorosis y Esmalte Veteado

El fluoruro es la maravilla dental de nuestra vida y un beneficio definitivo a la salud oral de nuestra nación. ¡Pero demasiado de algo bueno puede causar problemas! La fluorosis de los dientes y el esmalte veteado puede ocurrir cuando hay demasiada absorción de fluoruro por los dientes mientras se están formando. Normalmente se dan vitaminas recetadas de fluoruro de la dosis correcta a los niños. Pero un niño puede recibir demasiado fluoruro si está disponible de fuentes múltiples. Los niños con acceso a un sistema público de agua que contiene fluoruro pueden también recibir suplementos recetados de fluoruro o pueden tragar las pastas de dientes con fluoruro, los enjuagues bucales o ciertas bebidas frutales que también contienen fluoruro, lo que puede aumentar su absorción a un nivel por encima de lo recomendado. La fluorosis es una condición en la cual se forman manchas oscuras antiestéticas en los dientes. Algunos medicamentos y enfermedades también pueden causar un problema similar. Estas manchas oscuras, que se ven más frecuentemente en los dientes permanentes, no son más propensas al deterioro, sólo no son atractivas. Uno, varios o todos los dientes pueden estar afectados. El cambio de color (generalmente marrón/anaranjado o blanco mate/opaco) puede ser poco, moderado o severo.

Opciones de Tratamiento

Generalmente, tres soluciones son posibles. A veces la mancha es muy superficial y se puede eliminar con el pulido. No regresa. No hay dolor envuelto en este procedimiento. Sencillamente se pule el esmalte y se hace liso nuevamente.

Muchas veces es bastante fácil blanquear las manchas marrones para que sean del mismo color de los dientes a su alrededor. Generalmente esto es un procedimiento en la oficina (contrario al blanqueo de dientes amarillos, que se puede hacer en casa con cubetas para blanquear dientes hechas a la medida). Se colocan unos químicos fuertes de blanqueo en el área oscura y se activan con luz o calor o los dos. Se hacen varias aplicaciones (en la misma visita), ¡y la mancha generalmente desaparece en una visita!

Si la mancha es muy oscura o se extiende profundamente en el esmalte, el blanqueo puede funcionar, pero no lo suficiente para eliminar el desteñimiento total. En esta instancia, una combinación de blanqueo y una restauración adherida del color del diente resolverá el problema. Se blanquea el diente, entonces se prepara (se taladra) el área oscura restante para que reciba una empastadura de tipo adherida. Se tinta una resina del mismo color natural del diente y se pega en la sección preparada.
La igualación de color puede ser casi perfecta, y los pacientes ven una mejoría grande sobre lo que estaba allí anteriormente.

Manchas Blancas

Las manchas blancas también pueden ser el resultado de demasiado fluoruro, una enfermedad, un medicamento o una interrupción de la formación correcta del esmalte. Las manchas pueden ser apenas visibles o pueden contrastar con los dientes a su alrededor. Si los dientes se secan, como en el caso de un paciente que generalmente respira por su boca, las manchas blancas se vuelven prominentes. La mayoría de las veces, se pueden eliminar estas manchas con el pulido. Si están muy adentro del diente, sin embargo, hay que restaurarlas con una preparación del diente y la adhesión con un material del color del diente. Una vez que se eliminan, no regresan. Las manchas blancas afectan los dientes permanentes más que los dientes de leche. Aunque no se pueden blanquear como los desteñimientos causados por el fluoruro, el blanqueo de todos los dientes puede hacerlas menos notables.

Durante su examen se hablará sobre la mejor solución para su problema.

Si usted tiene cualquier pregunta sobre la fluorosis, el esmalte veteado o las manchas blancas, favor de sentirse libre de preguntarnos.

Incisivos Laterales Coniformes

A veces, por varias razones, los incisivos laterales maxilares no se forman correctamente. Los incisivos laterales maxilares son los dientes más pequeños a cada lado de los dos dientes frontales superiores. Esta malformación del diente está determinada por la genética. La malformación puede tomar varias apariencias diferentes y puede afectar los dos dientes o sólo un diente. Los dientes pueden ser más cortos de altura o menos anchos o una combinación de los dos. Esta clase de desviación de la forma normal del diente se llama un incisivo lateral coniforme. La solución para este problema cosmético puede ser sencilla o complicada, dependiendo de la forma del diente cuando se diagnóstico y cuando se comienza el tratamiento.

Posibilidades Restaurativas

Si el incisivo lateral coniforme (o los incisivos) es sólo un poco más estrecho de lo normal y hay espacio disponible a uno de los lados o a los dos lados, se puede hacer una adhesión con una restauración compuesta colocada directamente en el diente. Esto es el tratamiento más común. Los resultados son muy positivos y pueden durar mucho tiempo. No es difícil conseguir una igualación de color. El procedimiento es similar al de cerrar un diastema (un espacio que ocurre naturalmente entre los dientes).

Si no hay suficiente espacio en uno de los lados para poner el material compuesto, se podría requerir un tratamiento de ortodoncia para proveer espacio para la adhesión. Cuando se diagnóstica temprano, no es un problema hacer esto. Si el paciente espera hasta la adultez para el tratamiento de ortodoncia, el movimiento de los dientes pueden haber empujado al incisivo lateral coniforme fuera de su lugar, y se necesitará una ortodoncia más extensiva.

Si el incisivo lateral coniforme es demasiado pequeño tanto en su altura como en su ancho y queda a un espacio adecuado, todavía se puede reconstruir el diente con un compuesto. Sin embargo, si el paciente no es joven y hay que reemplazar una cantidad significativa del diente, una restauración de porcelana puede ser más apropiada. Esta restauración se hace en un laboratorio con resultados estéticos excelentes. Durará mucho tiempo. Es más costosa de llevar a cabo, y no se colocará hasta que la boca se haya desarrollado totalmente y los dientes y el tejido de las encías estén en su posición "adulta"—en algún momento después de los 18 años.

En resumen, la restauración de un incisivo lateral coniforme se puede hacer con la resina compuesta (en todas las edades) o la porcelana (después de los 18 años). El tamaño y la posición de los dientes determinarán lo que se va a hacer y cuándo se hace. Tan pronto como se observe, se deben hacer los planes para la restauración eventual. Es importante asegurar que haya suficiente espacio para la adhesión apropiada en el largo y en el ancho. Este espacio puede ocurrir naturalmente o puede requerir la asistencia ortodóntica.

Si usted tiene cualquier pregunta sobre los incisivos laterales coniformes y su restauración, favor de sentirse libre de preguntarnos.

Restauraciones de Resina Adherida: Empastaduras del Color del Diente para los Dientes Posteriores

En la ortodoncia se han usado las empastaduras del color del diente por muchos años, especialmente para restaurar los dientes frontales. Los materiales más recientes de empastaduras (las resinas) y del color del diente se usan con éxito para restaurar cavidades en los dientes de atrás. Estos materiales del color del diente son especialmente útiles cuando la restauración será visible cuando usted hable o sonría. Se puede esperar que estas resinas posteriores (de atrás) del color del diente duren varios años. En este momento un estimado razonable es de aproximadamente 10 a 12 años o más. El largo del tiempo que duran las empastaduras de resina (y las empastaduras de plata) depende de la posición y del tamaño de la empastadura, el cuidado que el paciente le da y las comidas que el paciente come.

Las restauraciones de resina en los dientes de atrás requieren menos uso del taladro que las empastaduras de plata; y cuanto menos el dentista tiene que taladrar su diente, mejor está usted y son menos los problemas dentales que usted desarrollará en el futuro. Cuando se taladra un diente para prepararlo, se pone más débil y la restauración con una resina adherida ayudará a fortalecerlo de nuevo. Las ventajas de las restauraciones de resina incluyen una apariencia final natural similar a la de su diente y la eliminación más conservadora de la estructura del diente. Requieren sólo una cita para terminarlas.

Las desventajas de las empastaduras del color del diente en los dientes posteriores incluyen la dificultad de colocarlas. Cuestan aproximadamente 50% más que las empastaduras de plata. Se pueden usar sólo raramente en los pacientes que tienen un hábito de rechinar o bruxismo (apretar); no se pueden usar en las áreas donde no hay una cantidad suficiente de la estructura del diente original; requieren más tiempo para terminarse.

Las restauraciones de resina están entre las restauraciones más conservadoras en la ortodoncia actual. Requieren la menos cantidad de taladrado. Mientras más pequeña puede ser cualquier empastadura, más tiempo durará. Son mejores para las empastaduras de tamaño pequeño a mediana. En las áreas donde el despliegue de metal de una empastadura de plata sería antiestético, son de gran importancia cosmética.

Si usted tiene cualquier pregunta sobre las restauraciones de resina adherida, favor de sentirse libre de preguntarnos.

Odontología Cosmética

La meta de la odontología cosmética es aumentar, mejorar o cambiar la apariencia de sus dientes. En la sociedad de hoy, su apariencia es muy importante. Aunque un juicio basado sólo en su apariencia puede ser superficial y no reflejar quién usted es de verdad, todavía puede afectar como las personas piensan de usted. Cuando usted habla, las personas se concentran en su cara, sus ojos y sus dientes. Las personas se fijan en lo natural de una boca, los dientes y la sonrisa. También se fijan en una boca antiestética debido a las cavidades visibles, las empastaduras defectuosas, la enfermedad de las encías o los dientes virados o malformados. Frecuentemente las personas formarán sus opiniones de usted basado en lo que ven.

Usted puede obtener una idea objetiva de cómo las otras personas le ven. Párese más o menos a 18 pulgadas de un espejo. Esto es más o menos cuan cerca la mayoría de las personas se le acercan cuando usted habla con ellos. Si usted se acerca más al espejo, la luz no será correcta y no se obtendrá una imagen de cómo se ven sus dientes. Sonría, hable, ríase, observe cuáles dientes están visibles y cómo se ven. Entonces pregúntese, "Si yo pudiera pasar una varita mágica sobre mis dientes y cambiar cualquier cosa que no me gustara, ¿qué cambiaría?" Apúntelo, entonces siga leyendo.

Muchas personas creen que la odontología se limita al arreglo de cavidades, canales radiculares, caperuzas y enfermedad de las encías. Pero usted estará fascinado por lo que podemos hacer para mejorar su apariencia. Aquí hay sólo una lista parcial de procedimientos que pueden mejorar la manera en que sus dientes se ven.

- ❑ Reemplazar las empastaduras desteñidas en los dientes frontales
- ❑ Blanquear los dientes a un color más blanco/claro
- ❑ Enderezar los dientes virados con la ortodoncia o reformar su esmalte natural
- ❑ Cerrar los espacios entre los dientes
- ❑ Laminados de porcelana o resina para cambiar la forma y la alineación de los dientes (adhesión)
- ❑ Colocar empastaduras del color del diente en los dientes de atrás (en vez de las empastaduras de plata/metal)
- ❑ Inlays u onlays de porcelana para los dientes de atrás
- ❑ Cirugía periodontal cosmética para igualar el tejido virado de las encías
- ❑ Restauración de dientes gastados y cortos a su forma apropiada
- ❑ Llenar las muescas de la abrasión del cepillo del diente
- ❑ Cubrir el lugar donde falta el tejido de las encías debido a la recesión con injertos del tejido suave
- ❑ Reemplazar los dientes que faltan con puentes o implantes
- ❑ Reemplazar las coronas (caperuzas) defectuosas y antiestéticas
- ❑ Cubrir las superficies manchadas de las raíces
- ❑ Remover del esmalte las líneas manchadas de fractura
- ❑ Restaurar los dientes agrietados (adhesión)
- ❑ Hacer que los dientes parezcan más largos
- ❑ Hacer que los dientes parezcan más cortos

Los costos por estos procedimientos varían según el grado del tratamiento. Díganos como usted desea que se vea su sonrisa. Entonces podemos decirle lo que podemos hacer, cuánto tiempo tomará y lo que costará. En la mayoría de los casos, las personas se sorprenden agradablemente al encontrar que el costo no es tanto como creían. Si usted tiene un seguro dental, frecuentemente puede encontrar que algunos de los procedimientos son parte de su conjunto de beneficios.

Si tiene cualquier pregunta sobre la mejoría de su apariencia con la odontología cosmética, favor de sentirse libre de preguntarnos.

Ilustración en CD-ROM

Recontorno del Tejido Cosméticamente

No es raro para nosotros sugerirle a un paciente que no tiene absolutamente ninguna señal de enfermedad periodontal (de las encías) que considere que se le hagan unos procedimientos periodontales electivos. En estos casos, los procedimientos casi siempre se necesitan para mejorar la apariencia. A veces se sugieren para promover la salud periodontal futura o para atender un problema potencial que puede desarrollarse.

Cuando usted sonríe o habla, sus dientes están enmarcados por sus labios y el tejido de encías visible. Las personas que le miran se dan cuenta de sus dientes. Las personas notan los dientes que faltan, la alineación de los dientes, el color de las encías, las empastaduras desteñidas, las empastaduras de plata, el color de los dientes y cuánto de sus dientes realmente se ven. Si todo está bien integrado y se ve natural, las personas dicen que usted tiene una sonrisa agradable. Si algo no se ve natural, puede ser fácil de definirlo, tales como los dientes virados, manchados o amarillos; la enfermedad periodontal evidenciada por el tejido de encía enrojecido o empastaduras desteñidas. O puede ser algo que no se determina tan fácilmente. Sólo es algo que no se ve bien.

Ese "algo" puede estar relacionado a la arquitectura de los dientes y de la encía. La posición de las encías donde se encuentran con los dientes es importante estéticamente. Si los dientes parecen ser demasiados cortos, puede ser que les cubra más tejido de la encía de lo que se considera atractivo. Usted puede enseñar demasiado tejido de la encía cuando sonríe. Puede haber una diferencia en la altura de la encía de un diente versus la de un diente adyacente o su pareja en el otro lado de la boca. Esto podría ser el resultado de la recesión causada por el cepillado demasiado fuerte; por enfermedad de las encías; por restauraciones defectuosas, especialmente las coronas o sólo por un problema con la manera que el diente hizo su erupción en el lugar. Todo esto puede disminuir su apariencia.

Varios procedimientos periodontales diferentes, fáciles de lograr, pueden corregir la mayoría de estos problemas rutinarios. Algunos implican la recesión indeseada del tejido; algunos implican el injerto de tejido. La ortodoncia puede ser provechosa en algunos casos. Los procedimientos más extensos requerirán enviarlo a especialistas.

En un tipo común de cirugía plástica periodontal cosmética, el tejido de las encías se reforma y recontorna sin el uso de suturas (puntos). Este procedimiento se hace en la oficina. Un diente o varios dientes pueden beneficiarse del tratamiento. El malestar postoperatorio es generalmente menor. Puede haber una sensibilidad del diente cuando se remueve el tejido de la encía, pero generalmente esto desaparece. La mejoría generada por este tipo de procedimiento puede ser asombrante.

Le mostraremos y describiremos con detalles cómo usted puede beneficiarse de los procedimientos periodontales cosméticos. En muchos casos, la cirugía periodontal cosmética completará el tratamiento que usted necesita. En algunos casos, será parte de un plan de tratamiento mayor que incluye las coronas, los laminados y las restauraciones adhesivas.

Si usted tiene cualquier pregunta sobre la cirugía cosmética periodontal electiva, favor de sentirse libre de preguntarnos.

Recontorno del Esmalte

La mayoría de las personas desean dientes derechos, maravillosamente alineados y blancos. Desgraciadamente, la mayoría de las personas no tienen esa suerte. Cuando los dientes están pobremente alineados, rotados, inclinados y/o apiñados, la manera más obvia para corregirlos es con la ortodoncia (los frenillos o los alineadores Invisalign). Sin embargo, hay situaciones en las cuales no puede ser posible ni deseable el uso de los frenillos para enderezar los dientes. Usted puede creer que es demasiado viejo (aunque esto es raramente el caso), el costo de la ortodoncia puede estar más allá de sus medios actuales, puede que usted no desee usar frenillos o tal vez sólo hay algunas áreas que necesitan atención y sencillamente la ortodoncia completa no sería apropiada.

En ciertos casos, la apariencia de sus dientes superiores e inferiores se puede mejorar poca o dramáticamente con el recontorno del esmalte. Los cuatro incisivos superiores y los cuatro inferiores se pueden alterar rutinariamente. A veces los dientes que están más atrás en su boca también se pueden mejorar cosméticamente. El recontorno es útil cuando hay superposición leve a moderada de los dientes frontales, un desgaste no igual o unos dientes que no tienen sus bordes de la mordida e incisión en armonía, lo que crea una apariencia no igual de "cerca de estacas puntiagudas".

El recontorno del esmalte generalmente es un procedimiento sin dolor y no se necesita anestesia local. El esmalte que está superpuesto o mal formado se remueve, se recontorna y se pule. Dependiendo de sus necesidades individuales, uno o varios dientes pueden requerir alguna reformación. Se pueden remover cantidades diferentes de esmalte de diversos dientes. Los dientes reformados no son más propensos al deterioro, no se ponen más sensibles a los cambios de temperatura y no son significativamente más débiles o dañados por el procedimiento.

Muchas veces, el recontorno es todo lo que se necesita para mejorar su apariencia significativamente. Otras veces, cuando la pobre alineación es más pronunciada, se puede hacer en conjunto con la adhesión de resina o porcelana a los dientes. Su tratamiento dependerá de sus condiciones actuales y de lo que le gustaría ver cambiado.

El procedimiento no es difícil para el paciente y muchas veces se puede hacer en sólo una cita. El cambio es inmediato y permanente. Requiere cierto don artístico por parte del dentista para ver cuáles son las posibilidades de cambio. Necesitamos determinar qué cantidad de esmalte necesita removerse, dónde debemos añadir material y dónde la ortodoncia es el mejor tratamiento. Los honorarios son razonables y dependen del grado del tratamiento.

Si usted tiene cualquier pregunta sobre el recontorno del esmalte, favor de sentirse libre de preguntarnos.

Laminados de Porcelana y Resina: Adhesión

Cuando las personas hablan de "adherir" algo a sus dientes para que se vean mejor, normalmente hacen referencia a los laminados de porcelana o resina. Los laminados cubren sólo la parte exterior del diente, la parte que se ve cuando usted sonríe. De hecho, todos los materiales restaurativos dentales de color son adheridos, no importa si la restauración está en un diente frontal o en un diente de atrás. En sentido estricto, en la odontología, la *adhesión* se refiere sólo a la unión, por medio de adhesivos, de dos materiales diferentes. Se pueden adherir (o fundir) tanto las empastaduras como las coronas (caperuzas).

Los laminados de porcelana y resina se colocan para corregir los defectos leves o severos en la alineación, la forma o el color de los dientes. También se colocan cuando los dientes se han restaurado moderadamente y se han debilitado los dientes. Se hace esto cuando todavía queda suficiente esmalte para que la adhesión sea exitosa. Si los dientes están muy mal alineados o no queda suficiente esmalte, la adhesión para mejorar la apariencia no es posible. Entonces hay que considerar las coronas de cobertura completa o la ortodoncia. El uso más común para los laminados de adhesión, o porcelana o resina, es para mejorar la apariencia cosmética del paciente.

Sin duda, los laminados de porcelana se ven mejor y duran más. Se indican cuando los dientes están en una alineación regular a buena. Usualmente no se usan con los pacientes menores de 16 años de edad. El procedimiento generalmente requiere alguna preparación (taladrado) leve a moderada. La anestesia local es usualmente necesaria. Para completarse el procedimiento se requieren 2 citas con una separación de aproximadamente 10 días laborales. Esto se debe al hecho que los laminados se construyen en un laboratorio externo. Una vez que se adhieren en su lugar, los laminados de porcelana se ponen muy sólidos. Su razón de éxito es alto y pueden durar hasta 12 años o más. Cualquier cosa que romperá sus dientes naturales puede romper los laminados de porcelana, por ejemplo, dulces duros o barras de caramelo congeladas. Los laminados son altamente resistentes a las manchas. Son una buena selección de tratamiento cuando se van a restaurar todos los dientes frontales. Son más costosos que los laminados de resina pero duran más tiempo y se ven mejor que la resina. Las superficies de mordida de porcelana pueden causar desgaste más rápido de los dientes opuestos naturales.

Los laminados de resina también están disponibles. El dentista los coloca en una visita a la oficina. Se usan los laminados de resina en situaciones similares a las del uso de la porcelana. Sin embargo, duran sólo la mitad de tiempo antes de requerir la reparación o el reemplazo. Se aconsejan para los pacientes que todavía están creciendo. Se ven muy bien pero no tan bien como la porcelana. Aunque las reparaciones de los laminados de resina no son muy difíciles, tienen una tendencia de agrietarse más que los laminados de porcelana.

Básicamente, la porcelana se ve mejor, dura más, es más fuerte y más costosa y requiere 2 citas dentales para terminarse. Los laminados de resina son menos costosos, más fáciles de reparar y son mejores para los niños o si hay consideraciones financieras.

Es muy importante venir para citas de cuidado repetido regular para la limpieza y un examen si se coloca cualquier tipo de laminado. De esta manera seremos capaces de corregir más rápidamente cualquier problema que se desarrolle. Un intervalo de 3 a 4 meses entre las citas es habitual.

Si usted tiene cualquier pregunta sobre los laminados de porcelana y resina, favor de sentirse libre de preguntarnos.

Inlays y Onlays de Porcelana

Porcelana

Cuando un diente se ha destruido moderada a extensivamente por el deterioro, el taladrado o la fractura pero todavía queda suficiente esmalte, una manera innovadora de restaurarlo es con un inlay u onlay de porcelana. Un inlay es una restauración en la cual una porción de la superficie oclusal (de mordida) se reemplaza con porcelana. Un onlay restaurará una porción más grande de la superficie de mordida del diente. Se consideran que éstas son restauraciones muy conservadoras. La porcelana permite un resultado estético excelente. Se adhiere al diente usando un procedimiento de adhesión, que lo convierte en un diente muy fuerte. Se puede usar con resultados magníficos en las restauraciones pequeñas, medianas y aun grandes y dura más de 12 años, relativamente sin problemas.

Un laboratorio dental está envuelto en la construcción de la restauración. Hay una demora de 2 a 3 semanas mientras se hace el inlay u onlay, por eso el diente tiene que llevar colocada una restauración temporal durante este tiempo.

Tienen algunas desventajas. Son de moderadamente a muy costosos para hacer y colocar. Toman dos citas para terminarse. Hay que ajustarlos y pulirlos bien, si no pueden causar el desgaste del esmalte contrario, similar a la porcelana fundida a una corona de metal. Por supuesto, aseguramos que están bien ajustados y bien pulidos desde el comienzo. Las superficies de mordida de porcelana pueden causar más desgaste rápido de los dientes opuestos naturales, especialmente en las áreas posteriores donde una superficie de mordida sería recomendada.

Las ventajas incluyen la estética excelente, la alta solidez, la longevidad predicha y preparación conservadora, es decir, menos taladrado que una corona. Si la porcelana se agrieta, se puede reparar. Sin embargo, usted no debe masticar cubos de hielo, caramelos muy duros y dulces duros con estos ni con cualquier otro tipo de restauración.

Para las personas que desean la restauración más fuerte, más duradera y más conservadora que iguala bien el color del diente, la porcelana es posiblemente la mejor selección. Una vez se haya terminado, el diente, si se cuida apropiadamente, no debe requerir otra restauración por años. Esto sí permite la conservación de la mayor parte del diente natural.

Resina

Los inlays y onlays de resina se usan en las mismas áreas como los inlays y onlays de porcelana. Son muy naturales en su apariencia y, como la porcelana, se adhieren en su lugar. Se consideran ser una restauración extremamente conservadora. Se requieren 2 citas separadas por aproximadamente 2 semanas, para fabricar el inlay/onlay de resina. Se protege el diente con una empastadura temporal mientras se hace la restauración final. El desgaste de la resina es similar al del esmalte. Así que, distinto de la porcelana, no tendrá la tendencia de desgastar la estructura natural contraria.

La resina se puede considerar un poco "más débil" que la porcelana. Sin embargo, la porcelana es más quebradiza y más difícil de reparar. La diferencia en la solidez no es significativa. La resina es más indulgente y se retoca o repara más fácilmente y es más fácil para trabajar con ella.

Con los dos tipos de materiales, la porcelana o la resina, usted puede desarrollar un deterioro en las superficies no restauradas, de modo que se requiere un excelente cuidado oral de sí mismo. Ninguno de los materiales se aconseja para los pacientes que tienen un hábito de bruxismo (rechinar) o apretar a menos que le haya construido un protector bucal para usted.

A menos que usted tenga una preferencia, seleccionaremos el material más apropiado para sus necesidades dentales. El costo de cada uno es similar. Los dos son selecciones excelentes y se consideran altamente conservadoras en la cantidad de taladrado requerido.

Si usted tiene cualquier pregunta sobre los inlays y onlays de porcelana o resina, favor de sentirse libre de preguntarnos.

Reemplazar Restauraciones Antiestéticas

Todo tiene una expectativa de vida, aun los materiales de empastaduras dentales. Los materiales dentales parecen tener dos clases diferentes de expectativas de vida—una funcional y una estética. Mientras mejor es el material original de restauración dental y la habilidad del operador, más tiempo durará la restauración. Los materiales procesados en el laboratorio generalmente durarán más tiempo que los que se colocan directamente.

El *largo de vida funcional* se define como la cantidad de tiempo que un material durará antes que deje de funcionar correctamente. Este fallo o (a) debilitará el diente o (b) permitirá el comienzo del deterioro o de la enfermedad de las encías. Por ejemplo, cuando se rompe un pedazo de empastadura (o frecuentemente en el caso de una empastadura de amalgama (metal de plata), causa que se rompa un pedazo del diente) el diente requiere una restauración nueva.

El *largo de vida estético* es un poco diferente. En el caso de las restauraciones adhesivas y del color del diente, significa que el material, aunque posiblemente todavía funcione, se ha comenzado a degradar. Una empastadura puede haber igualado al diente hermosamente cuando fue colocada, pero con el pasar del tiempo los cambios en el color del material de empastadura, al igual que los cambios reales del color del diente, causan que el diente y el material de empastadura no sean iguales. Como el material restaurativo no tiene las mismas propiedades que el esmalte del diente, se desgastará con un poco de diferencia. La forma también cambiará con el tiempo. Afortunadamente, el proceso es muy lento.

Con las restauraciones procesadas en el laboratorio, las coronas y los puentes, la corona puede todavía trabajar bien, pero la edad y los cambios en su boca hacen que ella y los tejidos que la rodean se vean menos aceptables de cuando se colocaron al principio. De nuevo, esto ocurre lentamente, con el paso de muchos años.

Otros problemas estéticos que se pueden corregir incluyen las muescas en las empastaduras o debajo de las coronas que son causadas por el cepillado incorrecto (o el deterioro), la recesión del tejido de la encía que expone las superficies más oscuras alrededor de las coronas o las empastaduras, las coronas de porcelana ("caperuzas") que ya no igualan a los dientes adyacentes y los márgenes de metal de las coronas que son visibles debido a la recesión de la encía (y esto es bastante común).

Cuando usted puede ver estos tipos de cambios, puede estar seguro que otros que le miran cuando usted habla o sonríe, también los verán. Si usted aprecia mucho su apariencia personal, ya es hora de considerar el reemplazo de las restauraciones con materiales más nuevos. Los materiales nuevos de restauración dental se ven mejor, duran más tiempo y son más de un color más estable y más resistentes al desgaste que los materiales adhesivos de las generaciones pasadas. Usted puede esperar que se vean bien por muchos años.

En nuestra opinión, las empastaduras de metal de plata nunca se ven "bien". Aun en su mejor punto, pulidas y brilladas, no representan una imagen de buena salud. Cuando el metal envejece, se corroe, se marca y se oscurece. Su constante expansión y contracción debido a las comidas calientes y frías que comemos debilita al diente. El oscurecimiento de una empastadura puede causar el oscurecimiento del diente mismo. Después de un tiempo, el diente se pondrá de un gris oscuro permanentemente. Mientras más ancha sea su sonrisa (y más dientes usted muestra cuando habla y sonríe), mayor puede ser el problema.

Las empastaduras rotas, manchadas, gastadas y visibles detraen de su apariencia. Cuando usted observa un diente (desde una distancia de más o menos 2 píes) que se ha restaurado, no debe ver la empastadura. Aunque estos tipos de problemas, por supuesto, no amenazan la vida, considere la posibilidad de atenderlos antes de que se empeoren—y sean más difíciles y más costosos de corregir.

En nuestra oficina, valoramos mucho la apariencia de sus dientes y cómo usted se siente en cuanto a su sonrisa. Queremos que usted luzca bien. Usamos los mejores materiales y técnicas disponibles en la odontología de hoy para asegurar una sonrisa saludable. Estaremos contentos de evaluar su condición en particular y hablar con usted de las opciones.

Si usted tiene cualquier pregunta sobre el reemplazo de restauraciones antiestéticas, favor de sentirse libre de preguntarnos.

La Sonrisa Perfecta

Casi todos pueden tener la sonrisa perfecta de sus sueños. Pero la sonrisa perfecta envuelve mucho más que los dientes blancos. La mayoría de las personas que miran a una sonrisa mirarán al color y la alineación de los dientes superiores e inferiores y se darán cuenta si los dientes están virados. También podrían prestar atención a una empastadura o corona que no es igual a la estructura natural del diente. Pero los dientes son sólo uno de tres componentes igualmente importantes para una sonrisa perfecta. La boca humana es un escenario y es enmarcada por los labios y el tejido suave (las encías) que rodean los dientes. Si cualquiera de estos se desvían de la norma aceptada, aun si los dientes son derechos y blancos, la sonrisa puede aparecer antiestética.

Sus labios enmarcan sus encías y sus dientes. No hay mucho que puede hacer un dentista en cuanto a los músculos y los vínculos de los labios. Pero los labios tienen un papel dominante en su sonrisa perfecta. La línea de los labios se divide en tres tipos—baja, mediana y alta. Una línea del labio *baja* quiere decir que usted muestra poca o ninguna estructura del diente cuando habla o sonríe. Hoy en los Estados Unidos, se considera que esto es la apariencia de una persona mayor. La piel y los músculos de la cara humana se bajan aproximadamente 1 mm cada 10 años, comenzando alrededor de los 40 años de edad. Esto se debe a la gravedad y la pérdida de elasticidad del tejido. Cuando los músculos y la piel se bajan, se ve menos estructura del diente, lo que contribuye a una apariencia de mayor edad, asociada con una línea del labio baja. Mientras mayor sea usted, se verá menos de los dientes superiores y más de los dientes inferiores. Una línea del labio *mediana* es aquella en que se ve el diente entero cuando usted habla o sonríe. La línea de los dientes generalmente sigue las líneas de los labios inferiores y superiores. Esta apariencia, junto con los dientes frontales dominantes, se considera como el tipo de sonrisa más deseable. Una línea *alta* es aquella en que se ven todos los dientes frontales y el tejido de la encía que está encima de ellos. Puede oscilar desde la visibilidad de un poco de encía hasta la visibilidad de una cantidad grande de encía. Esto se considera como una apariencia menos agradable.

El tejido de la encía rodea los dientes. El tejido de la encía debe llenar el espacio entre los dientes que se tocan, de modo que todo lo que usted ve es encía y dientes—sin espacios. Donde el diente parece salir de la encía, la encía debe tener una apariencia en forma de concha (de ondas). La encía debe estar ubicada más alta en los incisivos centrales (los dos dientes frontales), más baja en los incisivos laterales (los dos dientes más pequeños que están al lado) y de nuevo más alta en los dos colmillos. Usualmente, el tejido de la encía es más alto alrededor de los colmillos que de los dos dientes frontales. Y, por supuesto, el lado izquierdo y el derecho deben ser como reflejos el uno del otro. Esta forma de concha debe seguir la línea del labio superior. La apariencia correcta aquí tiene una importancia fundamental en el desarrollo de una sonrisa perfecta. Si la altura de la encía es demasiada baja o demasiada alta alrededor de un diente específico o de varios dientes, aun si los dientes son derechos, se verán "mal". Se pueden (y se deben) corregir los defectos en la posición de la encía antes de hacer cualquier restauración mayor de los dientes frontales. El tratamiento puede ser mínimo o mayor, dependiendo de la cantidad de dientes y el tipo del problema existente.

Generalmente los dientes mismos deben seguir la línea del labio desde la izquierda hasta la derecha. Deben ser proporcionales entre sí y para sí mismos. Comúnmente, una razón de 1.6:1 de largo a ancho es deseable. Los dientes adyacentes también siguen una razón proporcional similar cuando se ven directamente. Si los dientes individuales son demasiado largos o anchos o no están proporcionados el uno al otro o no son como reflejos de espejo de izquierda a derecha, los resultados son los problemas estéticos.

Podemos reconocer estos problemas y ofrecer sugerencias para mejorar la estética. Usted puede mirarse y no saber qué está mal con su sonrisa – pero sí sabe que no tiene la sonrisa que desea. Puede no ser sólo los dientes. La manera en que sus labios enmarcan los dientes y la arquitectura y posición de las encías que los rodean son dos variables en una ecuación de tres partes para una sonrisa perfecta—¡la suya!

Si usted tiene cualquier pregunta sobre su sonrisa perfecta, favor de sentirse libre de preguntarnos.

Blanquear los Dientes:
Visión General y Opciones

Usted ha expresado un interés en hacer más blancos sus dientes. Las siguientes son consideraciones importantes para que usted determine cuál método es mejor para usted:

- Un 97 por ciento de los pacientes que blanquean sus dientes tienen éxito.
- El proceso no daña los dientes.
- Es imposible predecir el grado de blanqueo antes del tratamiento.
- La enfermedad de las encías activa, el deterioro y la patología dental tienen que corregirse antes de comenzar el proceso de blanqueo.
- Los dientes tienen que estar limpios. Si han pasado más de 3 meses desde su última limpieza dental profesional, aconsejemos que ésta se haga primero. Mientras más limpios estén los dientes, mejor blanquean.
- Si usted tiene restauraciones (empastaduras) del color del diente, coronas de porcelana ("caperuzas") o una dentadura parcial removible con dientes que están visibles, esté consciente que estos materiales **no** cambiarán de color como lo harán sus dientes. Es posible que estas restauraciones necesiten ser reemplazadas o modificadas después de terminar el blanqueo. Esto se debe hacer después que pase 1 mes para que el color se estabilice.
- Mientras más amarillos están sus dientes inicialmente, más cambio de color (más claro/blanco) se notará después del blanqueo. Mientras más blancos/más claros están sus dientes al comienzo, menos cambio de color se notará.
- Las investigaciones indican que los dientes pueden blanquearse sólo "al máximo que les sea posible". El color es una función de las propiedades físicas de los dientes. Más blanqueo después de llegar a este punto no tendrá un efecto notable.
- Los dientes con desteñimiento por la tetraciclina probablemente necesitarán múltiples tratamientos de blanqueo.
- Si usted ha blanqueado sus dientes anteriormente (con soluciones y cubetas profesionales), habrá un cambio de color menos notable.
- La diferencia entre el blanqueo en la oficina y el blanqueo casero parece ser sólo en la cantidad de tiempo que se necesita para alcanzar el cambio de color. El procedimiento en la oficina es más rápido; la técnica casera es más lenta (y requiere más compromiso de tiempo por parte suya). El proceso en la oficina usa una solución de blanqueo más concentrada que las soluciones caseras.
- El proceso de blanqueo continúa por 2 días después del blanqueo en la oficina. Usted no debe tomar té, café, bebidas de cola o fumar durante esas 48 horas.
- Es posible que haya un "rebote" en el cambio de color después de concluir el blanqueo. Será entre un tono y un tono y medio según lo observado en las guías de tonos comúnmente usada. En la combinación de la técnica casera de cubeta, el rebote se minimiza o se elimina.
- Algunas personas experimentan sensibilidad después del procedimiento. Esta sensibilidad no es permanente y desaparecerá rápidamente. Se pueden prescribir geles de fluoruro en este caso.
- El cambio de color se mantiene satisfactorio por aproximadamente 3 a 7 años. Sus hábitos de comer/beber contribuyen a la posibilidad de que sus dientes se amarillecen en el futuro.
- Se puede repetir el proceso de blanquear los dientes cuando se oscurecen de nuevo.

Hay tres posibles combinaciones de blanqueo disponibles en esta oficina:

1. Técnica en la oficina solamente. Envuelve 6 a 10 dientes frontales superiores e inferiores; 12 a 20 en total. La cantidad total de dientes blanqueados depende de las condiciones existentes. Aunque los dientes se aíslan y se protegen los tejidos suaves, es posible que alguna de la solución de blanqueo pueda entrar en contacto con los tejidos. Los tejidos pueden ponerse blancos temporalmente y ser sensitivos. Esto pasará en algunas horas, como máximo. Este procedimiento se termina en una cita. Algún rebote de color postoperatorio es posible.
2. Blanqueo casero con el sistema de cubetas solamente. Las cubetas cubren todos los dientes superiores e inferiores. Normalmente se necesita un caja de la solución de blanqueo (posiblemente dos). Usted se puede poner las cubetas mientras duerme o durante el día. Esta técnica puede tomar varias semanas para completarse. Las cubetas se pueden guardar y usar en el futuro, con sólo una jeringuilla del gel de blanqueo para retocar los dientes antes de los eventos importantes. La comida y la bebida pondrán amarillos los dientes con el paso del tiempo.
3. Una combinación del blanqueo en la oficina y casera es lo más rápido, más efectivo y lo mejor por el precio. El blanqueo en la oficina se hace en una cita. Las cubetas estabilizan el color, reducen el rebote y están disponibles para el futuro.

Honorario—Opción 1: $ Honorario—Opción 2: $ Honorario—Opción 3: $

¡Usted Puede Tener Dientes Más Blancos!

La manera menos dañina y más conservadora de blanquear sus dientes es con el uso de una solución de blanqueo. Al contrario de lo que usted podría pensar, el cepillar sus dientes más fuertemente con una pasta de dientes abrasiva no blanqueará sus dientes sino puede causar que se oscurezcan más rápido. El concepto de blanquear los dientes ha existido por muchos años y las técnicas se han hecho más fáciles y menos costosas de llevar a cabo. Se notó el blanqueo de dientes en la literatura dental de los 1920. La técnica se ha hecho más fácil y el costo ha disminuido. Hoy hay dos métodos convenientes para blanquear los dientes oscuros: El Blanqueo Casero y el Blanqueo en la Oficina.

¿Por Qué los Dientes se Ponen Amarillos?

El color intrínseco (normal) de sus dientes está relacionado al color y el grosor del esmalte y la dentina y también a los tipos de comidas y líquidos que usted ingiere. Mientras más fino el esmalte, más oscura será la dentina subyacente; y mientras más café, té, bebidas de cola y vino tinto usted tome, más oscuros estarán sus dientes. Las grietas que comúnmente se encuentran en el esmalte de sus dientes pueden proveer un camino por el cual los fluidos descolorantes alcanzan la dentina subyacente.

Si usted tiene un tono amarillo, marrón o anaranjado en sus dientes, en la mayoría de los casos se pueden blanquear con el procedimiento de blanqueo. El blanqueo trabaja muy bien para remover el oscurecimiento de sus dientes relacionado a la edad. Este oscurecimiento relacionado a la edad probablemente se debe a los años de beber las bebidas oscurecíentes u otros factores del ambiente y no a la genética. No se requiere el taladrado ni la anestesia para el blanqueo. Sus dientes no se debilitarán. Como la mineralización de los dientes varía tanto de una persona a otra, no hay manera de determinar cuántas visitas a la oficina se necesitarán para efectuar el cambio de color ni cuán blancos los dientes se pondrán. Mientras más oscuros estén sus dientes, más tiempo se requiere para el cambio y más distintivo será el cambio de color.

El procedimiento de blanqueo también trabajará con un grado menor en los dientes desteñidos por la tetraciclina. Hemos visto unos resultados regulares a buenos tanto del blanqueo en la oficina como del casero. Sí toma más tiempo para lograr buenos resultados con este tipo de mancha, pero desgraciadamente, a veces el cambio es menor.

Dos Técnicas Disponibles

Hay dos tipos de blanqueo disponible. Uno se hace por el paciente en su casa y el otro lo hacemos nosotros durante una visita a la oficina. Se pueden hacer por separado o conjuntamente. La técnica casera envuelve el uso de un protector bucal suave, delgado y cómodo similar a una cubeta. Se hace una impresión de sus dientes y se fabrican unas cubetas de blanqueo hechas a la medida. Entonces en casa, usted coloca la solución de blanqueo en las cubetas y las pone por 1 ó 2 horas diarias o duerme con ellas puestas toda la noche. Con el blanqueo en la oficina, usted viene a la oficina por 1 ó 2 horas y aplicamos una solución de blanqueo más fuerte que se activa durante este tiempo. Normalmente se requiere sólo una visita.

El cambio de color debe durar por 3 a 7 años en la mayoría de las personas. El cambio de color que usted ve inmediatamente después de concluir el blanqueo regresará por un tono durante el paso de 1 a 3 meses, con la mayor parte del cambio durante la primera semana. Si usted toma mucho café, té, gaseosas de cola, vino tinto o si fuma los dientes pueden comenzar a oscurecerse de nuevo. Cuando pasa esto, se puede repetir el proceso de blanqueo.

Los posibles efectos secundarios incluyen un desteñimiento blanco temporal del tejido de las encías si la solución de blanqueo en la oficina toca la encía. Esto desaparece rápidamente. Los dientes se pueden poner un poco sensitivos a los cambios de temperatura por poco tiempo. Esto también desaparece rápidamente. El proceso de blanqueo **no** daña el esmalte del diente ni la dentina ni la pulpa. Las empastaduras y las coronas no emblanquecen. Cuando sus dientes cambian a un color más claro, usted puede necesitar que se rehagan esas empastaduras y/o coronas. Le dejaremos saber si esto es una posibilidad antes de que blanquear sus dientes. No hay otros efectos adversos conocidos.

Los dientes que se ven cuando usted habla, sonríe o come son los dientes que más beneficiarían a su apariencia si se blanquean. Normalmente se blanquean los dientes superiores porque son mucho más visibles que los dientes inferiores, pero se pueden blanquear los dos arcos con éxito. Los dientes inferiores toman más o menos tres veces más tiempo para alcanzar el cambio de color de los dientes superiores.

Si usted tiene cualquier pregunta sobre los dientes más blancos, favor de sentirse libre de preguntarnos.

Opciones Caseras para Blanquear los Dientes

La selección de uno de los muchos sistemas diferentes de blanquear los dientes puede ser muy confusa. Hay pastas de dientes que blanquean, gomas de masticar que blanquean, materiales que se usan con cubetas, tiras de blanqueo, geles de blanqueo, sistemas profesionales de blanquear con cubetas similares a los protectores bucales y procedimientos profesionales de blanqueo en la oficina. Para simplificar todos estos hemos limitado el campo a tres opciones muy diferentes y muy prácticas—Crest Professional Strength Whitestrips, los sistemas de blanqueo casero con cubetas hechas a la medida y los geles que se compran sin receta médica. Todos tienen ventajas y desventajas y todos tienen el potencial de blanquear sus dientes. La siguiente presentación debe darle una visión general justa de cada tipo y ayudarle a tomar una decisión informada sobre el sistema que es apropiado para usted.

El blanqueo casero de dientes con cubetas similares a los protectores bucales ha estado disponible por más tiempo. Es más apropiado para las personas que tienen 18 años o más. Se hacen impresiones de sus dientes (tanto los superiores como los inferiores), se hacen modelos en piedra de estas impresiones y se moldea un protector bucal que iguala sus dientes exactamente. Se le suple la solución de blanqueo en contenedores de jeringuillas. Usted repartirá una cantidad pequeña en el lugar para cada diente en la cubeta del protector bucal y pondrá la cubeta sobre sus dientes. Sólo se necesita una cantidad pequeña del material de blanqueo. Se usan las cubetas por alrededor de una hora diaria. Se puede notar un cambio de color en 3 a 5 días, pero el proceso completo puede tomar 2 a 3 semanas, dependiendo del color original de los dientes.

Los dientes quedarán blancos por 12 a 24 meses y usted puede retener el color nuevo por más tiempo al "retocarlos" con una aplicación del blanqueo por uno o dos días una vez al año. El tiempo ideal para el retoque es después de hacer que se limpien sus dientes profesionalmente. Tenemos unos tubos del blanqueo de retoque disponibles para la compra. Este proceso no daña los dientes de ninguna manera. La desventaja con esta técnica es el costo. El costo total de las impresiones, los modelos, las cubetas hechas a la medida y el suministro inicial de blanqueo es \$_____ .

Las Tiras de Blanqueo de Fuerza Profesional de Crest (Crest Professional Strength Whitestrips) son una nueva opción de blanqueo. Se ponen tiras transparentes que contienen la solución de blanqueo sobre los dientes superiores e inferiores dos veces al día por 30 minutes al día, por 21 días. El equipo profesional también contiene un cepillo de dientes y una pasta de dientes que blanquea. La versión profesional es 42% más efectiva que los Whitestrips que se compran sin receta médica. Los Crest Professional Strength Whitestrips son útiles para las personas que tienen preocupaciones financieras y para los adolescentes. El costo de los Crest Professional Strength Whitestrips es bastante permisible a \$_____ por un juego de materiales. Las desventajas son que las tiras no están hechas a la medida de modo que no cubren tantos dientes ni se ajusten tan bien ni tan cómodamente como el sistema de cubetas. Las tiras trabajan mejor para los dientes que están bien alineados. Según el manufacturero pueden necesitar otro tratamiento de blanqueo en intervalos de seis meses— hemos encontrado que el blanqueo dura satisfactoriamente por más tiempo.

Nuevos geles están disponibles que se compran sin receta médica y se pueden pintar en la superficie del diente. Colgate Simply White, Crest Night Effects y Ampollas de Go Smile son algunos de los productos que están disponibles actualmente. Estas fórmulas de geles claras se aplican a los dientes dos veces al día por 2 semanas. Los geles trabajarán efectivamente para blanquear sus dientes hasta que la saliva los quita. Como no hay manera de determinar y comparar el flujo de saliva de los pacientes, no podemos determinar cuán efectivamente trabajará para usted el gel puesto con cepillo. Este método es ideal para los adolescentes y los adultos jóvenes que pueden desear sólo un cambio leve de color. Estos geles que se compran sin receta médica son los menos costoso de todos los métodos pero también producirán los resultados de blanqueo menos dramáticos.

Cualquiera de los sistemas descritos puede trabajar. El grado de cambio de color dependerá del color original de sus dientes y cuán fielmente usted siga el proceso de tratamiento. Las cubetas hechas a la medida son el método más confiable, con un cambio de color que dura por mucho tiempo, pero son el más costoso de los tres métodos. Los Crest Professional Strength Whitestrips también pueden producir resultados, pero el cambio de color podrá no durar tanto tiempo y puede requerir unos retoques más frecuentes, pero es económico.

Instrucciones para el Sistema Casero para Blanquear los Dientes con Cubetas

Nombre del Paciente:_____   **Fecha:**_____

Ahora hay una técnica casera disponible para blanquear sus dientes. El procedimiento de blanqueo trabaja mejor para los dientes que tienen un tono amarillo, aunque puede trabajar en un grado inferior con los dientes que tienen un tono gris o un desteñimiento por la tetraciclina. Se construirá un protector bucal de una impresión que se hace de sus dientes. Esto mantendrá la solución de blanqueo en contacto con sus dientes. Las instrucciones generales para el blanqueo de dientes con el protector bucal son las siguientes. Las podemos variar un poco según sus necesidades particulares.

1. Antes de usar el gel de blanquear los dientes, cepille sus dientes y use el hilo dental. Enjuague su boca.
2. Como se ha demostrado, coloque una cantidad pequeña del gel blanqueador en cada diente que será blanqueado.
3. Inserte el protector bucal como se le ha enseñado, dejando salir el material en exceso. Escupa la solución en exceso. Si hay mucha para escupir, ponga menos blanqueador en la cubeta en la próxima aplicación.
4. Póngase el protector bucal como se le ha enseñado. Mantenga el protector bucal en su lugar por 1 a 2 horas. Siga esta rutina diariamente hasta que se acaba el gel blanqueador que le hemos suministrado. Usted puede ponerse las cubetas con la solución blanqueadora durante el día o puede optar de usarlas mientras duerme. El flujo disminuido de saliva mientras duerme mantendrá activo el gel blanqueador por más tiempo. Cuánto tiempo o cuánto usted puede usar la cubeta depende enteramente de su comodidad. Si no hay sensibilidad en los dientes, usted puede usar las cubetas tan frecuentemente como usted desee. Si es que usted comienza a desarrollar una sensibilidad en los dientes, **deje** de usar las cubetas hasta que la sensibilidad haya desaparecido (uno o dos días al máximo) y después comience de nuevo.
5. No coma ni beba por 30 minutos después de que se haya quitado el protector bucal y terminar la sesión de blanqueo. Después de cada uso, enjuague el protector bucal con agua, séquelo y guárdelo en un lugar seguro.
6. Regrese a la oficina para que se evalúe el progreso del blanqueo después de _____días de blanqueo.
7. Observe cualquier cambio que usted vea en sus encías y asegúrese de informarnos inmediatamente. Cualquier sensibilidad o alteración en su apariencia es temporal.
8. **Se debe hacer el blanqueo casero con el protector bucal sólo bajo la supervisión de un dentista.**
9. Como la mineralización de los dientes varía tanto de una persona a otra, no hay absolutamente ninguna manera de determinar cuánto cambio de color se puede esperar ni cuánto tiempo puede tomar para alcanzar el cambio de color. Piense que puede tomar tan poco como 2 a 3 horas y tan largo como 6 semanas para los dientes que están especialmente oscuros. Este marco de tiempo, por supuesto, depende de cuán frecuentemente usted use las cubetas llenadas con el gel blanqueador. Si hace el procedimiento por 1 hora cada dos días, tomará el doble del tiempo para terminarlo que si lo hace por 1 hora diaria. Si salta algunos días, esto no afectará el resultado final. El cambio de color final será igual no importa si usted toma 1 semana o 1 mes o más. Lo importante es el tiempo de contacto de la cubeta y el gel con los dientes que se blanquean.
10. El color más claro que usted ve inmediatamente después de terminar el proceso de blanqueo regresará a un tono más oscuro durante 1 a 3 meses, con la mayor parte de la regresión evidente después de la primera semana. Los dientes inferiores pueden tomar más tiempo para blanquearse que los dientes superiores.
11. Sus hábitos de comer y beber y las bacterias cromogénicas determinarán la duración del efecto de blanqueo. La mayoría de los pacientes mantienen un resultado satisfactorio por 3 a 7 años. Si usted fuma, bebe mucho té, café, colas, vino tinto, etc. sus dientes se oscurecerán de nuevo con el tiempo. **Mantenga sus cubetas de blanqueo en un lugar seguro.** En algún momento usted puede decidir "retocar" sus dientes con el blanqueo por un tiempo corto. Los retoques no toman tanto tiempo ni requieren tanto producto de blanqueo.
12. Si usted va a tener un reemplazo de empastaduras, debe esperar por lo menos 2 semanas después de terminar el blanqueo para que el color de los dientes se establezca antes de que se coloquen las restauraciones nuevas.

Otras instrucciones:

El costo del **blanqueo con protector bucal** es $_____ por un arco; $_____ por dos arcos.

Si usted tiene cualquier pregunta sobre el blanqueo de dientes con un protector bucal, favor de sentirse libre de preguntarnos.

Técnica Potente de Blanqueo de Dientes en la Oficina sin Activación de Luz

Los dientes frontales, los 6 a 10 dientes que se ven más fácilmente cuanto usted habla o sonríe, son los dientes que pueden más beneficiarse del blanqueo de dientes "potente". Al igual que los dientes de atrás, si hay empastaduras de tamaño mediano a grande en los dientes, es probablemente mejor si se protegen estos dientes con coronas. El procedimiento del blanqueo potente en la oficina es uno de los métodos más conservadores y menos costosos para intentar aclarar el color y regresarlo a una apariencia más aceptable.

El procedimiento envuelve el aislamiento de los dientes que se blanquearán y la protección de los tejidos de las encías y los labios. Entonces se mezcla una solución blanqueadora y se aplica a los dientes. El tipo de aplicación y el número de citas depende del tipo de sistema de blanqueo que creamos sea el mejor en su situación.

La mayoría de los pacientes demuestran una gran mejoría después de un sólo tratamiento. Como la bio-película protectora que normalmente cubre el esmalte del diente se remueve durante el procedimiento de blanqueo, usted debe evitar fumar y beber líquidos pigmentados (café, té, vino tinto) por alrededor de 24 horas después de terminar el blanqueo. Después de 24 horas, la bio-película normalmente regresa a su lugar. El color final normalmente regresará un tono durante los primeros tres meses, con la mayor parte del cambio ocurriendo en la primera semana. Algunos dientes pueden necesitar una segunda cita (o una combinación del procedimiento en la oficina y el sistema de blanqueo con cubeta casero) para alcanzar el resultado deseado. El grado de blanqueo para cualquier diente es variable e imposible de predecir. Sin embargo, los estudios recientes muestran que 97% de todos los pacientes que blanquean sus dientes están contentos con el resultado. El cambio de color debe ser satisfactorio por 3 a 7 años.

Si usted tiene restauraciones dentales (coronas, adhesión), los plásticos y la porcelana no cambiarán de color. Usted puede necesitar que le rehagan algunas empastaduras debido al cambio de color. Le dejaremos saber si usted puede esperar el tener algunas empastaduras reemplazadas debido al cambio en color. Si usted va a reemplazar las empastaduras, debe esperar por lo menos 2 semanas después de terminar el blanqueo para que el color del diente se establezca antes de que se coloquen las restauraciones nuevas. Alguna sensibilidad postoperatoria es posible, pero normalmente ésta desaparece rápidamente. El proceso de blanqueo no daña el esmalte ni la dentina.

Hablaremos de sus necesidades particulares y haremos las recomendaciones sobre el tratamiento apropiado.

Si usted tiene cualquier pregunta sobre la técnica potente de blanqueo en la oficina, favor de sentirse libre de preguntarnos.

Técnica Potente de Blanqueo de Dientes en la Oficina con Activación de Luz

Los dientes frontales, los 6 a 10 dientes que se ven más fácilmente cuanto usted habla o sonríe, son los dientes que pueden más beneficiarse del blanqueo de dientes "potente". Al igual que con los dientes de atrás, si hay empastaduras de tamaño mediano a grande en los dientes, es probablemente mejor si se protegen estos dientes con coronas. El procedimiento del blanqueo potente en la oficina es uno de los métodos más conservadores y menos costosos para intentar aclarar el color y regresarlo a una apariencia más aceptable.

El procedimiento envuelve el aislamiento de los dientes que se blanquearán y la protección de los tejidos de las encías y los labios. Entonces se mezcla una solución blanqueadora y se aplica a los dientes. Se pondrá una luz especial sobre cada diente particular por varios minutos. La luz proveerá la energía para activar la reacción química. Se repetirá este procedimiento más o menos tres veces para cada diente durante la cita de 60 a 90 minutos.

La mayoría de los pacientes demuestran una gran mejoría después de un sólo tratamiento. Como la bio-película protectora que normalmente cubre el esmalte del diente se remueve durante el procedimiento de blanqueo, usted debe evitar de fumar y beber líquidos pigmentados (café, té, vino tinto) por alrededor de 24 horas después de terminar el blanqueo. Después de 24 horas, la bio-película normalmente regresa a su lugar. El color final normalmente regresará un tono durante los primeros tres meses, con la mayor parte del cambio ocurriendo en la primera semana. Algunos dientes pueden necesitar una segunda cita (o una combinación del procedimiento en la oficina y el sistema de blanqueo con cubeta) para alcanzar el resultado deseado. El grado de blanqueo para cualquier diente es variable e imposible de predecir. Sin embargo, los estudios recientes muestran que 97% de todos los pacientes que blanquean sus dientes están contentos con el resultado. El cambio de color debe ser satisfactorio por 3 a 7 años.

Si usted tiene restauraciones dentales (coronas, adhesión), los plásticos y la porcelana no cambiarán de color. Usted puede necesitar que le rehagan algunas empastaduras debido al cambio de color. Le dejaremos saber si usted puede esperar el tener algunas empastaduras reemplazadas debido al cambio en color. Si usted va a reemplazar las empastaduras, debe esperar por lo menos dos semanas después de terminar el blanqueo para que el color del diente se establezca antes de que se coloquen las restauraciones nuevas. Alguna sensibilidad postoperatoria es posible, pero normalmente ésta desaparece rápidamente. El proceso de blanqueo no daña el esmalte ni la dentina.

Hablaremos de sus necesidades particulares y haremos las recomendaciones sobre el tratamiento apropiado.

Si usted tiene cualquier pregunta sobre el blanqueo potente en la oficina, favor de sentirse libre de preguntarnos.

Instrucciones Postoperatorias para el Blanqueo de Dientes en la Oficina

Nombre del Paciente:_____   **Fecha:**_____

Usted acaba de terminar el blanqueo "potente" de sus dientes. Debe tener muy pocos problemas después del procedimiento. Aquí hay algunas cosas que usted debe recordar:

- Favor de no fumar o beber bebidas muy pigmentadas (café, té, colas, vino tinto) durante las próximas 24 horas.
- El cambio de color final regresará aproximadamente un tono durante los próximos 1 a 3 meses, con la mayor parte del cambio ocurriendo en la primera semana después del blanqueo.
- Usted puede experimentar alguna sensibilidad después del procedimiento causada por el calor y los químicos usados en el proceso. Ésta desaparecerá después de algunos días, a lo máximo. Si usted desea, puede usar una pasta de dientes desensibilizadora. También podemos prescribir una pasta de dientes con fluoruro que trabaja bien en esta situación.
- Como se estiraron sus labios por alrededor de 60 a 90 minutos, espere que se sientan adoloridos o diferentes por algunas horas.
- Aunque se tomó mucho cuidado para que la solución blanqueadora no hiciera contacto con el tejido de sus encías, no es raro que algunas áreas pequeñas estuviesen en contacto con el material blanqueador. En esas áreas, las encías se pondrán blancas por algunas horas. Pueden estar un poco adoloridas. Tanto el blanqueo como el dolor son temporales y desaparecerán después de poco tiempo.
- Usted puede usar cualquier pasta de dientes no abrasiva para limpiar sus dientes y remover las manchas superficiales. Si desea usar una pasta de dientes blanqueadora para ayudar a mantener el color, siéntase libre de hacerlo.
- Si usted ha decidido usar la combinación de blanqueo potente en la oficina/técnica de blanqueo casero con sistema de cubetas, use el protector bucal como se le ha enseñado.
- Si usted va a reemplazar las empastaduras, debe esperar por lo menos 2 semanas después de terminar el blanqueo para que el color del diente se establezca antes de que se coloquen las restauraciones nuevas.

Si usted tiene cualquier pregunta sobre estas instrucciones, favor de sentirse libre de preguntarnos.

Opciones No Vitales para Blanquear los Dientes

Cuando un nervio en el diente se muere, el diente necesita un tratamiento endodóntico (canal radicular). El diente que se ha tratado endodónticamente puede, sin embargo, oscurecerse lentamente con el tiempo. El cambio de color puede variar de un gris claro a un negro oscuro. Este cambio de color no es cosméticamente agradable.

Para los dientes de atrás, los molares y los premolares, este cambio de color puede no ser ofensivo. El diente puede no ser visible cuando usted habla o sonríe. Usualmente, un diente de atrás estará protegido y cubierto con una corona de cerámica o de porcelana a metal. Se hace el color de la corona para igualar su color de diente natural.

Los dientes frontales, o los dientes que se ven fácilmente cuando usted habla o sonríe, son los dientes que más se benefician del blanqueo no vital. Al igual que los dientes de atrás, cuando está presente una empastadura de tamaño mediano a grande, probablemente es mejor proteger el diente con una corona. Sin embargo, muchas veces los dientes frontales que han tenido una terapia de canal radicular tienen restauraciones de un tamaño más pequeño. Cuando estos dientes se tornan de un color más oscuro que el normal, el resultado es un problema cosmético. El procedimiento de blanqueo no vital es el método más conservador y menos costoso para intentar cambiar el color no deseado a una apariencia más aceptable.

El procedimiento envuelve el acceso a la preparación original hecha para el canal radicular y la eliminación de parte de la empastadura y cualquier escombro remanente. Se remueve una porción pequeña del canal radicular existente para permitir que se ponga un material sellador nuevo sobre la empastadura restante del canal radicular para protegerlo de la solución blanqueadora. Dependiendo de su situación particular, se puede entonces blanquear el diente internamente, externamente o hacer los dos en la misma visita. Por lo general, mientras más tiempo el diente ha estado oscuro, más tiempo toma para blanquearlo.

Hay tres métodos disponibles para blanquear el diente tratado endodónticamente: el blanqueo potente, blanquear y caminar o el blanqueo aplicado por el paciente.

El blanqueo potente envuelve la aplicación de una solución blanqueadora a la superficie exterior e internamente (donde la empastadura se ha removido parcialmente). La mayoría de los pacientes demuestran una gran mejoría después de sólo un tratamiento.

El blanquear y caminar envuelve el colocar la solución blanqueadora en la apertura del diente y sellarla en su lugar temporalmente. Quedará allí por alrededor de 1 semana. Entonces se re-evalúa el color del diente para determinar si otra aplicación de la solución blanqueadora es necesaria.

El proceso aplicado por el paciente requerirá que usted coloque la solución blanqueadora en el acceso abierto en su diente. Se mantiene en su lugar con una bolita de algodón. Usted quitará el algodón y la solución después de aproximadamente 1 hora. Repetirá este proceso diariamente hasta que el diente haya alcanzado el tono deseado.

Algunos dientes pueden no responder y necesitarán laminados de porcelana o coronas completas para llegar a ser atractivos de nuevo. Es imposible predecir el grado de blanqueo para cualquier diente. Es posible que después de algún tiempo, el diente comience a oscurecerse de nuevo y se necesite repetir el proceso de blanqueo.

Hay un honorario asociado con la apertura del acceso inicial del diente y la limpieza y el sellado de las partes internas del diente.

En muchos casos la mejoría en la apariencia del diente oscurecido es bastante notable. Ciertamente es la manera más sencilla y mejor por el costo para corregir este tipo de problema.

Hablaremos sus necesidades particulares y haremos las recomendaciones sobre el tratamiento apropiado.

Si usted tiene cualquier pregunta sobre el blanqueo no vital de los dientes, favor de sentirse libre de preguntarnos.

Dientes Desteñidos por Tetraciclina: Opciones para la Mejoría Cosmética

Cuando los dientes permanentes se están formando en la mandíbula de un niño joven (antes de que salgan del tejido de las encías y se puedan ver), pueden ser positivamente afectados por los fluoruros sistémicos controlados (hechos más fuertes y más resistentes al deterioro dental). Pueden ser adversamente afectados por las fiebres altas, la malnutrición y los medicamentos con receta—especialmente los antibióticos en la clase de tetraciclina. Las tetraciclinas se dan a los niños que han demostrado una reacción a la penicilina o que tienen un problema médico que se puede tratar mejor con las tetraciclinas.

Dependiendo de la edad del paciente, la etapa de desarrollo de los dientes permanentes y el tipo y la dosis del medicamento, el cambio en el color del diente (tanto en la dentina como en el esmalte) puede ser poco, moderado o bastante desfigurante. El color de los dientes puede cambiar del amarillo/blanco homogéneo normal al gris claro u oscuro, amarillo o aun morado/azul. Es más frecuente, que el color no es uniforme a través de todo el diente. Pueden haber rayas horizontales o franjas de color que son visibles. Si alguna vez usted ha visto una fotografía del planeta Júpiter, con las franjas horizontales de color brillante que marcan las diferentes zonas de viento, sería similar a las franjas de tetraciclina y los colores que se ven en los dientes permanentes.

Mejorar la Apariencia de los Dientes
El cambio de color debido a las manchas por la tetraciclina no es un problema superficial o de la superficie. La dentina (la capa de diente debajo del esmalte) es normalmente más oscura que el esmalte y da su color al diente. El cepillar los dientes con más fuerza o el uso de una pasta de dientes blanqueadora no mejorará el color. Hoy en día se puede mejorar la apariencia de los dientes desteñidos a través del blanqueo de dientes, los laminados de porcelana o cerámica adherida, los laminados de resina o las coronas completas.

Lo Que Sea Mejor para Usted
Lo que sea mejor para usted depende de la cantidad y tipo de desteñimiento, la velocidad con la cual usted desea la mejoría y sus finanzas. Para los desteñimientos leves a moderados, un proceso de blanqueo puede mejorar la apariencia de los dientes significativamente. Una combinación del blanqueo en la oficina y casero trabaja bien. Con el proceso de blanqueo "potente" se aplica una solución a sus dientes. Esta solución se activa por la energía de la luz y se deja en cada diente que se blanqueará por varios minutos. Si creemos que es apropiado para usted y si usted necesitara aun más blanqueo, podemos sugerir que usted continúe el proceso de blanqueo en su casa con una técnica de blanqueo con un protector bucal. Con esta técnica, se fabrican cubetas especiales similares a un protector bucal hechas a la medida para que se ajusten a sus dientes. Le daremos una solución blanqueadora para poner en las cubetas y ponerse por la noche hasta que ocurra el cambio de color deseado. El tiempo requerido para alcanzar el efecto deseado depende del grado de desteñimiento. Usualmente el proceso de blanqueo casero necesitará ser realizado por al menos 6 meses para que sea efectivo. Éste es el método menos invasivo y menos costoso para mejorar el color del diente.

Los laminados de porcelana hechos a la medida requieren la preparación del diente y el procesamiento por un laboratorio dental. Los laminados son más rápidos pero más costosos y los requisitos de mantenimiento son más complejos. Se puede esperar que los laminados duren 8 a 15 años, tal vez más. Los laminados directos de resina se colocan en los dientes en una visita. Son menos costosos que los laminados procesados en el laboratorio. Los laminados directos de resina se pueden ver casi tan bien como la resina procesada en el laboratorio, pero no se ven tan naturales como la porcelana. Durarán más o menos 5 años antes de necesitar un reemplazo o un retoque. Si usted está considerando los laminados, todavía podríamos recomendar algún grado de blanqueo antes de hacerlos porque mientras más oscuros están los dientes, más difícil es opacar u ocultar el color subyacente, que es el propósito primario de poner los laminados. El laminado que puede transmitir parte del color subyacente tiende a verse mejor que uno totalmente opaco. Como alternativa, se puede hacer más preparación del diente para permitir que una capa opaca se cubra por una porcelana estética más gruesa. Cada caso es diferente, pero una apariencia mejorada es posible. En el caso de los desteñimientos más oscuros, la única solución cosmética efectiva puede ser una corona completa.

Si usted tiene cualquier pregunta sobre el tratamiento para los dientes desteñidos por tetraciclina, favor de sentirse libre de preguntarnos.

Endodoncia

Revisión del Contenido: Endodoncia

Apicectomía
Explica las indicaciones y los procedimientos para la apicectomía. Incluye información postoperatoria para el paciente.

Síndrome de Periodoncia-Endodoncia
Describe el síndrome de Periodoncia-Endodoncia, su diagnóstico y opciones de tratamiento.

Terapia Endodóntica: Una Visión General
Explica la terapia endodóntica, porqué puede ser necesaria y qué el procedimiento exige.

Terapia Endodóntica: Procedimiento
Quita la confusión de la terapia endodóntica. Presenta lo que cubre el honorario por el procedimiento endodóntico.

Retratamiento de los Canales Radiculares
Explica porqué un diente puede requerir retratamiento endodóntico, el procedimiento y los posibles problemas que pueden presentarse mientras se vuelve a tratar.

Hemisecciones y Amputaciones Radiculares
Las razones y los procedimientos para hemisecciones y amputaciones radiculares son explicados.

Apicectomía

Indicaciones

Aunque el tratamiento endodóntico tiene un índice de éxito extremadamente alto, no es 100% eficaz. Algunos dientes pueden no responder según lo esperado a la terapia del canal radicular. A veces, está claro desde el principio que el canal radicular no está trabajando como se planifico. Otras veces, años más tarde se presenta la necesidad de otro tratamiento. El primer y más deseable método para solucionar este problema es el retratamiento del canal radicular en una o más raíces. En otras palabras, el tratamiento del canal radicular se vuelve a hacer con un método similar a la terapia original. Si es posible el re-tratamiento del canal radicular con este acercamiento no quirúrgico, es lo mejor. Si no, una forma de tratamiento diferente, la *apicectomía*, se debe considerar.

Los dientes que tienen raíces estrechas, dobladas, "obstrucciones" del canal, resorción de la raíz, infecciones persistentes, fracturas, un ápice ancho abierto y los quistes asociados son algunos de los problemas que se pueden corregir con una "apicectomía". Puede haber razones para no realizar la "apicectomía", tales como inaccesibilidad quirúrgica, pobre o carencia del soporte del hueso, raíces cortas o fractura vertical de la raíz.

El Procedimiento

La raíz o las raíces que van a recibir la apicectomía son medidas con las radiografías, y la localización aproximada de la punta de la raíz es estimada. El área que va a ser tratada se anestesia con un anestésico local. Se hace una incisión en la encía sobre la punta de la raíz y la encía es echada hacia los lados. El acceso se hace a través del hueso, la punta o el ápice de la raíz entonces se puede ver a través de esta "ventana" en el hueso. La punta de la raíz es usualmente removida, y un sellador para empastadura es colocado en la punta que queda. El tejido entonces se sutura nuevamente en su lugar. El diente no pierde estabilidad significativa por este procedimiento.

No hay dolor durante la cirugía. El malestar postoperatorio será eliminado con medicación anti-inflamatoria y analgésica. Hay usualmente cierta hinchazón leve en el lugar de la cirugía. La hinchazón es temporal y desaparecerá después de algunos días.

Cuando se comienza la "apicectomía" y el diente puede ser visto, otro tipo de problema puede ser observado. El problema puede ser una raíz fracturada, y una "apicectomía" no trabajaría y el diente tendría que ser sacado.

Este procedimiento puede ser completado por un dentista general, pero frecuentemente es enviado a un endodontista (un especialista en canal radicular) para evaluación y tratamiento.

Si usted tiene cualquier pregunta sobre la apicectomía, favor de sentirse libre de preguntarnos.

Síndrome de Periodoncia-Endodoncia

El síndrome de periodoncia-endodoncia es un problema dental combinado. El término *endodoncia* se refiere al interior del diente, y el término *periodoncia* se refiere a los tejidos y al hueso alrededor del diente. En este problema dental, el nervio en un diente está muerto o apostemado y la destrucción del hueso ha ocurrido alrededor del diente.

El deteriro o trauma de un diente puede causar que el nervio en el diente se muera. La enfermedad periodontal (de la encía) severa y la pérdida significativa del hueso pueden exponer un nervio accesorio de un diente, también causando la muerte del nervio. Más frecuente, un nervio muerto en un diente es la causa del síndrome de periodoncia-endodoncia. Usted puede o no experimentar algún síntoma con cualquiera de estas condiciones.

Este tipo de destrucción del hueso se caracteriza por un sistema de drenaje entre la raíz apostemada y los surcos (espacio entre la encía y el diente). Los surcos de un diente se pueden representar como el collar del tejido alrededor del diente donde el diente y la encía se encuentran visiblemente. Es normalmente solamente alrededor de 3 milímetros de profundidad. Un absceso se forma en la punta de la raíz y esta infección puede regarse, moviéndose por la raíz hacia la corona del diente. La infección puede drenar en el surco y entrar en su boca. Usted puede que incluso note un mal sabor en su boca cuando esto sucede.

Una vez el sistema de drenaje es establecido, y no hay un aumento en la presión del absceso, el diente puede estar sin síntomas. Usted incluso puede que no experimente un mal sabor en su boca.

Diagnóstico y Tratamiento

El síndrome de periodoncia-endodoncia es diagnósticado por el uso de radiografías y de una sonda periodontal. El tratamiento primero implicará el tratamiento endodóntico tradicional (terapia del canal radicular) para eliminar la causa de la infección. Antibióticos pueden ser recetados para ayudar a eliminar la infección. Esto se debe comenzar tan pronto como sea posible.

Luego de la terminación del canal radicular, el sistema de drenaje debe empezar a desaparecer y el hueso empieza a llenarse. Este proceso puede tomar de 3 a 4 meses. Mientras más tiempo la infección estuvo activa antes de que fuera tratada, más tiempo le tomará al hueso volver a llenarse. En circunstancias severas, el hueso puede que no llene y el diente puede necesitar ser sacado.

Si el hueso no se está llenando bien, otra evaluación será hecha. Esta evaluación puede ser realizada por un periodontista (un especialista que trata problemas asociados con las encías y el hueso de soporte). El periodontista puede sugerir tratamiento adicional para rellenar en las áreas dañadas del hueso. Si el procedimiento de rellenar el hueso no es exitoso, o si la infección vuelve, esto puede indicar problemas adicionales con el diente. Una grieta de línea capilar de la raíz, canales adicionales que no pueden ser visualizados o llenados o los canales accesorios microscópicos que son intratables pueden ser la razón. En estos casos es posible que el diente no pueda ser salvado.

El síndrome de periodoncia-endodoncia no es infrecuente en la odontología. Puede ocurrir alrededor de cualquier diente. Cuando es tratado en una manera oportuna, el problema se resuelve generalmente de una manera satisfactoria. Cuando se deja sin tratar durante mucho tiempo, el diente puede llegar a no tener salvación.

Si usted tiene cualquier pregunta sobre el síndrome de periodoncia-endodoncia, favor de sentirse libre de preguntarnos.

Terapia Endodóntica: Una Visión General

CANAL RADICULAR

La pulpa de su diente, la cual contiene el nervio y los vasos sanguíneos pequeños, puede infectarse. La pulpa tiene una capacidad limitada de curarse por sí misma. Esta infección puede ser causada por una cavidad profunda que alcanza el centro del diente lo que causa que la pulpa se muera, una lesión traumática al diente o una preparación extensa (taladrado) del diente. La preparación extensa se pudo haber hecho para preparar el diente para una corona u otra preparación grande para una restauración. La pulpa puede o no haber creado el absceso inmediatamente en estos casos. Puede tomar años para que un problema se desarrolle. El tejido infectado de la pulpa puede o no ser doloroso. Puede o no ser visible en una radiografía dental. Un diente con este tipo de absceso no es extraído generalmente porque la infección puede ser tratada con terapia endodóntica en el diente. Este procedimiento rutinario puede salvar el diente y ayudarlo a evitar los efectos dañinos de la pérdida del diente. Es exitoso en más de un 90% de los dientes en los cuales se termina el tratamiento.

El tratamiento endodóntico puede tomar de una a tres citas para terminarse. Los dientes pueden tener de uno a cuatro canales que necesiten ser tratados. Una abertura es creada para tener acceso al nervio, y el nervio apostemado es removido de la raíz o de las raíces. Los canales donde los nervios han sido localizados son limpiados y formados y un medicamento puede ser colocado en el canal para promover una mejor curación.

Cuando se ha determinado que los canales están libres de infección, estos son llenados con un material especial parecido a la goma y sellados con un medio de cementación. El área apostemada asociada al diente entonces comenzará a curarse. Puede tomar varios meses antes de que la curación se complete y para que el diente se vuelva asintomático, esto es, para que cualquier dolor en el área desaparezca.

Una vez la terapia endodóntica se ha completado, el diente se restaura generalmente con una corona de molde u onlay. Esto se hace para proteger el diente y para evitar que se fracture. El no seguir con los procedimientos restaurativos obligatorios que siguen la terapia endodóntica en un diente que no ha sido previamente coronado puede resultar en una fractura vertical. Si lo que queda es una estructura del diente muy pequeña, podemos también aconsejar el uso de un poste y una base para ayudar a que el diente pueda retener su restauración final. Discutiremos con usted el tipo exacto de restauración que usted necesitará.

Por favor entienda que esta infección puede causar malestar entre las citas para el canal radicular. Esto es normal y generalmente no es causa de ninguna preocupación. Contacte esta oficina si hay dolor y/o hinchazón. Recuerde evitar el morder en el diente hasta que se termine el canal radicular y se haya colcado la restauración final. Usted puede que no haya tenido ningún malestar en el diente antes del tratamiento del canal radicular o no estaba enterado de que usted incluso tenía un absceso. Sin embargo, usted puede experimentar dolor o hinchazón después de que el tratamiento del canal radicular ha comenzado.

Si hemos recetado antibióticos para el absceso, asegurese de comprar la receta y tomarla hasta que se termine. Es importante que usted haga esto para controlar rápidamente la infección. Si usted no toma la medicación recetada, la resolución del absceso puede ser retrasada y los problemas con el dolor postoperatorio son más probables.

Si usted tiene cualquier pregunta sobre el procedimiento del canal radicular o la restauración final del diente, favor de sentirse libre de preguntarnos.

Terapia Endodóntica: Procedimiento

Aunque hacemos un gran esfuerzo para explicar el tratamiento específico y los honorarios relacionados, encontramos que referente a la endodoncia (terapia del canal radicular) en particular, sigue habiendo cierta confunsión a veces Por favor lea cuidadosamente lo siguiente para que usted se entere de lo que es incluido en los honorarios para el procedimiento y dónde otros honorarios pueden ser autorizados.

Tratamiento Endodóntico (Canal Radicular)

El honorario por el tratamiento endodóntico para cada diente incluye:

❑ Todas las radiografías
- las radiografías de diagnóstico iniciales
- radiografías de funcionamiento y medida
- radiografías del canal radicular terminado para su historial y, donde lo indique, para la verificación del tratamiento para el portador de seguro

❑ Toda la anestesia (local) necesaria para "adormecer" el diente

❑ Acceso al diente

❑ Extracción del tejido del nervio

❑ Limpieza y formación de los canales

❑ Irrigación de los canales con soluciones medicinales

❑ Colocación de preparaciones medicinales donde se necesite

❑ Relleno de los canales con los materiales de relleno para canal radicular

❑ Una empastadura temporal en la abertura de acceso entre citas o cuando se complete el canal radicular

❑ Cualquier visita de emergencia necesaria durante el tratamiento del canal radicular para el diente que se está tratando

❑ Un año de chequeo postoperatorio y las radiografías necesarias. El honorario NO cubre:
- Medicamentos recetados (escribiremos una receta que se debe comprar en una farmacia)
- La restauración final, la cual es siempre un honorario separado

La restauración final que usted necesitará después que se termine el canal radicular dependerá de qué diente se está tratando y de cuanto diente natural quede y que tan fuerte parezca. Usted será informado de la posible restauración que usted necesitará y su costo, antes de que se comienze el canal radicular. Una vez más, este honorario es separado de los honorarios del canal radicular.

Si usted tiene cualquier pregunta sobre lo que esta incluido en los honorarios para la terapia endodóntica, favor de sentirse libre de preguntarnos, antes de que el tratamiento comienze, si es posible.

Retratamiento de los Canales Radiculares

El tratamiento endodóntico es una de las formas de terapia dental más exitosas que están disponibles en estos momentos. Pero aproximadamente 10% de los dientes que se tratan nunca se curarán totalmente o desarrollarán problemas más adelante. Usted tiene una situación que cae en este 10%.

Hay varias posibles indicaciones de que hay un problema. Usted puede experimentar dolor o sensibilidad en el diente tratado cuando muerde o aplica presión sobre él. Puede haber hinchazón leve o severa en el área tratada. Una fístula (sistema de drenaje) puede desarrollarse, o nunca cerrarse completamente. Este lugar de drenaje tendrá pus que se puede exprimir a través de él. O usted puede que no sienta nada. El problema puede ser algo que fue descubierto a través de una radiografía postoperatoria. El hueso alrededor del diente puede que no haya crecido nuevamente, o se puede ver más destrucción del hueso.

Estos problemas ocurren por una variedad de razones. Una infección pre-existente, la razón para el canal radicular en primer lugar, puede haber dejado efectos residuales, que nunca desaparecieron enteramente y comenzaron a actuar nuevamente. Es también probable que el relleno original del canal radicualr no era clínicamente el ideal. Esto sucede debido a cualquiera de varios factores por ejemplo raíces torcidas o curvadas; canales pequeños, adicionales; instrumentos separados del canal radicular; derrubio del cemento y otros. A veces, no hay una razón clara que se pueda considerar para el fracaso del canal radicular. Sólo sucede.

Incluso si el problema no ha sido notado por usted, no es prudente dejar una infección activa en su cuerpo. Un procedimiento no quirúrgico para retratamiento quitará los materiales de relleno del canal radicular, limpiará y volverá a limar el canal radicular, para entonces rellenar los canales. El retratamiento es generalmente más difícil y consume más tiempo que el primer canal radicular. Es más difícil remover el material del canal radicular que se encuentra condensado y cementado, los postes cementados y las resinas adheridas o cementadas para el retratamientode los canales. Los intentos para remover estos materiales pueden causar la fractura del diente y llegar a la desesperación. Puede que no sea posible la re-intrumentación del diente, dependiendo de lo que haya en él. Esto puede que no se conozca hasta que se haya comenzado el tratamiento. Es también posible que el retratamiento no trabaje.

A pesar de estos posibles problemas, el retratamiento es el enfoque más conservador y generalmente el menos costoso. Cuando se presenta la situación, es éste el método a escoger. Se realiza en un diente que usted necesita conservar. Si el retratamiento no se pude hacer, el problema debe ser tratado quirúrgicamente o el diente tendrá que ser sacado. Un procedimiento quirúrgico de endodoncia, llamado una *apectomía,* puede ser requerido si el retratamiento no trabaja.

Si usted tiene cualquier pregunta sobre el retratamiento de los canales radiculares, favor de sentirse libre de preguntarnos.

Hemisecciones y Amputaciones Radiculares

Indicaciones

Ocasionalmente, una porción de un molar es dañado incurablemente, pero todavía queda una parte del diente saludable. Dependiendo del problema individual, puede ser posible y deseable conservar la parte buena del diente y sacar la porción dañada. Los dientes de atrás tiene dos (en la parte inferior) o tres (en la parte superior) raíces. Una de las raíces puede estar seriamente deteriorada, periodontalmente implicado o partida. Lo más común, es una raíz partida, el diente ya ha tenido terapia endodóntica (tratamiento del canal radicular). Si el problema es deterioro, puede que no haya canal radicular en ese diente y necesitará un canal radicular en las raíces que serán conservadas.

Procedimiento

Un amputation radicualr es el retiro de parte o de toda una raíz individual. Una hemisección radicular es la división del diente por la mitad para hacer dos raícer por separado, y dos dientes separados de lo que era un solo diente con dos raíces unidas. Este procedimiento se realiza más frecuentemente en los molares inferiores.

El procedimiento para cualquiera es similar. Si un canal radicular no fue terminado, se comienza y se termina en la raíz o las raíces que quedan. El área es accesada quirúrgicamente para alcanzar una visión directa y la sección radicular incurable es removida o el diente es divido. Generalmente, la remoción de la raíz no es muy difícil de hacer. El seccionar la raíz se hace con una pieza de mano dental de alta velocidad.

El área es entonces cerrada, suturada y se deja curar de 6 a 8 semanas. Cuando está suficientemente curada, la raíz restante es finalmente restaurada. Casi 100% del tiempo, el diente necesitará una restauración de molde. Para una resección de la raíz, en la cual el diente molar se ha dividido en dos porciones de tamaño premolar, las raíces recibirán un poste y una base y luego coronas féruladas. Si es necesario, otros dientes pueden ser coronados, también, y añadidos al molar hemiseccionado para apoyo adicional. En un diente que ha tenido una amputación radicular, una sola corona se puede colocar o puede ser unido a otro diente para soporte adicional. Sus necesidades individuales dictarán qué es lo mejor para usted.

Los aspectos críticos para el éxito de estos procedimientos son el diagnóstico y la ejecución del tratamiento. Postes y bases pueden ser necesarios. Frecuentemente, los dientes tratados deben ser férulados a los dientes adyacentes. Las raíces y las coronas de molde deben ser formadas perfectamente para asegurar que las partes restantes puedan ser limpiadas fácilmente y completamente con un cepillo de dientes e hilo dental.

En muchos casos, la invención de procedimientos exitosos de implante han reemplazado la hemisección y la amputación radicular. Su situación en particular puede indicar que cualquiera de éstas es la mejor para usted.

Si usted tiene cualquier pregunta sobre la hemisección o la amputación radicular, favor de sentirse libre de preguntarnos.

Revisión del Contenido: Odontología en General

General
Estos documentos incluyen la información general en cuanto a los procedimientos y conceptos en la odontología en general.

Antes de Comenzar el Tratamiento
Ayuda a clarificar las metas del tratamiento, compromiso financiero y de tiempo y los requisitos del cuidado oral de sí mismo para el paciente antes de la comenzar el tratamiento.

Anatomía Dental y Oral
Ayuda al paciente a entender las partes del ambiente oral y como trabajan juntos.

Obtenga la Odontología Que Usted Necesita, Quiere y Se Merece
Ayuda a los pacientes a entender por qué pueden haber opciones de tratamiento, escrito desde el punto de vista financiero.

Procedimientos de Control de Infecciones
Al explicar los procedimientos de esterilización, alivia las preocupaciones de los pacientes en cuanto a la posibilidad de que la oficina dental sea una fuente de infección.

Examen Oral Inicial
Prepare a los pacientes para un examen oral inicial con esta visión general de los procedimientos envueltos. Informa al paciente de cuán extensivo será el proceso de examen.

Medicamentos Recetados
Recuerda a los pacientes la necesidad de tomar la medicación recetada exactamente como se ha recetado. Incluye una descripción breve de los medicamentos que un profesional del cuidado de la salud oral probablemente recetará.

Ejemplo de Folleto para el Paciente
Un ejemplo de un folleto para la educación del paciente para penicilina V potásica.

Antibióticos Profilácticos para la Premedicación
Asegura la cooperación del paciente al proveer razones para la premedicación y una descripción breve de los medicamentos que probablemente se usarán en esta capacidad.

Línea de la Sonrisa (Labio)
Una explicación de cómo el labio contribuye a la estética general de la sonrisa del paciente y las maneras en que se puede alterar este componente.

Quedando Bien: Cómo Mantener Su Boca Saludable
Sugerencias de cómo un paciente puede tener una magnífica salud oral durante toda su vida.

Tratar a un Paciente Adulto
Información general de los cambios en las necesidades dentales de los pacientes adultos. Incluye comentarios sobre el envejecimiento, las restauraciones, la terapia endodóntica, la fractura del diente y la prevención de problemas.

Prevención
Al detallar los conceptos de prevención, estos documentos resumen conceptos claves como piedras angulares en la práctica.

Para una Vida con una Magnífica Salud Oral
Recomendaciones punto por punto para mantener una magnífica salud oral en los pacientes.

¡Como Cepillarse! ¡Como Limpiarse con Hilo Dental!
Descripción de la técnica de cepillar y limpiarse con el hilo dental, usada para recordar a los pacientes de lo que han aprendido durante su cita de higiene.

Alerta de Bebidas Chatarras
Notifica a los pacientes de una posible amenaza nueva a su salud oral y recomienda soluciones para el problema.

Prevención del Deterioro
Dirigida a las causas bacterianas de las infecciones y su prevención tanto en los infantes como los adultos.

Revisión del Contenido: Odontología en General—continuación

Cuándo las Radiografías Son Necesarias
Discute la necesidad de radiografías y medidas de seguridad.

Dar Marcha Atrás al Deterioro
Repasa el proceso de desmineralización y las maneras para parar el problema o darle marcha atrás.

Selladores y Fluoruro: Beneficios para los Pacientes Adultos
Explica la necesidad de los adultos de los selladores y el fluoruro tópico.

Fluoruro Tópico: En el Hogar y en la Oficina Dental
Exhorta a los pacientes que se aprovechen del uso de fluoruro en el hogar y/o en la oficina. Incluye instrucciones específicas para los procedimientos de aplicación de fluoruro por medio de cubeta.

Problemas: Causas y Curas
Cada documento describe una condición dental específica y las posibles opciones de tratamiento.

Abfracción: Un Nuevo Término Dental
Explica la abfracción, sus causas y las posibles opciones de tratamiento.

Reflujo Ácido (Enfermedad de Reflujo Gastroesofágico)
Explica la enfermedad de reflujo gastroesofágico y su impacto en la cavidad oral.

Atrición y Abrasión
Cubre el por qué del desgaste de los dientes, los hábitos de rechinar y apretar, la abrasión de la dentina y las opciones de tratamiento.

Mal Aliento
Discute la prevención y el tratamiento del mal aliento crónico.

Síndrome de Diente Fraccionado
Una visión general del síndrome del diente fraccionado, sus causas, el diagnóstico, las opciones de tratamiento y las consecuencias de no tratarlo.

Síndrome de Diente Fraccionado: Instrucciones Postoperatorias
Instrucciones postoperatorias para el tratamiento del síndrome del diente fraccionado por medio de ajuste ocluso, el reemplazo de una restauración o el colocar una corona provisional.

Deterioro de la Dentina
Explicación, detección y tratamiento del deterioro de la dentina, con información para la prevención.

Displasia del Esmalte
Se define la displasia del esmalte, y se explican las causas y los procedimientos correctivos. También se da información sobre la decalcificación del esmalte, la cual los pacientes pueden confundir con la displasia del esmalte.

Desgaste Excesivo
Un documento alterno sobre la abrasión, concentrado sólo en la abrasión sus causas, consecuencias y tratamiento.

Extracción
Una visión general breve de las razones para la extracción como también de lo que el paciente puede esperar después de la operación.

Extracción: Instrucciones Postoperatorias
Cuidado de seguimiento general y específico para los pacientes después de una extracción dental.

Dolores de Cabeza: La Conexión Dental
Explica la relación causal importante entre los dolores de cabeza y la disfunción de la articulación temporomandibular (DTM).

Cómo Fomentar el Deterioro de los Dientes (Humor)
Un repaso humorístico de la mejor manera de animar el deterioro de los dientes.

Siga

Revisión del Contenido: Odontología en General—continuación

Dientes Impactados
Una explicación de la impacción y de cuáles dientes se afectan comúnmente.

Grietas Inducidas en el Esmalte por las Empastaduras de Metal
Discute la posibilidad de remover las amalgamas cuando la aleación está causando fracciones o grietas en el esmalte. Posible precursor al síndrome de diente fraccionado.

Sensibilidad al Metal
Explica la detección de la sensibilidad al metal y la adaptación para pacientes sensibles al metal.

Protectores Oclusos (de Mordida)
Se clarifica la fabricación y los usos de aparatos antibruxismo/antirechinar.

Pericoronitis
Una descripción de la infección asociada comúnmente con los terceros molares y su posible tratamiento.

Caries en la Superficie Radicular
Discute los factores que contribuyen al deterioro de la raíz, el tratamiento y la prevención.

Dientes Sensibles
Describe las causas y el tratamiento para los dientes sensibles.

Cuestionario de Disfunción de la Articulación Temporomandibular (DTM)
Un cuestionario para que los profesionales del cuidado de la salud para usar en el diagnóstico de la disfunción de la articulación temporomandibular.

Síndrome de Disfunción de la Articulación Temporomandibular (DTM)
Describe el síndrome de disfunción de la articulación temporomandibular y las posibles opciones de tratamiento.

Abrasión por el Cepillo de Dientes: Evitando la Destrucción del Diente
Ayuda a los pacientes a comprender los efectos del cepillado incorrecto.

Oclusión Traumática: Equilibración Oclusal o Ajuste de la Mordida
Información acerca de las causas y tratamiento de la oclusión traumática.

Muelas Cordales (Terceros Molares)
Reafirma la confianza de los pacientes con un entendimiento de las muelas cordales, por qué las tenemos, los problemas que éstas causan y las razones para la extracción.

Xerostomía: Síndrome de Sequedad en la Boca
Provee una explicación de la xerostomía, sus consecuencias y la prevención de estas consecuencias.

Antes de Comenzar el Tratamiento

Mientras considera el tener un tratamiento dental extenso, puede ser beneficioso que repase los siguientes puntos:

- *Compromiso del Tiempo.* Debido a la naturaleza de las citas dentales, puede ser necesario que usted tome tiempo libre del trabajo. Algunas citas más largas son generalmente más eficientes y menos incómodas que muchas citas cortas. Esto reducirá su tiempo en la oficina. Usualmente, el mejor tiempo para tener una cita larga es por la mañana. Una vez que el tratamiento ha comenzado, necesita terminarse en una manera oportuna. Si el tratamiento se retrasa o pierde, podría cambiar el plan de tratamiento propuesto. Esto podría afectar desfavorablemente el costo total para usted.

- *La odontología es un arte y una ciencia.* En casos complicados y técnicamente difíciles, y debido a nuestros altos criterios, puede ser necesario rehacer una porción o volver para atrás o volver a tomar impresiones o volver a hacer las coronas, etc.

- *Asegúrese de que está enterado de qué tratamiento es requerido y las metas del tratamiento.* Si usted no entiende por qué hemos hecho una recomendación en particular o la secuencia del tratamiento o el largo del tratamiento requerido, por favor pídanos que le aclaremos antes de que el tratamiento comience. Es posible que problemas dentales previamente no detectados serán descubiertos una vez la preparación del diente ha comenzado. Cuando esto ocurre después de que se ha desarrollado el plan de tratamiento, usted será informado inmediatamente.

- *Usted debe estar cómodo con todos los arreglos financieros antes que se comience cualquier tratamiento.* El pre-estimado enviado al portador de seguro puede ayudarle a aproximar sus costos no pagados por el portador de seguro. Establezca su presupuesto dental. Esto determinará cuánto y qué tan rápido el tratamiento puede proceder. Entienda que usted, y no su portador de seguro, es en última instancia responsable por el costo total del tratamiento. Si usted quiere tener más tratamiento en una sola vez del que usted puede pagar con facilidad, los procedimientos dentales se pueden hacer en fases que pueden durar meses o años. Esto también permitirá que usted utilice sus beneficios del seguro al máximo permitido. El pago es esperado mientras se completa el trabajo.

- *El cuidado oral de sí mismo completo es muy importante, tanto al principio del tratamiento como después.* Mientras mejor es su salud oral, más fácil será el proceso de restauración. Se le puede pedir que utilice un enjuague bucal antimicrobiano recetado 2 semanas antes de que comencemos el tratamiento hasta después que todo el tratamiento restaurativo se termine. Por favor, siga estas instrucciones.

- *Aunque las restauraciones dentales funcionan bien por años de servicio, nada dura por siempre.* Ni nosotros, ni las restauraciones dentales. Nosotros utilizamos los mejores materiales y técnicas dentales disponibles, pero la realidad es que algunas restauraciones duran más tiempo que otras. Hoy en día, con una duración de vida más larga, ¡la restauración puede que incluso se gaste! Mientras mejor usted mantiene sus restauraciones dentales, más tiempo le durarán. Como con cualquier otra cosa, mantenimiento apropiado es requerido.

- *Antes de comenzar el tratamiento, entienda claramente qué será requerido por su parte para su cuidado oral diario, sus citas periódicas de cuidado con profesionales de la higiene dental y las limitaciones de las restauraciones y prótesis dentales que usted recibirá.* Esto significa que usted debe cepillar y limpiar con hilo dental sus dientes como se le enseñó todos los días. Cuando se completa un tratamiento odontológico extenso, se aconseja fuertemente un intervalo de 3 a 4 meses para las citas dentales periódicas de higiene de cuidado repetido.

- *Las restauraciones dentales están sujetas al mismo abuso físico que los dientes naturales.* Cualesquiera de los hábitos orales que romperán un diente natural, sin taladrar, sin daño—por ejemplo masticar hielo, morderse las uñas, objetos duros, etc.—probablemente pueden romper una restauración también. La expansión y las contracciones debido a los líquidos calientes y los alimentos fríos pueden causar daño, al igual que el ambiente oral húmedo, oscuro y lleno de bacterias de la cavidad oval.

- *Si usted ha considerado alguna vez el blanquear sus dientes, el tiempo para hacer esto es antes de que las restauraciones dentales se coloquen en los dientes que son visibles cuando usted habla o sonríe.* ¡Si usted está interesado en el blanqueo de dientes, pregúntenos ahora!

Anatomía Dental y Oral

La Anatomía de los Dientes

Corona: la parte del diente que es visible sobre el borde de la encía

Raíz: la parte del diente que no es visible normalmente y que está debajo del borde de la encía

Esmalte: la cubierta externa de la corona del diente

Los dientes son una de las sustancias más duras que ocurren naturalmente en el cuerpo. Son lo suficientemente fuertes para resistir adecuadamente el uso normal que ocurre a lo largo de la vida masticando alimentos. Los dientes se componen de varias partes diferentes—esmalte, dentina, cemento y tejido de la pulpa (nervio). El esmalte es la cubierta exterior del diente. Es la parte del diente que usted normalmente ve cuando una persona sonríe. Aunque el esmalte es muy duro, es también muy frágil. Es mayormente de naturaleza inorgánica. Cuando el fluoruro es incorporado en el esmalte, (sistemáticamente cuando el esmalte se está formando, tópicamente cuando el diente está en la boca), llega a ser más resistente al ataque de los ácidos y al deterioro. El esmalte del diente cubre las capas internas de la parte de la corona del diente.

Dentina: la capa debajo del esmalte

La dentina normalmente no es visible. Solamente cuando un diente se parte o se gasta, puede ser notada. La dentina es de color más oscuro, más suave y más flexible que el esmalte. Las fibras pequeñas del nervio que van de la dentina a la pulpa pueden hacer el diente sensible a los cambios de temperatura o a otros estímulos cuando la dentina está expuestas a la cavidad bucal. Si un diente es sensible, la dentina expuesta muchas veces es la razón. La dentina, cuando está expuesta a la cavidad bucal, se gastara más rápidamente que el esmalte y esto puede conducir a otros problemas dentales.

Pulpa: la capa más interna del diente

La pulpa del diente se compone de material suave, altamente orgánico—mayormente fibras del nervio y vasos sanguíneos. Cuando la pulpa se daña por deterioro profundo u otros problemas dentales, puede volverse apostemada y debe entonces ser tratada con terapia endodóntica (canal radicular) o ser extraída.

Cemento: la cubierta externa de la raíz del diente

La raíz de un diente no se ve normalmente. Es rodeada y cubierta por hueso y tejido de la encía. La raíz está cubierta por una capa delgada de cemento. El cemento es similar a la dentina en la composición y puede deteriorarse o gastarse si está expuesto en la boca. Las fibras que unen el diente al hueso se encajan en la raíz del cemento y sirven como amortiguadores durante el funcionamiento normal, tal como masticación.

Hueso: la estructura que hace las mandíbulas

El hueso que rodea cada diente es menos denso en la mandíbula superior y más denso en la mandíbula inferior. Como con el hueso en otras partes del cuerpo, puede experimentar resorción y reparación. Los espacios en los cuales los dientes descansan, llamados *alvéolos,* proporcionan los caminos para una fuente rica de sangre y nutrientes y de otros líquidos vitales para alcanzar los dientes.

Con el cuidado y la atención apropiada, sus dientes le servirán bien toda la vida. Cepíllese y límpiese con hilo dental, diariamente. Véanos para los exámenes periódicos y las citas de higiene dental (limpieza) preventiva tres veces al año. Investigaciones demuestran que un intervalo de 3 a 4 meses promoverá la **prevención** de la enfermedad oral con más eficacia que un programa de dos veces al año. Su meta y nuestra meta es prevenir la enfermedad oral.

Si usted tiene cualquier pregunta sobre la anatomía dental y oral, favor de sentirse libre de preguntarnos.

Obtenga la Odontología Que Usted Necesita, Quiere y Se Merece

Se le ha dado la información verbal y escrita que describe detalladamente sus problemas dentales y las alternativas de tratamiento disponibles para eliminar estos problemas. Usted necesita esta información para basar su decisión en hechos. Como su dentista nosotros debemos, por ley, informarle sus problemas dentales y las alternativas de tratamientos que podemos proporcionar. Usted debe también entender la responsabilidad financiera implicada, porque usted tendrá que hacer arreglos financieros para pagar todos los procedimientos.

Cómo Saber Que Es lo Mejor

Una manera de determinar la mejor manera de proceder en la restauración de su boca para una salud oral óptima es decidiendo cuánto tiempo usted desea que las restauraciones duren antes de que tengan que ser reemplazadas. Es un hecho de la vida que casi cualquier cosa que un dentista hace para usted (cualquier tipo de empastadura o restauración colocada) eventualmente necesitará ser reemplazada. Las leyes de la física y química no pueden ser simplemente suspendidas. Todos los materiales de empastadura están sujetos a fatiga. Cuando la fatiga alcanza cierto punto, la empastadura se rompe y el diente se debe restaurar otra vez.

Usted tiene gran control sobre el intervalo al cual las empastaduras deben ser reemplazadas. En resumen, usted obtiene por lo que usted paga. Las restauraciones que durarán por más tiempo y protegen el diente costarán más inicialmente. Si examinamos esta opción a largo plazo, usted terminará pagando menos dinero por la empastadura del diente porque la misma restauración no tendrá que ser reemplazada, y pagada, repetidas veces.

Las restauraciones menos costosas pueden trabajar muy bien, pero generalmente por un tiempo más corto. La mayoría de las restauraciones menos costosas necesitarán ser reemplazadas en al menos de 5 a 12 años. Las coronas, puentes y inlays y onlays en oro o porcelana procesados o fabricados en el laboratorio pueden durar mucho más tiempo. No es inusual para un inlay de oro durar 25 años o más. Pero, nuevamente, este tipo de restauración costará más inicialmente.

La experiencia del dentista, así como la calidad de los materiales, es un aspecto importante a considerar cuando toma sus decisiones de tratamiento. Pero el mejor dentista no puede hacer que un material menos costoso, colocado directamente dure tanto tiempo o proteja el diente tan bien como el material más costoso procesado en un laboratorio.

Nuestra Recomendación

Lo que recomendamos es que el mejor material o restauración más duradera sea colocado primero. Hágalo bien la primera vez y no tendrá que ser hecho otra vez—tan pronto. Si su situación financiera y la cantidad de tratamiento dental dictan que usted no puede completar inmediatamente toda la odontología deseada, entonces el tratamiento se puede hacer en fases de semanas, meses o años. De esta manera, sobre el curso del tiempo, usted puede tener la odontología que usted necesita, desea y se merece.

Le haremos sugerencias indicando lo que pensamos es el mejor curso del tratamiento para usted. También le aconsejaremos tratamientos alternos y le diremos las ventajas y desventajas de las posibilidades. La decisión final es suya. Aunque no forzaremos nuestras recomendaciones sobre usted, si deseamos proveerle las mejores restauraciones, más duraderas y de mejor protección que la odontología tiene que ofrecer, incluso si no se pueden hacer todas de una vez.

Si usted tiene cualquier pregunta sobre sus necesidades dentales, favor de sentirse libre de preguntarnos.

Procedimientos de Control de Infecciones

Si usted ha sido un paciente de esta oficina por cualquier periodo tiempo, usted sabe que hemos estado preocupados con los procedimientos apropiados del control de infección mucho antes de que se convirtió en una regulación para la odontología. Usamos guantes para cada paciente. Los guantes se utilizan una vez y después se botan. Desde la década del 1970, hemos utilizado protección para los ojos, batas y máscaras para los procedimientos durante los cuales puede haber un aerosol atomizador o salpicadura de materiales potencialmente infecciosos. Esto fue mucho tiempo antes de que se convirtiera en un requisito. Hemos usado batas clínicas por años. Cambiamos nuestra ropa de la calle cuando entramos en la oficina, y cambiamos nuestra vestimenta de la clínica cuando salimos. Si usted es nuevo en la oficina, conozca por favor que hemos tomado siempre el control de infección y su seguridad, así como la nuestra, seriamente.

Todos los instrumentos que deben ser reutilizados se limpian correctamente según el protocolo más reciente aprobado para la odontología. Los instrumentos son colocados en bolsas y después se esterilizan. Las bolsas se abren en la presencia del paciente sólo cuando son necesarias para un procedimiento dental. Hemos estado esterilizando los instrumentos de esta manera por años - mucho antes que cualquiera de las regulaciones gubernamentales.

Cuando es posible, compramos artículos desechables que pueden ser usados una sola vez, los cuales se desechan correctamente después de usarlos una vez. El costo de artículos desechables es mayor que el costo de productos y de instrumentos dentales reutilizables.

Las piezas de mano han sido siempre desinfectadas y esterilizadas de acuerdo a las instrucciones del fabricante. Todas las piezas de mano se esterilizan después de cada uso. Cada año, gastamos miles de dólares en nuevas piezas de mano y en la reparación las piezas de mano dañadas por el proceso de la esterilización.

Siempre hemos estado preocupados por la esterilización apropiada: esto no es nuevo para esta oficina. Lo que es nuevo es el costo. Con una mayor demanda por los productos de esterilización y desinfección, universalmente, el costo para nosotros se ha elevado dramáticamente. Los cálculos demuestran que los procedimientos de esterilización agregan un costo considerable a la visita del paciente—entre 8 y 15 dólares **por visita del paciente**. Este costo estimado cubre los costos de los artículos de esterilización y desinfección aumento de costos por compras y reparaciones más frecuentes de piezas de mano dentales, y el costo del tiempo (aproximadamente de 12 a 15 minutos) para limpiar debidamente el cuarto de tratamiento después de cada uso. Está también el costo del sueldo pagado a los miembros del equipo dental que pasan más tiempo con procedimientos de control de infecciones mandatarios, por lo tanto, menos tiempo con el tratamiento dental del paciente. Estos costos añadidos son considerables. Los portadores de seguro dental todavía no han aumentado los pagos para reflejar el aumento en los costos.

No estamos dispuestos a comprometer su salud y nuestra salud por no seguir las pautas apropiadas del control de infección. Seguimos las guías del Acto de Seguridad y Salud Ocupacional (OSHA, por sus siglas en inglés) (para el empleado y el lugar de trabajo) y las guías del Centro para el Control de Enfermedad (CDC, por sus siglas en inglés) (para el paciente). Con excepción de la nueva montaña de papeleo requerida, nuestra oficina no tuvo que realizar ningún cambio para cumplir con las guías del CDC: ya estábamos siguiendo todas las guías y procedimientos para el control de infección.

Si usted tiene cualquier pregunta sobre los procedimientos de control de infecciones, favor de sentirse libre de preguntarnos.

Examen Oral Inicial

Una de las partes más importantes del tratamiento dental exitoso es el **examen oral inicial** completo. Para poder hacer una diagnóstico preciso, y luego un plan de tratamiento apropiado para usted, debemos saber la naturaleza exacta de cualquier patología (enfermedad) presente en su boca. Incluso si no hay enfermedad dental presente al momento del examen oral inicial, es extremadamente importante el registrar el aspecto normal de su boca, de modo que en si acontece un cambio, podamos hacer un diagnóstico apropiado. Esta línea basal en el registro hace posible el poder juzgar más precisamente el progreso y la severidad del cambio que ha ocurrido.

El examen oral inicial incluye la inspección de su cabeza, cuello y estructuras faciales, y la palpitación de los nódulos linfáticos en el cuello. Examinamos su articulación temporomandibular (articulación de la mandíbula o ATM) para un funcionamiento apropiado. Observamos la condición de sus labios, el interior de sus cachetes, la lengua, glándulas y las aperturas de los conductos de las glándulas, ligamentos del músculo y el paladar duro y suave. Esto todo ocurre antes de que incluso miremos sus dientes y encías.

Al examinar sus dientes, registramos en la gráfica dental cuántos dientes hay y cuáles faltan. Miramos la alineación del diente y el estado del deterioro. Además, registramos en la gráfica dental las restauraciones existentes y que restauraciones pueden estar rotas o defectuosas y necesitan ser reemplazadas. Si usted tiene dientes de reemplazo, ya sean dentaduras parciales (las cuales son removibles) o coronas fijas, determinamos su condición y función actual. Si le faltan dientes, comenzamos a determinar si considerar su reemplazo es lo mejor para su salud dental.

También miramos la apariencia de sus dientes, la posición de sus dientes, como se ve cuando sonríe; en resumen, como otras personas ven sus dientes. Anotamos irregularidades en la alineación de los dientes y los desteñimientos en los dientes y las empastaduras que pueden disminuir su apariencia.

Examinamos el soporte para sus dientes, encías y hueso. Vemos el color, contorno, textura y consistencia del tejido de la encía rodeando el diente. Cuidadosamente determinamos si hay sangrado de las encías. Anotamos cualquier recesión del tejido donde el tejido de la encía ha sido sacado de su posición original contra el diente. Utilizamos una sonda periodontal para ayudar a medir y a cuantificar la salud de sus encías, mientras verificamos la profundidad sulcular (bolsillos periodontales) alrededor del diente. La movilidad de los dientes también se verifica. Señales de la enfermedad de las encías incluye, pero no están limitadas a, sangrado espontáneo de las encías o cuando son sondeadas, recesión de las encías, enrojecimiento e hinchazón, exudado (pus) y movilidad de los dientes.

Para ser completo, el examen debe también incluir una evaluación de radiografías recientes (rayos-X) de la calidad de diagnóstico. Dependiendo de la condición de su boca, podemos necesitar de 14 a 20 radiografías recientes. De las radiografías, podemos examinar más directamente la salud del hueso que en última instancia soporta los dientes. Inspeccionamos para dientes que no han salido o retenidos, deterioro que puede estar presente debajo de empastaduras viejas o entre los dientes y áreas de infección alrededor de las raíces que pueden requerir terapia endodóntica (tratamiento del canal radicular). Un estimado de la altura del hueso alrededor del diente y anormalidades que pueden existir son también anotadas. Un diagnóstico completo no se puede hacer sin esta herramienta de diagnóstico, tomamos solamente el número necesario de radiografías de sus dientes. Estamos bien enterados de los peligros que enfrentan el paciente y la persona que hace las exposiciones radiográficas. La práctica segura para la toma de radiografías es extremadamente importante para nosotros.

Para ciertos tipos de tratamiento, podemos también necesitar tomar fotografías intraorales, imágenes de video, impresiones para los modelos de estudio de las relaciones de los dientes y la mordida (arco).

Algunas partes del examen serán terminadas y registradas por el personal auxiliar dental entrenado y licenciado tal como higienistas dentales y ayudantes dentales.

Usando los resultados de los hallazgos del diagnóstico y sus preocupaciones expresadas, llegaremos al diagnóstico de su condición dental. Podemos entonces formular planes de tratamiento con las opciones apropiadas que tratarán todas sus necesidades. Solamente cuando esto es realizado su tratamiento dental puede comenzar.

Debido a las muchas facetas de un examen oral inicial completo, usted puede ver que no puede ser realizado adecuadamente en 10 minutos. Mientras más su boca se desvía de lo ideal (todos los dientes en su lugar, alineación perfecta, sin restauraciones [empastaduras] y sin enfermedad de las encías), más tiempo el examen tomará. Si su boca se ha descuidado o se ha cuidado incorrectamente, el examen podría tomar más de una hora para completarse. Deseamos proveerle el mejor cuidado oral posible y éste comienza con en examen dental completo.

Si usted tiene cualquier pregunta sobre el examen oral inicial, favor de sentirse libre de preguntarnos.

Medicamentos Recetados

La Dosis Correcta Es Importante

La parte más importante cuando se toman medicamentos recetados es estar seguro que se toman según lo indicado. No se diagnostique y no se trate usted mismo decidiendo que usted no necesita continuar tomando su medicación (especialmente antibióticos) cuando comienza a sentirse mejor. Los medicamentos se diseñan para ser tomados en dosis específicas por largos de tiempo específicos para curar o aliviar problemas específicos. Cambiando la cantidad que usted está tomando o el largo de tiempo que usted está tomando la medicación recetada podría anular su efecto.

Mantenga a Su Equipo Dental Informado

Es también importante que su equipo dental esté informado de todos los medicamentos que usted está tomando actualmente. Los medicamentos interactúan y la interacción podría ser indeseable. Deberíamos también estar informados de cualquier problema que usted ha tenido con algún medicamento recetado en el pasado. Éstos pueden incluir, pero no están limitados a, reacciones alérgicas, malestar estomacal, erupciones, ronchas, dificultad para respirar, náusea y picazón.

Analgésicos **No Opioides** acetaminofeno (Tylenol) aspirina (Zorprim, Ascriptin)	**Cefalosporinas** cefaclor (Ceclor) cefalexina (Keflex)

Analgésicos **Opioides**
 acetaminofeno con codeína
    (Tylenol con codeína números
    2, 3, ó 4)
 meperidina (Demerol)
 propoxifena clorhidrato (Darvon)
 napsilato de propoxifena (Darvon-N)
	Fluoroquinolonas
	 ciprofloxacina (Cipro)
	
	 Drogas No Esteroide Antiinflamatorias Drogas
	 (NSAIDs siglas en inglés)
	 celecoxib (Celebrex)
	 diflunisal (Dolobid)
	 etodolac (Lodine)
	 ibuprofen (Motrin)
	 naproxen sodio (Anaprox)
	 rofecoxib (Vioxx)

Ansiolítico/Sedante-Antihipnóticas diazepam (Valium)	
Antiinfectivos eritromicina (Erytroderm)	**Penicilinas** amoxicilina (Amoxil) penicilina V potásica (V-Cillin K)
Antivirales (topicas) penciclovir (Denavir)	**Tetraciclinas** doxiciclina (Atridox, Periostat, Vibramycin) minociclina (Minocin, Arestin) tetraciclina (Achromycin)
Antiulcerativo amlexanox (Aphthasol): usada para tratar estomatitis eftosa	

Por favor vea las dos páginas siguientes (pp. 491-492) para ver un folleto para la educación del paciente para V-Cillin K. El CD que acompaña este libro provee folletos para la educación del paciente para **todos** de los medicamentos enumerados arriba que pueden adaptarse para su oficina. Para obtener acceso a los folletos de educación del paciente para drogas adicionales recetadas a los pacientes dentales, véase por favor el CD que acompaña Gage TW, Pickett FA: *Mosby's Dental Drug Reference, ed 6.* St. Louis, 2003, Mosby, Inc. o visite **www.mosby.com/dental** para información para comprarlo.

Información técnica obtenida de *Mosby's Drug Consult 2003,* en línea www.mosbysdrugconsult.com y Gage TW, Pickett FA: *Mosby's Dental Drug Reference,* ed 6, St. Louis, 2003, Mosby, Inc.

Favor de informarnos sobre cualquier medicamento que usted está tomando, (incluyendo medicamentos no recetados) para poder verificar las posibles interacciones de drogas antes de escribir una receta para un nuevo medicamento.

Ejemplo de Folleto para el Paciente

Nombre:_____

Este medicamento es recetado para:_____

Dosis y hora para tomarlo:_____

ID Genérico #: d001971

Forma—Oral

Nombre Genérico:

Penicilina V Potásica (pe nee see leé nah vay po tah'see kah)

Otros nombres
Pen-Vee K
V-Cillin K

¿Qué Es Penicilina V Potásica?

Penicilina V es usada para:

- Tratar diferentes clases de infecciones (incluyendo infecciones de los oídos, nariz, garganta, piel y tracto respiratorio).
- Prevenir fiebre reumática y gonorrea en personas que han tenido estos problemas antes.

¿Cómo Utilizo la Penicilina V Potásica?

- Tome este medicamento por la boca.
- Tome este medicamento alrededor de la misma hora cada día.
- Si olvida tomar una dosis, salte esa dosis y tome la próxima dosis a la hora regular.
- Tome este medicamento hasta se acabe todo, aun si se siente mejor.
- Mida la forma liquida de este medicamento usando una cuchara de medir o un gotero, no con una cuchara de cocina.

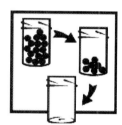

Tome este medicamento hasta
que se acabe todo, aun si se siente mejor.

Efectos Secundarios

Diga a su doctor sobre cualquier efecto secundario que le suceda.

Posibles Efectos Secundarios

- Vómitos
- Diarrea espesa
- Dolor de estómago
- Lengua negra y lanuda

Efectos Secundarios Raros/Severos

- Ronchas
- Picazón

Busque atención médica inmediata si cualesquiera de estos efectos secundarios le suceden.

- Problemas para tragar
- Dificultad para respirar
- Problemas para respirar
- La sensación mareo o desmayo
- Mareo cuando está parado
- Mareo cuando está sentado

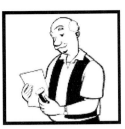

Tome este medicamento exactamente como su doctor le diga.

Hacer

- Tome este medicamento exactamente como su doctor le diga.
- Hable con su doctor o farmacéutico si usted tiene algunas preguntas o preocupaciones acerca de este medicamento.
- Diga a su doctor si usted ha tenido una reacción a este medicamento o a cualquier otro medicamento.
- Mantenga este medicamento en un lugar fresco, seco ausente de la luz del sol.
- Mantenga la forma líquida de este medicamento en el refrigerador.
- Agite bien siempre la forma líquida de este medicamento antes de usarlo.
- Enjuague la cuchara de medir o el gotero después de usar la forma líquida de este medicamento.
- Tire cualquier medicamento líquido que quede después de 14 días.

No Hacer

- No tome más de una dosis a la vez.
- No aumente la cantidad de la dosis a menos que esté dirigido por su doctor.
- No comience a tomar ningún medicamento nuevo (incluyendo píldoras para el control de la natalidad) sin primero decirle a su doctor o farmacéutico.
- No mantenga este medicamento en el baño debido al calor y la humedad.

Este folleto no contiene todas los posibles usos, acciones, precauciones, efectos secundarios o interacciones de este medicamento y está destinado a ser un resumen de la información solamente. Por favor, contacte a su médico o farmacéutico directamente, si usted tiene algunas preguntas o preocupaciones.

Instrucciones especiales

Antibióticos Profilácticos para la Premedicación

Hay ciertas condiciones de salud que pueden conducir a la debilitación de una válvula en su corazón. Si las bacterias se introducen en su corriente sanguínea, hay un riesgo de que estas bacterias pueden alojarse en esa válvula débil y causar una inflamación del revestimiento de su corazón. Ésta es una condición seria llamada la *endocarditis infecciosa,* la cual puede tener consecuencias significativas en la su salud. **Por esta razón, si lo han diagnosticado con cualesquiera de las siguientes condiciones, usted necesitará estar premedicado antes de algunos o de todos los tipos de tratamiento dental:**

- a un historial médico de prolapso de la válvula mitral con regurcitación valvular y/o aletas gruesas
- válvula prostética del corazón incluyendo las válvulas bioprostéticas y homoinjertos valvulares
- reemplazo de las coyunturas tales como caderas o rodillas
- enfermedad cardíaca congénita compleja cianótica
- enfermedad cardíaca reumática
- cardiomiopatía hipertrófica
- reemplazo con injertos de tejidos animal
- endocarditis bacteriana subaguda
- dispositivos intravasculares de acceso (para quimioterapia, hemodialisis, hiperalimentación)
- desviaciones del líquido cerebroespinal

Antes de poder comenzar el tratamiento en algunos casos, debemos consultar con su médico para determinar que premedicación es recomendada para su condición específica. Cuando se ha determinado que usted necesita premedicación antes de los procedimientos dentales, le preguntaremos antes de cada cita dental si usted ha tomado la premedicación.

Cuando su médico, cirujano o cardiólogo determina que lo mejor para usted es que sea premedicado antes de ciertos procedimientos dentales, usted debe tomar el premedicamento. Su médico puede recetar un antibiótico diferente de los enumerados abajo.

Si usted no lo ha tomado según recetado, no podremos realizar ningún tratamiento dental. No hay excepciones. El resultado puede ser una enfermedad seria con una estancia prolongada en el hospital.

Régimen Estándar Recomendado para la Prevención de Endocarditis
Adultos

Situación	Agente	Régimen
Profilaxis general estándar	Amoxicilina	2.0 g oral 1 hora antes del procedimientos
Incapaz de tomar la medicación oralmente	Ampicilina	2.0 g intramuscular (IM) o intravenosa (IV) en el plazo de 30 minutos antes del procedimiento
Alérgico a la penicilina	Clindamicina o	600 mg oral 1 hora antes del procedimiento
	Cefalexina[†] o cefadroxil[†] o	2.0 g oral 1 hora antes del procedimiento
	Azithromicina o clarithromicina	500 mg oral 1 hora antes del procedimiento
Alérgico a la penicilina e incapaz de tomar la medicación oralmente	Clindamicina o	600 mg IV en el plazo de 30 minutos antes del procedimiento
	Cefazolina	1.0 g IM o IV en el plazo de 30 minutos antesdel procedimiento

[†]*Las cefalosporinas no deben utilizarse en personas con reacción de hipersensibilidad de tipo inmediato (urticaria, edema angioneurótico, anafilaxis) a la penicilina.*

Siga

Régimen Estándar Recomendado para la Prevención de Endocarditis—continuación
Niños

Situación	Agente	Régimen*
Profilaxis general estándar	Amoxicilina	50 mg/kg** 1 hora antes del procedimiento
Incapaz de tomar la medicación oralmente	Ampicilina	50 mg/kg** IM o IV en el plazo de 30 minutos antes del procedimiento
Alérgico a la penicilina	Clindamicina o	20 mg/kg** 1 hora antes del procedimiento
	Cefalexina[†] o cefadroxil[†] o	50 mg/kg** 1 hora antes del procedimiento
	Azithromicina o clarithromicina	15 mg/kg** 1 hora antes del procedimiento
Alérgico a la penicilina e incapaz de tomar la medicación oralmente	Clindamicina o	20 mg/kg** IV en el plazo de 30 minutos antes del procedimiento
	Cefazolina[†]	25 mg/kg** IM o IV en el plazo de 30 minutos antes del procedimiento

*La dosis total de los niños no debe exceder la dosis del adulto.
**Conversión de kilogramos a libras: 1kg = 2.2 lb.
[†]Las cephalosporinas no deben utilizarse en personas con reacción de hipersensibilidad de tipo inmediato (urticaria, edema angioneurótico, anafilaxis) a la penicilina.

Si usted tiene cualquier pregunta sobre los antibióticos profilácticos para la premedicación, favor de sentirse libre de preguntarnos.

Línea de la Sonrisa (Labio)

Cuántos dientes usted enseña cuando sonríe o habla, y cuánto de cada diente (longitud) se exhibe cuando usted sonríe ampliamente o (en el lado opuesto del espectro) cuando sus labios están en reposo es una función de donde su labio superior está conectado a su cara—y cuántos años usted tiene.

Hay tres clasificaciones de la "línea de la sonrisa" que los dentistas utilizan—baja, mediana y alta. Una línea de la sonrisa *baja* es una en la cual muy poco de sus dientes es visible cuando usted habla o sonríe. Alguien con una línea de la sonrisa baja demostrará, como mucho, un milímetro o dos del borde de la mordida del diente. Una línea de la sonrisa *mediana* hará visible la mayoría del diente, hasta e incluyendo un milímetro o dos del tejido de la encía. Una persona con una línea la de sonrisa *alta* demostrará todos los dientes delanteros superiores y una cantidad significativa del tejido de la encía al hablar o sonreír.

Los dentistas (y cirujanos plásticos) no han sido muy exitosos cambiando quirúrgicamente la línea de la sonrisa baja, mediana o alta. Hay algunos 'trucos' dentales que se pueden utilizar en situaciones limitadas para reducir la cantidad de exhibición de la encía evidente con una línea de la sonrisa alta. La mayoría de los procedimientos correctivos para mejorar la estética en esta situación requieren inversiones significativas de tiempo y dinero. La cirugía periodontal (de la encía), solamente o en conjunto con laminados de porcelana o coronas de cerámica, es lo más común. En casos extremos la única opción puede ser volver a colocar quirúrgicamente la maxilar entera (con o sin ortodoncia). Inversamente, la apariencia de no demostrar ningún diente al hablar o sonreír está asociada con el envejecimiento avanzado.

Hay otro componente de cuánto de sus dientes enseña cuando sus labios están en reposo—y esto tiene ver con gravedad y tiempo. Su cara y labios se componen de tejido suave que está bajo desafío constante de la gravedad. La gravedad siempre gana, si se le da suficiente tiempo. Los tejidos de la piel y de la piel secundaria caen con el pasar de los años. Si, con sus labios en reposo, usted enseñaba alrededor de 3mm de los bordes de mordida en los dos dientes delanteros superiores cuando usted tenía 20 años de edad, para el momento en que usted tenga 40, usted puede demostrar solamente 2mm del borde. Alguien de 50 años de edad puede enseñar 1mm, y a los 60 años ningún diente es visto cuando los labios están en reposo. Los tejidos de la cara humana caerán cerca de 1mm cada 10 años, comenzando alrededor de los cuarenta años. A medida que tejidos faciales pierden elasticidad, caen lentamente. Obviamente, algunas personas afortunadas tiene una mejor genética y sus caras permanecerán firmes y el tejido caerá más lentamente. El corregir el tejido de la caída relacionada con la edad se puede hacer con cirugía plástica—el estiramiento facial común.

¿Genética o Gravedad? Si usted está leyendo esto, entonces usted ha hecho preguntas sobre su sonrisa y la línea de la sonrisa o este problema se ha tratado en un contexto más amplio de los procedimientos cosméticos de la odontología que usted requiere. Después de un examen cuidadoso, nosotros explicaremos qué situación usted tiene y qué medidas correctivas son posibles.

Si usted tiene cualquier pregunta sobre su línea de la sonrisa, favor de sentirse libre de preguntarnos.

Quedando Bien: Cómo Mantener Su Boca Saludable

¡Felicitaciones! Usted ha terminado todo el tratamiento dental necesario hasta este punto. Si usted sigue las sugerencias mencionadas, usted tendrá la mejor oportunidad de mantener su salud oral óptima por un tiempo más largo. Si usted esta inseguro sobre cualquier cosa de lo que usted debe hacer, por favor pídanos instrucción adicional.

Cepille, limpie con hilo dental y use las de ayudas dentales de limpieza recomendadas correctamente, por lo menos una vez cada día. Utilice un enjuague bucal con fluoruro (no una medicación de recetada) por lo menos una vez cada día.

POR FAVOR venga a la oficina para las citas de cuidado repetido de la higiene, en los intervalos específicos que recomendamos. Esto es muy importante. Cada boca es diferente. De acuerdo con el número de restauraciones dentales que usted tiene, el número y la alineación de sus dientes, su habilidad aparente en este momento para mantener sus dientes limpios y su historial médico, recomendamos que el intervalo no sea más largo de _____ meses. Con este intervalo, hay una mejor oportunidad de prevenir la enfermedad o de corregir los problemas encontrados temprano, cuando son pequeños, más fáciles y menos costosos de tratar.

Cada vez que usted venga para la limpieza y examen de sus dientes, haga su próxima cita de cuidado repetido antes de salir de la oficina. De esta manera usted permanecerá en el "sistema" y no se perderá. Pero por favor intente recordar cuando es su cita. No importa cuan atractiva hacemos nuestras tarjetas de recordatorio, parecen tener el hábito mezclarse con el correo de los anuncios y ser botadas sin ser notadas.

Si usted ha seguido nuestro consejo, hemos utilizado los procedimientos y materiales mejores y más apropiados para usted. Usted debe recibir años de servicio exitoso de ellos. Los dientes naturales y los materiales restaurativos están sujetos a gran tensión diariamente. Por favor no ponga cosas en su boca que no pertenecen allí. Esto acortará enormemente la vida útil de sus dientes y restauraciones.

No mastique hielo o barras congeladas de dulces, bombones o mantenga bombones o mentas para aliento en su boca como una rutina diaria. Cualquier alimento azucarado que usted mantenga su boca durante mucho tiempo (mientras se disuelve) puede fácilmente y rápidamente causar deterioro del diente.

Si usted fuma, pare. Si usted no puede parar, recuerde que el fumar tiene un efecto negativo en sus tejidos de las encías y en su salud en general.

El fumar, el café, el té y las bebidas de cola tienen la tendencia a manchar o a obscurecer los dientes con el pasar del tiempo. Esto se puede evitar con una higiene dental de cuidado repetido regular, y si es necesario, procedimientos para blanquear los dientes no invasivos.

Si usted está teniendo su tratamiento dental por fases ya sea por razones de tiempo o financieras, por favor haga una nota para usted para continuar cuando hemos discutido.

Si usted tiene un protector bucal (para proteger restauraciones nuevas o reducir los efectos de bruxismo/habito de rechinar), por favor úselo como se le indicó.

Hemos utilizado el conocimiento del diagnóstico y tratamiento, procedimientos y los materiales disponibles más apropiados para su tratamiento. Como cualquier pieza de una maquinaria, el servicio rutinario es necesario si la máquina (o sus dientes y restauraciones) va a durar el mayor tiempo posible. Los dientes y las restauraciones se pueden romper por fuerza excesiva o trauma. Si usted cuida su carro, durará más que si nunca le cambia el aceite, fluidos, etc., y le costará mucho menos para que siga funcionando. Sus dientes y encías necesitan cuidado regular también. Ningún tratamiento individual cuesta tanto como su carro, pero con el cuidado adecuado, usted probablemente seguirá teniendo restauraciones hasta mucho después que el carro sea historia. Gracias por darnos la oportunidad de servirle, y esperamos verle pronto.

Tratar a un Paciente Adulto

La Edad Afecta las Necesidades

Las necesidades de tratamiento dental cambian a medida que usted envejece. De nuestros años de experiencia dental, hemos encontrado que las necesidades dentales de un paciente adulto caen en dos categorías diferentes: aquellos que no tienen un historial de muchas restauraciones (empastaduras) y aquellos que han tenido sus dientes taladrados y empastados repetidas veces al pasar de los años.

El primer grupo es afortunado. Aunque el deterioro nuevo puede comenzar en cualquier momento, mientras más usted envejece, es menos la probabilidad de que le den caries nuevas. Cuando esos adultos que han tenido pocas empastaduras se cepillan y se limpian con hilo dental para prevenir la enfermedad periodontal, ellos probablemente desarrollen menos problemas dentales nuevos. Restauraciones viejas no necesitan reemplazo frecuente (especialmente si las empastaduras son solamente empastaduras pequeñas). La necesidad para coronas, puentes, implantes o tratamiento endodóntico (terapia del canal radicular) es mínima.

Restauraciones Múltiples

Aquellos que han tenido numerosas empastaduras al pasar de los años probablemente experimenten más necesidades dentales que el primer grupo. Las restauraciones existentes grandes tienen la tendencia a romperse más frecuentemente que las empastaduras pequeñas. Cuando un diente tiene una empastadura grande, esto significa que queda menos diente natural, lo que puede llevar a fracturas. Las empastaduras de plata son mantenidas en su lugar por el diente alrededor. Cuando no queda diente suficiente, las empastaduras de plata no duran por mucho tiempo. El segundo grupo puede esperar que los dientes empastados pesadamente se partan y hasta que una restauración de molde (corona o inlay) sea necesaria para restaurar el diente.

Restauraciones de Molde

Las restauraciones de molde procesadas en el laboratorio duraran más que los materiales colocados directamente (empastaduras de plata). De hecho, sería inteligente el considerar la colocación de restauraciones de molde (cuando es indicado) temprano mejor que tarde. Esto puede eliminar el tener que taladrar en el futuro y el empeoramientodel paciente.

Terapia Endodóntica

El paciente adulto que ha tenido historia de deterioro de restauraciones de moderadas a severas puede también requerir más tratamiento endodóntico (canales radiculares) que un adulto que tiene pocas empastaduras. Las restauraciones más grandes son más propensas a estar situadas muy cerca al nervio de la raíz. Al pasar del tiempo, el nervio del diente puede morir cuando una restauración es colocada muy cerca del nervio u ocasionalmente se vuelve evidente cuando el diente es preparado para una corona o una restauración de molde. La única alternativa al tratamiento endodóntico es sacar el diente—no una solución que nosotros recomendamos.

Diente Fracturado

Cualquier diente que ha sido taladrado y empastado también puede estar sujeto a una fractura. Mientras más vieja y grande la empastadura, más probable es a fracturarse. Si la encía ha sido retirada debido a hábitos de cepillado incorrectos o enfermedad periodontal, las raíces sensitivas o el deterioro de la superficie de la raíz puede volverse evidente. El deterioro de la superficie de la raíz puede dañar el diente mucho más rápido que el deterioro del esmalte.

La Prevención Sigue Siendo un Elemento Clave para una Buena Salud Oral

Hay un lado brillante. Muchos problemas pueden ser evitados o resueltos rápidamente con el tratamiento adecuado. Un tratamiento adecuado incluye sus buenos hábitos de cuidado oral de sí mismo, citas con nosotros para examen periodontico y profilaxis (limpieza) en los intervalos basados en sus necesidades individuales (no basados en los beneficios del seguro dental) y pronta atención a problemas que se están desarrollando.

Prevenga que el problema comience: **cepillando y limpiando con hilo dental.** Una vez note el síntoma, consiga que el problema sea diagnosticado y trate el área de preocupación cuando es pequeña. **Véanos en los intervalos recomendados.** Arregle el problema de manera que se quede arreglado por el mayor tiempo posible y que no cause más problemas. **Menos taladrado es mejor que más. La restauración más duradera debe ser su elección de restauración.**

Si usted tiene cualquier pregunta sobre el tratamiento dental para un paciente adulto, favor de sentirse libre de preguntarnos.

Para una Vida con una Magnífica Salud Oral

La prevención es la clave para una magnífica salud oral. Una mejor dieta, cuidado médico y otros factores nos permiten vivir vidas más largas. Desgraciadamente, nuestros dientes no se han adaptado a que tengamos una vida más larga. Si usted quiere tener sus dientes por toda su vida, aquí está lo que debe hacer:

- Cepille, limpie con hilo dental y el use las ayudas dentales recomendadas correctamente, por lo menos una vez cada día. Utilice un enjuague bucal con fluoruro, diariamente.

- Venga a la oficina para las citas de higiene de cuidado repetido, en los intervalos específicos que recomendamos. Permítanos proveerle un tratamiento de fluoruro tópico fuerte recetado en cada cita de cuidado repetido.

- Déjenos tomar radiografías cuando creemos que son necesarias.

- Los dientes se envejecerán y gastarán, como el resto de nuestro cuerpo. La cubierta externa del esmalte duro puede volverse delgada, romperse o gastarse y exponer la dentina más suave. La dentina se erosiona muy rápidamente. Cuando veamos la dentina expuesta, déjenos cubrirla y protegerla.

- El colocar selladores en todos los dientes puede ser beneficioso para ellos.

- No nos pida que "remendemos" nada. La ortodoncia de remiendos es contraria al concepto de mantener sus dientes libres de problemas de por vida. Si las reparaciones pequeñas son posibles y apropiadas, nosotros le diremos.

- Escoja el procedimiento o material restaurativo que le durará más tiempo. Todos los materiales dentales tienen un largo de vida esperado, y deben ser reparados. Cada vez que un diente se vuelve a taladrar, se hace más débil. Solamente oro amarillo sólido puede durar por toda la vida. Cerámicas del color del diente y porcelana pueden durar por mucho tiempo. Es su elección.

- Restauraciones adheridas (última tecnología) requieren menos taladrar que las empastaduras de plata. El diente conserva más fuerza y la restauración dura más. Déjenos utilizar las mejores cosas.

- La enfermedad de las encías puede comenzar en cualquier momento. La genética, dieta, cuidado oral de sí mismo, medicamentos y la salud en general pueden todos tener una influencia. La enfermedad de las encías puede ser en un lugar específico (más frecuentemente comienza en un área localizada) y episódica (puede comenzar en cualquier momento). Es también sin dolor en sus primeras etapas. Le diremos tan pronto como encontremos enfermedad de las encías. Necesitará ser tratada correctamente e inmediatamente.

- Nuestras recomendaciones de tratamiento se basan siempre en sus necesidades, no en los deseos o el balance de su compañía de seguro. Hay docenas de procedimientos dentales comunes que no son parte del paquete beneficios. Los portadores de seguro dental están en el negocio para hacer dinero. Desean pagar lo menos posible tan tarde como sea posible. La actitud de "si mi compañía de seguro no paga por ello, no lo quiero", solo le hace daño a usted y a SU salud oral.

- Hemos escuchado lo que usted desea, examinado su boca y sabemos sus necesidades dentales. La mayoría de los pacientes pueden tener la mejor odontología que desean y se merecen. Sólo toma planear un poco. Podemos ayudarle con eso también. Si usted desea todos sus dientes, toda su vida, siga las recomendaciones mencionadas y hágalo bien de la primera vez.

¡Cómo Cepillarse! ¡Cómo Limpiarse con Hilo Dental!

Una vieja expresión humorística afirma, "Usted no tiene que cepillar todos sus dientes todos los días. ¡Solamente los que usted desea mantener!". Y mientras que nos reímos de estas palabras, el mensaje no puede estar más correcto. Para mantener una buena salud oral, cada diente debe ser limpiado completamente cada día. Un buen método para cepillar es llamado *la técnica modificada de Bass*. Es fácil y bastante efectiva. Podemos darle instrucciones de cómo cepillar correctamente. Ciertamente es más fácil ver como se hace que leerlo e imaginárselo. Pero esto le ayudará a comenzar.

Utilice un cepillo de dientes copetudo con cerdas suaves de nilón. Los cepillos de dientes con cerdas duras pueden dañar fácilmente sus dientes y encías. Los cepillos de dientes de cerdas suaves duran alrededor 3 meses antes de que necesiten ser reemplazados. No se quede con un cepillo de dientes por un período de tiempo extendido. Cuando las cerdas del cepillo de dientes se gastan, no le darán el mejor funcionamiento posible. Los cepillos medianos y duros durarán más tiempo, pero casi todas las personas se cepillan demasiado fuerte para utilizar estos cepillos. Si usted utiliza cepillos medianos y duros, o se cepilla incorrectamente con cualquier cepillo de dientes, usted puede causar daño permanente a su tejido de las encías, causando desgaste. Esto también puede causar cortes en el diente mismo, exponiendo la dentina. En ambos casos, se puede desarrollar sensibilidad severa del diente.

El Método Bass
- Las cerdas del cepillo deben estar alineadas hacia el área donde el diente se encuentra con la encía, aproximadamente a un ángulo de 45 grados.
- Las cerdas del cepillo deben poder resbalar suavemente debajo del tejido de la encía. Mueva el cepillo suavemente hacia adelante y hacia atrás de modo que haya un movimiento vibratorio, **no un movimiento de fregado.** La cabeza del cepillo debe poder cubrir y limpiar cerca de dos dientes a la vez.
- Cepille cada área por aproximadamente 10 segundos, después rude las cerdas hacia la superficie de mordida. Mueva la cabeza del cepillo de modo que recubra una porción pequeña del diente que apenas cepillo y los dientes adyacentes. Repita hasta que todos los dientes estén cepillados.

Cepille todos los dientes. Comience en el lado del cachete en los dientes de atrás, en una esquina de su boca, cepillando mientras se mueve a través de la boca hasta la esquina opuesta. Entonces cambie al interior (lado del paladar o de la lengua) y cepille otra vez de una esquina a la otra. Cepille los dientes superiores e inferiores usando el movimiento vibratorio hacia adelante y hacia atrás.

Algunas áreas requerirán cambiar el cepillo a un ángulo diferente como para el interior (de la lengua y el lado del paladar) en la parte superior e inferior de los dientes delanteros. Usar la punta o el extremo pequeño del cepillo ayudará a cepillar alrededor de esta área curvada. Utilice el mismo tipo de movimiento vibratorio con el cepillo, moviendo hacia arriba y hacia abajo contra el diente.

Cepillar la superficie de mordida de los dientes es fácil. Coloque las cerdas en la superficie de mordida de los dientes en los surcos y cepille hacia adelante y hacia atrás. Asegúrese de cepillar las superficies de mordida en el lado izquierdo y lado derecho, dientes superiores e inferiores.

Uso del Hilo Dental
Comience con un pedazo de hilo dental de 14 a 16 pulgadas. Está bien usar cualquier tipo de hilo dental. El tipo que no se desmenuza es el más fácil de utilizar. Es más fino y la mayoría de las personas lo encuentran más fácil de usar. Envuelva ligeramente el hilo dental alrededor de los índices de cada mano hasta que un pedazo de 1 a 1.5 pulgadas disponibles entre los dedos. ¡No lo envuelva tan apretado que usted se corte la circulación y sus dedos se pongan azules! Usando sus pulgares e índices, coloque el hilo dental sobre el punto donde dos dientes se encuentran. Con un movimiento de pulido sutil, hacia adelante y hacia atrás, mueva el hilo dental entre los dientes y resbálelo primero debajo de la encía alrededor de uno de los dientes en forma de U. Mueva el hilo dental hacia arriba y abajo algunas veces, entonces haga la U en dirección contraria y limpie con hilo dental el otro diente. El hilo dental necesita llegar debajo de la encía. Después quite el hilo dental y colóquelo entre los siguientes dos próximos dientes. Aguantar el hilo dental tenso entre sus dedos le dará más control, y el limpiarse con hilo dental será más fácil.

Cuando usted puede realizar estos procedimientos diarios con eficacia, usted reducirá significativamente su riesgo de enfermedad de la encía y deterioro y los gastos asociados al tratamiento. Hay otras ayudas para limpiarse con hilo dental disponibles si usted tiene problemas usando sus manos. Déjenos saber sobre estos problemas. Los cepillos de dientes eléctricos o mecánicos pueden también ser utilizados. Una vez más, háblenos de estos aparatos. Mantener sus dientes sanos por el resto de su vida puede lograrse—un día a la vez.

Si usted tiene cualquier pregunta sobre cómo cepillarse o limpiarse con hilo dental, favor de sentirse libre de preguntarnos.

Alerta de Bebidas Chatarras

Hemos notado recientemente el desarrollo de un problema de deterioro serio. Lo que estamos viendo en nuestra práctica dental es un deterioro del diente que progresa mucho más rápidamente de lo que estamos acostumbrados a ver. Este deterioro es visto alrededor de las orillas de las restauraciones (empastaduras) y coronas donde el diente y el material restaurativo se encuentran. En algunas personas estas restauraciones fueron colocadas hace poco tiempo. De la discusión con los pacientes que presentaron este tipo extremo e inusual de deterioro, parece haber dos factores comunes. Primero, la mayoría de estas personas son mujeres, y en segundo lugar, todas ellas beben bebidas de dieta, sobre todo soda y té helado en botella. Sus hábitos de cepillado y limpieza con hilo dental parecen ser adecuados. No están tomando ninguna medicación especial. El rango de edad va de 12 a 55 años. Todas parecen estar preocupadas por su peso—por lo cual están bebiendo bebidas de dieta.

Años atrás, este tipo de deterioro era visto en pacientes que mantenían dulces, mentas u otros refrescantes de alientos en sus bocas por horas, causando deterioro en los bordes de las encías de los dientes. Aunque otro factor o factores pueden ser reales o contribuyentes a la causa de este problema, las únicas causas actualmente detectadas son las bebidas de dieta y el té helado en botella endulzado artificialmente.

El azúcar en alimentos y bebidas alimenta las bacterias presentes en la placa dental, permitiendo que las bacterias produzcan ácido láctico. El ácido láctico rompe los minerales en el esmalte del diente, lo que causa las cavidades. Aunque las bebidas de dieta son sin azúcar, son también muy ácidas. Este ácido también rompe los minerales en el esmalte del diente, causando las cavidades. Para el momento en que la saliva diluya estos ácidos lo suficiente para traer la boca de nuevo a su acidez apropiada, deterioro nuevo o adicional puede ya estar en marcha. O peor, antes de que la boca recupere su equilibrio ácido apropiado, ¡el paciente está destapando ya otra botella de bebida de dieta!

Sugerencias para la reducción o eliminación de este tipo de deterioro incluyen la reducción o cesación de la ingestión de bebidas de dieta, enjuagar su boca con agua cuanto antes después del contacto con la bebida, usar un enjuague bucal con fluoruro y un tratamiento de fluoruro tópico fuerte recetado tanto en la oficina (4 veces al año) y en el hogar. Podemos incluso necesitar recomendar el uso de cubetas especiales para administrar fluoruro para aumentar el tiempo que el fluoruro puede estar en contacto con los dientes. Esto ayudará a hacer el esmalte de los dientes más fuertes para resistir el ataque ácido que comienza el deterioro. También promoverá un mejor equilibrio en el proceso constante de desmineralización/remineralización del esmalte que ocurre en boca de todos. Las lesiones de deterioro en las etapas tempranas se pueden parar e incluso curar de esta manera.

Aunque la mayoría de nosotros podríamos perder unas pocas libras, esté enterado de que algunas de las cosas que usted pone en su boca, con las esperanzas de perder peso, pueden realmente tener el efecto desfavorable de perder los dientes.

Si usted tiene cualquier pregunta sobre este deterioro acelerado, favor de sentirse libre de preguntarnos.

Prevención del Deterioro

Deterioro Dental

Las caries dentales (deterioro) es una infección bacteriana, primero del esmalte, luego de la dentina del diente. La tradición en odontología ha sido quitar quirúrgicamente la porción enferma del diente "taladrando" el deterioro, y luego rellenando el hueco en el diente con algún material inerte. Como la mayoría de los adultos saben, este procedimiento será realizado una y otra vez cuando nuevo deterioro comienza, o cuando la empastadura (frecuentemente plata) se rompe o el diente se fractura.

¿No sería mejor eliminar la causa de la infección y no ser forzado a tener huecos grandes perforados dentro de los dientes? Creemos que la causa bacteriana de la infección debe ser tratada.

Prevención del Riesgo del Deterioro Dental

Hay varias medidas positivas que usted puede tomar para reducir su riesgo del deterioro dental. Primero, todo el deterioro activo en su boca se debe tratar inmediatamente. Después, todos los dientes que se beneficiarían de los **selladores** (vea el folleto adicional) deben ser tratados. Esto evitaría que la bacteria alcance los hoyos y las ranuras que normalmente existen en las superficies oclusales (de mordida) de los dientes. Cualquier bacteria que puedan todavía en el área sellada son efectivamente separadas de su fuente de alimento y se vuelven inactivas. Aunque los selladores son más eficaces en los dientes que no se han restaurado previamente, pueden ser colocados con éxito en los dientes empastados con empastaduras adheridas.

La infección se puede tratar con antimicrobianos. Creemos que el uso de un enjuague bucal con fluoruro usado dos veces al día o el uso de un dentífrico con fluoruro recetado proporciona una gran ventaja. El fluoruro no solamente es eficaz contra bacterias, sino que también crea un ambiente que promueve la remineralización del esmalte levemente dañado. Se invierte el proceso del deterioro y el diente puede que no necesite ser taladrado. También podemos recetar un enjuague bucal de clorhexidina, un enjuague oral antimicrobiano que tiene un gran efecto en mutantes estreptococos.

Su dieta y cuidado oral de sí mismo son importantes en la prevención del deterioro dental. Cuando usted come y bebe alimentos chatarra y líquidos azucarados, sus dientes están más propensos al deterioro. Mientras más frecuente usted come meriendas, más propensos serán sus dientes al deterioro. Si la manera en que cepilla y limpia con hilo dental no es eficaz, más propensos serán sus dientes al deterioro. Cuando usted no puede cepillarse después de una comida, enjuague por lo menos su boca con agua en un plazo de 15 minutos para diluir los ácidos que se forman del alimento injerido o de la bebida. Si usted tiene un flujo salival disminuido, tome sorbos frecuentes de agua durante el día para ayudar a diluir los ácidos producidos por las bacterias.

Si usted tiene un problema continuo con deterioro activo, recomendamos citas preventivas de cuidado repetido más frecuentes. Se ha demostrado en varias ocasiones que los pacientes que tienen buen cuidado oral de sí mismo y mantienen un intervalo de cuidado repetido de 3 a 4 meses tienen menos problemas dentales relacionados (cavidades o enfermedad de las encías).

El intervalo rutinario de cuidado repetido de 6 meses no es recomendado en nuestro programa. Sería personalmente feliz si nunca más escuchara la frase de "vea a su dentista cada seis meses". ¡Ese intervalo fue basado en una vieja filosofía de hace 50 años que nunca ha tenido base científica! Los tiempos han cambiado. La práctica dental actual se basa en la información científica probada. Puede que usted necesite que sus dientes sean limpiados por el higienista dos veces cada año o usted puede necesitar ser visto más con frecuencia.

Para algunas personas, también sugerimos la prueba de los niveles bacterianos orales para determinar la magnitud y la presencia de mutantes de infección estreptococos y para determinar su nivel de riesgo para enfermedad dental futura.

Si usted tiene cualquier pregunta sobre la prevención del deterioro dental, favor de sentirse libre de preguntarnos.

Cuándo las Radiografías Son Necesarias

Solamente tomamos las radiografías necesarias en esta oficina. Una radiografía necesaria es una que se utiliza para diagnosticar el grado de un problema dental que ya sabemos que existe, como por ejemplo un diente partido, una cavidad o un absceso. También debemos utilizar radiografías como parte de un examen oral inicial o periódico. En estos exámenes, las radiografías se utilizan para determinar si hay problemas en una etapa inicial que no pueden ser vistos simplemente mirando el diente o el área.

Podemos ver solamente cerca de un 50% de sus condiciones orales sin las radiografías. Las radiografías permiten que veamos, entre otras cosas, entre los dientes, en y debajo de las orillas de las empastaduras y coronas y la localización y la densidad del hueso que soporta sus dientes. Con esta información podemos hacer un diagnóstico completo, tratando problemas pequeños u ocultos antes de que se conviertan en problemas realmente grandes. Las radiografías **no** se consideran una medida preventiva. Sin embargo, permiten que diagnostiquemos y tratemos un problema temprano, previniendo así que llegue a ser peor.

A veces debemos tomar varias radiografías de un área en particular. Las radiografías son solamente una representación de dos dimensiones, en blanco y negro de un diente y hueso con color tridimensional. Las radiografías tomadas de diversos ángulos dan una apariencia más tridimensional y por lo tanto más verdadera de las características anatómicas. Tendremos un cuadro mucho más claro de la clase, tamaño y localización de cualquier problema.

Cuanto más sana su boca es, y más extraordinaria su historia dental es, menos radiografías necesitamos recomendar. Mientras más problemas dentales usted tenga, más supervisión y por lo tanto más las radiografías necesitaremos. Sin embargo, si no tomamos las radiografías, el problema crecerá desapercibido y aún más radiografías que las que aconsejamos originalmente pueden ser necesarias.

Seguridad para la Radiación
Somos cuidadosos con la seguridad para la radiación. La protección apropiada como protectores de plomo son **siempre** provistos. Trabajamos en la oficina alrededor de las unidades de radiografía todo el día, todos lo días. Tenemos interés en tomar solamente las radiografías necesarias para su salud y la nuestra. Esté seguro de que las únicas radiografías que recomendamos son ésas que necesitamos para diagnosticar y tratar.

Si usted tiene cualquier pregunta sobre las radiografías, favor de sentirse libre de preguntarnos.

Dar Marcha Atrás al Deterioro

Si le pidieran que describa una cavidad, usted diría probablemente que el proceso es similar a enmohecer—algo que sucede en el exterior del diente que hace el diente blando y crea un hueco eventualmente será visible. Usted puede que incluso tenga la noción de que las bacterias están implicadas. Y, usted tendría razón en ambos casos.

El proceso del deterioro es una interacción complicada de un equilibrio ácido y básico de la química en la boca. El flujo y contenido salival, la presencia de bacterias que causan deterioro, la edad de los dientes, la dieta y el nivel de la placa todo desempeña un papel en el deterioro (desmineralización) así como el proceso de reconstrucción (remineralización) implicado en el deterioro de los dientes.

Desmineralización

En la etapa inicial del proceso de deterioro, no hay un "hueco" real en el diente. Hay, sin embargo, una alteración del contenido mineral del esmalte. Esta etapa de deterioro es totalmente invisible al ojo. No puede ser detectado por una radiografía. Éste es un cambio microscópico donde, debido al nivel de ácido en el área inmediata, los bloques que constituyen el esmalte (calcio y fosfato) se comienzan a disolver en un nivel microscópico. Cuando el ambiente ácido se deja sin verificar (se permite que la placa se acumule tranquilamente contra la superficie del diente), más y más de los enlaces entre el calcio y el fosfato se disuelven. Éste es un proceso llamado *desmineralización*. Si el desafío del ácido llega a ser severo y más de la estructura subyacente del diente se comienza a disolver, la superficie externa se queda sin apoyo. Es en este momento que el hueco real, o lo qué usted llama una *cavidad,* aparece.

Remineralización

Cuando la superficie externa del esmalte sigue estando intacta, sin que se perciba ninguna rotura, hay una oportunidad para volver a unir los enlaces entre el calcio y fosfato en un proceso llamado *remineralización.* Y las buenas noticias son que la ciencia dental ha descubierto que, en la presencia de fluoruro, estos enlaces llegan a ser realmente más fuertes que lo que eran inicialmente. Y es de esta manera que una cavidad en su etapa inicial puede ser invertida. Cuando sucede esto, el diente no necesita ser taladrado y empastado. El proceso de desmineralización y de remineralizacion se puede considerar como un tira y jala a nivel molecular de todas las superficies de todos sus dientes, ¡todo el tiempo!

Cómo Usted Puede Promover la Remineralización

Hay varios pasos que usted puede tomar diariamente para ayudar a asegurar que usted está promoviendo la remineralización: Estos son:

- Controle su dieta: vigile el tipo de alimentos que promueven el deterioro que usted come y la cantidad
- Mejore su cuidado oral de sí mismo cepillando y limpiando con hilo dental todos lo días
- Utilice el fluoruro tópico diariamente
- Utilice los agentes antimicrobianos y otros agentes anticaries según lo dirigido regularmente
- Mantenga su programa de higiene dental de cuidado repetido

Las primeras etapas del deterioro dental SE PUEDEN invertir sin la pérdida de la estructura del diente, y usted puede ayudar a promover una boca sana siguiendo apenas algunas reglas simples.

Si usted tiene cualquier pregunta sobre el proceso de deterioro, favor de sentirse libre de preguntarnos.

Selladores y Fluoruro: Beneficios para los Pacientes Adultos

El deterioro dental puede desarrollarse en cualquier momento, sin importar la edad de las personas. Un cambio en la dieta, cambio en el estilo de vida, cambio en los hábitos de cuidado oral de sí mismo, el uso de medicamentos recetados o un cambio en la salud sistemática debido al proceso normal de envejecimiento, todos éstos pueden afectar la susceptibilidad a caries (deterioro). Pocas personas permanecen totalmente libres de deterioro. Cuidado oral de sí mismo apropiado por su parte y citas de higiene dental para prevención espaciadas correctamente lo llevarán por un largo camino para reducir la oportunidad de que comience nuevo deterioro.

A medida que usted envejece, es posible que algunos de sus tejidos de las encías retrocedan, exponiendo las superficies de las raíces de sus dientes. Esta recesión de las encías puede ocurrir por cepillar incorrectamente (cepillar demasiado fuerte con un cepillo de cerdas duras) o como resultado de problemas periodontales pasados. Cuanto más de un diente y las raíces está expuesto, mayor es el área superficial que usted tendrá que mantener limpia. Los dientes con las raíces expuestas son a veces muy difíciles de mantener limpios. Estas raíces pueden ser sensibles a los cambios de temperatura, y son a menudo incómodas para cepillar. El flujo salival disminuido ayuda a crear un ambiente fértil para que las bacterias se acumulen en el esmalte y especialmente en la superficie de la raíz. ¡Y el deterioro de las raíces progresa generalmente bastante rápido!

Meta de la Prevención
Su meta debe ser evitar que el dentista taladre sus dientes. Cualquier medida preventiva razonable que esté disponible debe ser considerada seriamente. Cuando el dentista taladra, usted pierde. Cuando el dentista no taladra, usted gana.

Selladores Dentales
Por favor vea el folleto de **selladores**. Aunque los selladores están diseñados mayormente para niños, los adultos que tienen un historial de deterioro activo deben considerar el colocar selladores en la parte de atrás cuando sea indicado. Le diremos dónde es posible colocar selladores. Incluso si usted no ha tenido una cavidad durante mucho tiempo considere el uso de un sellador como una póliza de seguro barata para sus dientes. Quizás usted nunca tendrá deterioro en las superficies sin sellar. Pero, de la misma manera como usted asegura su hogar contra la destrucción por el fuego, un sellador asegura la superficie del diente del deterioro. Las medidas preventivas pueden permitir que usted evite tener sus dientes taladrados. ¡Usted gana!

Fluoruro Tópico
Por una razón similar, aconsejamos el uso de tratamientos tópicos de fluoruro para los adultos. La efectividad del fluoruro sistémico y tópico en la prevención del deterioro está bien documentada. Cuando una cavidad comienza, el uso del fluoruro puede (dependiendo de cuando se utiliza) reducir o eliminar la necesidad de taladrar.

Una alternativa al tratamiento de fluoruro que podemos proporcionar en nuestra oficina es un enjuague diario. Si usted se puede enjuagar con un enjuague bucal vendido sin receta que contiene fluoruro **cada noche** según lo indicado en la etiqueta del enjuague, usted no necesita el tratamiento tópico de fluoruro en la oficina. Si usted no puede enjuagarse **diariamente** según indicado, usted necesitará el beneficio del tratamiento tópico de fluoruro más fuerte aplicado en la oficina. Su salud oral se beneficiará mas de los incrementos pequeños de fluoruro que se aplican **diariamente** que de una concentración más grande cada 6 meses. Sin embargo, solamente usted sabe si usted será fiel a su rutina de enjuague. Si tiene duda, permítanos hacerlo aquí.

Usted ha seleccionado nuestra oficina para administrar sus necesidades dentales. Si usted ha sido un paciente aquí por cualquier largo de tiempo, usted sabe que enfatizamos la **prevención** de la enfermedad dental sobretodo. Los selladores y los tratamientos tópicos de fluoruro son dos de las medidas de prevención dental más importantes de las cuáles creemos pueden realzar significativamente su salud oral.

Si usted tiene cualquier pregunta sobre selladores y fluoruro, favor de sentirse libre de preguntarnos.

Ilustración en CD-ROM

Fluoruro Tópico: En el Hogar y en la Oficina Dental

¿Por Qué el Fluoruro Tópico?

La mayoría de nosotros estamos familiarizados con las ventajas dentales de los suplementos de fluoruro que se administran a los niños sistemáticamente mientras sus dientes se están formando. La investigación de este tipo de tratamiento de fluoruro demuestra una reducción de un 35% en el deterioro de los dientes. El uso del fluoruro para reducir y eliminar el deterioro es una de las medidas de salud pública más estudiada y documentada. En nuestra oficina, recomendamos un tratamiento de fluoruro con cubeta por 4 minutos por lo menos dos veces al año, normalmente después de una cita de cuidado repetido de higiene dental periódico. Hemos encontrado que este tipo de ayuda preventiva hace cuatro cosas:

- Reduce la solubilidad del esmalte al ataque ácido, haciendo que los dientes sean más resistentes al deterioro.
- Ayuda con la remineralización del esmalte del diente donde ha acabado de comenzar el deterioro.
- Con el uso diario por más tiempo, reduce la sensibilidad del diente a los cambios de temperatura.
- Reduce la tensión de la superficie del esmalte de modo que la placa no se adhiere fácilmente al diente.

La investigación reciente también ha demostrado que usted puede beneficiarse de los enjuagues de fluoruro tópico sin receta, especialmente si usted los usa fielmente todos los días. Usted puede esperar una reducción adicional en el deterioro cuando también aplicamos un fluoruro tópico en la oficina. Se aplica cuatro veces al año. ¡La reducción del deterioro puede ser tan alta como un 30%! Si usted ha tenido un deterioro activo recientemente, no importa su edad, le recomendaremos esta rutina de fluoruro.

Aplicaciones Especiales de Fluoruro

Otra opción para el fluoruro tópico está disponible para los pacientes que experimentan la sensibilidad de un diente o una raíz, niveles de deterioro más altos y/o crónicos, deterioro en la superficie de la raíz o el síndrome de sequedad de la boca (xerostomía). Si le han diagnosticado con cualquiera de estos problemas dentales, le haremos unas cubetas de fluoruro a la medida. Luego le recetaremos o dispensaremos un producto con una alta concentración de fluoruro para que lo use en las cubetas durante las noches.

Las instrucciones son simples. Seque los dientes lo más posible, con una gasa cuadrada o un paño o succionando el aire a través de sus dientes. El fluoruro trabajará mejor si los dientes no están tan mojados. Como las cubetas se ajustan bien a los dientes, ponga sólo una cantidad pequeña del gel de fluoruro en la cubeta para cada grupo de dientes. Escupa el exceso. Si usted observa que sobra mucho fluoruro después de terminar el tratamiento, sencillamente reduzca la cantidad que pone en las cubetas. Déjelas puestas por _____ minutos. Entonces, saque las cubetas. Escupa la saliva y el fluoruro restante. **No coma ni beba por _____ minutos**.

La cantidad de semanas que usted necesitará hacer este procedimiento de cubeta de fluoruro depende de su condición específica. Si usted tiene un flujo de saliva disminuido con deterioro aumentado o la posibilidad de un deterioro aumentado, necesitará seguir esta rutina de fluoruro hasta que el flujo de saliva regrese a lo normal. En el caso de las raíces o los dientes sensibles, usted necesitará seguir esta rutina hasta que la sensibilidad se haya reducido. Comentario: la reducción de la sensibilidad es normalmente un proceso gradual—no espere una mejoría rápida. Desensibilizar las raíces puede también requerir que se coloquen otros materiales sobre el área como un procedimiento adjunto.

Si usted tiene cualquier pregunta sobre el uso de los fluoruros tópicos en el hogar o en la oficina dental, favor de sentirse libre de preguntarnos.

Abfracción: Un Nuevo Término Dental

Abfracción—Un término nuevo para un "viejo" problema

Usted probablemente no ha escuchado este término antes porque es relativamente nuevo para la odontología. Éste describe un problema recientemente reconocido que comúnmente ha sido confundido con abrasión en el pasado. Hasta recientemente, se creía que la **abfracción** era causada por técnicas incorrectas de cepillado.

Ahora se sabe que una lesión de abfracción es la pérdida de la estructura del diente vista clínicamente en el lado del cachete de un diente cerca y frecuentemente debajo del borde de la encía. Se puede identificar por su corte horizontal agudamente marcado. Aunque se puede desarrollar una caries en el área debido a la dentina expuesta, el proceso de deterioro no es responsable por la abfracción.

La Causa

La abfracción es causada cuando dos dientes opuestos—un diente superior y un diente inferior—se encuentran incorrectamente mientras se mastica o por los hábitos de rechinar o apretar los dientes. En este punto de estrés, el diente se "dobla" un poco. Cuando una relación de mordida no es correcta, el diente está bajo fuerzas de compresión y tensión por el diente opuesto. De esta manera, el diente es doblado un poco cada vez que los dientes están completamente cerrados.

Este doblaje crónico del diente causa la pérdida de la sustancia del diente (esmalte y dentina) en el borde de la encía donde el esmalte es más fino. El esmalte es frágil y no puede doblarse fácilmente. A medida que el diente se mueve de atrás para adelante (debido a la mordida o porque rechina sus dientes), piezas de esmalte se fracturan. La dentina, o la estructura subyacente del diente, es más elástica y se puede doblar un poco. El doblaje del diente dañará lentamente el diente y el corte eventualmente será visible.

Una característica de la abfracción que puede hacer el diagnóstico difícil es que puede estar parcialmente o enteramente debajo de los tejidos de las encías. En un momento dado, se pensó que este tipo de corte del diente era causado por hábitos de cepillado incorrectos, como el restregar con fuerza hacia adelante y hacia atrás contra el cuello del diente. Auque es cierto que usted realmente puede gastar un corte en el diente cepillándose muy fuerte en una manera de sube y baja, el primer tejido que se gasta bajo esas condiciones es el tejido de la encía. Contrario a la abfracción, la abrasión ocurre sobre el borde de la encía. En contraste, una abfracción ocurre muchas veces debajo de la encía o es cubierto parcialmente por el tejido de la encía.

Opciones de Tratamiento

Su oclusión (mordida) debe ser verificada y ajustada de modo que sus dientes se encuentren correctamente en todos los movimientos de la mandíbula. Este ajuste de la mordida puede requerir más de una cita para completarse con éxito, dependiendo de la naturaleza específica del problema oclusal.

Segundo, el corte en el diente debe ser tratado. El esmalte que falta y la dentina subyacente expuesta necesitan ser reemplazadas y cubiertas. La dentina no está diseñada para estar expuesta al ambiente oral—es por eso que está cubierta naturalmente con esmalte. Aun cuando los factores que inicialmente causaron el corte han sido eliminados, la dentina expuesta se puede continuar desgastando porque la dentina es suave. Esta dentina expuesta puede deteriorase. El diente también puede llegar a ser sensible a los cambios de temperatura y puede llegar a ser más débil.

Una resina adherida del color del diente es frecuentemente colocada para restaurar el diente cortado, y es una restauración relativamente fácil de realizar. Si el corte se extiende profundamente debajo del borde de la encía, puede ser necesario quitar el tejido para exponer el área del corte para restaurarlo.

Si todos los procedimientos son exitosos, el corte de la abfracción será restaurado para igualar exactamente la estructura natural del diente y la mordida será ajustada de modo que los dientes se encuentren correctamente. Por favor esté enterado que si los dientes cambian de lugar levemente, o si usted continúa rechinando sus dientes, el diente restaurado puede comenzar a doblarse otra vez y la restauración puede ser eliminada. También, otros dientes pueden comenzar a exhibir el mismo tipo de pérdida del esmalte. Si ocurre esto, la mordida puede ser ajustada nuevamente y se puede colocar una nueva restauración.

Si usted tiene cualquier pregunta sobre la abfracción, favor de sentirse libre de preguntarnos.

Reflujo Ácido (Enfermedad de Reflujo Gastroesofágico)

Los dientes son tan duros que usted pensaría que son indestructibles y que no serían afectados adversamente por nada. Debido a la solidez del esmalte y del hueso, deben seguir siendo iguales desde del día que los dientes salen en la boca hasta el día que ya no se necesitan. Desgraciadamente, esto está lejos de la verdad. Mientras que quisiéramos pensar en los dientes como fuertes y sin cambios, la mayoría de las personas saben que los dientes se pueden dañar por el deterioro dental—causando bacterias. Sabemos, también, que los dientes se pueden dañar por medios mecánicos—atrición causada por el rechinar los dientes y abrasión causada por cepillar los dientes incorrectamente. Sin embargo, pocas personas saben que hay un tercer factor que puede destruir los dientes—la erosión química.

La erosión química es causada por exceso de ácido entrando en contacto con un diente por períodos de tiempo extendidos. El ataque ácido puede ser autoinducido (bulimia) o más comúnmente por un problema con reflujo ácido. En reflujo (gástrico) ácido, el contenido ácido y parcialmente digerido del estómago vuelve nuevamente dentro de la garganta y de la cavidad bucal. Normalmente, el músculo del esfínter del esófago inferior, que conecta el esófago con el estómago, se cierra una vez que el alimento pasa al estómago. Este cierre evita que el contenido del estómago fluya nuevamente hacia el esófago. El reflujo ácido ocurre cuando el esfínter no trabaja correctamente y permite que el líquido ácido vuelva al esófago y más arriba—la boca.

Esta condición puede ser observada por un dentista mucho antes que es reconocida por un paciente o un médico. El dentista verá una erosión lisa y circular en las puntas de los primeros molares inferiores. Las puntas (las protuberancias del diente) pierden sus picos, se aplanan y se vuelven cóncavas. Pronto el esmalte que cubre es penetrado y la dentina inferior es expuesta. Debido a que la dentina es más "suave" que el esmalte, la erosión puede progresar mas rápidamente. Esta erosión ácida tiene un aspecto muy diferente a la pérdida del diente debido a una etiología mecánica. La atrición y la abrasión tienen un aspecto muy afilado y bien delineado. La erosión química tiene una presentación más suave y redondeada y es localizada primero en los primeros molares inferiores (los primeros molares inferiores son los primeros molares permanentes en erupcionar en la boca) por lo tanto los dientes permanentes tienen el potencial de exposición más largo. Cuando el ácido refluye (regresa) a la boca, se acumula mayormente alrededor de los primeros molares inferiores. Éste es el área con más características erosivas.

Una porción significativa de la población experimenta reflujo ácido al menos una vez al mes. Alrededor del 25% de aquellos que están afectados están inconscientes de su problema. Los infantes y los niños pueden ser afectados, y puede haber un componente genético a esta enfermedad. Un diagnóstico temprano de la erosión de los primeros molares permanentes inferiores se puede hacer desde la edad de los 7 ó 8 años. Una hernia hiatal puede debilitar el esfínter del esófago inferior y causar reflujo. La dieta y el estilo de vida contribuyen al reflujo ácido. El chocolate, la hierbabuena, la fruta cítrica, los tomates, los alimentos fritos o grasosos, el café (especialmente café ácido), las bebidas alcohólicas, el ajo y las cebollas son alimentos a evitar. El aumento de peso (también el aumento de peso asociado con el embarazo) y el fumar (relaja el esfínter del esófago inferior) pueden ser factores que contribuyen. Información adicional se puede obtener del Internet entrando a un lugar de búsqueda y escribiendo "reflujo ácido", "reflujo gástrico" o "enfermedad de reflujo gastroesofágico".

Al igual que la mayoría de los problemas médicos y dentales, mientras más temprano se hace el diagnóstico, más fácil es de tratar. Si hemos traído esta condición a su atención, le pedimos que usted hable con su médico. Los factores variables incluyen la naturaleza y severidad del problema, así como la frecuencia y el tipo de líquido que refluye del estómago. Un cambio en la dieta, en los hábitos alimenticios y/o medicamentos (sin receta o recetados) pueden ser efectivos. Dentalmente, una vez que el esmalte es penetrado y la dentina llega a ser visible, se recomienda que las áreas afectadas sean protegidas cubriéndolas con un reemplazo de esmalte—un material adherido del color del diente. Este material no sólo protege a la dentina y al esmalte, es más resistente al ácido que la dentina en su estado natural. En muchas ocasiones, la preparación con taladro no es necesaria.

Si usted tiene cualquier pregunta sobre el reflujo ácido, favor de sentirse libre de preguntarnos.

Atrición y Abrasión

Por Qué los Dientes se Desgastan

La fricción natural de los dientes moviéndose contra ellos mismos produce desgaste del esmalte. Esto es considerado un proceso natural que ocurre a través de los años, así que los cambios son muy graduales. La atrición (desgaste o pérdida de la sustancia del diente) de las superficies de mordida de los dientes ocurre en uno de cuatro adultos en los Estados Unidos, o aproximadamente 25% de la población.

Usted puede haber notado estos tipos de cambios observando que sus dientes delanteros aparecen estar astillados. Estos dientes pueden parecer más cortos y los bordes de mordida pueden aparecer desteñidos, especialmente en los dientes delanteros inferiores. Este proceso puede ocurrir más rápidamente cuando usted tiene una mordida no útil o no bien dirigida, hábito de rechinar o de apretar que puede hacer que los dientes estén en contacto más de tiempo y más poderosamente, ya sea durante el día o mientras duerme.

Hábitos de Rechinar y Apretar

Los hábitos de rechinar y apretar son generalmente una expresión física de la tensión sicológica o emocional. Muchas veces, los pacientes están totalmente inconscientes de sus hábitos de rechinar, apretar o morder. Típicamente, este hábito destructivo ocurre durante el sueño, y los pacientes niegan comúnmente el saber que ocurre. Estos hábitos pueden ocurrir durante períodos de alta tensión u ocasionalmente por la alta demanda personal. Siempre que ocurre desgaste no funcional de los dientes, el esmalte se desgasta mucho más rápido de lo normal. Cuando esto sucede, el esmalte dental subyacente del diente se expone, y esto crea un problema.

Atrición de la Dentina

El esmalte es absolutamente duro y resistente al desgaste. La dentina, por otra parte, tiene un componente orgánico más alto y no maneja las fuerzas de fricción de rechinar, apretar y morder muy bien. Por lo tanto, la cubierta externa del diente (esmalte) se desgasta, la dentina subyacente comenzará a desgastarse más rápidamente, exponiendo aún más la dentina a la cavidad bucal. El diente se puede astillar y fracturar. La dentina también tiene una tendencia de demostrar más manchas del fumar, alimento y/o bebidas. El café, té, bebidas de cola y el vino rojo son notables por causar una mancha fea marrón/anaranjada en la dentina.

Incluso cuando usted elimina el hábito que lo causa, una vez que se expone la dentina, ésta continuará desgastándose más rápidamente que el esmalte circundante. Esto causará un área en forma de plato o dona que progresará en defectos más grandes. Al menos, es mejor restaurar las áreas cuanto antes (incluso si no son problemas cosméticos todavía) para prevenir el deterioro adicional de la estructura del diente.

Opciones de Tratamiento

Hay varias soluciones posibles a los problemas de atrición y abrasión, dependiendo del nivel de desgaste del diente. Usted puede elegir no hacer nada. Sus dientes probablemente continuarán desgastándose, manchándose y tornándose cada vez más feos mientras pierden su forma apropiada, se rompen, se agrietan y/o se destiñen. Pueden llegar a ser más sensibles a los cambios de temperatura. El desgaste excesivo puede incluso requerir tratamiento endodóntico (terapia del canal radicular). En los casos más avanzados, los dientes traseros se gastan hasta quedar planos y las relaciones de la mandíbula cambian hasta el punto que la articulación de la mandíbula (articulación temporomandibular) no funciona apropiadamente, causando dolor.

- Puede hacerse un protector bucal o protector de mordida que evita que sus dientes entren en contacto cuando usted aprieta o rechina. Se usa en momentos de mucha tensión cuando es más probable que usted apriete y rechine.
- Los dientes posteriores (traseros) fracturados y desgastados pueden ser restaurados. Las restauraciones de molde pueden ser utilizadas para restaurar y mantener una relación de la mandíbula apropiada. El oro de molde es generalmente el material que se escoge para los pacientes que sufren de hábitos de apretar y rechinar. La decisión final sobre los materiales será tomada a base de una evaluación de cada situación individual.
- La dentina expuesta en los dientes delanteros se puede restaurar con una resina del color del diente adherida directamente a las áreas.
- Identifique y elimine la causa de su tensión.

Desgraciadamente, una vez el diente se ha desgastado, no crecerá nuevamente. Solamente puede ser reparado. Es mucho mejor detener el progreso de la atrición. ¿Cuándo es el mejor momento para comenzar el tratamiento para el hábito de bruxismo y rechinar? Tan pronto como se diagnostique el problema.

Si usted tiene cualquier pregunta sobre la atrición o la abrasión, favor de sentirse libre de preguntarnos.

Mal Aliento

De vez en cuando, todos experimentamos mal aliento. Ciertas comidas—con mucho ajo, cebollas o especies—pueden dejar un olor persistente, pero es solamente un problema temporal. El mal aliento crónico es otro problema diferente. Puede ser causado por la enfermedad periodontal, deterioro en los dientes, deterioro debajo de las empastaduras o coronas, así como por problemas del sistema digestivo o seno. El mal aliento causado por cualesquiera de estas condiciones necesita ser corregido por su dentista o médico.

Aunque pueden haber problemas médicos y/o sistémicos que causan el mal aliento, la mayoría de las veces el mal aliento es el resultado de cosas dejadas en y alrededor de sus dientes. Su boca es caliente, húmeda y oscura—el lugar perfecto para que las bacterias crezcan y se descompongan. Cuando sucede esto y los dientes no se limpian correctamente diariamente, un olor crónico puede resultar. El mal aliento se puede eliminar bastante fácil, o por lo menos controlarlo, removiendo los residuos de comida, placa o cálculos, reemplazando las empastaduras rotas que causan que el alimento quede atrapado, restaurando las áreas de deterioro y/o eliminando la enfermedad de la encía. La placa que se acumula en o alrededor del borde de las encías puede también encontrar la manera de llegar a los recesos en la superficie de su lengua, contribuyendo también al mal aliento.

El cepillarse los dientes, limpiarse la lengua y limpiarse con hilo dental correctamente, por lo menos una vez al día, son la mejor prevención y cura para el mal aliento. Estos procedimientos no solamente prevendrán la enfermedad periodontal y el deterioro removiendo las bacterias, sino también removerán todos los residuos de alimento. Los fabricantes de pastas de dientes, cepillos de dientes, hilo dental y enjuagues bucales reclaman que ayudan a prevenir el mal aliento y pueden proporcionar un alivio temporal de ese síntoma. No importa qué producto usted utiliza, asegúrese de quitar la placa bacteriana diariamente.

La clave para prevenir problemas dentales y mal aliento es el limpiar sus dientes correctamente cada día. La mejor manera de aprender cómo limpiar sus dientes es visitándonos. Usted tiene la capacidad de tomar buen cuidado de su boca; es solo cuestión de practicar las habilidades correctas que mejor satisfagan sus condiciones orales únicas. Ya sea que usted tenga muchas empastaduras, coronas o puentes, dentaduras removibles parciales o completas, implantes, frenillos u otros aparatos en su boca, hay un método o una herramienta que funcionará para usted.

También, para asegurar un aliento fresco, tenga sus dientes limpiados profesionalmente, por nosotros, regularmente. La meta aquí no es solamente corregir cualquier problema relacionado a una enfermedad, sino también evitar que cualquier problema comience en el primer lugar.

Su problema de mal aliento no tiene que ser una fuente crónica de vergüenza. A menudo es un síntoma de un problema dental. Mientras más pronto se trate, más fácil y menos costoso será arreglarlo.

Si usted tiene cualquier pregunta sobre el mal aliento, favor de sentirse libre de preguntarnos.

Síndrome de Diente Fraccionado (SDF)

Definición de Síndrome de Diente Fraccionado (SDF)

Cuando los dientes se han rellenado mucho, no es inusual que se desarrolle el síndrome de diente fraccionado (o partido). Los síntomas incluyen un dolor agudo cuando muerde algo duro. Cuando abre su boca, y los dientes ya no están tocándose, el dolor se va.

Las áreas más comunes donde ocurre el SDF son los premolares y molares—los dientes traseros que muelen y machacan el alimento. Frecuentemente el diente tiene una empastadura extensa (usualmente amalgama de plata) que ha estado en su lugar por un largo tiempo. De vez en cuando, el SDF ocurre en un diente que se ha taladrado recientemente y una gran cantidad de la estructura del diente se ha perdido. Sin embargo, el síndrome de diente fraccionado puede ocurrir en dientes que tienen una empastadura de plata pequeña. En la mayoría de los casos, la empastadura ha debilitado el diente justo lo suficiente que cuando usted mastica o muerde, el diente y la empastadura se separan levemente (doblan), causando dolor inmediato y, a veces, severo. El dolor no persiste generalmente después de que se termina de morder.

El hecho de que usted siente dolor cuando se aplica presión al diente significa que el nervio está afectado. Si el problema no se soluciona rápidamente, el nervio puede morir y el diente entonces requerirá tratamiento endodóntico (canal radicular).

Tratamiento

El tratamiento implicará por lo menos una radiografía para asistir el diagnóstico para ayudar a eliminar otras causas. Intentaremos encontrar la sección del diente que está causando el problema empujando en varias secciones del diente, o haciendo que usted muerda un objeto duro. Cuando la sección del diente que está agrietada se encuentra, hace el tratamiento más fácil. Primero, se anestesia el diente y se remueve la empastadura vieja. Luego, examinamos cuidadosamente el área para determinar si la sección agrietada se puede ver. Muy frecuentemente es visible en este momento. El siguiente paso es considerar si el área partida se puede arreglar con un relleno directo (adherido). Ésta es la situación ideal si la grieta es pequeña. Desgraciadamente, esto raramente ocurre. Más a menudo (más de un 95% del tiempo), las superficies de mordida del diente se deben cubrir y proteger completamente primero, con una corona u onlay provisional (temporal). Si esto es exitoso en la eliminación del dolor (esperamos generalmente algunas semanas para estar seguros que el problema está resuelto), se hace una impresión para un molde fabricado en el laboratorio—ya sea un onlay de porcelana o de resina o una corona. Si queda una estructura del diente adecuada, una restauración de cobertura parcial—un onlay—es preferida. Si el diente se ha agrietado gravemente o si no queda mucho del diente, entonces una corona será necesaria. El propósito de cualquier tipo de restauración es unir todas las secciones del diente de manera que no puede moverse o separarse bajo las fuerzas normales de morder. Si la restauración provisional es exitosa eliminando el dolor, esperamos que la corona de molde final u onlay corrija el problema.

Retrasar el Tratamiento

¿Qué sucede si el SDF no se trata rápidamente? Lo mejor que usted puede esperar es que el diente le continúe molestando solamente cuando usted mastica o muerde. Esto no sucede frecuentemente. Generalmente, la sección agrietada del diente se hace más débil y más débil hasta que se fractura. Además, si la grieta se hace más profunda en el diente, el nervio morirá y el diente necesitará tratamiento endodóntico antes de colocar la corona u onlay. En algunas ocasiones el nervio se afecta inmediatamente por la grieta inicial y muere. Esto puede ocurrir rápido o puede tomar años antes de que sea evidente. Cada caso de SDF es único. Si es de alguna consolación, el diente fraccionado no es su culpa. Es el resultado de que su diente se ha taladrado y rellenado con grandes empastaduras de plata usted cuando era más joven. Vemos este problema dental en particular en pacientes entre los 25 y 45 años.

Desgraciadamente, un diente fraccionado no desaparece. Muchas veces, solamente duele cuando usted muerde en ellos en un ángulo particular. Si al segmento fracturado no se le aplica tensión, el diente se siente normal. Puede ser que también usted pueda "entrenarse" a masticar en diversos dientes y evitar el diente fraccionado. En el mejor de los casos, usted pospone el tratamiento necesario mientras el nervio puede morir lentamente.

Si usted tiene cualquier pregunta sobre el síndrome de diente fraccionado, favor de sentirse libre de preguntarnos.

Ilustración en CD-ROM

Síndrome de Diente Fraccionado (SDF): Instrucciones Postoperatorias

Nombre del Paciente:_____   **Fecha:**_____

❑ Su diente ha sido diagnosticado con el **"síndrome de diente fraccionado"**. Debido a la naturaleza de la apariencia clínica de la fractura, hemos tratado de disminuir los síntomas ajustando su oclusión (mordida) en el diente. Éste puede ser el único tratamiento que usted necesitará. **Si el malestar que usted siente cuando muerde no se elimina en el plazo de una semana, por favor llame a la oficina y déjenos saber.** Si la partición sigue presente, se debe tratar un enfoque diferente. Dele al diente algunos días para "calmarse" antes que intente morder alimentos duros.

❑ El diente partido ha sido tratado quitando la restauración vieja y colocando una empastadura adherida en su lugar. Si la partidura, es pequeña esto puede eliminar el problema. No muerda duro sobre el diente por algunos días, luego coloque más presión gradualmente en el diente. **Llame a la oficina en una semana y déjenos saber como se siente.** Si la partición sigue presente, se debe tratar un enfoque diferente. Si se deja sin tratar, el diente se puede partir más y puede que necesite tratamiento endodóntico y una corona. Si el diente se parte severamente, puede que necesite ser sacado.

❑ Una corona temporal ha sido cementada sobre el diente fraccionado con un cemento temporal. Debido a que la grieta era tan severa, utilizaremos este procedimiento para determinar si el diente se puede o no tratar sin un canal radicular. **Por favor dele al diente algunos días para descansar antes de que intente morder alimentos duros.** Espere que el diente esté sensible por algunos días después de que se coloque el temporal. Esto es normal. Aplique gradualmente más fuerza cuando muerde los alimentos. Espere que la corona temporal permanezca en su lugar por varias semanas, hasta que se pueda determinar si el problema está o no resuelto.

Cuanto antes se diagnostica y trata un diente fraccionado, mayor es el éxito del tratamiento. Si la partición es severa, un canal radicular puede ser necesario para salvar el diente. Dependiendo de los síntomas que usted describa, podemos elegir tratarlo como un ajuste de mordida, una empastadura pequeña o una preparación grande para un onlay o corona. Si esto no trabaja, el plan de tratamiento será modificado. Si se deja sin tratar, el diente se puede perder eventualmente. Puede también ser posible que la partición inicial sea de tal magnitud que el diente no pueda ser salvado, a pesar de nuestros mejores esfuerzos.

Si usted tiene cualquier pregunta sobre estas instrucciones postoperatorias para el síndrome de diente fraccionado, favor de sentirse libre de preguntarnos.

Deterioro de la Dentina

Generalmente, el deterioro de la dentina es bastante fácil de detectar. Cuando una caries está comenzando, se identifica típicamente por un color marrón o blanco o un cambio en la translucidez del esmalte del diente. El dentista o higienista dental usa un instrumento dental especial llamado un *explorador* para sentir el área sospechada y verificar su dureza. Si el área es dura, en otras palabras, si no hay rotura en la capa del esmalte perceptible; creemos que no hay caries presente. Si, sin embargo, la superficie se siente suave y el explorador se "atasca" en el sitio sospechado, creemos que hay una caries presente.

Debido al extenso uso y la disponibilidad del fluoruro en nuestra agua potable, alimentos y productos del cuidado oral, estamos viendo un patrón diferente de deterioro. La apariencia es diferente del patrón típico de deterioro y es más difícil de detectar. Como la superficie externa del esmalte absorbe el fluoruro (de la pasta de dientes, por ejemplo), el esmalte llega a ser muy resistente a la desmineralización y al deterioro eventual. Si hay una rotura pequeña en la integridad del esmalte, un hoyo o una ranura donde las bacterias que causan el deterioro pueden vivir, las bacterias pueden disolver el esmalte de tal manera que el hoyo en el esmalte no puede ser detectado. Una vez que las bacterias que causan el deterioro alcanzan la dentina subyacente, los ácidos se comen la sustancia y rápidamente hacen una caries grande—pero una que todavía no puede ser vista o detectada fácilmente. De esta manera el esmalte se socava. Un dentista que mira una caries tan pequeña pensaría que es muy fácil restaurar. Sin embargo, una vez la porción deteriorada del esmalte se quita y la dentina llega a ser visible, el grado verdadero del daño llega a ser obvio. La caries pequeña se convierte en una caries grande.

Detección y Tratamiento

Uno de los problemas principales con el deterioro que aparenta ocurrir solamente en la dentina es en la detección. Si una radiografía se toma como parte del proceso periódico del examen, puede que veamos el deterioro de la dentina si es moderado a extenso. El deterioro que se ve en las radiografías es típicamente dos a siete veces mayor en el diente. La película radiográfica de alta velocidad moderna y la radiografía de exposición reducida hace más difícil de detectar el deterioro temprano en radiografías.

Prevención

La aplicación concienzuda de una fuente de fluoruro tópico—mediante un dentífrico sin receta o un producto de fluoruro recetado—y la remoción de la placa son esenciales. Los **selladores** adheridos son una protección eficaz contra el deterioro de la dentina. **Aconsejamos enfáticamente estos procedimientos.** Los exámenes periódicos en los intervalos recomendados por el dentista pueden detectar el deterioro cuanto antes. Ésta es la única manera de mantener problemas pequeños de convertirse en problemas más grandes.

Si usted tiene cualquier pregunta sobre el deterioro de la dentina, favor de sentirse libre de preguntarnos.

Displasia del Esmalte

Definición

La palabra *esmalte,* probablemente le es familiar a usted como la cubierta externa dura de la corona del diente. La palabra *displasia,* es probablemente menos familiar. La *displasia del esmalte* es un término dental que discute un número de problemas dentales, tanto cosméticos y estructurales. La condición puede afectar solamente la superficie del diente y aparecer como hoyos pequeños en el esmalte o como una malformación gruesa del esmalte y de la forma del diente. La displasia del esmalte puede extenderse de leve a severa con todos los grados en el medio.

Causas

Las causas de la displasia son numerosas, pero ocurre durante una etapa crítica del esmalte/de la formación del diente. La fiebre, la enfermedad, la medicación, el cambio en nutrición o la medicación recetada todos han sido mencionados como causas.

Procedimientos Correctivos

Raramente estas condiciones hacen el diente más débil o más propenso al deterioro. Los dientes con displasia no son "suaves". ¡En realidad, muchas veces estos dientes afectados exhiben menos incidencia de deterioro que los dientes que tienen forma, color, contorno y textura normales!

Todos están de acuerdo que la displasia del esmalte es fea y la corrección del problema es necesaria. La solución depende del tipo de defecto y del grado al cual los dientes están implicados. Si la mancha es superficial, muchas veces el diente puede ser pulido— y nunca regresa. Esto se hace con un taladro o con los compuestos especiales de pulir o ambos. A veces un agente que blanquea es también usado. No se requiere un anestésico local porque no hay dolor implicado. Una restauración (empastadura) no es necesaria para corregir una displasia superficial.

Cuando el defecto es más profundo en el diente, el defecto puede necesitar ser quitado mecánicamente (taladrado) y una restauración adherida del color del diente será colocada. A veces una inyección de un anestésico local es necesaria para corregir un defecto más profundo. La empastadura debe durar por muchos años antes de que necesite ser substituida. La igualación de color es generalmente perfecta.

Alisar el defecto del esmalte o sustituir el área con una empastadura pequeña es a menudo todo lo que es necesario. Cuando el defecto es más severo, sin embargo, la reconstrucción del diente con onlays o coronas adheridos es necesario. Le diremos qué es lo indicado después de examinar su boca y de determinar el grado de su problema.

Descalcificación del Esmalte

Hay un tipo de mancha o línea blanca que se forma en un diente que no es realmente displasia del esmalte pero parece que es. Esto aparece como línea blanca a lo largo del borde de la encía y es causada por una descalcificación del esmalte debido a placa o desechos que se acumulan en el diente. En resumen, el área no está siendo cepillada correctamente y una caries se ha comenzado a formar. Cuando un paciente tiene frenillos ortodónticos, la limpieza del espacio entre la banda ortodóntica y el borde de la encía puede ser un problema. El cuidado oral de sí mismo apropiado es esencial para los pacientes que están bajo terapia ortodóntica.

El tratamiento, con excepción de algunos tratamientos con fluoruro tópico, puede no ser necesario si la descalcificación del esmalte se descubre en la etapa temprana. Cuando la línea blanca es suave o la descalcificación ha invadido la dentina subyacente, el taladrar y la restauración serán necesarios.

Si usted tiene cualquier pregunta sobre la displasia del esmalte, favor de sentirse libre de preguntarnos.

Desgaste Excesivo

CONTACTO DE DIENTE CON DIENTE

Cuando dos superficies se frotan una contra la otra, las superficies eventualmente se gastaran. Cuán rápidamente esto ocurre y cuánta área superficial se pierde depende de la dureza de la superficie (resistencia a la abrasión), y cuánto tiempo la fuerza (acción abrasiva) continúa.

Cómo Ocurre la Abrasión

El esmalte es una sustancia extremadamente dura. En realidad, pocas sustancias son más duras. Debido a la dureza, el esmalte puede resistir desgaste y durar por una vida de masticar el alimento. Éste protege y cubre la sustancia interna subyacente del diente mucho más suave, la dentina y el tejido del nervio.

Aunque el esmalte es muy resistente a la abrasión, sí ocurre. He aquí cómo: la abrasión más común que vemos es cuando los dientes delanteros inferiores frotan contra los dientes delanteros superiores. El esmalte en las superficies de mordida de estos dientes es moderadamente grueso, hasta aproximadamente 2 mm. Sobre el curso de la vida de una persona, estos dientes entrarán en contacto y el esmalte se perderá lentamente. Normalmente, esto sucede lentamente. Este tipo de desgaste no es para preocuparse. El problema con el desgaste excesivo comienza cuando un paciente rechina o aprieta los dientes, poniendo más fuerza sobre los dientes o trabajándolos juntos por períodos largos de tiempo. Aunque el esmalte es muy duro, si se "abusa" por suficiente tiempo, se gastara. El desgaste ocurre más rápidamente cuando un diente natural está opuesto a una corona de porcelana. La porcelana es mucho más dura que el esmalte y puede gastar el esmalte aun bajo uso normal. En este caso es crítico que la mordida esté ajustada correctamente para reducir esta posibilidad.

Consecuencia de la Abrasión

¿Por qué es el desgaste acelerado del esmalte un problema? Aunque el desgaste continúa en todos los dientes, es más visible en los dientes delanteros inferiores. Los dientes delanteros inferiores pueden ser los dientes más importantes de su boca puesto, que controlan las relaciones de la mordida de su mandíbula inferior y superior.

Una vez el esmalte se gasta, dos cosas indeseables pueden suceder. Primero, la dentina expuesta puede llegar a ser sensible a los cambios del aire o de temperatura. En segundo lugar, cuando no es apoyado por dentina resistente, el esmalte se puede romper y el diente llegará a ser más pequeño. Mientras esto sucede, el movimiento natural del diente empuja el diente más hacia fuera de su hueco. El diente ahora más corto para solamente cuando se encuentra con el diente opuesto. Además, la dentina tiende a mancharse más fácilmente que el esmalte, así que habrá un aspecto cosmético distinto y desagradable que llegará a ser excesivo con el pasar del tiempo.

Tratamiento para la Abrasión

El tratamiento del desgaste excesivo depende de cuánto diente falta. Si solamente el esmalte es afectado, se recomienda un protector bucal. Si una cantidad de pequeña a moderada de la dentina está expuesta, puede ser cubierta fácilmente con una resina adherida del color del diente. La resina, aunque no es tan resistente como el esmalte original, sigue siendo mucho más dura que la dentina. Si usted todavía continúa rechinando o apretando sus dientes, la resina será la única estructura del diente ahora afectada. En casos extremos del desgaste excesivo, los laminados de porcelana o las coronas completas pueden ser los únicos medios de restauración.

El desgaste excesivo es difícil de diagnosticar en las primeras etapas. Puede tomar meses y años para que llegue a ser evidente. No sucede de la noche a la mañana. Cuando es observado, es mejor tratarlo temprano cuando hay menos cantidad de pérdida de diente y hay una mayor oportunidad de una solución duradera, conservadora.

Si usted tiene cualquier pregunta sobre el desgaste excesivo, favor de sentirse libre de preguntarnos.

Extracción

Razones para la Recomendación de la Extracción del Diente

Los dientes pueden necesitar ser extraídos por varias razones, incluyendo, pero no está limitado a:

- enfermedad periodontal severa
- daños irreversibles al tejido del nervio dentro del diente (y el paciente está en contra de salvar el diente)
- fallo de la terapia endodóntica
- fractura o deterioro extremo de la estructura del diente
- colocación incorrecta del diente o para los propósitos ortodónticos

En gran parte, la razón de la extracción influenciará la cantidad de malestar que usted puede experimentar después del procedimiento. Cuando el diente debe ser extraído por razones periodontales, habrá menos soporte del hueso para el diente y el diente se puede extraer más fácilmente que si hubiese soporte completo del hueso. En este caso puede haber menos malestar después de la extracción.

Después de la Extracción

Le diremos la razón para la extracción y le dejaremos saber qué esperar después del procedimiento. Por favor siga las instrucciones dadas a usted. Si se le recetan antibióticos, tómelos hasta que la receta se acabe *totalmente*. Si se receta medicamentos para el dolor, *tómelos solamente si es necesario*. Si la medicación recetada contiene un componente narcótico, tal como codeína, no conduzca un vehículo de motor u opere maquinaria que podría ocasionar daños a usted o a otros. **Espere que cierto sangrado ocurra en el lugar de la extracción por las primeras 24 horas.** Recuerde, que ahora hay un hueco en su mandíbula de donde se ha extraído el diente, y el hueco puede ser bastante grande. Se debe esperar cierto sangrado.

Algunas complicaciones infrecuentes de procedimientos quirúrgicos orales rutinarios incluyen (pero no están limitadas a):

- fractura de dientes adyacentes o de restauraciones (lo que por supuesto significa que éstas áreas afectadas se deben restaurar a la función normal después de la curación del lugar de la extracción)
- puntas de la raíz o fragmentos de la raíz separados
- daño del nervio del área temporal o permanente, como resultado de la anestesia o parestesia (adormecimiento)
- curación incompleta, resultando en dolor severo —un "alveolo seco"
- fractura del hueso circundante.

Si usted tiene cualquier pregunta sobre las razones para una extracción dental, favor de sentirse libre de preguntarnos.

Extracción: Instrucciones Postoperatorias

Nombre del Paciente:_____   **Fecha:**_____

Si estas instrucciones no se siguen, el lugar de la extracción puede que no se cure correctamente y el tiempo necesario para la curación apropiada aumentará.

- Mantenga su boca cerrada firmemente sobre la gasa por _____ minutos. Entonces, quite la gasa.
- No cambie la gasa a menos que sea mandado por el dentista.
- No escupa, enjuague o fume por 24 horas.
- Sería una buena idea no cepillar cerca del lugar de la extracción por un día o dos.
- Cuando cepille y limpie con hilo dental el área, ¡sea cuidadoso!
- Por 24 horas después de la extracción, intente masticar el alimento lejos del lugar de la extracción.
- Se debe esperar una leve hinchazón en el área, especialmente si la extracción fue difícil.
- Si se colocan suturas, regrese para quitárselas.
- Si se han recetado medicamentos para el posible malestar después de la extracción, tómelo según dirigido.
- Si NO se han recetado medicamentos, usted debe tomar su aliviador de dolor normal que consigue sin receta.
- Vuelva en _____ semanas para que el dentista pueda evaluar la curación del lugar de la extracción.

Notifíquenos por favor sí:

- Si hay un sangrado extendido del lugar de la extracción. Sangrado leve por varias horas es normal.
- Cualquier cosa con excepción de hinchazón leve ocurre.
- El malestar continúa por más de 24 horas, especialmente si no es aliviado con aliviadores de dolor que se consiguen sin receta.

Instrucciones especiales:_____

_____

Diente(s) # a ser extraído: , conocido comúnmente como

Comentarios:_____

_____

He leído y entiendo esta información sobre la extracción dental y consiento a tener el procedimiento realizado en esta oficina. No tengo ninguna otra pregunta sobre el procedimiento o del cuidado postoperatorio.

_____   _____
Firma del paciente o guardián   Fecha

Dolores de Cabeza: La Conexión Dental

Usted probablemente recuerda la vieja canción "... el hueso de la rodilla está conectado con el hueso de la pierna; el hueso de la pierna está conectado con el hueso de la cadera ... etc". Su hueso de la mandíbula (inferior) está conectado con su 'hueso de la cabeza'—y está conectado por músculos, ligamentos y tendones. Esta área se conoce como la *articulación temporomandibular* o *ATM*. Cuando la mandíbula inferior se alinea perfectamente con la mandíbula superior y todo funciona normalmente, todo está bien. Si la mandíbula inferior no se alinea correctamente o, quizás más importante, si hay tensión anormal presente cuando la mandíbula inferior entra en contacto con la mandíbula superior, los problemas pueden ocurrir. La tensión anormal generalmente es el apretar o rechinar de los dientes y puede ocurrir en cualquier momento, día o noche, despierto o dormido. Cuando esto sucede, una persona puede desarrollar dolores de cabeza de migraña regulares o crónicos, dolor muscular o sensibilidad en los músculos de las articulaciones de la mandíbula o disfunción de la articulación temporomandibular (DTM). Cuarenta y cuatro millones de americanos sufren del apretar y rechinar los dientes crónicamente resultando en daño del diente, y 23 millones sufren de migraña.

Aunque los protectores bucales se han utilizado con cierto éxito para tratar a pacientes con DTM, un nuevo dispositivo aprobado por la FDA parece ofrecer una razón de éxito mayor en la eliminación de problemas de ATM. Este dispositivo tiene una ventaja adicional ya fue diseñado para reducir los hábitos de apretar que conducen a menudo a los dolores de cabeza crónicos y de migraña. Este dispositivo evita que los dientes superiores e inferiores entren en contacto. Los estudios han demostrado que evitando el apretón de alta intensidad (y la irritación muscular que conduce al dolor de migraña, DTM y dolor de cabeza crónico), el 82% de las víctimas de migraña y de dolor de cabeza han tenido una reducción del 77% en los incidentes de migraña. En resumen, la frecuencia e intensidad de los episodios de dolor de cabeza y la sensibilidad del músculo se pueden reducir con el uso de un protector bucal.

Un sistema de supresión de tensión es otra forma eficaz de protector bucal que puede tratar la DTM. Este dispositivo pequeño removible, hecho en la oficina, puede ser usado de día y/o noche y ha sido demostrado que reduce la intensidad del apretar en un 66%. Éste aprovecha un reflejo naturalmente protector que suprime los poderosos músculos de masticación activos durante el apretar. Para aquellos preocupados sobre la cobertura del seguro, el costo de este dispositivo se somete primero al seguro médico para la evaluación del beneficio de la cobertura. La mayoría de los portadores de seguro consideran este dispositivo un beneficio pagable.

¿Cuán importante es la reducción de la tensión del apretón? Intente esta demostración simple. Ponga un lápiz entre los últimos molares superiores e inferiores en un lado y muerda fuerte. Recuerde cuán fuerte usted mordió. Después tome el lápiz y colóquelo entre los dientes delanteros superiores e inferiores y muerda fuerte otra vez. Usted no podrá morder tan fuerte cuando está mordiendo en los dientes delanteros. Usted debe poder detectar una gran diferencia entre morder (apretar) en los últimos dientes y los dientes delanteros solamente. Intente otra prueba: coloque ligeramente sus yemas de los dedos de cualquier lado de su cabeza en el área temporal (sobre y delante de los oídos). Apriete sus dientes y sienta los músculos a cualquier lado de la cabeza hincharse. Luego, tome un lápiz, colóquelo entre los dientes delanteros superiores e inferiores, y muerda otra vez. Usted sentirá fácilmente que no se hinchan tanto los músculos temporales, significando que no es posible tanta compresión del apretón.

Si usted tiene cualquier pregunta sobre la conexión entre dolores de cabeza y sus dientes, favor de sentirse libre de preguntarnos.

Cómo Fomentar el Deterioro de los Dientes

UN MANUAL DE CÓMO CONSEGUIR TODOS LOS DIENTES DETERIORADOS QUE USTED DESEA Y SE MERECE...

El deterioro comienza en los dientes en localizaciones específicas en una manera que casi enteramente depende sobre lo que usted hace. Este manual describirá diversos tipos de caries y qué USTED puede hacer para asegurar conseguir todos los dientes podridos que usted desea.

1. Las caries pueden comenzar en las superficies de mordida de los dientes. Para conseguir deterioro en estas áreas, haga lo siguiente:
   a. Ya sea un niño, un adolescente o un adulto, no coloque selladores protectores sin dolor en sus dientes.
   b. Diariamente y tan frecuentemente como sea posible, coma y beba alimentos que tengan un alto contenido de azúcar.
   c. Coma dulces pegajosos tan a menudo como sea posible.
   d. NO cepille sus dientes diariamente. NO utilice un enjuague bucal que tenga fluoruro.

2. Las caries pueden comenzar entre los dientes. Éstas se llaman las *caries de no limpiarse con hilo dental.* Para conseguir este tipo específico de deterioro:
   a. NO limpie con hilo dental sus dientes correctamente cada día. Racionalice y encuentre las excusas para no limpiar con hilo dental sus dientes. Si esto se hace muy difícil, sólo limpie con hilo dental los dientes usted desea mantener.
   b. NO utilice diariamente un enjuague bucal que tenga fluoruro.

3. Las caries pueden comenzar a lo largo del borde de la encía (donde el diente aparece salir del tejido de la encía). Éstas son un tipo especial de caries. ¡Pueden progresar muy rápidamente hasta el punto que usted hasta puede necesitar un canal radicular! Para conseguir caries rápidas y grandes en estas áreas (especialmente en los dientes traseros):
   a. Asegúrese de chupar caramelos duros ricos en azúcar, bombones para la tos y mentas para el aliento. Haga esto a menudo durante el día.
   b. NO cepille correctamente sus dientes. Cerciórese que las cerdas del cepillo de dientes no entren en contacto con la conexión entre el diente y la encía. Si usted encuentra esto muy difícil de hacer, deje que el higienista dental le demuestre como hacerlo correctamente y después haga lo contrario de lo que le digan.
   c. NO utilice un enjuague bucal que tenga fluoruro.

4. Si le faltan dientes:
   a. NO los sustituya en una manera oportuna. Los dientes adyacentes y opuestos entonces podrán moverse a las nuevas áreas que son difíciles de limpiar y serán más propensos, no solamente al deterioro, pero a problemas de la encía y mordida también.

5. NO vea al dentista y al higienista dental rutinariamente (2–4 veces por año, dependiendo de su situación individual) para examinar y limpiar sus dientes. Si usted va, los profesionales dentales pueden encontrar y tratar los dientes deteriorados cuando el deterioro es mínimo. Ellos no están inclinados a dejar que las caries crezcan correctamente. En realidad, si encontramos el deterioro cuando es realmente pequeño, puede que podamos tratar y remineralizar el incipiente (comienzo) del deterioro ¡sin incluso usar un taladro o poner una inyección!

Bajo ninguna circunstancia utilice la goma de mascar o las mentas sin azúcar. Algunos de estos productos tienen un aditivo (RECALDENT) que se ha demostrado que hace al esmalte más fuerte y más resistente al deterioro. El RECALDENT promueve la remineralización del esmalte. Esto podía retrasar el proceso de deterioro o aun prevenir la formación de algunas caries.

Si usted sigue terminantemente las reglas antedichas, usted asegurará conseguir las caries más grandes que usted pueda.
La responsabilidad de hacer crecer las caries es suya solamente.

Dientes Impactados

Un diente impactado es un diente que no ha salido (emergido completamente en la cavidad bucal). El diente impactado puede estar completamente rodeado por hueso (una impacción huesuda completa), puede estar rodeado parcialmente por hueso (una impacción huesuda parcial) o puede solamente estar rodeado por tejido suave de la encía (una impacción del tejido suave).

Tradicionalmente, el término de *diente impactado* generalmente se refiere a las muelas cordales (los terceros molares, los dientes más atrás en la boca). Las muelas cordales superiores e inferiores pueden estar impactadas. Muchas veces si no parecen estar causando problemas al paciente, estos no se tocan. Si están posicionados en una manera que parecen estar empujándose contra las raíces de los segundos molares (el siguiente diente) o si están causando problemas periodontales (de la encía), estos necesitarán ser removidos. Aunque casi todos los dentistas generales se sienten cómodos removiendo dientes, los pacientes con dientes impactados son generalmente referidos a un especialista (cirujano oral) para removerlos.

Las muelas cordales no son los únicos dientes que pueden estar impactados. Cada diente permanente puede estar impactado. Si la impacción no parece afectar el diente adyacente, ningún tratamiento puede ser requerido. Si afecta otros dientes, pueden necesitar ser extraídos.

No es raro para un 'colmillo' (diente canino) estar impactado. Esto se descubre generalmente temprano en la vida, y se harán recomendaciones para el tratamiento ortodóntico ('frenillos'). Frecuentemente, estos dientes impactados no son removidos, sino que son expuestos quirúrgicamente y movidos ortodónticamente por varios meses a su posición correcta. La detección y el diagnóstico temprano son importantes para el tratamiento exitoso de esta situación.

Normalmente, hay hueso separando las raíces del diente de los dientes adyacentes. Si el diente impactado, debido a su ángulo y posición, consigue acercarse mucho a las raíces del siguiente diente, el hueso entre los dos dientes se disolverá. Si esto sucede, es posible que se forme un bolsillo periodontal patológico profundo. La deterioración adicional de los tejidos periodontales que rodean el diente en la posición normal puede poner en peligro su salud y conducir a tratamiento dental adicional. Para evitar que esto suceda, el diente afectado se extrae. Si la impacción es profunda y difícil acercarse, y hay cuatro muelas cordales que se extraerán al mismo tiempo, el dentista puede elegir realizar el procedimiento en un hospital o centro quirúrgico.

Mientras más hueso rodea el diente impactado, más difícil es extraerlo. La posición del diente cerca de otros dientes o nervios y la manera en la cual el diente impactado está inclinado en el hueso también afecta el nivel de dificultad de la extracción. Cuanto más joven el paciente, mejor y más fácil parece ser la curación. Si se quita una gran parte del hueso para poder extraer el diente impactado, el dentista puede elegir colocar algún material de 'relleno de hueso' en el lugar donde estaba el diente (el hueco) para promover una mejor curación del hueso.

Si usted tiene cualquier pregunta sobre los dientes impactados, favor de sentirse libre de preguntarnos.

Grietas Inducidas en el Esmalte por las Empastaduras de Metal

Le han diagnosticado con grietas en uno o más dientes que fueron restaurados previamente con un material de empastadura de amalgama (metal) de plata. Quizás le demostramos, con la cámara de vídeo intraoral, que algunos de los dientes tienen estas grietas, y dónde en los dientes están localizadas las grietas. Generalmente, las grietas se manchan fácilmente y se ven fácilmente.

Aunque el esmalte del diente es duro y frágil, con el pasar del tiempo pequeñas microgrietas aparecerán en el esmalte. Esto se piensa que es debido a los ciclos termales por los que pasa el esmalte debido a los artículos que usted come y bebe que son más calientes o más fríos que la temperatura del ambiente. Una vez más, con el pasar del tiempo, la expansión y contracción del esmalte hace aparecer las grietas. Esto no se considera un problema dental y generalmente no se trata. Sin embargo, los dientes que se restauran con las empastaduras de metal son otra historia. Las empastaduras de amalgama (metal) de plata se componen no solamente de plata, pero de otros metales también. Uno de los metales es mercurio. La mayoría de los materiales de empastadura son por lo menos 30%, y algunos son tan altos como 50%, mercurio. Además de ser clasificado como un metal pesado, el mercurio es líquido a temperatura ambiente (aunque no es líquido en el material de empastadura) y se expande y contrae rápidamente cuando se sube y baja su temperatura.

Cómo Ocurren las Grietas

La temperatura de su boca es de cerca de 98.6 grados. Cuando usted toma café caliente, seguido por helado, la temperatura de su boca aumentará unos 20 a 30 grados, entonces bajará unos 60 a 70 grados, entonces vuelve a 98.6 grados. Esto sucede cada vez que usted come o bebe algo que no es de la misma temperatura que su boca. Debido a la expansión del componente de mercurio y de los otros metales del material de empastadura, esta expansión y contracción de la empastadura causará una presión hacia fuera en el esmalte y la dentina. Cuanto más grande la empastadura es al comienzo, y más fino es el esmalte, más propenso es el diente a desarrollar grietas. Las grietas también proporcionan un camino para el ingreso de líquidos y bacterias—un camino para que comience una caries profundamente en el diente. Como si esto no fuese suficientemente malo, el metal absorberá algo de la humedad presente en su boca, y con el tiempo, aumentará de volumen. A medida que se expande, aplica presión hacia fuera en las paredes de la empastadura original. Esto también promueve el desarrollo de grietas en el diente.

Hay dos diversas trayectorias por las cuales la empastadura de metal puede romper los dientes. Viéndose que las empastaduras están cambiando. El que fue metal liso y brillante en algún momento se torna negro, opaco, con hoyos y áspero. Hay una fatiga del metal. Cuanto más vieja es la empastadura, más probable es que esto suceda. Usted puede tener cierta sensibilidad del diente con los líquidos o dulces. Ésta es una indicación adicional de que la empastadura puede estar filtrándose o fallando. Si el diente empastado le duele cuando usted muerde, el diente puede estar partido y pudieron haber ocurrido daños al nervio, o puede ser un problema totalmente diferente y más serio. Las empastaduras de metal colocadas directamente son una técnica anticuada con un material que ha estado sin cambios por casi 180 años.

Opciones de Tratamiento

Usted tiene una opción. Usted puede esperar hasta que las grietas lleguen a ser serias y dolorosas, y luego hacer el trabajo restaurativo aún más extenso, o usted puede comenzar, enseguida, a sustituir las empastaduras de metal donde las grietas son evidentes. Algunas veces, las grietas no se hacen más grandes o causan problemas; sin embargo, muchas grietas sí. Durante los años, el metal se fatiga más y más, y la grieta se agranda. En la mayoría de los casos una resina adherida del color del diente se puede usar para sustituir el metal. Ésta sella mejor a su diente y no se ha demostrado que agrieta los dientes como lo hacen las empastaduras de metal. Si la grieta existente o la empastadura es de moderada a grande, un inlay/onlay de oro, resina o cerámica será recomendado para el material de reemplazo.

Si usted tiene cualquier pregunta sobre las grietas inducidas en el esmalte por las empastaduras de metal, favor de sentirse libre de preguntarnos.

Sensibilidad al Metal

Se ha hecho claro que muchas personas pueden desarrollar sensibilidad a algunos de los metales usados comúnmente en las restauraciones dentales. Esto pudo o no haber sido el caso en los pasados años. Quizás los pacientes no eran sensibles a los metales en ese entonces, o quizás la sensibilidad no fue reconocida y diagnosticada correctamente. Hay muchas clases de metales usados en la odontología. Nosotros en esta oficina hemos, por años, limitado su exposición a posibles problemas usando materiales que tienen pocas combinaciones de metales, o metales que tienen un potencial muy bajo para reacciones de sensibilidad.

Las mujeres parecen tener más reacciones a los metales que los hombres. Los estudios indican que por lo menos una mujer de cada siete tiene una reacción adversa a los metales. Puede estar relacionado con la joyería que las mujeres usan—especialmente las pantallas para las orejas perforadas. Los postes pueden estar hechos de acero inoxidable que contienen níquel. Usted puede entonces notar, después de cierto tiempo usando la joyería, que sus lóbulos de las orejas se ponen rojos, resecos o le pican. También se puede ver en cualquier lugar que la joyería entra en contacto con su piel—muñeca, cuello, dedos, etc. Si éste es su caso, usted está teniendo una reacción de sensibilidad al metal. Si usted tiene cualesquiera de estos problemas, probablemente es recomendable que usted limite el contacto con los metales problemáticos. Esto puede incluir los metales usados en la restauración de sus dientes.

Ocasionalmente, usted podría notar un sabor metálico en su boca. Esto puede venir de las empastaduras de amalgama de plata que se utilizan comúnmente. Algunos estudios demuestran la filtración del metal a través del diente hasta las estructuras que soportan el diente (ligamento periodontal) proveniente de los postes adheridos en el diente después del tratamiento de canal radicular. Estos postes están rodeados enteramente por diente o restauraciones y no están para nada en contacto con el ambiente oral. Otros síntomas orales de sensibilidad al metal incluyen tejido de la encía que permanece crónicamente rojo e hinchado o que sangra fácilmente cuando entra en contacto con la corona de metal o la empastadura.

¿Qué metales se utilizan en la odontología? Las empastaduras de plata (disponible desde aproximadamente 1816) pueden tener cobre, plata, zinc, mercurio y otros metales. Hoy en día, sabemos que varios países han obligado a reducir el uso de las empastaduras de plata debido a las preocupaciones de salud. Las coronas están compuestas de oro, plata, paladio de platino y de otros metales. Un poste usado para fortalecer un diente después del canal radicular es de acero inoxidable o titanio. La sensibilidad a cada uno de estos metales se ha visto—algunos más que otros. El oro y titanio ocupan un nivel bajo. El titanio se ha utilizado por años para reemplazos de articulaciones. El oro puro es demasiado blando para ser utilizado en restauraciones dentales y el titanio es demasiado frágil. Si usted tiene sensibilidad al metal y necesita una corona, puede ser mejor utilizar un metal que sea solamente oro y platino—o quizás un material de cerámica adherida. Aunque estas opciones pueden ser más costosas que otras, la sensibilidad al metal debe ser evitada.

Alternativas No en Metal

Las alternativas a las restauraciones de metal incluyen las resinas, cerámica y porcelana adherida. Aunque es posible que usted sea sensible a algunos de los materiales adheridos, estos tipos de sensibilidades no son comunes. Las ventajas de las empastaduras de plata son que son rápidas para colocar y bastante baratas. Las ventajas de los moldes de metal usados debajo de las coronas de porcelana son similares; las coronas de metal/porcelana son menos costosas de hacer y más fáciles de colocar que las variedades de cerámica completas.

Preferiríamos no utilizar empastaduras de plata/mercurio, especialmente en niños y mujeres que planean tener niños. Las resinas adheridas del color del diente reducen significativamente la necesidad de taladrar un diente. Éstas se ven mejor y mantienen el diente más fuerte que las empastaduras de plata. Si le han diagnosticado con sensibilidad al metal, automáticamente escogeremos materiales con menos potencial para causarle problemas.

Si usted tiene cualquier pregunta sobre la sensibilidad al metal, favor de sentirse libre de preguntarnos.

Protectores Oclusos (de Mordida)

Fabricación de un Aparato Protector de Mordida

El aparato construido para eliminar o reducir los efectos adversos de el/los hábito(s) de bruxismo y/o rechinar está hecho de un plástico rígido. Está hecho a la medida para que se ajuste a su boca exactamente. Tomará dos visitas para completarse. Puede ser insertado de una sola forma, no permanecerá en su lugar si es insertado incorrectamente. En la primera visita haremos impresiones de sus dientes superiores e inferiores y registraremos la relación oclusal (mordida) de sus mandíbulas. Después que se hace el protector para la mordida, usted volverá para una segunda visita en una o dos semanas para ajustes y entrega. En la segunda cita, el aparato ajustará de modo que sus dientes se encuentren correctamente con el plástico. El aparato encaja justo alrededor de las superficies de mordida de los dientes de la mandíbula superior. No cubrirá el cielo de su boca.

Después de que se haya entregado el aparato, se espera que usted vuelva en algunas semanas con el aparato para observación y posibles ajustes adicionales. Usted no debe, en ningún momento, tener algún dolor o inflamación en los músculos o articulaciones alrededor de su cara u oídos, esté o no usando el protector de mordida. Está hecho para proteger sus dientes naturales (esmalte y dentina) del desgaste no natural, patológico causado por los hábitos de bruxismo y rechinar. Debido a que el plástico del aparato es más "suave" que lo que queda de su esmalte, el plástico se desgastará por el bruxismo o rechinar. Espere que el plástico dure alrededor de 2 años—más tiempo si usted no tiene un problema severo, menos si los hábitos son muy abusivos.

Usando Su Aparato

Después de que reciba su protector, úselo por favor según indicado. Si usted rechina o sufre de bruxismo en las noches mientras duerme (muy común), use el protector mientras duerme. Si usted sufre de bruxismo o rechina durante el día, trate de identificar cuándo durante el día usted tiene el problema (atrapado en el tráfico, hablando por teléfono, trabajando en el escritorio) y use el protector en ese momento. El estar enterado de los tiempos del día o de las tensiones que le causan que rechine o apriete, puede ayudarle a romper con el hábito.

Si en cualquier momento, usted desarrolla hinchazón de los músculos alrededor de la articulación temporomandíbular o ATM (articulación de la mandíbula), deje de usar el protector de mordida y llame a la oficina. La articulación temporomandíbular es la articulación en bisagra delante de cada oído; usted puede sentirlas cuando abre y cierra su boca. No use el protector de mordida otra vez hasta que tengamos la oportunidad de evaluar su situación.

Duración del Tratamiento

¿Cuánto tiempo usted debe usar el aparato protector? Todo depende de la naturaleza de su problema. Si este aparato se está utilizando para prevenir el desgaste anormal de sus dientes relacionado a la tensión, entonces usted necesitará usarlo hasta que no esté cargado por mucha tensión. Cuando la fuente del problema se elimina o resuelve, el problema puede desaparecer y usted no necesitara usar más el aparato. Evaluaremos periódicamente su condición.

Cuando usted no está usando su protector de mordida, debe limpiarlo con agua y un cepillo de dientes suave para remover cualquier placa y guardarlo en un lugar seco.

Por favor traiga su protector de mordida cuando asista a su cita de higiene dental rutinaria de la limpieza de modo que podamos verificar su aparato y estar seguros de que está funcionando bien. Permanezca siempre en el intervalo cuidado repetido que hemos diseñado para usted. Cuando los problemas dentales se diagnostican en las primeras etapas, el tratamiento generalmente es más fácil (y menos costoso).

Mantenga el protector de mordida limpio. Cuando termine de usar el aparato, cepíllelo con un cepillo de dientes y pasta dientes, enjuáguelo, séquelo y guárdelo en el envase proporcionado. Si no puede ser cepillado inmediatamente, enjuáguelo por lo menos con agua limpia para quitar cualquier saliva o desechos.

Si usted tiene cualquier pregunta sobre los aparatos antibruxismo/antirechinar, favor de sentirse libre de preguntarnos.

Pericoronitis

La periocoronitis es una inflamación (infección) de los tejidos suaves de las encías que rodean la parte de la corona (parte cubierta por el esmalte) de un diente. Puede estar asociada con la salida de un diente, pero más frecuentemente es asociado con las muelas cordales (inferiores). La periocoronitis alrededor de las muelas cordales es el tema de esta corta explicación.

A través de miles de años, la dieta de los seres humanos se ha vuelto más suave y requiere menos masticación. Nuestro tamaño disminuido de la mandíbula y la necesidad reducida de las muelas cordales refleja esta tendencia. Desgraciadamente, nuestras mandíbulas se están contrayendo más rápidamente de lo que están desapareciendo nuestras muelas cordales. Como resultado, particularmente en la mandíbula inferior, las muelas cordales no tienen espacio suficiente para crecer completamente (salir) en la boca. Aunque muchas encuentran su manera para tener la posición apropiada y no causar daño alguno, es demasiado frecuente que las muelas cordales aparezcan parcialmente cubiertas con tejidos de la encía. Esto causa una situación en la cual es difícil, sino imposible, para que las muelas cordales y la encía que las rodean sean limpiadas efectivamente diariamente. Hay un alto riesgo para que las infecciones de la encía se repitan. Si el diente y la encía no se pueden limpiar diariamente, los desechos se acumulan debajo del tejido de la encía que cubre parcialmente las muelas cordales. Los desechos y los productos derivados se deterioran y causan una respuesta inflamatoria en el tejido circundante. La encía se infecta e hincha. Si se hincha bastante, usted puede que no pueda evitar morderse cada vez que trata de masticar la comida o hasta al tragar.

Estas infecciones pueden ser de naturaleza leve, moderada o severa. Pueden suceder solamente una vez o ser un problema continuo. Puede haber poco dolor, o tanto dolor que usted no puede ni siquiera abrir su boca. Puede que le dé fiebre, dolor de garganta o hinchazón de las glándulas en el lado de su cuello.

Hay varias soluciones posibles a este problema. Usted puede hacer que le extraigan la muela cordal, y el problema nunca ocurrirá otra vez. Dependiendo de la posición de los dientes, esto puede ser hecho en esta oficina o puede ser enviado a un especialista. Si usted decide no extraer el diente, podemos irrigar el área alrededor y debajo de la encía con una solución medicada y limpiar los desechos con instrumentos especiales. Entonces recetaremos un enjuague bucal específico para usar después del procedimiento por varios días. Si la infección no es demasiado severa, esto resolverá frecuentemente la situación inmediata. Sin embargo, ¡puede ocurrir de nuevo! En algunas personas, el que vuelva a ocurrir es frecuente; en otras, ocurre solamente una vez y nunca vuelve a suceder. Es muy difícil de predecir. Mientras más efectivamente usted pueda limpiar el área, menos probable es que tenga la infección otra vez.

Después de una evaluación de su problema, le sugeriremos la opción apropiada para usted. Recuerde por favor que mientras mejor usted siga nuestras recomendaciones específicas en el cepillar y limpiar con hilo dental sus dientes diariamente, y manteniendo sus intervalos de tiempo entre sus citas periódicas de higiene de cuidado repetido, menos probable será que usted tenga cualquier problema de pericoronitis.

Los siguientes procedimientos fueron realizados hoy:

❏ Extracción del diente #_____ con anestesia local
❏ Irrigación del diente afectado/bolsillo infectado con_____
❏ Instrumentación manual y/o ultrasónica del bolsillo infectado
❏ Receta para   ❏ Antibiótico:_____   ❏ Analgésico_____   ❏ Enjuague Peridex_____
❏ Envío a un cirujano oral para la extracción del diente #_____

Si usted tiene cualquier pregunta sobre la pericoronitis, favor de sentirse libre de preguntarnos.

Caries en la Superficie Radicular

Causas

En una boca normal, una pequeña porción del esmalte está cubierto con el tejido de las encías. La sección de la raíz del diente (la parte que no está cubierta por el esmalte) está incrustada en el hueso y queda cubierta por el tejido de la encía. Al pasar de los años, el tejido de la encía se aleja de corona del diente, y la estructura de la raíz queda expuesta. Esto puede ocurrir debido a técnicas incorrectas de cepillado, enfermedad de la encía, la reposición quirúrgica del tejido de la encía, deterioro o sólo por envejecimiento.

El esmalte de un diente absorbe fácilmente el fluoruro y llega a ser duro y resistente al ataque de ácidos causantes de deterioro. La raíz, sin embargo, está cubierta con cemento y/o dentina. Ambos son muy suaves comparados con el esmalte. Al alejarse las encías, el cemento y la dentina quedan desprotegidos del ataque de los ácidos, y están propensos a deteriorase. Hay problemas adicionales. La cubierta de la raíz no es tan gruesa como el esmalte, permitiendo que el deterioro comience más cerca al nervio. Esto aumenta la sensibilidad del diente y la oportunidad para la muerte del nervio, que conduce a la necesidad de terapia del canal radicular. El deterioro de la raíz puede conducir a la carencia de soporte para la porción de la corona del diente, resultando en fracturas si el diente tiene empastaduras de metal. Si el diente comienza a fracturarse, puede requerir una corona preparada en el laboratorio.

Otros factores que pueden contribuir al deterioro de la raíz: un cuidado oral de sí mismo pobre, exposición de la raíz y disminución del flujo salival lo cuál puede ser debido a muchos factores como medicamentos, radioterapia, el proceso natural de envejecimiento y quimioterapia. La saliva proporciona productos químicos que remineralizan los dientes después de la exposición al ácido, y puede proteger contra concentraciones ácidas destructivas. Sin un flujo salival normal, el deterioro de la raíz tiene un potencial más alto para comenzar.

Tratamiento

El tratamiento para el deterioro de la raíz implica quitar la porción deteriorada y restaurar el diente. Podemos utilizar un material de empastadura del color del diente que lentamente suelta fluoruro. Un deterioro de la raíz más serio puede requerir tratamiento con terapia endodóntica y una corona de molde.

Prevención

Las medidas preventivas incluyen un mejor cuidado oral de sí mismo. Esto puede incluir el uso de una pasta de dientes con fluoruro, ya sea una pasta sin receta o una con un nivel de fluoruro mayor receta, un enjuague tópico de fluoruro sin receta, medicamentos y el uso todas las noches de una cubeta de fluoruro. Una aplicación de fluoruro tópico y citas más frecuentes de higiene de cuidado repetido son también medidas preventivas apropiadas.

Si usted tiene cualquier pregunta sobre el deterioro de la raíz, favor de sentirse libre de preguntarnos.

Ilustración en CD-ROM

Dientes Sensibles

Los dientes pueden llegar a ser sensibles por muchas razones. Algunas veces la sensibilidad es una indicación de un problema potencialmente serio. Otras veces, el problema dental relacionado puede ser pequeño pero los efectos (la sensibilidad) son extremadamente graves. Un diente puede llegar a ser sensibles después que ha sido preparado (taladrado) para una restauración (empastadura). Usted pudo haber sido anestesiado durante el procedimiento, así que no sintió ningún malestar cuando el nervio en el diente reaccionó al calor generado por el taladro. Cuanto más se acerca el taladro al nervio, más probable es que cause un problema de sensibilidad. La rotación de alta velocidad del taladro genera calor, y la respuesta del nervio al calor es inflamación. Esta inflamación usted la siente como "sensibilidad". Si el deterioro, la fractura o el taladrar no fue demasiado profundo, esta sensibilidad disminuirá con el pasar del tiempo. De una semana a un mes o dos no es un tiempo inusual para que la sensibilidad desaparezca. Una buena señal es que continúe disminuyendo la sensibilidad. Sin embargo, si la oclusión (mordida) está fuera de lugar después de que se haya colocado la restauración, el diente puede llegar a ser sensible o puede permanecer sensible. Una vez se ajuste la mordida, la sensibilidad debe desaparecer.

Las razones adicionales para la sensibilidad de un solo diente son el deterioro, una restauración defectuosa o un diente fracturado. Cuando se deteriora un diente, los cambios de temperatura y los dulces lo harán sensible. Si una empastadura está defectuosa o cayéndose, la filtración alrededor la empastadura puede causar que el diente sea sensible. En ambos casos, la solución puede ser tan simple como quitar el deterioro o la empastadura defectuosa, y colocar una restauración apropiada. Si el diente está fracturado, usted puede ser sensible a los cambios de temperatura o al masticar alimentos. Esta condición de la fractura puede ser difícil de diagnosticar. Si usted piensa que puede tener este tipo de sensibilidad, pida por favor el folleto separado que explica el "síndrome de diente fraccionado" con más detalles.

La sensibilidad del diente puede también ser causada por un nervio muerto. Ésta puede ser el resultado de una caries profunda. Comúnmente, el diente sensible tiene una empastadura grande y vieja. El nervio se pudo haber dañado cuando se taladró y el nervio ha estado muriendo gradualmente desde entonces. Si éste es el problema, el diente necesitará tratamiento endodóntico.

Otras dos razones para la sensibilidad del diente están relacionadas. Uno es una muesca inadvertida de la superficie del diente y/o el retiro del tejido de la encía (exponiendo la superficie de la raíz del diente) causado por el cepillado incorrecto: ya sea cepillando demasiado fuerte, cepillando con un cepillo de dientes demasiado duro o con una técnica de cepillado incorrecta. Esta sensibilidad puede ir de leve a extrema, el grado de sensibilidad no parece estar relacionado con el tamaño de la exposición de la raíz o la muesca. Finalmente, el colocar de nuevo a propósito el tejido de la encía durante cirugía puede también puede conducir a la sensibilidad del diente. Aunque la retirada del tejido de la encía por cepillarse es lenta, la retirada de la encía después de la reposición de la encía ocurre rápidamente. La porción del diente una vez cubierta con encía y hueso ahora puede estar expuesta. La sensibilidad de la raíz en estos casos puede ser bastante severa e inmediata. A veces puede durar por meses o años si no es tratada.

Opciones de Tratamiento

El tratamiento en estos dos últimos casos es similar. Si hay una muesca en el diente, o la forma del defecto es apropiada, se restaurá el defecto (se empasta) con un material adherido. Esto puede dar alivio inmediato—a veces parcialmente, a veces completamente. Cuando no hay defecto para restaurar, las superficies de la raíz expuestas y sensibles son cubiertas con una dentina adherida u otro material. Este material es invisible y no es muy grueso, así que usted no nota ningún cambio en la apariencia del diente, pero funciona. Puede que necesite ser reaplicado después de varios meses porque el material adherido se ha desgastado por el cepillado.

Si usted tiene cualquier pregunta sobre la sensibilidad de los dientes, favor de sentirse libre de preguntarnos.

Cuestionario de Disfunción de la Articulación Temporomandibular (DTM)

Paciente: _____

Fecha del examen: _____

Queja principal del paciente: _____

	Sí	No
¿Usted tiene dificultad abriendo su boca?	❏	❏
¿Es doloroso para usted abrir su boca grande?	❏	❏
¿Usted nota cualquier chasquido, estallido u otros ruidos cuando abre?	❏	❏
¿Usted tiene dolores de cabeza frecuentes?	❏	❏

¿Dónde están localizados? _____
_____

	Sí	No
¿Usted tiene dolores de oído o cuello frecuentes?	❏	❏
¿Usted tiene dificultad masticando alimentos duros?	❏	❏
¿Usted tiene dificultad masticando alimentos blandos?	❏	❏
¿Su mandíbula se ha quedado alguna vez en la posición abierta?	❏	❏

Explique por favor: _____
_____

	Sí	No
¿Usted aprieta sus dientes?	❏	❏
¿Usted rechina sus dientes?	❏	❏
¿Durante el día?	❏	❏
¿Mientras duerme?	❏	❏
¿Usted alguna vez ha despertado en la mañana y ha encontrado que los músculos de su mandíbula están adoloridos o cansados?	❏	❏

Explique por favor: _____
_____

Para el doctor:

Capacidad de movimiento: Vertical _____ Horizontal _____

Desviación de la abertura: Izquierda _____ Derecha _____ Grado _____

Abertura oclusal máxima: _____

Sensibilidad anormal al tacto: _____

Diagnóstico: _____
_____
_____

Síndrome de Disfunción de la Articulación Temporomandibular (DTM)

Causas y Síntomas

La disfunción de la articulación temporomandibular (ATM), o DTM, puede ser un problema complicado y complejo. La ATM está localizada enfrente de cada oído y es responsable, con los ligamentos asociados, tendones, discos y músculos, de todos los movimientos de la mandíbula. Los problemas con la articulación se refieren como *DTM*. Pueden ser manifestados en varias maneras incluyendo dolores de cabeza, dolores de oído, zumbido en los oídos, problemas con la abertura o el cierre de la mandíbula, sensibilidad de los músculos de la mandíbula, ruidos de chasquido o estallidos cuando se abre o cierra la mandíbula, dolor de cuello y dolor en parte alta de la espalda.

Cuando la articulación de la mandíbula no funciona correctamente, puede haber dolor y espasmos musculares. Sin embargo, se debe aclarar que los espasmos musculares y el dolor resultante no tienen nada que ver con la articulación de la mandíbula. La articulación temporomandibular es esencial para todos los movimientos que envuelven la mandíbula. El dolor puede ser leve, moderado o severo. Puede ser esporádico o constante e incluso debilitante. Es común para un paciente con DTM tener dificultad masticando alimentos duros o abriendo la boca grande sin sentir malestar. Algunos pacientes pueden tener problema masticando alimentos blandos. La función normal de la articulación se puede afectar por un trauma (accidente), posición incorrecta de los dientes, enfermedad (artritis) y hábitos relacionados a la tensión como lo son apretar y rechinar.

La disfunción de la ATM ha sido llamada *La Gran Impostora* porque imita otros problemas. A veces es difícil de diagnosticar; a veces es fácil de determinar. Muchas veces, radiografías especiales son absolutamente necesarias para ver la naturaleza del problema.

Opciones de Tratamiento

Una vez se diagnostica el problema, se consideran los posibles tratamientos. El método usual de tratamiento es muy conservador: protectores bucales y varios aparatos específicamente construidos para usted. Estos permiten que el área de la articulación descanse y le dan la oportunidad de curarse. Estas terapias son relativamente económicas. La duración del tratamiento varía considerablemente entre pacientes. Algunos pueden conseguir alivio en pocos días; otros pueden necesitar meses. Algunos quizás necesiten usar el aparato todo el tiempo; algunos, solamente durante la noche. Otro tratamiento puede incluir medicamentos recetados, aparatos para romper el hábito, ortodoncia de ATM, terapia física, biorretroalimentación y psicoterapia y cirugía correctiva ortodóntica.

Dependiendo de la naturaleza exacta de su problema de DTM, podemos decidir tratarle aquí o enviarlo a un dentista que se especialice en este tratamiento. El tratamiento temprano puede ayudarle a tener una mejor oportunidad para un resultado exitoso. Esto es especialmente cierto si la naturaleza del problema es degenerativa, y no relacionada con el apretar o rechinar. Aunque el diagnóstico de los problemas de DTM es frecuentemente fácil, la naturaleza exacta del tratamiento necesario para obtener alivio puede ser difícil.

Si usted tiene cualquier pregunta sobre la disfunción de la articulación temporomandibular, favor de sentirse libre de preguntarnos.

Abrasión por el Cepillo de Dientes: Evitando la Destrucción del Diente

La Causa

El cepillar incorrectamente (especialmente con un cepillo de dientes de cerdas duras) puede causar erosión/abrasión de su diente o dientes. Esto es un problema muy común. Comienza como una pequeña área de desgaste en forma de V o U cerca de los tejidos gingivales (de la encía) justo al lado del diente, generalmente donde el diente y la encía se encuentran. El cepillar incorrectamente causa que el tejido de la encía se aleje; y que el diente llegue a ser sensible al estímulo del calor, frío o aire. Con el tiempo, más esmalte se desgasta y una muesca horizontal pequeña se ve en el diente en el borde de la encía. Ésta no es un área de deterioro, sino una "caries" mecánica cortada en el diente. Eventualmente el esmalte se desgasta totalmente y la dentina queda expuesta. Cuando esto ocurre, algunas personas experimentan sensibilidad severa en el diente. Puede ser tan severa que es doloroso beber líquidos fríos, respirar aire o simplemente cepillar sus dientes. Sin embargo, otros experimentan poca a ninguna sensibilidad adicional en el diente.

Una vez se ha removido bastante de la encía, la raíz del diente queda expuesta. La superficie de la raíz no está cubierta por el esmalte y es mucho más blanda que el esmalte. Puede también ser feo el tener el tejido alejado de la encía. Debido a que la superficie de la raíz no está protegida por el esmalte duro, si el cepillado incorrecto continúa, el cemento de la raíz será desgastado y se hará una muesca en la dentina. Esta muesca aumentará de tamaño, debilitando el diente y a veces haciendo el área más propensa al deterioro.

Sensibilidad del Diente

Algunos pacientes con muy poca pérdida de la estructura del diente experimentan sensibilidad extrema. Este problema se puede corregir generalmente con el uso de un material de dentina adherido u otros productos químicos de desensibilización. El problema de sensibilidad frecuentemente se cura totalmente. El tratamiento puede durar (dependiendo de sus hábitos de cepillado) por 6 meses o más. Si es necesario, el diente puede ser tratado otra vez si la sensibilidad vuelve.

Algunos pacientes con una pérdida enorme de la estructura del diente notan muy poca sensibilidad del diente. Estén los dientes sensibles o no, es recomendable corregir el problema de cepillado para retrasar o eliminar el proceso de desgaste. También se recomienda que las muescas sean restauradas con un material de empastadura del color del diente. Esto restaurará la apariencia del diente y protegerá la dentina previamente expuesta. En esta manera, aún si usted continúa cepillando incorrectamente, el diente estará protegido.

En casos de menos sensibilidad, podríamos recomendar el uso de una pasta dental desensibilizadora como una alternativa económica a la colocación de materiales adheridos. Algunos casos se pueden manejar también con el uso de aplicaciones de fluoruro tópico.

Prevención de la Abrasión

Los problemas del cepillado de dientes incorrecto se corrigen fácilmente y económicamente cuando se diagnostican en las primeras etapas del desarrollo. Si se permite que progresen, el daño del diente aumentará, así como el costo de reparación. ¡La mejor solución es la **prevención!**

Cepille sus dientes minuciosamente pero no abusivamente. No los restriegue o cepille cruzado (un movimiento exagerado de cepillado horizontal). Seleccionaremos un método de cepillado de dientes que mejor cumpla con sus necesidades y le enseñaremos a cuidar su boca. Utilice un cepillo de dientes suave. Cambie a un cepillo nuevo cada 3 meses. Pero si sucede que usted está creando el problema de la abrasión del cepillo de dientes, corríjalo tan pronto como se diagnostique.

Si usted tiene cualquier pregunta sobre la erosión o abrasión por el cepillo de dientes, favor de sentirse libre de preguntarnos.

Oclusión Traumática: Equilibración Oclusal o Ajuste de la Mordida

La Relación Normal de la Mordida

En una boca normal, sana, los dientes se deben encontrar sin colocar tensión adicional sobre cualquier diente individual. Los dientes que engranan y se encuentran correctamente son similares a ruedas de engranes de metal que, al rotar juntas, tienen la punta (o *diente* como se llama) de un engranaje encajando perfectamente y suavemente en la depresión del otro engranaje. Si por alguna razón los dientes de los dos engranajes no se encuentran exactamente, las puntas en ambos chocarán y habrá una interferencia indeseada. Esta interferencia puede hacer que partes de los dientes del engranaje se astillen, fracturen o desgasten anormalmente causando facetas en los dientes de metal. Si la interferencia continúa por un período largo de tiempo o la interferencia es severa, los dientes del engranaje serán más propensos a romperse, y la rotura puede ser más severa. Las ruedas de engrane podrían también aflojarse de su eje y comenzar a bambolear al rotar.

Aunque los dientes no están hechos de metal, existen semejanzas con los engranajes. La superficie exterior que normalmente entra en contacto con el diente opuesto está hecha de esmalte—duro pero frágil. Sus dientes están sostenidos en su lugar y son apoyados por el hueso que rodea los dientes. Cuando su oclusión (mordida) cambia, evitando el engranaje de sus dientes al unísono, el esmalte podría comenzar a astillarse o desgastarse. Cuando se han restaurado estos dientes, estas restauraciones podrían fracturarse. En los casos más severos, los dientes se aflojarán. Usted también puede encontrar que el esmalte se desgasta anormalmente bastante rápido y los dientes cambian de forma y se ponen más cortos.

Oclusión Traumática

Todos los problemas antes mencionados podrían ser síntomas de la oclusión traumática. Los dientes que se encuentran incorrectamente pueden dañarse cada vez que cierre su boca. Un diente o todos sus dientes pueden ser afectados. Frecuentemente, usted no sabe que existe un problema porque usted experimenta poco o nada de dolor hasta que alcanza una etapa muy avanzada. Si usted tiene dientes que han dañado el soporte del hueso debido a enfermedad periodontal activa o pasada, los dientes tendrán una tendencia de moverse levemente, lo que podría colocarlos en oclusión traumática. La "mordida" no tiene que estar fuera de lugar por mucho antes que ocurra un problema. Un movimiento fuera de la posición apropiada por no más que el grueso de un pedazo de papel es frecuentemente suficiente para causar un problema. Si usted tiene un hábito de apretar o rechinar relacionado con la tensión, usted puede inducir una oclusión traumática.

Tratamiento

Una vez que se haya diagnosticado el problema, debe ser tratado rápidamente. El tratamiento puede ser simple o complejo. Implicará el determinar qué dientes no se están encontrando correctamente cuando usted cierra los dientes. Si solamente un diente está en una posición incorrecta, puede poder ser corregido con una cita. Si más de un diente está implicado, o si los dientes están flojos, varias citas pueden ser necesarias para corregir el problema. Sus dientes pueden ser levemente sensibles a los cambios de temperatura por un tiempo después de que se termine el ajuste oclusal.

Si usted tiene cualquier pregunta sobre la oclusión traumática, favor de sentirse libre de preguntarnos.

Muelas Cordales (Terceros Molares)

Los seres humanos tienen más dientes que los que realmente necesitan: cuatro dientes de más, para ser exactos. Los terceros molares (muelas cordales) son los últimos dientes a cada lado y en cada arco de la boca. Si no los necesitamos, entonces ¿por qué los tenemos? Miles de años atrás, nuestros antepasados no lucían como nosotros lucimos hoy en día. Tenían cuerpos más pequeños pero mandíbulas más grandes y fuertes. Su dieta dictó esta estructura de la mandíbula y el número de dientes. Nuestros antepasados comían un tipo de alimento más duro y abrasivo. No estaba bien cocinado, y no estaba bien molido. Habían muchos granos duros y alimentos que requerían mucha masticación. Las mandíbulas grandes eran capaces de sostener más dientes para esta masticación.

Hoy en día, no necesitamos la capacidad de moler que los seres humanos de antes tenían. El alimento es más fácil de comer, menos abrasivo y mucho más blando. La evolución está reaccionando (lentamente) a este hecho disminuyendo el tamaño de nuestros huesos de la mandíbula y los músculos de masticar. La mandíbula humana que una vez sostuvo cómodamente 12 muelas (32 dientes en total) ahora frecuentemente es solamente suficientemente grande para sostener ocho muelas (28 dientes en total). Desgraciadamente, nuestras mandíbulas se están poniendo más pequeñas más rápido que lo que están desapareciendo nuestras muelas cordales. Las muelas cordales frecuentemente no tienen suficiente espacio para crecer correctamente. Eventualmente, dentro de miles de años, los seres humanos no tendrán muelas cordales. Han perdido su función y están desapareciendo gradualmente, igual que el apéndice.

Debido a que la mandíbula es demasiado pequeña (para la mayoría de las personas) para acomodar a los terceros molares, estos salen en la boca parcialmente, en mala posición o no salen. Estos pueden salir completamente, parcialmente, con una impacción del tejido suave, con una impacción huesuda parcial o con una impacción huesuda completa. Si los dientes salen bien y usted puede mantenerlos limpios, los dejamos solos. Si están apiñados o colocados incorrectamente y no pueden ser mantenidos limpios, son como un accidente esperando suceder. Es probable que ocurra deterioro e infección de la encía. Generalmente, estos dientes son extraídos—idealmente antes que comiencen a causar problemas grandes con los segundos molares que están directamente delante de ellos. Los dientes que salen parcialmente deben ser extraídos siempre: hay demasiada oportunidad para que comience la infección de la encía. Si los dientes no pueden ser limpiados, una inflamación crónica dolorosa puede ocurrir (pericoronitis). Cuanto antes se quiten, mejor será su curación.

Las extracciones menos complejas (dientes que han salido completamente o impacciones parciales del tejido suave) pueden ser hechas por un dentista general. Referiremos las extracciones difíciles a un cirujano oral para tratamiento. Dependiendo del tipo de extracción y del historial médico del paciente, las extracciones pueden hacerse en una oficina o en el hospital. Esto será determinado después de ver las radiografías de los dientes. El extraer las cuatro muelas cordales al mismo tiempo es una práctica común. El malestar postoperatorio puede ser de mínimo a extremo—en el caso impacciones huesudas completas difíciles. Medicamentos antiinflamatorios y para aliviar el dolor son recetados apropiadamente.

No necesitamos las muelas cordales para comer bien. Si necesitan salir, es mejor que salgan (1) antes que causen problemas con los dientes adyacentes que usted realmente necesita y (2) cuando usted es más joven y cura bien. Si usted necesita que le extraigan una muela cordal, también haga que le extraigan la muela cordal opuesta. Cuando un diente no encuentra un diente de oposición, éste "sale de más" o continua creciendo fuera de la posición normal. Cuando se deja por cierto tiempo, el diente que queda puede desarrollar deterioro y hacer que le suceda lo mismo al diente delante de él.

Si usted tiene cualquier pregunta sobre sus muelas cordales, favor de sentirse libre de preguntarnos.

Xerostomía: Síndrome de Sequedad en la Boca

La xerostomía (sequedad de la boca) no es una condición que todas las personas deben esperar. Usted puede notarlo a medida que usted envejece debido a un cambio en hormonas, medicación y/o radioterapia en la región de la cabeza y del cuello.

Por Qué la Xerostomía Es un Problema

La saliva es importante para la salud oral por varias razones. El flujo de la saliva ayuda a limpiar los desperdicios de la cavidad bucal. Éste proporciona los minerales necesarios para ayudar el proceso de remineralización. El esmalte del diente diariamente experimenta ataques ácidos que remueven los minerales inorgánicos. Esto es llamado desmineralización. La remineralización es lo opuesto de desmineralización. Ésta ocurre cuando moléculas inorgánicas fluyen a la región débil del esmalte y lo hacen fuerte.

Cuando se reduce el flujo salival, ocurren una cadena de acontecimientos. La acción natural de limpieza se disminuye, al igual que las características de regulación y remineralización de la saliva. Las personas con un flujo salival disminuido tienen un índice de deterioro muy rápido, muchas veces más rápido y a través de varios dientes. Este tipo de deterioro dental se observa típicamente a lo largo del borde de la encía, alrededor del trabajo dental existente y en las superficies de la raíz expuestas.

Prevención

Usted puede ayudar a prevenir el deterioro dental que puede resultar de la xerostomía.

- Cepillando y limpiando con hilo dental correctamente por lo menos una vez al día es muy importante.
- Sorbos frecuentes de agua durante el día pueden ayudar a humedecer la boca y a la limpiar los desechos.
- El uso diario de un enjuague bucal que contenga fluoruro puede ayudar a remineralizar los dientes.
- Utilice una pasta dental que contenga fluoruro de sodio.
- Recomendamos el cepillado diario con una pasta o gel recetado, con una alta concentración de fluoruro de sodio. Dispensaremos esto o le daremos una receta.
- Mastique goma de mascar sin azúcar o una goma elástica para ayudar a estimular el flujo salival.
- En casos de moderados a severos, se pueden hacer cubetas especiales para la aplicación de fluoruro para que usted las utilice en el hogar. Éstas mantendrán el fluoruro de alta concentración en una posición para "remojar" sus dientes con el fluoruro por varios minutos a la vez.
- Recomendamos que usted tenga sus dientes limpiados, pulidos y un tratamiento aplicado en la oficina de fluoruro tópico cada 3 meses mientras persista la condición.

La sequedad de la boca puede tener consecuencias dentales serias y se debe tratar por consiguiente.

Si usted tiene cualquier pregunta sobre la xerostomía, favor de sentirse libre de preguntarnos.

Ortodoncia

Revisión del Contenido: Ortodoncia

Cuidado de los Frenillos
Discute el cuidado oral de sí mismo apropiado; incluye una lista de verificación de las recomendaciones para el paciente individual.

Dientes Que Faltan Congénitamente
Alerta al paciente de los problemas asociados con los dientes que faltan congénitamente y el tratamiento necesario.

Ortodoncia Fija y Removible
Compara ambos métodos para la terapia ortodóntica, destacando los beneficios de ambos.

Ortodoncia (Frenillos)
Una visión general de la necesidad para la ortodoncia, el horario y el cuidado oral de sí mismo durante la fase activa.

Enderezar los Molares Inclinados
Una explicación de los cambios en la alineación de los dientes que son posibles como resultado del no reemplazar los dientes extraídos.

Cuidado de los Frenillos

Si usted está recibiendo un tratamiento ortodóntico, probablemente siente que tiene muchas "cosas" en su boca. La odontología tiene nombres para los diferentes tipos de accesorios: bandas, brackets, arco de alambres, ligaduras, elásticos, etc. Lo que esto significa para usted es que cualquier tipo de aparato ortodóntico cementado y/o adherido a sus dientes hace más difícil que usted limpie sus dientes correctamente. Usted encontrará que tiene más restos de comida atrapados alrededor de sus dientes y accesorios ortodónticos que antes. Es más difícil y toma más tiempo para limpiarlos y remover los restos.

Es muy importante mantener sus dientes inmaculados mientras estén puestos los frenillos. La comida adicional que se puede atrapar fácilmente alrededor de la banda, los brackets y los alambres se descompondrá con el tiempo y puede causar el deterioro de las encías y posiblemente la enfermedad de las encías. Es bastante devastador ver que los dientes están todos deteriorados o desfigurados cuando se quitan los frenillos de los dientes recién enderezados. Es aún más deprimente tener unas restauraciones puestas en estos dientes bellos y rectos. Afortunadamente, esto puede evitarse con el cuidado oral de sí mismo y el mantenimiento apropiado.

Pasaremos tanto tiempo como usted necesite en enseñarle cómo mantener sus dientes limpios y sus encías saludables. Hay ayudas de limpieza disponibles para ayudar a mantener el cuidado oral de sí mismo apropiado mientras usted está bajo la terapia ortodóntica activa. Le demostraremos su uso o los proveeremos para usted o le informaremos dónde los puede comprar.

Le aconsejamos que usted regrese a la **oficina cada tres meses** mientras tenga puestos los frenillos para que un higienista dental limpie sus dientes y para que reciba un tratamiento de fluoruro tópico. Encontramos que con este intervalo de cuidado preventivo repetido, usted tiene menos posibilidad de desarrollar problemas periodontales (de las encías) alrededor de los frenillos y deterioro debajo y alrededor de los aparatos ortodónticos.

Aquí una lista de varios consejos adicionales para el cuidado de sus frenillos:

- ❏ Use una pasta de dientes que contenga fluoruro cuando usted cepilla sus dientes.

- ❏ Use un enhebrador de hilo dental tal como le hemos enseñado y demostrado para limpiar debajo de los arcos de alambre todas las noches.

- ❏ Enjuáguese con un enjuague que contenga fluoruro por lo menos una vez al día. Siga las instrucciones que acompañan el enjuague. El uso del enjuague con fluoruro ayudará a reducir la posibilidad de deterioro o descalcificación (manchas blancas o lugares blandos en el esmalte) debajo de las bandas y los brackets cementados o adheridos. Lo consideramos una ayuda de prevención muy importante.

- ❏ Use un irrigador como se le ha demostrado para ayudar a remover los restos de alrededor de los frenillos. **Esto de ninguna manera sustituye el cepillado y el uso del hilo dental correcto.** Es una ayuda de cuidado oral de sí mismo adjunta.

- ❏ Use un cepillo eléctrico como se la ha enseñado.

Cuide sus dientes apropiadamente mientras los frenillos estén puestos. Usted estará contento de haberlo hecho.

Si usted tiene cualquier pregunta sobre el cuidado dental ortodóntico y preventivo, favor de sentirse libre de preguntarnos.

Dientes Que Faltan Congénitamente

Algunos de nosotros tendremos 32 dientes desarrollados durante nuestra vida. Esto se ha considerado como un conjunto normal de dientes en un adulto. Sin embargo, con la evolución del ser humano vemos menos adultos con un juego completo de 32 dientes. Es común que a las personas les falte uno o más de los terceros molares, también llamados *muelas cordales.* Los tamaños de la mandíbula del ser humano moderno son tales que muchas veces sencillamente no hay espacio en la boca para la ubicación correcta de los terceros molares y normalmente hay que extraerlos. Todos conocemos a personas que han tenido muelas cordales retenidas que necesitaban ser sacadas.

No tan común, pero tampoco raro, es la persona que nunca desarrolla algún otro diente permanente. Cuando esto ocurre, frecuentemente envuelve uno o dos de los incisivos superiores laterales, que son los dientes más pequeños a los lados de los dos dientes frontales superiores. Con menos frecuencia no se desarrollarán los colmillos (caninos) o premolares.

El problema que resulta debido a los dientes que faltan congénitamente se debe al espacio donde el diente (los dientes) debería estar. Esto es un problema cosmético muy serio. Los otros dientes alrededor del espacio se moverán a posiciones diferentes.

Los problemas que pueden resultar de los dientes permanentes que faltan se pueden reducir o eliminar con la detección temprana y un plan futuro de restauración. El tratamiento común envuelve la ortodoncia para mover los dientes permanentes a una posición mejor o para mantener los dientes permanentes en su lugar correcto. Vemos los incisivos laterales que faltan tan a menudo que la rutina de tratamiento está bien establecida. Se alcanza la mejor estética, la apariencia más natural, al dejar los incisivos centrales permanentes y los caninos contiguos en su lugares habituales. El mantenimiento de la posición correcta del diente es muy importante para la futura apariencia del reemplazo.

La secuencia de tratamiento es la ortodoncia tan temprano como sea necesario para mantener el espacio. Si los dientes se han movido demasiado, más tratamiento ortodóntico será necesario. Entonces mientras crecen el niño y su boca, se hace un reemplazo removible. Éste se usa hasta que los dientes estén listos para recibir el implante o el puente, más o menos después de la edad de los 18 años.

Es menos común que falten los dientes permanentes en la parte más atrás de la boca. Es común que se retengan los dientes de leche en estas áreas cuando no salen los dientes permanentes. A veces los dientes de leche pueden durar por años pero no tienen la estructura de la raíz para quedarse estables durante toda la vida. Si se deterioran y se empastan, se vuelven débiles y más propensos a las fracturas. Si usted tiene suerte, tienen suficiente raíz para funcionar y se ven mejor a través del uso de las resinas y la porcelana adheridas. Como los dientes de leche retenidos son apropiados para una boca pequeña, éstos no pueden funcionar de la misma manera que los dientes permanentes. Cuando se pierden, un diente de leche sobre retenido se puede reemplazar con un implante o un puente. Su propia situación particular determinará el mejor desarrollo del tratamiento.

Si usted tiene cualquier pregunta sobre los dientes que faltan congénitamente favor de sentirse libre de preguntarnos.

Ortodoncia Fija y Removible

La visión tradicional y estereotípica del tratamiento ortodóntico dada en las películas, la televisión y los comerciales es una de yardas de alambre de metal atados a los dientes que están tan cubiertos con bandas y brackets de plata que lo blanco de los dientes es apenas visible. Con la tecnología dental avanzada actual, este cuadro está lejos de ser exacto.

Los cambios en la alineación del diente se pueden lograr de diversas maneras. Cuando son apropiados, lo expansores del arco superior e inferior se pueden utilizar para aumentar la curvatura de las estructuras de soporte del diente. Estos expansores se cementan en lugar y no pueden ser quitados por el paciente. Los expansores son a menudo un preludio de las bandas de metal fijas. Estos pueden ser cementados a los dientes así como también a los alambres y resortes longitudinales del arco y todavía ser utilizados para mover los dientes.

Hace algún tiempo atrás, el deseo de los pacientes de demostrar menos metal dio lugar al desarrollo de los brackets adheridos del color del diente y transparentes (opuesto a las bandas de metal que rodean totalmente un diente). Estos brackets cubren solamente 25% de la superficie del diente y están adheridos en lugar. El trueque con los brackets más estéticos adheridos es un porcentaje más alto desalojamiento del bracket, lo que requiere visitas adicionales a la oficina para la reparación y el reemplazo. Los alambres y los resortes se cambian periódicamente para lograr las varias etapas del movimiento. Los componentes de metal permanecen en su lugar hasta que se acaba el movimiento del diente. Algunas condiciones dentales decretan el uso de este proceso ortodóntico tradicional.

No es siempre necesario utilizar los aparatos fijos para mover los dientes. Un movimiento menos agresivo del diente puede ser hecho con los aparatos removibles por los pacientes. Algunos se hacen de un material del color de la encía en acrílico rosa con los alambres y los resortes de metal encajados en ellos. Éstos son usados por el paciente excepto cuando come, se cepilla y se limpia con hilo dental. Los aparatos de metal y de plástico no enseñan tanto metal así que son un poco más aceptables. El trueque con los aparatos removibles es que trabajan solamente cuando están en la boca de los pacientes, lo que hace el cumplimiento apropiado del paciente un punto decisivo grande. Si usted no los usa, los dientes no se moverán tal y como se planificó. Los aparatos de metal y de plástico se utilizan en lo que se llama un movimiento *menor* del diente. Muchos casos ortodónticos no son apropiados para la terapia de aparatos removibles.

Hace varios años, un nuevo tipo de terapia de aparato removible fue desarrollado y patentado. Align Technology tiene un producto llamado Invisalign®. Los alineadores plásticos claros, finos (posicionadores) se colocan consecutivamente para mover los dientes en una manera exacta. Los alineadores son dejados en la boca tanto como sea posible y removidos solamente para comer, beber y limpiar los dientes. Nuevamente, si usted no los utiliza, los dientes no se moverán. Los alineadores son casi invisibles cuando están colocados y son extraordinariamente aceptados estéticamente. Están indicados para adultos y para pacientes mayores de 14 años que tiene todos los dientes permanentes incluyendo los segundos molares completamente brotados. Pueden ser usados para tratar problemas de alineación desde muy simples a bastante extensivos. La mayoría de los casos son completados en alrededor de 12 meses. La investigación sigue en proceso para determinar los límites de este proceso.

El doctor que estará realizando el tratamiento ortodóntico tomará estas diferentes modalidades en consideración y desarrollará un plan de tratamiento que se ajuste bien a sus necesidades. La edad del paciente, número de dientes involucrados y la extensión del movimiento son los factores fundamentales en el proceso de tomar la decisión. Por favor esté seguro de preguntar por qué o por qué no una técnica fue sugerida en vez de la otra.

Si usted tiene cualquier pregunta sobre su tratamiento ortodóntico, favor de sentirse libre de preguntarnos.

Ortodoncia (Frenillos)

Si sus dientes están mal alineados, puede ser que usted enfrente un problema funcional o cosmético. La ortodoncia (los frenillos) puede eliminarle este problema. Una de las primeras cosas que las personas ven de usted es su sonrisa y cómo se ven sus dientes. Usted no tiene que ser dentista para reconocer dientes mal posicionados o virados. En la cultura de hoy, los dientes virados no se consideran ni atractivos ni deseables. La mayoría de las personas, cuando se les pregunta, dicen que les gustaría tener dientes rectos. Dientes rectos y blancos son las mejorías cosméticas dentales más pedidas por los pacientes.

Es mejor que descubra la necesidad para la ortodoncia mientras usted es joven. Un dentista tendrá una buena indicación de si sus dientes serán rectos cuando le ve como un niño de 6 a 8 años de edad. Normalmente no se comenzaría el tratamiento hasta que un paciente tenga 8 años, aunque en algunos casos se puede comenzar la ortodoncia más temprano.

Es más fácil dirigir el movimiento de los dientes en un niño. La guía temprana de los dientes es una fase muy importante del cuidado ortodóntico, que puede darse aunque todos los dientes permanentes todavía no estén en su lugar. Ciertos problemas son muchos más fáciles de corregir en esta etapa de "dentición mixta" de dientes de leche y dientes permanentes. Cuando se requiere más tratamiento que la simple guía temprana del diente, un caso promedio puede durar de 18 a 24 meses.

Aunque la verdad es que la terapia ortodóntica es más fácil en pacientes niños, usted nunca está demasiado viejo para comenzar la ortodoncia. La cantidad de adultos que buscan el tratamiento ortodóntico ha crecido dramáticamente durante la década pasada. Mientras usted tenga un sostén de hueso saludable para sus dientes, usted puede recibir la terapia ortodóntica. La mayoría de los casos adultos toman de 18 a 24 meses para terminarse.

Una vez se remueven los frenillos, normalmente es necesario poner un retenedor. Este retenedor mantendrá la nueva alineación de los dientes hasta que tengan la oportunidad de fijarse firmemente en su nueva posición. Este retenedor puede ser removible o fijo.

Mientras el tratamiento ortodóntico está en la fase activa, es decir, mientras los frenillos están puestos en sus dientes, usted tiene que ser muy diligente en mantener sus dientes limpios. Esto será más difícil y un poco diferente a la limpieza de sus dientes sin frenillos. Se le instruirá en el uso de las ayudas necesarias para la limpieza. Éstas pueden incluir los enhebradores de hilo dental, un irrigador para lavar los restos a chorro, los hábitos correctos de cepillado, los enjuagues bucales de fluoruro y las ayudas periodontales. Usted **tiene que** seguir su rutina apropiada de cuidado oral de sí mismo cada noche para evitar el deterioro, la descalcificación de los dientes y la enfermedad de las encías.

También se pueden sugerir los frenillos para corregir un problema dental específico que sólo afecta uno o varios dientes. Esto no es una reposición de dientes cosmética sino un movimiento de dientes funcional. Ocasionalmente, para terminar con un caso ortodóntico correctamente, el ortodoncista puede pedir al dentista que ajuste el esmalte de algunos dientes o que adhiera una resina a algunos dientes para mejorar la oclusión (alineación de la mordida) o para aumentar la apariencia cosmética. Se hablará de esto con usted tan pronto sea evidente.

En resumen, recuérdese que usted nunca está demasiado viejo para comenzar un tratamiento ortodóntico.
- Tal vez sea más fácil y menos costoso tratarse en una edad temprana (más o menos a los 8 años).
- Usted tiene que seguir su rutina apropiada de cuidado oral de sí mismo cada noche.
- Consiga que un higienista dental limpie sus dientes profesionalmente cada tres meses para reducir la ocurrencia de deterioro y enfermedad de las encías.

La ortodoncia puede mejorar dramáticamente su apariencia, su vida y cómo usted piensa de sí mismo.

Si usted tiene cualquier pregunta sobre la ortodoncia, favor de sentirse libre de preguntarnos.

Enderezar los Molares Inclinados

Una de las condiciones más comunes en un adulto que ha experimentado una pérdida temprana de un molar anterior o un premolar es el desplazamiento o la inclinación hacia el frente de los primeros o segundos molares. Este desplazamiento o inclinación causará que los dientes se muevan fuera de sus posiciones verticales y horizontales normales. Los dientes se mueven a un paso muy lento, así que puede tomar muchos años para que usted se dé cuenta de este movimiento. Normalmente los dientes se mantienen en su posición por el contacto con los dientes adyacentes y opuestos. Cuando se cambia este contacto u oclusión a causa de una extracción, los dientes migrarán hacia el frente de la boca. A causa de las fuerzas de oclusión, comenzarán a inclinarse y moverse al espacio creado por la extracción. A causa del cambio, el diente que se ha movido será más propenso al comienzo del deterioro entre él y el diente que está detrás. También habrá una tendencia a un cambio adverso en la posición del hueso y la arquitectura de la encía y el cambio no es hacia lo mejor. A causa del cambio en la manera en que la comida se encuentra con el diente y se desvía y las acciones y fuerzas diferentes en la raíz, los bolsillos periodontales patológicos pueden desarrollarse y normalmente sí se desarrollan. Cuando un diente comienza a moverse, los otros dientes alrededor también comienzan a cambiar de posición. Mientras más cerca están del diente al lado del espacio, más se mueven. Esto puede afectar fácilmente tres, cuatro, cinco dientes o más.

Como normalmente esto no es una situación estable ni buena, le aconsejamos que usted considere su corrección. La solución más fácil cuando sólo falta un diente y sólo un diente se ha movido hacia delante y se ha inclinado es enderezar el diente mal posicionado ortodónticamente. Normalmente esto se puede hacer en algunos meses. Una vez que se ha regresado el diente a su posición, usted tiene que estabilizarlo para que no vuelva a desplazarse hacia el espacio. Si se puede mover el diente hacia delante de modo que esté en contacto con el diente anterior, la estabilización puede incluir algún tipo de retenedor nocturno por varios meses. Si hay un espacio anterior al diente movido, eso es, que el diente se movió hacia atrás en el proceso de enderezarlo, usted debe considerar el reemplazo del diente que falta con un puente fijo convencional, un puente adherido, un implante o una dentadura parcial removible. Todas estas opciones se deben considerar y la selección se debe hacer antes de comenzar el tratamiento ortodóntico.

Si se ha movido más de un diente, la corrección ortodóntica será más complicada y envolverá más tiempo y más dientes. Se pueden mover algunos dientes hacia delante y algunos hacia atrás. Los dientes contrarios se pueden haber extruído al espacio y necesitar una intrusión para regresarlos a su alvéolo. Similar al movimiento de un solo diente, hay que determinar el plan prostético final antes de comenzar cualquier trabajo. Hay que comenzar la estabilización y la restauración lo antes posible después de mover los dientes correctamente, si no, se moverán de nuevo.

La prevención es el mejor tratamiento. Los dentistas recomiendan la retención de los dientes. Si ha tenido un diente extirpado, reemplácelo lo antes posible, así evitará el movimiento incorrecto futuro y la mala alineación. Pero si usted tiene la mala fortuna de haber tenido un diente de atrás extirpado a una edad temprana y los dientes están comenzando a moverse, considere la ortodoncia para enderezar y reposicionar los dientes. Si no lo hace, usted podría esperar problemas futuros con el deterioro y con sus tejidos de sostén periodontal. ¡El movimiento continuado hasta puede causar la pérdida de más dientes!

Si usted tiene cualquier pregunta sobre el enderezar de los dientes, favor de sentirse libre de preguntarnos.

Odontología Pediátrica

Revisión del Contenido: Odontología Pediátrica

La Primera Visita del Niño al Dentista
Explica a los padres cuándo y cómo preparar a su niño para la primera visita del niño al dentista.

Caries Tempranas en la Infancia
Explica el "cariado de bebé por la botella" y provee sugerencias para prevención.

Patrones de Erupción de los Dientes
Informa a los padres cómo y cuándo los dientes se forman y eventualmente salen en los niños.

Prevención de la Enfermedad Dental en Infantes y Niños
Específica las sugerencias para prevenir la enfermedad dental en infantes y niños.

Selladores
Discute los selladores para la prevención de la enfermedad oral.

Garantía del Sellador
Asegura a sus pacientes la necesidad y la integridad de los selladores con una garantía del sellador.

Fluoruro Suplementario
Asegura que el niño recibe la cantidad correcta de fluoruro con una tabla para agua con fluoruro.

Fluoruro Tópico: En el Hogar y en la Oficina Dental
Anima a los pacientes a aprovecharse de la entrega de fluoruro ya sea en el hogar y/o en la oficina. Incluye instrucciones específicas para los procedimientos de fluoruro de cubeta.

La Primera Visita del Niño al Dentista

Prepararse

La primera visita del niño al dentista debe ser a una edad mucho más temprana de lo que los padres creen—y por una razón diferente. La primera visita dental debe ocurrir en la infancia, cuando los dientes comienzan a salir. Durante esta visita, le dejaremos saber cómo cuidar los dientes de su niño y cuáles medidas preventivas usted debe tomar para su bebé en esta etapa temprana. Se pueden interceptar muchos problemas dentales cuando tenemos la oportunidad de examinar a su niño y hablar con usted en las etapas tempranas de desarrollo.

La primera limpieza para su niño (profilaxis pedodontica) debe ser hecha alrededor de los 2 a 2$^{1}/_{2}$ años de edad, dependiendo de la conducta del niño. Es importante que ésta no sea la primera vez que el niño visite nuestra oficina. Antes de esta visita, nos gustaría que el niño venga con un padre que está recibiendo una profilaxis preventiva rutinaria. Tenemos muchos juguetes, libros de colorear, libros y películas para niños que se pueden ver. De esta manera los niños van a conocer a la oficina dental como una experiencia muy agradable, y no amenazante. Con un poco de suerte, cuando vienen para su propia profilaxis, habrán estado en la oficina varias veces. Conocen al dentista, al higienista dental y la manera en que se ve la oficina y el equipo dental. Tendrán una buena idea de lo que se espera de ellos. Habrán tenido sólo experiencias buenas con todas estas personas en este lugar. Usualmente, cuando se presenta la odontología a los niños de esta manera, están emocionados de tener sus propias citas dentales.

Es importante que los padres siempre hablen positivamente de ir a una cita dental y también después de que ocurra la cita dental. Los niños son muy listos. Podrán no saber lo que significan algunas palabras, pero pueden entender como usted se siente sobre ello. Usted debe intentar no usar palabras cerca de ellos que puedan tener una connotación desagradable: dolor de muelas, taladrado, tirar, doler, dolor, infeliz, etc. Siempre hable de cuán contento usted está de ir al dentista y cuán magnífica fue la experiencia. Si su cita no fue magnífica, hable de esto en privado donde el niño no puede escucharle. Si es necesario, y si su niño pregunta, dígale cuán contento(a) usted está de que el dentista está haciendo que su boca se sienta bien de nuevo, sin mencionar nada de la incomodidad.

También es importante que los niños no se sientan amenazados al hacer que el dentista sea el "cuco". No le diga los niños, por ejemplo, que si come dulce tendrá que ir al dentista para que taladren y pongan empastaduras a sus dientes. Entonces los niños pensarán que la oficina del dentista es un lugar donde le castigan por hacer algo malo. Queremos que los niños se sientan completamente cómodos y que no se preocupen cuando sea hora para una cita dental.

La Visita

La primera vez que se hace un procedimiento dental al niño, a los 2 a 2$^{1}/_{2}$ años de edad, normalmente será muy sencillo, rápido y totalmente sin dolor. Por supuesto, asumimos que usted habrá seguido todas las sugerencias preventivas que le habíamos dado: vitaminas de fluoruro, si son apropiadas, cepillar los dientes del niño, no poner nada en la botella nocturna excepto agua y así sucesivamente.

Primero, pasaremos un poco de tiempo con el niño en el modo de mostrar y explicar. Le mostremos al niño los instrumentos: los pulidores, los espejos, el Señor Sed (el expulsador de saliva), la pistola de agua (siringe de aire/agua), y así sucesivamente. El higienista dental también comenzará a instruir al niño en la técnica correcta para cepillarse. A esta edad tierna, los niños no manipulan el hilo dental y el cepillo correctamente. Esto es un proyecto para el padre. Como los niños admiran y tratan de imitar a los padres, su buen ejemplo diario del cepillado y el uso del hilo dental ayudará tremendamente en esta área. Los niños verán que esto es algo que usted hace y tratará de imitarlo.

También durante esta visita, el dentista "contará" los dientes del niño mientras busca el deterioro u otros problemas. Luego el higienista dental "hará cosquillas" (limpiar y pulir) a los dientes. Se quitarán fácilmente las manchas y la placa que pueden haberse acumulado. Es muy raro que un niño tenga problemas periodontales mayores.

Si se ha preparado al niño correctamente, la primera visita al dentista para un tratamiento se anticipará sin ansiedad, procederá sin problemas y el niño se animará a regresar. Lo que usted hace en la casa para prepararle para esta visita es muy importante para su éxito. ¡Buena suerte!

Si usted tiene cualquier pregunta sobre la primera visita del niño al dentista, favor de sentirse libre de preguntarnos.

Caries Tempranas en la Infancia

¿Qué Son las Caries Tempranas en la Infancia?

Las caries tempranas en la infancia, que antes se llamaban "cariado de bebé por la botella" y "caries del amamantado", es una forma severa del deterioro dental que se encuentra en los niños muy jóvenes que probablemente se duermen con cualquier líquido en la botella que no sea agua. Los niños que experimentan el amantado prolongado a gusto tienen los mismos patrones de deterioro en los dientes. Muchas veces, el deterioro está muy avanzado antes de que el padre se dé cuenta del problema. Ésta es otra razón por la que queremos ver a su niño(a) para su primera visita dental mientras esos dientes nuevos todavía están en la fase de salir.

¿Cómo se Desarrollan las Caries Tempranas en la Infancia?

Los dientes más afectados por las caries tempranas en la infancia son los dientes frontales superiores. Mientras el niño se duerme con una botella que contiene cualquier líquido que no sea agua (o en el pecho), las charcas de líquido azucarado se juntan al lado de las superficies de los dientes. Estos azúcares alimentan las bacterias que se encuentran en las placas de bacterias para producir un ácido que comienza el proceso de deterioro. Cuando el proceso de desmineralización no es detenido a través de la prevención correcta, las coronas de los dientes se pueden destruir hasta el borde de las encías; se pueden desarrollar abscesos, y el niño puede experimentar dolor severo e incomodidad.

¿Cuál Es la Mejor Prevención?

Cuando las bacterias orales se alimentan con el azúcar líquido por un período de tiempo prolongado, el ácido resultante puede ser muy dañino a la estructura de los dientes. Del mismo modo, cuando las bacterias orales se alimentan con un poco de líquido azucarado, sin parar, por un día, los resultados pueden ser bastante dañinos a la estructura de los dientes.

Creemos que la mejor prevención para este tipo de problema comienza con el entendimiento del proceso de deterioro y cómo usted puede pararlo aun antes de que comience. Recomendamos que usted traiga a sus niños al dentista cuando están en la etapa de infancia de modo que podamos hacer un examen oral del infante y hablar con el niño sobre el cuidado oral de sí mismo, incluyendo:

- Los niños no se deben dormir con una botella de líquido azucarado. Ni leche. Ni jugo. Ni soda. Solamente agua pura.
- Los niños, incluyendo los infantes, requieren una limpieza oral diaria. Si no hay dientes, se deben limpiar las encías suavemente con un paño mojado.
- Cuando hay dientes, se deben cepillar con una pasta de dientes con fluoruro, pero sólo con una *cantidad muy pequeña*—del tamaño de un guisante (chícharo) o menos.
- Los líquidos azucarados y los otros carbohidratos fáciles de fermentar, como el pan, tortas o galletas dulces o saladas, se deben dar con las comidas y no como "meriendas".
- El nivel apropiado de fluoruro sistémico debe estar fijo cuando su niño tiene 6 meses. Hablaremos con usted del régimen de fluoruro específico a su localización y las edades de sus niños.

Si usted tiene cualquier pregunta sobre las caries tempranas en la infancia, favor de sentirse libre de preguntarnos.

Patrones de Erupción de los Dientes

Los dientes comienzan a formarse muy temprano en la vida de los niños, tan temprano como el primer mes del segundo trimestre del embarazo. Por esto es tan importante que las mujeres embarazadas sigan una dieta correcta. No sólo es para tener un bebé saludable sino para asegurar la formación correcta de los dientes. Cuando se forma el tejido duro (el futuro esmalte) del diente, los dientes toman los minerales y los nutrientes y los incorpora en la estructura del esmalte. La buena nutrición fortalecerá los dientes. La malnutrición puede interferir con la formación correcta del esmalte. Coma prudentemente. Consulte a su médico sobre los suplementos de vitaminas necesarios y antes de tomar cualquier medicamento.

Esta referencia le ayudará a saber cuando los dientes de leche, también llamados dientes deciduos, deben salir y eventualmente caerse cuando salen los dientes permanentes. Los dientes de las niñas suelen salir antes que los dientes de los niños. Hay un margen de 6 a 8 meses que se considera una variación normal para cualquier lado de la edad en la cual los dientes salen en la boca. En algunos niños los dientes pueden salir aun más temprano o más tarde que esto. Todo depende de sus patrones de crecimiento. Quisiéramos ver que los dientes salieran más tarde en vez de más temprano. Cuando los dientes salen más tarde, hay una buena posibilidad que la boca estará más grande de modo que los dientes tienen el espacio necesario para salir derechos. Mientras mayor sea el niño cuando le sale el diente, más destreza manual tendrá para cepillarse y para usar el hilo dental para mantenerlo limpio y sin enfermedad.

La dentición normal del niño tendrá 20 dientes de leche. Los adultos típicamente tienen 32 dientes, aunque hay evidencia que muchos adultos no tienen los primordios dentales para las cuatro muelas cordales.

Dientes Primarios

Los primeros dientes comienzan a formarse a los 4 a 6 meses en el útero, durante el segundo trimestre del embarazo. Después de nacer el bebé, los dientes siguen creciendo y salen en la boca.

incisivos centrales inferiores	6 meses
incisivos laterales inferiores	7 meses
incisivos centrales superiores	7.5 meses
incisivos laterales superiores	9 meses
colmillos y caninos inferiores	16 meses
segundos molares inferiores	20 meses
segundos molares superiores	24 meses

Dientes Permanentes

El esmalte de los dientes permanentes realmente comienza a formarse a los 3 a 4 meses de edad. Si su agua no tiene fluoruro, asegúrese que su bebé reciba los suplementos de fluoruro necesarios. Los dientes permanentes salen debajo de los dientes de leche. La presión del movimiento hacia arriba del diente permanente causa una resorción de la raíz del diente de leche. Cuando la raíz desaparece, el diente se afloja y eventualmente se cae. Si el diente permanente no sale directamente debajo del diente de leche, la raíz del diente de leche no se resorbe y no se afloja. El segundo diente saldrá al frente o detrás del diente de leche. Esto es común. Cuando ocurre, vea al dentista para determinar si se debe o no remover el diente de leche para permitir que el diente permanente se posicione correctamente.

incisivos centrales inferiores	6–7 años
primer molar inferior	6–7 años
primer molar superior	6–7 años
incisivos centrales superiores	7–8 años
incisivos laterales inferiores	7–8 años
incisivos laterales superiores	8–9 años
caninos inferiores	9–10 años
primeros premolares superiores	10–11 años
primeros premolares inferiores	10–11 años
caninos superiores	11–12 años
segundo premolares inferiores	11–12 años
segundo molar inferior	11–13 años
segundo molar superior	12–12 años
muelas cordales	17–22 años

¡Asegúrese de recordar los selladores para los molares y los premolares!

Si usted tiene cualquier pregunta sobre la formación de los dientes, favor de sentirse libre de preguntarnos.

Prevención de la Enfermedad Dental en Infantes y Niños

Hay varios pasos positivos que usted puede tomar para asegurar que su niño tenga pocos, si algunos, cavidades y problemas relacionados a los dientes. Una rutina diaria de cuidado oral de sí mismo efectiva y correcta (cepillado de dientes y uso del hilo dental) es la parte más importante de la prevención. Visitas programadas con el dentista y el higienista dental para los exámenes y los procedimientos de profilaxis (limpieza) también son muy importantes para el bienestar dental de su niño. Estas sugerencias ayudarán a mantener los dientes y las encías de su niño sin enfermedad dental.

1. Limpie los dientes de su infante diariamente con un paño mojado o una gasa mojada de dos pulgadas cuadradas.
2. Use el hilo dental en los dientes de su niño diariamente hasta que el niño pueda desarrollar la habilidad de hacerlo solo. Esto puede no ser una transición fácil pero el esfuerzo vale la pena.
3. Después de notar que los dientes están saliendo por el tejido de las encías, las botellas nocturnas deben contener sólo agua. Los fluidos de las botellas nocturnas forman charcos detrás de los dientes mientras el infante duerme. Las botellas nocturnas que contienen leche, jugo, ponche, soda, etc. pueden causar deterioro **extensivo.**
4. Si usted no vive en un área con agua con fluoruro, el infante debe recibir un suplemento de vitaminas con fluoruro. La dosis depende de la edad y el peso del infante. Esto debe continuar hasta que el niño desarrolle las muelas cordales—en los años de la adolescencia. Su pediatra o su dentista puede escribir una receta para estas vitaminas de fluoruro sistémico tan importantes.
5. Los niños no desarrollan la destreza para cepillarse y usar el hilo dental correctamente en sus propios dientes hasta más o menos la edad de 6 ó 7 años. Usted tiene que asegurarse que esto se hace bien, aun si significa que usted tenga que hacer el cuidado oral de sí mismo para ellos. Su buen ejemplo de cepillarse y usar el hilo dental diario aumentará mucho la voluntad y la habilidad de su niño en esta área.
6. La primera visita al dentista debe ser en la infancia, en el momento cuando los dientes comienzan a salir. Durante esta visita le daremos unas guías de lo que usted puede esperar en cuanto al desarrollo oral y sugerencias sobre el tipo de nutrición y cuidado oral de sí mismo son apropiados para su niño.
7. La primera visita al dentista para un tratamiento debe tomar lugar en la edad de 2½ años. En este momento se hará un examen, limpieza y tratamiento de fluoruro.
8. El tratamiento de fluoruro tópico que se da en la cita regular de limpieza es importante. Ayuda a hacer que los dientes que ya están en la boca sean más fuertes y más resistentes al deterioro y a la acumulación de la placa. Las vitaminas de fluoruro sistémico fortalecen el esmalte de los dientes que no han salido. El fluoruro tópico asume la responsabilidad después de esto.
9. Una capa de plástico conocida como un *sellador* puede ser colocada en las superficies de mordida de los dientes de atrás. Este sellador puede reducir por un 90% la incidencia de deterioro en las superficies tratadas. Se debe colocar en la mayoría de los dientes de atrás, tanto los premolares como los molares, tan pronto como sea posible para mantener estos dientes suficientemente secos para que el sellador se adhiera en su lugar. A veces se coloca en los dientes de leche en situaciones especiales. Hay una hoja informativa disponible que cubrirá este tema en más detalle. Normalmente se aplican los selladores cuando los niños tienen 6 años de edad. El dentista o el higienista le aconsejará cuando creen que se puede colocar el sellador con éxito.
10. Cuando su niño puede entender y hacer la rutina de "enjuagar y escupir", es hora de comenzar a usar el enjuague bucal con fluoruro. Éste no un enjuague bucal usado para cubrir el mal aliento. Realmente es un suplemento nocturno a los tratamientos de fluoruro tópico que su niño recibe en la oficina del dentista. Sin embargo, no es tan fuerte como la versión de la oficina. No es un medicamento con receta.

Si usted sigue estas sugerencias fielmente, su niño podrá nunca desarrollar ningún deterioro. Si el deterioro comenzara, será pequeño y fácil de tratar. Nada reemplaza el cepillado el uso del hilo dental diario concienzudo, ni los buenos hábitos de comida. Las citas rutinarias para el examen y limpieza dental son vitales. Usted encontrará que seguir estas instrucciones será muy efectivo en ayudar a su niño a mantener una salud dental óptima.

Si usted tiene cualquier pregunta sobre la prevención de la enfermedad dental, favor de sentirse libre de preguntarnos.

Selladores

¿Por Qué Selladores?

El deterioro en los dientes de atrás, los premolares y los molares generalmente comienza en las ranuras y las fisuras que normalmente existen en las superficies de mordida de los dientes de atrás. Los selladores dentales, disponibles desde los 1960, son unas capas de plástico claro que se pueden colocar en las superficies de los dientes posteriores. Estos selladores evitan la formación de deterioro en las superficies tratadas. Los selladores hasta se pueden colocar en los dientes con áreas pequeñas de deterioro conocidas como *lesiones cariosas incipientes.* Los selladores pararán el progreso habitual de la destrucción del diente. Puede quedarse en el diente desde 3 hasta más de 20 años, dependiendo del diente, el tipo de sellador usado y los hábitos de comer del paciente. Se pueden colocar sólo en los dientes que no hayan sido restaurados previamente.

El sellador se coloca en el diente a través de un procedimiento de unión químico/mecánico. No se requiere taladrado ni anestesia local para el procedimiento de aplicar el sellador. Es completamente sin dolor.

En esta oficina, estamos dedicados a la prevención de la enfermedad oral. Es claro que si se previene el comienzo del deterioro inicial o si la caries es suficientemente pequeña, hay un gran ahorro de tiempo, dinero, incomodidad y estructura dental. El deterioro del diente hay que removerlo con taladrado, luego hay que colocar una empastadura. Es posible que haya que hacer el taladrado y colocar la empastadura varias veces durante la vida del paciente cuando se envejece la empastadura y necesita un reemplazo. Sugerimos enfáticamente que los pacientes con dientes que se pueden proteger con un material sellador consideren que se les haga este procedimiento lo antes posible.

Selladores y Prevención

Aconsejamos especialmente que los niños tengan el sellador aplicado a sus dientes tan pronto los dientes salen por la encía y las superficies de los dientes ya no estén cubiertas con el tejido de la encía. Si no se pueden aislar los dientes totalmente de la humedad en la boca durante el proceso de adhesión, es probable que el sellador no se quedará en el diente por tanto tiempo como lo esperado. Generalmente se aplica el sellador a los dientes permanentes, pero a veces surge una situación en la cual será beneficioso aplicarlo a un diente primario.

Un estudio terminado en 1991 encontró que una aplicación de sellador redujo el deterioro de la superficie de mordida por un 52% sobre un período de 15 años. Otro estudio terminado en 1990 demostró que se podía reducir el deterioro en las superficies de mordida por un 95% sobre 10 años al reparar rutinariamente 2% a 4% de los selladores cada año. Esperamos que los selladores duren muchos años. El reemplazo o arreglo progresivo, como sea necesario, dará la mejor protección.

Un sellador no es un sustituto de los hábitos correctos de cepillado y uso del hilo dental. La efectividad del sellador se reduce con la negligencia del cuidado oral de sí mismo. También, aún se pueden formar caries en las superficies no tratadas. Por eso, un tratamiento de fluoruro tópico queda como una ayuda preventiva esencial y necesaria.

Tanto en 1984 como en 1994, el Servicio de Salud Pública de los Estados Unidos y el Cirujano General de los Estados Unidos, entre otros, han recomendado los selladores. Sabemos que los selladores son uno de los tratamientos disponibles más importantes para la prevención del deterioro dental.

Si usted tiene cualquier pregunta sobre los selladores, favor de sentirse libre de preguntarnos.

Garantía del Sellador

Nombre del Paciente: _____   **Fecha:** _____

Creemos que los selladores son uno de los procedimientos dentales preventivos más importantes que usted puede obtener. Esto es cierto para los niños y para los adultos. Las caries pueden comenzar en casi todas las personas en casi cualquier edad.

La colocación de un sellador no requiere el taladrado. El costo de un sellador es menos de la mitad del costo para un diente que necesita prepararse y tener una restauración colocada. Cuando esta oficina coloca un sellador y usted sigue algunas instrucciones sencillas y beneficiosas, garantizamos que si alguna vez hay que reemplazar el sellador (mientras el Dr. _____ está en la práctica dental activa), reemplazaremos el sellador sin cargo adicional para usted ni para su portador de seguro. La razón por la cual haremos esto es para darle más incentivo de reemplazar el sellador.

Esta garantía estará vigente, todo el tiempo que usted viva en el área y visite esta oficina en los intervalos recomendados para el examen y la profilaxis (limpieza de dientes) periódicos. Para la mayoría de los pacientes este intervalo es cada 6 meses.

Diente #(s) sellado(s): _____

Fecha que se coloco el sellador: _____

Material usado: _____

Colocado por: _____

_____

(Nombre del dentista, credenciales)

Si usted tiene cualquier pregunta sobre la garantía del sellador, favor de preguntarnos.

Fluoruro Suplementario

Existen dos métodos por los cuales usted o su niño puede recibir el fluoruro. El método más común es una aplicación tópica. Estos incluyen: el fluoruro contenido en los enjuagues bucales, las pastas de dientes y los tratamientos profesionales de aplicar el fluoruro (aplicación con cubeta) en la oficina dental. Cada uno de estos artículos que contienen fluoruro tiene la intención de trabajar en el esmalte expuesto, superficial, desarrollado del diente que ya está en su lugar en la boca. El fluoruro hace que es esmalte sea más duro y provee la base para la remineralización. El fluoruro también puede inhibir el crecimiento de las bacterias. En los productos tópicos de cuidado oral sí mismo, la concentración de fluoruro es baja, pero la aplicación repetida y diaria del fluoruro puede ayudar a asegurar que sus dientes tengan menos caries. Este tipo de fluoruro no se traga.

Antes de que los dientes se puedan ver y mientras todavía se están desarrollando debajo de las encías, el uso de fluoruro puede hacer que los dientes sean más fuertes y más resistente al deterioro. Los fluoruros sistémicos se dispensan con una receta y se tragan. Fortalecen los dientes que están en desarrollo. Recomendamos enfáticamente que sus niños reciban los beneficios de este combatidor comprobado del deterioro.

La dosis del fluoruro sistémico recomendada por la Asociación Dental Americana (ADA) fue reducida en mayo del 1994. El uso de las vitaminas de fluoruro (sistémicas), conjunto con el trago por los pacientes jóvenes de las pastas de dientes que contenían el fluoruro resultó en demasiado de algo bueno. Muchos dentistas habían observado una mayor incidencia de manchas blancas pequeñas que se formaban en los dientes frontales. Aunque no eran un problema dental, estas manchas blancas podrían ser antiestéticas. Aunque las manchas blancas frecuentemente son fáciles de remover, la razón fundamental para cambiar la dosis es reducir su frecuencia de formación.

Las nuevas recomendaciones son las siguientes:

Concentración de Fluoruro en el Agua Potable (partes por millón [ppm])			
Edad	Menos de 0.3 ppm	0.3–0.6 ppm	Más de 6 ppm
6 meses – 3 años	0.25 mg	0	0
3 años – 6 años	0.50 mg	0.25 mg	0
6 años – 16 años	1.0 mg	0.50 mg	0

Si sus niños caen dentro de los grupos de edades anteriores, **y si usted no tiene una fuente de agua con fluoruro,** deben tomar un fluoruro suplementario. El fluoruro sistémico fortalece el esmalte y lo hace más resistente al ataque de bacterias y menos susceptible al deterioro. Es una de las acciones preventivas más importantes que usted puede tomar por sus niños. En nuestra opinión aun una carie es mucho. La mejor manera de preservar los dientes es mantenerlos sin taladrado y sin empastaduras. Esto requiere unas medidas preventivas serias: el cepillado, el uso del hilo dental, una buena dieta y un suplemento de fluoruro.

Si usted tiene cualquier pregunta sobre el fluoruro suplementario, favor de sentirse libre de preguntarnos.

Fluoruro Tópico: En el Hogar y en la Oficina Dental

¿Por Qué el Fluoruro Tópico?

La mayoría de nosotros estamos familiarizados con las ventajas dentales de los suplementos de fluoruro que se administran a los niños sistemáticamente mientras sus dientes se están formando. La investigación de este tipo de tratamiento de fluoruro demuestra una reducción de un 35% en el deterioro de los dientes. El uso del fluoruro para reducir y eliminar el deterioro es una de las medidas de salud pública más estudiada y documentada. En nuestra oficina, recomendamos un tratamiento de fluoruro con cubeta por 4 minutos por lo menos dos veces al año, normalmente después de una cita de cuidado repetido de higiene dental periódico. Hemos encontrado que este tipo de ayuda preventiva hace cuatro cosas:

- Reduce la solubilidad del esmalte al ataque ácido, haciendo que los dientes sean más resistentes al deterioro.
- Ayuda con la remineralización del esmalte del diente donde ha acabado de comenzar el deterioro.
- Con el uso diario por más tiempo, reduce la sensibilidad del diente a los cambios de temperatura.
- Reduce la tensión de la superficie del esmalte de modo que la placa no se adhiera fácilmente al diente.

La investigación reciente también ha demostrado que usted puede beneficiarse de los enjuagues de fluoruro tópico sin receta, especialmente si usted los usa fielmente todos los días. Usted puede esperar una reducción adicional en el deterioro cuando también aplicamos un fluoruro tópico en la oficina. Se aplica cuatro veces al año. ¡La reducción del deterioro puede ser tan alta como un 30%! Si usted ha tenido un deterioro activo recientemente, no importa su edad, le recomendaremos esta rutina de fluoruro.

Aplicaciones Especiales de Fluoruro

Otra opción para el fluoruro tópico está disponible para los pacientes que experimentan la sensibilidad de un diente o una raíz, niveles de deterioro más altos y/o crónicos, deterioro en la superficie de la raíz o el síndrome de sequedad de la boca (xerostomía). Si le han diagnosticado con cualquiera de estos problemas dentales, le haremos unas cubetas de fluoruro a la medida. Luego le recetaremos o dispensaremos un producto con una alta concentración de fluoruro para que lo use en las cubetas durante las noches.

Las instrucciones son simples. Seque los dientes lo más posible, con una gasa cuadrada o un paño o succionando el aire a través de sus dientes. El fluoruro trabajará mejor si los dientes no están tan mojados. Como las cubetas se ajustan bien a los dientes, ponga sólo una cantidad pequeña del gel de fluoruro en la cubeta para cada grupo de dientes. Escupa el exceso. Si usted observa que sobra mucho fluoruro después de terminar el tratamiento, sencillamente reduzca la cantidad que pone en la cubeta. Déjela puesta _____ minutos. Entonces, saque las cubetas. Escupa la saliva y el fluoruro restante. **No coma ni beba por___minutos.**

La cantidad de semanas que usted necesitará hacer este procedimiento de cubeta de fluoruro depende de su condición específica. Si usted tiene un flujo de saliva disminuido con deterioro aumentado o la posibilidad de un deterioro aumentado, necesitará seguir esta rutina de fluoruro hasta que el flujo de saliva regrese a lo normal. En el caso de las raíces o los dientes sensibles, usted necesitará seguir esta rutina hasta que la sensibilidad se haya reducido. *Comentario:* La reducción de la sensibilidad es normalmente un proceso gradual: no espere una mejoría rápida. Desensibilizar las raíces puede también requerir que se coloquen otros materiales sobre el área como un procedimiento adjunto.

Si usted tiene cualquier pregunta sobre el uso de los fluoruros tópicos en el hogar o en la oficina dental, favor de sentirse libre de preguntarnos.

Periodoncia

Revisión del Contenido: Periodoncia

Evaluación y Enfermedades

Clasificación de la Enfermedad Periodontal
Use para informar al paciente de su tipo de enfermedad periodontal usando las descripciones de la Academia Americana de Periodontología.

Señales Tempranas de la Enfermedad Periodontal
Explica al paciente cómo reconocer los cambios en sus tejidos que significan una enfermedad periodontal y cómo la oficina rutinariamente le examina para detectar estas señales tempranas.

Involucración de la Furcación
Una descripción de la furcación, la pérdida de hueso y sus implicaciones en la enfermedad periodontal.

Hiperplasia Gingival
Informa cómo ocurre la hiperplasia gingival, las opciones de tratamiento y la prevención.

Gingivitis
Provee información sobre las características, las consecuencias y el tratamiento de la gingivitis.

Gingiva Adherida Insuficiente
Define lo que es insuficiente encía adherida y los problemas orales que pueden resultar.

Enfermedad Periodontal Necrótica
Explica lo que es la gingivitis ulcerativa, cómo se desarrolla y los pasos del tratamiento profesional y cuidado de sí mismo.

Enfermedad Periodontal
Provee una visión general de la enfermedad periodontal, su etiología, progresión y prevención.

Enfermedad Periodontal y la Salud Sistémica
Enfatiza el aspecto de la enfermedad de las encías como infección y la correlación a la salud sistémica.

Recomendaciones para el Tratamiento Periodontal: Terapia Inicial
Lista de las clasificaciones de la enfermedad periodontal del paciente, el número esperado de visitas a la oficina, los procedimientos y los honorarios envueltos, con cuadros de verificación.

Medida de la Profundidad del Bolsillo
Describe el método de la hoja clínica periodontal y cómo los números están relacionados con los niveles de salud oral.

El Fumar y la Periodontitis del Adulto
Hace énfasis en la relación entre el fumar y la ocurrencia de la enfermedad periodontal.

Opciones de Tratamiento

Cirugía Plástica Periodontal Electiva Cosmética: Recontorno del Tejido
Aconseja de cómo la cirugía periodontal puede mejorar la apariencia de los dientes y de la arquitectura de las encías y las posibles vías de tratamiento.

Electrocirugía
Describe los procedimientos de la electrocirugía y su uso en la odontología.

Procedimientos de Colgajo
Informa acerca de las indicaciones y procedimientos para el procedimiento quirúrgico de colgajo periodontal.

Injertos Gingivales
Una descripción de las condiciones que requieren un injerto gingival y un repaso del procedimiento.

Procedimientos de Gingivectomía y Gingivoplastia
Se explican las indicaciones y el tratamiento para estos dos procedimientos.

Revisión del Contenido: Periodoncia—continuación

Desbridamiento Completo
Explica lo que es el desbridamiento completo y lo que pasará durante y después del procedimiento.

Cirugía Ósea
Informa acerca de las indicaciones y procedimientos asociados con la cirugía ósea periodontal.

Cirugía Periodontal
Provee a los pacientes un conocimiento general de la cirugía periodontal y los resultados probables.

Profilaxis
Una explicación de la importancia de la visita de profilaxis dental y los factores que se usan para determinar los intervalos recomendados.

Aumento de Reborde
Explica las indicaciones y las posibles opciones de tratamiento para el aumento del reborde.

Hemisecciones y Amputaciones Radiculares
Se explican las razones y los procedimientos para las hemisecciones y las amputaciones radiculares.

Raspado y Alisado Radicular
Informa acerca del propósito y los procedimientos envueltos en el raspado y alisado radicular.

Raspado y Alisado Radicular: Instrucciones para después del Procedimiento
Una lista de verificación para individualizar las instrucciones para el paciente para después del procedimiento.

Raspado y Alisado Radicular: Reevaluación
Informa del propósito y la importancia de la reevaluación después del raspado y alisado radicular.

Manejo del Tejido Suave
Información de la terapia periodontal inicial: por qué es necesaria; qué está envuelto y qué se puede hacer para prevenir la necesidad futura de ella.

Colocar Férulas en los Dientes
Información acerca de los procedimientos y la necesidad por colocar férulas en los dientes.

Agentes de Quimioterapia
Enjuague Oral de Gluconato de Clorhexidina 0.12%
Una visión general del enjuague recetado, gluconato de clorhexidina, y sus usos y precauciones.

Protocolo de Enjuague Oral
Instrucciones para un procedimiento de protocolo de enjuague suplementario para pacientes que rechazan la cirugía periodontal convencional.

Periostat: Dosis Submicrobiana Sistémica de Doxiciclina
Repaso de la dosis submicrobiana sistémica de doxiciclina como un suplemento al raspado y alisado radicular.

Terapia Antibiótica Específica al Lugar
Describe el uso de la terapia antibiótica específica al lugar, los procedimientos envueltos y los tipos de productos disponibles para esta terapia.

Irrigación Subgingival
Introduce la irrigación subgingival como una modalidad usada con varios otros procedimientos.

Clasificación de la Enfermedad Periodontal

Cualquier enfermedad periodontal no es deseable y, si se deja sin tratar o se ignora, puede conducir a una cantidad de problemas dentales serios. Si usted desea mantener sus dientes y encías (gingiva) en un estado saludable y sin enfermedad, es importante que cepille los dientes correctamente y use el hilo dental diariamente. Haga estos procedimientos tal como le hemos enseñado. Regrese para la higiene dental continua en los intervalos de tiempo que hemos recomendado. Estos intervalos de tiempo para sus citas de limpieza se han establecido para su condición dental existente. Los intervalos pueden fluctuar según su habilidad de cuidar sus dientes y encías. Una infección periodontal es específica al lugar y de naturaleza episódica. Cualquier demora en sus citas rutinarias de higiene dental de cuidado repetido podría resultar perjudicial a su salud oral.

Lo siguiente es una visión general breve de la clasificación de la Academia Americana de Periodontología de los tipos de enfermedad periodontal.

Tipo I.
   Enfermedades Gingivales: Una inflamación o lesión de la encía caracterizada por cambios de color, la forma gingival, la posición, la apariencia de la superficie y la presencia de sangrado y/o pus.

Tipo II.
   Periodontitis Crónica: Una inflamación de las estructuras que sostienen los dientes asociada con la placa y el cálculo; los factores locales, sistémicos o ambientales afectan la velocidad del progreso. Se puede clasificar como localizada o generalizada.

Tipo III.
   Periodontitis Agresiva: Caracterizada por el progreso rápido de la enfermedad periodontal en un individuo saludable en la ausencia de grandes acumulaciones de placa y/o cálculo. Se puede clasificar como localizada o generalizada.

Tipo IV.
   Periodontitis como Manifestación de Enfermedad Sistémica: Periodontitis asociada con los trastornos genéticos o de la sangre.

Tipo V.
   Enfermedad Periodontal Necrótica: Encías ulceradas y necróticas entre los dientes y en los márgenes de los dientes. Se puede clasificar como gingivitis ulcerativa necrótica o periodontitis ulcerativa necrótica.

Tipo VI.
   Abscesos del Periodonto: Una infección del tejido periodontal localizada y con pus.

Tipo VII.
   Periodontitis Asociada con Lesiones Endodónticas: Un bolsillo periodontal profundo y localizado que se extiende hasta la punta de la raíz del diente y envuelve la muerte de la pulpa.

Tipo VIII.
   Deformidades y Condiciones de Desarrollo o Adquiridas: La enfermedad gingival o la periodontitis comenzada por factores localizados relacionados al diente que lo modifican o lo hacen susceptible a la acumulación de la placa o a la prevención de medidas efectivas de cuidado oral.

Debido a la naturaleza de la enfermedad, la mayoría de las clasificaciones envolverán un diagnóstico general y uno localizado.

Si usted tiene cualquier pregunta sobre la clasificación de su enfermedad periodontal, favor de sentirse libre de preguntarnos.

Señales Tempranas de la Enfermedad Periodontal

Las señales tempranas de advertencia para cada enfermedad ocurren en un nivel microscópico. Las señales tempranas de advertencia no se pueden ver, sentir, tocar, diagnosticar ni descubrir. No se pueden notar por sus síntomas. Puede que los cambios tempranos se puedan detectar mediante análisis químicos o biológicos sofisticados, pero no por las medidas diagnósticas normales.

Cuando usted nota que sus encías sangran (gingivitis), la enfermedad ya ha estado presente por algún tiempo y no está en su etapa más temprana. No es raro escuchar "Mis encías siempre han sangrado así", pero no se busca tratamiento. Sin embargo, si nuestros ojos comenzaran a sangrar cuando nos lavamos la cara, generalmente, ¡correríamos a buscar tratamiento médico! Las encías que sangran no son normales ni saludables. Afortunadamente, en esta etapa la enfermedad periodontal es bastante fácil de tratar y es reversible. Cuando la enfermedad ha progresado más lejos de la etapa donde sangran las encías, usted puede notar algún dolor, el retiro de las encías, dientes que se aflojan y mal aliento. Si usted ha ignorado el sangrado de sus encías (posiblemente la señal más temprana de la enfermedad de las encías) porque cree que es normal tener un poco de color "rosa" en su cepillo, probablemente tendrá síntomas y condiciones adicionales asociados con el progreso de la enfermedad. En este punto, el hueso y las encías que sostienen los dientes pueden estar permanentemente alterados y disminuidos.

Se recomienda que usted se adhiera a los intervalos de tiempo sugeridos para sus citas de limpieza dental. Examinaremos sus encías durante sus citas dentales periódicas de limpieza para descubrir las señales tempranos de la enfermedad periodontal. Mientras limpiamos sus dientes notaremos las áreas donde le es difícil remover la placa o donde se forma el cálculo y las áreas de inflamación del tejido de las encías y registraremos las profundidades de la sonda que medirán su tejido de las encías para las señales de la enfermedad periodontal. Entonces podemos demostrar el cuidado efectivo de sí mismo para evitar que estas áreas progresen en enfermedad periodontal

Queremos enfatizar la prevención. No espere hasta que ocurran las señales tempranas de advertencia de la enfermedad de las encías antes de fijar su cita de higiene dental. Si usted tiene muy pocas empastaduras, no ha perdido ninguno de los dientes permanentes (fuera de las muelas cordales) y tiene un cuidado oral diario de sí mismo muy completo, un examen y una limpieza anual por el dentista y el higienista dental pueden ser adecuados. Si le han hecho mucho trabajo dental (puentes, coronas, empastaduras) o si tiene dientes que faltan que no se han reemplazado y usted no pasa tiempo con el cuidado oral de sí mismo adecuado, podría ser necesario visitar la oficina dental tres o cuatro veces al año. Le informaremos de lo que es apropiado para su condición oral individual.

Involucración de la Furcación

Las raíces de los dientes están cubiertas y rodeadas por tejidos del hueso y de las encías cuando están en su estado normal y han estado sin enfermedad. Sólo es visible la porción de la corona. Algunos dientes hacia la parte de atrás de la boca tienen dos o tres raíces que se extienden desde las coronas del diente hasta el hueso de la mandíbula. Esta área "en forma de V" donde el diente se divide o se bifurca en dos o tres raíces se llama la *furcación o la furca*. La furca también está cubierta con hueso y está ligada al diente por las fibras del ligamento periodontal.

Mientras la furcación de un diente con múltiples raíces esté cubierta con una cantidad normal de hueso y encía, todo está bien y la furca no presenta ningún interés excepcional para el dentista o el higienista dental. Cuando hay una alteración en la densidad del hueso de la furca o cuando realmente comienza a resorber (desaparecer debido a algún tipo de patología dental), el área de la furca se vuelve importante e interesante. La pérdida continua de hueso terminaría en la pérdida del diente.

La pérdida de hueso en el área de la furca podría estar relacionada a la enfermedad periodontal (enfermedad de las encías). La patología periodontal en la furca podría ser parte de un problema localizado—sólo presente en este lugar—o una señal de que hay un problema más extenso que necesita atención. La desintegración de hueso en la furcación también podría indicar que el nervio dentro del diente se está muriendo, y que el diente necesitará un canal radicular (tratamiento endodóntico).

Si la desintegración es específica al lugar en sólo este diente, el tratamiento sería localizado. El tipo de terapia recomendada dependería de la severidad de la desintegración. Una enfermedad mínima podría tratarse con una profilaxis dental (limpieza) y con un refuerzo del cuidado oral de sí mismo. El tratamiento de una desintegración más extensiva podría envolver procedimientos periodontales agresivos incluyendo, pero no están limitados a, cirugía periodontal y aumento del hueso. Le podríamos enviar a donde un periodontista para estos procedimientos.

Si la desintegración de la furca es señal de una enfermedad periodontal más extensa, se evaluará toda la boca y se harán recomendaciones de tratamiento específico.

Hay muchos nervios muy pequeños que salen a través de varias porciones del diente y un problema localizado de furcación podría indicar que el nervio de un diente está muerto o está muriendo y el diente puede requerir un canal radicular.

Usted puede creer que es difícil cepillar los dientes y usar el hilo dental cuando la alineación y la posición de las encías son ideales. Cuando hay pérdida de hueso en una furca, el cuidado oral diario de sí mismo se complica más. Una furca es un área difícil de limpiar—mientras más pérdida de hueso, más difícil será. En los casos extremos, que no queda ni hueso ni encía en la furca, y el paciente podría pasar una ayuda de limpieza interdental entre las raíces de un diente con dos raíces. Para un diente con tres raíces y una involucración de furcación, el proceso de limpieza es aun más problemático.

Usted ha sido diagnosticado con un problema de involucración de furcación. Después de un examen cuidadoso, se hará una recomendación de tratamiento. Nuestra recomendación se basará no sólo en el tratamiento del problema de furcación, sino también en la prevención de la extensión del área descubierta.

Si usted tiene cualquier pregunta sobre la involucración de la furcación, favor de sentirse libre de preguntarnos.

Ilustración en CD-ROM

Hiperplasia Gingival

Factores de Predisposición

La hiperplasia gingival es un crecimiento en el tamaño de los tejidos de la encía causado por el aumento en la cantidad y el arreglo normal de las células. Se caracteriza por la inflamación de los tejidos suaves alrededor de los dientes. Los tejidos de la encía parecerán brillantes e hinchados y de un color rojo oscuro hasta un poco morado. Los factores de predisposición en esta inflamación pueden incluir, pero no están limitados a los factores sistémicos (diabetes mellitus), los medicamentos anti-epilépticos (tales como DILANTIN®, MYSOLINE® y DEPAKENE®), los medicamentos inmunosupresores (ciclosporina), los bloqueadores del canal de calcio (PROCARDIA®, CALAN®, CARDIZEM®, y BAYOTENSIN®), otros medicamentos selectos, los cambios hormonales asociados con el embarazo, los contraceptivos orales o los tipos de cambios hormonales que experimentan los adolescentes jóvenes durante la pubertad. Normalmente vemos la hiperplasia asociada con el embarazo, la contracepción oral y la pubertad.

Estas condiciones **no** necesariamente causan que las encías se inflamen o se engrandezcan, sino que en la presencia de sólo cantidades pequeñas de placa y/o cálculo, la respuesta de los tejidos de las encías puede ser fuera de lo ordinario. La gingivitis hiperplásica también puede ocurrir sólo a causa de la presencia de mucha placa bacterial sin que ningunos de estos factores estén presentes.

Indicaciones

Si usted tiene cualquier de estos factores de predisposición o si toma ciertos medicamentos, hay un potencial de hiperplasia gingival. Desgraciadamente, la enfermedad de las encías no duele hasta que es demasiado tarde. Si usted tiene hiperplasia gingival, y si tiene suerte, notará probablemente que sus encías sangran probablemente cuando cepilla los dientes o usa hilo dental. El sangrado siempre es señal de enfermedad o infección.

Eliminación y/o Prevención

Para eliminar o prevenir estos problemas, su cuidado oral de sí mismo tiene que ser completo. Usted debe cepillar los dientes y usar el hilo dental y hacer cualquier otro procedimiento de cuidado oral que le han enseñado que haga todos los días. Esto puede eliminar el problema por completo. Si no, usted necesitará ajustar el intervalo entre las citas de cuidado repetido con el higienista dental. Un marco de tiempo de 2, 3 o 4 meses entre las limpiezas, dependiendo de la severidad del problema, será más apropiado para la prevención de la hiperplasia. Esto será necesario por tanto tiempo como existan los factores de predisposición. Si el medicamento es el factor, usted deberá de ver al higienista en el intervalo recomendado.

Si usted está embarazada, la hiperplasia gingival podría persistir hasta que los cambios hormonales asociados con el embarazo regresan a lo normal. Hasta entonces, usted necesita fijar sus citas de cuidado oral repetido con el higienista dental como se ha recomendado. Igualmente, si toma los contraceptivos orales y nota las señales recurrentes de las infecciones de las encías (el sangrado cuando cepilla los dientes y usa hilo dental), asumiendo que su cuidado oral de sí mismo es completo, puede ser necesario un programa de cuidado repetido más regular.

La hiperplasia gingival en los adolescentes jóvenes normalmente se ve cuando el cuidado oral de sí mismo no es adecuado. Un intervalo de tres meses es mejor en estas circunstancias. Algunos adolescentes tienen hábitos inadecuados de cuidado oral de sí mismo. La comida chatarra y las bebidas azucaradas (aun el jugo) junto con el cepillado y uso del hilo dental casi inexistentes causan la enfermedad seria de las encías, el mal aliento y el deterioro. Generalmente, el cambio hormonal se estabiliza y el problema agudo se resuelve. Para los jóvenes de esta edad, las cuestiones sociales de querer ser más atractivos muchas veces influyen en los hábitos de cuidado oral de sí mismo ¡cuando toda la atención dental del mundo no lo puede hacer!

Estas recomendaciones están diseñadas para prevenir los problemas de las encías. La prevención es mejor y mucho menos costoso que cualquier remedio. Si usted tiene seguro dental, probablemente **no** cubrirá el tratamiento dental adicional necesario. Aunque usted necesita mantener su salud oral, el portador piensa que estas situaciones no son usuales y generalmente no son procedimientos cubiertos.

Si usted tiene cualquier pregunta sobre la hiperplasia gingival, favor de sentirse libre de preguntarnos.

Gingivitis

Casi todos saben lo que es una caries. A causa del gran alcance de los anuncios de los manufactureros de las pastas de dientes y de los enjuagues orales, para el 2004 casi todos han oído hablar de la **gingivitis**. Lo que puede no estarle tan claro, sin embargo, es exactamente qué es la gingivitis. Usted puede reconocerla como un problema, pero sin saber el por qué ni cuán seria puede ser. Usted puede aun saber que es un tipo de enfermedad de las encías (periodontal). Puede también saber que de alguna manera está relacionada con la placa y el sarro (el cálculo) en los dientes. Pero ¿por qué se debe preocupar de tenerla?

La gingivitis es una infección de los tejidos de las encías alrededor de los dientes. Es una infección muy común que afecta casi 95% de la población mundial. Esta infección puede estar caracterizada por enrojecimiento y por la hinchazón y el sangrado de las encías alrededor de los dientes. Esta infección de las encías necesita absolutamente que se trate lo antes posible. Las infecciones de las encías se pueden evitar casi siempre con el cuidado oral responsable de sí mismo.

La gingivitis es la forma menos severa de la enfermedad periodontal y es reversible. Por su definición no hay pérdida del hueso que sostiene el diente. Si se trata temprano, la gingivitis se puede eliminar. Si no se trata, puede progresar a la forma más seria de la enfermedad periodontal llamada *periodontitis*. En su forma más seria, los tejidos del hueso y de las encías se pueden afectar permanentemente. Las encías que sangran, una de las señales de la gingivitis, son señal de una infección en la boca. Sus tejidos de las encías nunca deben sangrar. No es normal que haya sangre en su cepillo de dientes cuando usted termina de cepillarse los dientes. Generalmente la gingivitis no duele, por eso usted puede no saber que la tiene. Puede ser local (alrededor de algunos dientes) o generalizada (alrededor de casi todos o de todos los dientes). La gingivitis se ve más frecuentemente en los pacientes que no se cepillan bien los dientes y no usan el hilo dental diariamente, pero también puede estar relacionada al medicamento. El mal aliento puede ser otra señal de la gingivitis. Si usted usa un enjuague oral para eliminar el mal aliento, puede necesitar atención dental. Aunque el mal aliento puede estar relacionado con algunos problemas médicos, generalmente es sólo el resultado de los restos que permanecen en los dientes, las encías y la lengua no bien limpiados y que se están descomponiendo en el ambiente oscuro, tibio y húmedo de su boca—un lugar perfecto para criar gérmenes.

Si usted tiene encías que sangran debe preocuparse. El tejido saludable en cualquier lugar en nuestros cuerpos no sangra. Ahora, ¿qué puede usted hacer para detener el sangrado?

Podemos ayudarle a eliminar la gingivitis. Esto envuelve una buena limpieza profesional y buenos hábitos de cuidado oral de sí mismo. Hay que eliminar la placa (los restos blandos compuestos de bacterias) y el sarro (el cálculo o los restos endurecidos) antes que los tejidos de las encías puedan sanarse y se pueda eliminar la infección. Si ha pasado algún tiempo desde que limpiaron sus dientes correctamente, puede tomar más de una cita para ponerle en forma nuevamente.

Consiga que se limpien sus dientes y sus encías regularmente. Manténgalos limpios con el cepillado y el uso del hilo dental diarios. La infección que usted tiene se eliminará. Si usted mantiene limpios sus dientes y sus encías, ellos pueden ser saludables y sin problemas para toda su vida.

Ilustración en CD-ROM

Gingiva Adherida Insuficiente

Si usted mirara un corte transversal del diente y la mandíbula, vería lo siguiente desde la punta del diente hacia la gingiva (encía): la parte del diente cubierta de esmalte se pone más ancha, luego se pone más estrecha al acercarse al área gingival; el margen del tejido gingival (que está contiguo); el tejido gingival que está firmemente adherido al hueso subyacente y que no se puede mover, quizás con una apariencia granulada; y un tejido gingival que se ve más suave que es muy movible y que no está estrechamente adherido al hueso subyacente. La última área puede ser más rojiza en color que el otro tejido gingival descrito y se extiende hasta los cachetes y los labios.

El enfoque de este tema es la zona de la gingiva adherida. Como parte de su examen periodontal, usamos una sonda periodontal para medir y registrar la profundidad del surco. La profundidad sulcular es la profundidad del espacio entre la gingiva marginal y el diente. La sonda periodontal usada para medir este surco se inserta suavemente en al margen de la gingiva y se coloca en el surco hasta que la pare el tejido gingival que está más estrechamente adherido al hueso. Esta medida ayuda a determinar su salud periodontal. Se espera, que la profundidad del surco sea de 3 milímetros o menos. La zona del tejido gingival estrechamente adherida alrededor del diente es bastante importante.

Esta zona de gingiva adherida necesita estar intacta y de un ancho adecuado para proteger (porque separa) el tejido alrededor del diente. Si no es suficiente, el cepillado incorrecto (muy fuerte), o una unión del músculo que no está en una posición correcta, puede halar el tejido gingival adherido. Si lo tira suficiente, la profundidad normal de 1–3 milímetros puede aumentar a 4 milímetros o aun 6 milímetros o más. Esto no será un cambio estable ni saludable en su salud periodontal. El margen gingival normal (borde de la encía) tiene la forma de concha (como ondas pequeñas regulares). Si hay insuficiente gingiva adherida, la forma de concha se altera, y la gingiva se pondrá roja y sangrará fácilmente. El área tirada será más propensa a atrapar la placa bacterial y los restos de la comida, será más difícil de limpiar y siempre estará más inflamada e infectada. Si usted tiene este problema, quizás lo ha visto esto en sí mismo. Puede conducir a la pérdida temprana de dientes. La gingiva adherida insuficiente no es buena y necesita ser corregida.

Una vez se ha diagnosticado, la corrección es relativamente fácil. Esto requerirá cirugía periodontal menor. Normalmente, se le pedirá a un periodontista (especialista de las encías) que haga este procedimiento. Usted recibirá un anestésico local para adormecer el área y el área del tejido problemático se reformará y se reconstituirá para darle el ancho correcto del tejido gingival adherido.

Aunque éste es un problema relativamente común, los pacientes normalmente no lo reconocen. Si usted lo tiene diagnosticado, consiga que se lo arreglen lo antes posible. Usted se ahorrará muchos problemas en el futuro.

Si usted tiene cualquier pregunta sobre la gingiva adherida insuficiente, favor de sentirse libre de preguntarnos.

Enfermedad Periodontal Necrótica

La enfermedad periodontal necrótica es una enfermedad inflamatoria destructiva de los tejidos de las encías. Otros nombres que se han usado para describir el proceso de esta enfermedad son *boca de zanja, enfermedad* o *infección de Vincent, gingivitis necrótica ulcerativa* y *periodontitis necrótica ulcerativa*.

Síntomas

La enfermedad periodontal necrótica puede ocurrir a cualquier edad. Sin embargo, normalmente se ve en las personas jóvenes entre las edades de 15 a 30 años. Frecuentemente se ve en los estudiantes de escuela superior o de universidad, que están bajo estrés estudiando para los exámenes. Los hábitos pobres de dieta y la resistencia disminuida a la infección son factores significativos de predisposición. Las señales de la enfermedad periodontal necrótica pueden incluir:

- comienzo repentino
- dolor, hasta el punto que es difícil masticar normal
- sangrado espontáneo, aun con la menor presión
- sabor metálico o desagradable
- fiebre leve
- glándulas linfáticas hinchadas

Causas

La enfermedad periodontal necrótica es una enfermedad infecciosa causada por un complejo específico de microbios que se desarrollan y aumentan una vez que las defensas del cuerpo se han bajado. Los factores mayores de predisposición son el fumar, el estrés, el cuidado oral de sí mismo muy pobre y la nutrición pobre.

Tratamiento

El tratamiento para la enfermedad periodontal necrótica envuelve tanto a nuestro equipo dental como a usted. El tratamiento consiste de una evaluación cuidadosa de sus hábitos personales: lo qué usted come y cómo cuida su boca. Sacaremos las células bacteriales muertas acumuladas y la comida descompuesta de aquellas áreas infectadas y le instruiremos en los hábitos de cuidado oral de sí mismo que le ayudarán a eliminar la enfermedad y evitar su regreso. Su trabajo es asegurarse que siga esas instrucciones:

1. **Siga cuidadosamente todas las sugerencias de cuidado oral de sí mismo.** No permita que nadie que use su cepillo de dientes. Use sólo el cepillo de dientes más suave posible para limpiar sus dientes suavemente y minuciosamente. Permita que su cepillo se seque entre usos.
2. **Asista a todas sus citas.** Aunque usted ya no tenga el dolor severo esto no quiere decir que la infección haya desaparecido. La infección periodontal subyacente puede recurrir si no se trata completamente.
3. **Un enjuague con agua salada tibia** cada hora es aconsejable mientras existan los síntomas agudos.
4. **Evite el uso de los productos de tabaco** en cualquier forma.
5. **Balancee su dieta** con granos integrales, verduras, proteínas y frutas. Evite las comidas altamente sazonadas y las bebidas alcohólicas. Podremos también prescribirle una vitamina durante este tiempo.
6. **Descanse adecuadamente.** El cuerpo se sanará mucho más rápido cuando se ha descansado adecuadamente.
7. Si le han recetado algún enjuague o medicamento, asegúrese de usarlo siguiendo las instrucciones cuidadosamente.

La enfermedad periodontal necrótica puede ser una condición médica seria que necesitará ser vigilada muy de cerca. Como la enfermedad periodontal necrótica puede recurrir, es esencial que tengamos toda su cooperación y entendimiento del tratamiento antes de que comencemos.

Si usted tiene cualquier pregunta sobre la enfermedad periodontal necrótica, favor de sentirse libre de preguntarnos.

Enfermedad Periodontal

La enfermedad periodontal es un proceso infeccioso clasificado según la cantidad de daño hecho a las estructuras que rodean los dientes, principalmente la gingiva (las encías) y el hueso. **Es una infección en su boca.** Puede ocurrir en cualquier momento, alrededor de cualquier diente y afecta algunos o muchos de sus dientes en grados diferentes. Hay factores genéticos de predisposición a la enfermedad periodontal, y nuestros sistemas inmunes juegan un papel en la salud de las encías, pero normalmente está relacionado a cuán bien usted puede mantener limpios sus dientes mediante el cuidado oral de sí mismo apropiado. Mientras mejor usted limpie sus dientes para remover todas las bacterias de la placa, menos probable será que usted desarrolle la enfermedad periodontal.

Progreso de la Enfermedad

Las bacterias que causan esta enfermedad primero causan que el tejido de las encías se inflame y se retire de los dientes. Cuando el problema se pone más serio, el hueso que sostiene los dientes también se infecta y se comienza a descomponer y disolver. Entonces los dientes se aflojan. Una vez que el hueso ha desaparecido, es extremadamente difícil, si no imposible, que se reconstruya con hueso nuevo. El daño es permanente y se pondrán en peligro los dientes, el hueso alrededor y su salud general.

La enfermedad periodontal se clasifica en varios tipos. Se le dará un folleto aparte con la descripción apropiada de la severidad de su infección.

La forma menos severa de esta infección aparecerá en el tejido de las encías que está rojo e hinchado y sangra fácilmente. Es raro que haya algún dolor envuelto en esta etapa. Usted puede notar también que su aliento se pone ofensivo y siente que necesita usar un enjuague oral. Nuestro sentido de olor se hace inmune a los mismos olores, por eso podemos perder la habilidad de detectar nuestro aliento enfermo ofensivo. A medida que la enfermedad progresa, los tejidos de las encías se ponen más rojos y más hinchados, se puede ver más sangrado y los dientes comienzan a aflojarse. Esta movilidad de los dientes es señal de un problema severo. Todavía puede no haber ningún dolor en esta etapa avanzada. A medida que se pierde más y más hueso y más dientes se ven envueltos en la infección, el tratamiento se pone más difícil. En este punto, muchas veces, el manejo de su problema envuelve procedimientos quirúrgicos periodontales. Si éste es el caso, podemos enviarle a un periodontista (especialista de las encías) para más tratamiento. Generalmente la enfermedad periodontal comienza y continúa a causa de la negligencia. El cepillado y el uso del hilo dental no se están haciendo efectivamente todos los días. Usted puede haber sido negligente en conseguir que se examinen y limpien sus dientes dentro de los intervalos de tiempo que usted necesita. Una vez que hayamos diagnosticado esta enfermedad, le informaremos del problema y sugeriremos el tratamiento. Si no se termina el tratamiento, sin embargo, la enfermedad continuará progresando. Desgraciadamente, la enfermedad es bastante invisible para la mayoría de las personas hasta que ha ocurrido daño severo y posiblemente irreversible.

Solución

Si el problema se ha diagnosticado en las etapas tempranas y no ha progresado a la pérdida de hueso, una limpieza apropiada (profilaxis) lo resolverá. Los casos más avanzados pueden necesitar el raspado y el alisado radicular a través de citas múltiples. En la mayoría de los casos más avanzados, la cirugía periodontal y la pérdida de dientes son inevitables. Usted recibirá un estimado de los honorarios por el tratamiento recomendado.

La enfermedad periodontal es una condición que se debe tratar rápidamente. Creemos que si se trata la infección agresivamente en las etapas tempranas, un tratamiento periodontal conservador puede ser posible y efectivo. Aunque no rechazamos automáticamente la intervención de la cirugía periodontal, esperamos que usted pueda evitarla o reducir la cantidad que necesitará.

El tratamiento exitoso de su problema periodontal dependerá de varios factores. Pero el más importante de éstos es su habilidad de llevar a cabo un cuidado oral de sí mismo excelente—con el cepillado, el uso rutinario y diario del hilo dental y el uso de las ayudas periodontales. Sin esto, el tratamiento periodontal fracasará y regresará la enfermedad.

Si usted tiene cualquier pregunta sobre la enfermedad periodontal, favor de sentirse libre de preguntarnos.

Enfermedad Periodontal y la Salud Sistémica

Investigaciones demuestran claramente que hay una relación estrecha entre las infecciones orales (periodontales) y los problemas médicos generalizados (sistémicos). Hay más de 300 tipos diferentes de bacterias que se encuentran normalmente en la boca humana, y la boca está conectada a todo el cuerpo.

Una infección de las encías es similar a una infección que podría ocurrir en otra parte del cuerpo. Las bacterias están en todos los lugares, incluyendo a nuestras bocas. Cuando las bacterias se multiplican por encima de una cantidad crítica, comienzan los problemas. ¿Por qué cambiaría la cantidad de bacterias? El cuidado oral de sí mismo pobre, la genética, el medicamento recetado, la enfermedad o los problemas sistémicos podrían contribuir. Cuando el cuerpo reconoce los invasores bacteriales, el sistema inmune inicia una respuesta para combatir al invasor.

Usted podría decir, "Mis encías siempre han sangrado así", y no ha buscado tratamiento. Imagínese ver sangre saliendo a chorros de sus ojos cuando usted lava su cara. Usted buscaría atención médica de inmediato, ¡quizás hasta iría a la sala de emergencia!

La enfermedad de las encías es una infección en su boca, no es diferente a una infección en otra parte de su cuerpo. Las bacterias invaden los tejidos suaves, el hueso y se meten en la corriente sanguínea. De esta manera, pueden entonces circular a través del cuerpo entero. Junto con las bacterias están las células muertas, los productos metabólicos secundarios, las toxinas, los restos de la comida y los virus.

Tal como sabemos que el fumar tiene un efecto adverso en nuestra salud, la ciencia está examinando el vínculo entre la enfermedad de las encías y muchas condiciones sistémicas tales como la enfermedad cardiovascular y respiratoria, la enfermedad pulmonar obstructiva crónica, nacimientos prematuros y nacimientos de bebés de peso bajo, la apoplejía, la diabetes mellitus y posiblemente la artritis reumatoide. Aunque la información científica todavía no ha confirmado los vínculos con indicadores diagnósticos, es importante para nosotros reconocer las posibles implicaciones. La cavidad oral es parte de la biología humana unida a todos los otros sistemas del cuerpo y es un portal de entrada para una variedad de organismos infectivos. Sólo hace sentido mantenerla tan limpia como sea posible para reducir el riesgo de no sólo infección oral, sino también una posible inflamación sistémica.

El cuidado oral de sí mismo completo no tiene que ser difícil ni consumir mucho tiempo. Los beneficios son más que un aliento dulce y una sonrisa que se ve magnífica. El pasar sólo algunos minutos diarios en el cuidado de sus dientes y encías y el venir para las visitas de higiene profesional en los intervalos que aconsejamos pueden hacer la diferencia entre la salud de todo el cuerpo y la enfermedad. Después de todo, ¡los huesos de la mandíbula están conectados a todos nuestros otros huesos!

Recomendaciones para el Tratamiento Periodontal: Terapia Inicial

A usted se le ha diagnosticado enfermedad periodontal. Esta enfermedad y su proceso de infección se clasifica por su severidad. La cantidad de destrucción de las estructuras duras y suaves que sostienen los dientes también está indicada en la clasificación. La clasificación para su enfermedad periodontal es:

Tipo I	**Enfermedades Gingivales**
Tipo II	**Periodontitis Crónica**
Tipo III	**Periodontitis Agresiva**
Tipo IV	**Periodontitis como Manifestación de Enfermedad Sistémica**
Tipo V	**Enfermedad Periodontal Necrótica**
Tipo VI	**Abscesos del Periodonto**
Tipo VII	**Periodontitis Asociada con Lesiones Endodónticas**
Tipo VIII	**Deformidades y Condiciones de Desarrollo o Adquiridas**

La explicación escrita de su tipo de enfermedad periodontal le fue dada en una hoja aparte. Usted también ha recibido una explicación verbal de su diagnóstico periodontal.

La enfermedad periodontal es una infección del tejido gingival (de las encías) en su boca. El tratamiento de esta enfermedad depende de la extensión del problema, de la severidad y del largo de tiempo que ha estado presente. La enfermedad es específica al lugar y de naturaleza episódica, como se explicó previamente.

El tratamiento exitoso de su problema periodontal dependerá de varios factores. Estos factores incluyen la posición y la alineación de sus dientes, la pérdida del hueso que sostiene los dientes, la cantidad de placa y cálculo (sarro) que está presente, las restauraciones existentes, los dientes partidos, el deterioro y el estado actual de la inflamación de los tejidos periodontales. Probablemente el factor más importante en el tratamiento exitoso de su enfermedad periodontal es su habilidad de llevar a cabo los procedimientos apropiados de mantenimiento oral rutinariamente. Éstos incluyen el cepillado, el uso del hilo dental y el uso de las ayudas recomendadas para la limpieza periodontal como le hayan enseñado. Esto es de máxima importancia para el tratamiento exitoso de su enfermedad periodontal y la preservación de sus dientes.

Recomendamos que para el tratamiento de su enfermedad periodontal, usted consiga que le hagan los siguientes procedimientos. Tomaremos tiempo para explicarle cada procedimiento, incluyendo el tiempo y el honorario envuelto y para contestar todas sus preguntas.

Si usted ha sufrido daño severo y/o permanente a su tejido periodontal por esta enfermedad, es posible que requiera cirugía periodontal para corregir cualquier problema periodontal restante. La evaluación final para esto se hará después de la terapia periodontal inicial. En ese momento, si es apropiado, le enviaremos a un especialista periodontal. Si usted lo desea, el especialista puede hacer todos los procedimientos que hemos recomendados además de la cirugía misma.

Los honorarios son inclusivos y no importa la cantidad de visitas a la oficina ni el tiempo requerido para terminar toda la terapia periodontal inicial. La cantidad de visitas necesarias es el mínimo necesario probable.

Cantidad aproximada de visitas necesarias a la oficina: _____

❏ **Profilaxis** $
❏ **Pulido** $
❏ **Fluoruro tópico** $
❏ **Raspado y alisado radicular por:**
  ❏ **cuadrante**   ❏ **sextante**   ❏ **media boca**   ❏ **boca completa**   ❏ **diente** $
❏ **Anestesia local necesaria** $
❏ **Irrigación subgingival con una solución medicada** $
❏ **Instrucción y evaluación del cuidado oral de sí mismo** $
❏ **Gráfica periodontal y re-evaluación** $
❏ **Otro: _____** $

Honorario total por la terapia periodontal inicial: $

Si usted tiene cualquier pregunta sobre el tratamiento periodontal, favor de sentirse libre de preguntarnos.

Medida de la Profundidad del Bolsillo

Cuando un dentista o médico prepara una agenda de tratamiento para sanar una enfermedad, se analizan los resultados de las pruebas. Las decisiones de tratamiento para una potencial cura dependen de la información recopilada. Mientras más precisa sea la información para el diagnóstico, mejor serán el diagnóstico y el tratamiento. En el reino de la enfermedad periodontal, el diagnóstico está basado en parte en la colección y el análisis de muchos números, específicamente las medidas de la profundidad del surco (hendidura) del tejido de las encías que rodea cada diente.

La preparación de una gráfica periodontal generalmente consiste en tomar por lo menos seis medidas alrededor de cada diente. Las áreas donde hay sangrado también se registran. La evidencia del sangrado es significante. El tejido de las encías saludable no sangra cuando es sondeado suavemente. Hay ciertos factores, tales como los que se encuentran en los fumadores, que restringen el sangrado, por eso la falta de sangrado sólo no indica un lugar saludable.

Estas medidas (en milímetros) son una de las herramientas diagnósticas (junto con el color, la posición y la forma del tejido) que usan el dentista y el higienista dental para determinar la severidad de la enfermedad periodontal (de las encías). Las medidas generalmente varían desde 0 mm a 12 mm. El sondeo del surco alrededor del diente frecuentemente muestra profundidades normales de 1 mm a 2 mm con profundidades mayores entre los dientes donde estos se tocan versus las profundidades en el lado del cachete o de la lengua. Los números variarán de una posición a otra y de un diente a otro. Es raro que sean uniformes a través de toda la boca. Los números más altos indican una involucración más severa del tejido suave y duro, y mientras mayor sea el número de lecturas altas, más probable es que se necesite intervención quirúrgica.

> 0 mm a 3 mm **sin sangrado:** Cantidades grandes. La enfermedad periodontal no está presente.
>
> 1 mm a 3 mm **con sangrado:** Gingivitis (la forma menos severa de la enfermedad de las encías) está presente. Probablemente no hay pérdida de hueso. Normalmente se trata con una buena profilaxis (limpieza) profesional y un cuidado oral de sí mismo mejorado.
>
> 3 mm a 5 mm **sin sangrado:** La enfermedad de las encías puede o no estar presente. El fumar puede ser un factor en la falta de sangrado. Como un paciente no puede limpiar las áreas más profundas de 3 mm con seguridad y rutinariamente, hay un potencial alto para que comience la enfermedad de las encías. Se debe recomendar las visitas de cuidado repetido profesional 3 a 4 veces al año.
>
> 3 mm a 5 mm **con sangrado:** Enfermedad periodontal temprana moderadamente avanzada. El tratamiento es una profilaxis profesional que consiste del raspado y el alisado radicular y posiblemente antibióticos sistémicos y/o específicos al lugar y otros medicamentos. El hueso que sostiene los dientes puede estar envuelto. Se requieren citas de cuidado repetido más frecuentes y más extensivas. Alguna intervención quirúrgica es posible.
>
> 5 mm a 7 mm **con sangrado:** Daño al tejido suave y duro. La pérdida de hueso es probable. El tratamiento envolverá una profilaxis más agresiva—el raspado y el alisado radicular. Se necesitarán múltiples citas. La intervención quirúrgica localizada es probable. Normalmente se usan los medicamentos sistémicos y específicos al lugar. Los dientes pueden haber comenzado a aflojarse.
>
> 7 mm y más **con sangrado:** Enfermedad periodontal avanzada. Se requiere tratamiento agresivo si se van a salvar los dientes. Casi siempre requiere cirugía. Una co-consulta con un periodontista es común. Normalmente se usan los medicamentos sistémicos y específicos al lugar.
>
> En resumen, los números bajos son buenos, los números altos son malos. La presencia de bolsillos periodontales profundos corresponde a una enfermedad de las encías más extensiva y a la necesidad de más tratamiento periodontal.

El Fumar y la Periodontitis del Adulto

Si usted es fumador, usted está a mayor riesgo no sólo para los problemas pulmonares y circulatorios sino también para la enfermedad oral. El fumar causa la muerte de las células y puede ser responsable por más del 50% de los casos de periodontitis del adulto. Se ha reportado que más del 85% de todos los casos periodontales están presentes en las personas que fuman. Y más del 90% de las infecciones de las encías que parecen ser resistentes al tratamiento (enfermedad de las encías refractaria) se encuentran entre los fumadores. Los fumadores tienen 2.6 a 6 veces más probabilidad de tener enfermedad periodontal. Los que han dejado de fumar tienen más probabilidad de tener enfermedad periodontal. Una persona que fuma no sanará tan bien y no responde igual de bien a la terapia periodontal que un no fumador.

Miles de químicos se liberan cuando se fuma, lo que causa un efecto profundo en el sistema inmune que es responsable de ayudarnos a rechazar las infecciones. Y como ya sabemos que la enfermedad periodontal es una infección, es fácil hacer la conexión. Muchos fumadores exhiben pocas áreas de sangrado durante el registro en la gráfica periodontal porque uno de los efectos del fumar es circulación reducida.

Si usted está leyendo esto, probablemente es un fumador que tiene enfermedad periodontal. A muchos fumadores les gustaría dejar este hábito. Dejar de fumar no es tan difícil como usted puede imaginarse. La idea de hacerlo es probablemente el aspecto más difícil. Hoy en día hay muchas ayudas para ayudarnos a tomar ese gran paso de hacer una decisión saludable sobre nuestro bienestar dental y general. Nuestra oficina puede ser una gran fuente de sugerencias para ayudarle a dejar de fumar. Si le gustaría que hiciéramos sugerencias para un estilo de vida más saludable, ¡no vacile en hacer la pregunta!

Cirugía Plástica Periodontal Electiva Cosmética: Recontorno del Tejido

No es raro que le sugiriéramos a un paciente que no tiene absolutamente ninguna señal de enfermedad periodontal (de las encías) que considere seriamente que le hagan los procedimientos periodontales electivos. En estos casos, los procedimientos casi siempre se necesitan para mejorar la apariencia. A veces se sugieren para fomentar la salud periodontal futura o para atender un problema potencial que puede desarrollarse.

Cuando usted sonríe o habla, sus dientes están enmarcados por sus labios y el tejido de las encías visible. Las personas que le miran se dan cuenta de sus dientes. Las personas notan los dientes que faltan, la alineación de los dientes, el color de las encías, las empastaduras desteñidas, las empastaduras de plata, el color de los dientes y cuánto de sus dientes realmente se ven. Si todo está bien integrado y se ve natural, las personas dicen que usted tiene una sonrisa agradable. Si algo no se ve natural, puede ser fácil definirlo, tal como los dientes virados, manchados o amarillos, enfermedad periodontal evidenciada por el tejido de la encía enrojecido o empastaduras desteñidas. Quizás puede ser algo que no se determina tan fácilmente. Sólo es algo que no se ve bien.

Ese "algo" puede estar relacionado a la arquitectura de los dientes y de la encía. La posición de las encías donde se encuentran con los dientes es importante estéticamente. Si los dientes se ven muy cortos, puede ser que les cubra más tejido de encía de lo que se considera atractivo. Usted puede enseñar demasiado tejido de encía cuando sonríe. Puede haber una diferencia en la altura de la encía de un diente versus la de un diente adyacente o su compañero en el otro lado de la boca. Esto podría ser el resultado del retiro causado por cepillarse muy fuerte; por enfermedad de las encías; por restauraciones pobres o defectuosas, especialmente las coronas o sólo por un problema con la manera que el diente hizo su erupción en el lugar. Todo esto puede detraer de su apariencia.

Varios procedimientos periodontales diferentes sencillos pueden corregir la mayoría de estos problemas rutinarios. Algunos implican el retiro del tejido indeseado; algunos implican el injerto de tejido. La ortodoncia puede ser provechosa es algunos casos. Los procedimientos más extensos requerirán co-consultas con especialistas.

En un tipo común de cirugía plástica periodontal cosmética, el tejido de las encías se reforma y recontorna sin el uso de suturas (puntos). Este procedimiento se hace en la oficina dental. Un diente o varios dientes pueden beneficiarse del tratamiento. El malestar postoperatorio es generalmente mínimo. Puede haber una sensibilidad transitoria de los dientes si se remueve algún tejido. La mejoría generada por este tipo de procedimiento puede ser asombrante.

Le mostraremos y describiremos con detalles cómo usted puede beneficiarse de los procedimientos periodontales cosméticos. En muchos casos, la cirugía periodontal cosmética completará el tratamiento que usted necesita. En algunos casos, será parte de un plan de tratamiento mayor que incluye coronas, laminados y restauraciones adheridas.

Si usted tiene cualquier pregunta sobre la cirugía plástica periodontal electiva cosmética, favor de sentirse libre de preguntarnos.

Electrocirugía

La electrocirugía dental es un procedimiento quirúrgico para eliminar el tejido periodontal o suave. Usted puede estar más familiarizado con el procedimiento quirúrgico de bisturí y sutura. La electrocirugía consigue lo mismo pero de una manera diferente. Sus condiciones y necesidades particulares determinan la selección.

La electrocirugía se usa más frecuentemente para remover o reformar cantidades pequeñas del tejido gingival (de las encías), detener el sangrado menor de los tejidos suaves (antes de hacer impresiones para coronas o colocar restauraciones), y/o exponer la estructura del diente saludable cuando hay uno de los siguientes:

- Queda insuficiente estructura clínica del diente para permitir la retención correcta de una corona.
- La estructura saludable del diente está debajo del tejido gingival.
- El tejido gingival está en una posición o contorno pobre.

Se necesita la cirugía convencional cuando se requiere la eliminación de tejido, la reposición o la modificación más extensiva.

La electrocirugía se usa regularmente en la odontología. Antes de comenzar el procedimiento se administra un anestésico local. Se dirige una corriente eléctrica calibrada al lugar a través de un equipo manual especial y una selección de puntas de formas diferentes. Se usan las formas diferentes para lograr cosas diferentes. La punta del equipo manual de electrocirugía "dibuja" una línea en el tejido suave y el tejido suave "se cae". Normalmente hay muy poco sangrado postoperatorio asociado con los procedimientos electroquirúrgicos.

Generalmente hay muy poco dolor postoperatorio asociado con el procedimiento electroquirúrgico. La mayoría de los pacientes dicen que se siente como la quemazón del queso caliente en una pizza. Normalmente cualquier aliviador de dolor sin receta es adecuado para aliviar el dolor. La incomodidad postoperatoria causada por el alargamiento quirúrgico convencional de la corona también es normalmente mínima y el tiempo de sanarse es rápido.

Al igual que todas las alteraciones del tejido suave en los procedimientos de coronas y puentes, puede haber una demora inevitable antes de que se pueda tomar la impresión final. Esto es especialmente cierto cuando las coronas que se están preparando se ven fácilmente cuando usted habla o sonríe. Aunque el tejido suave parece sanarse en más o menos una semana, el tejido seguirá cambiando de posición lentamente y sanando más completamente por hasta 8 semanas. En este momento, el diente puede necesitar una leve reformación para compensar por el cambio antes de tomar la impresión. Esto es especialmente crítico para los dientes frontales superiores. Obviamente, mientras más tejido se elimine, más largo el tiempo curación será y más probable es que se tengan que posponer los procedimientos de la impresión final. Si el procedimiento se hace en un área no cosméticamente crítica, normalmente se hace la impresión en el mismo día.

A veces los cambios necesarios del tejido suave periodontal son tan extensivos que no se pueden hacer adecuadamente con la electrocirugía ni con un procedimiento quirúrgico convencional pequeño. Si éste es el caso suyo, se le enviará a un periodontista para el procedimiento. Habrá una demora inevitable en la restauración final mientras que el tejido se sana y madura. Una espera de 4 a 12 semanas o más no es rara.

Si usted tiene cualquier pregunta sobre la electrocirugía, favor de sentirse libre de preguntarnos.

Procedimientos de Colgajo

Los procedimientos de colgajo periodontal pueden ser los más universales y más frecuentemente usados de todas las técnicas quirúrgicas periodontales. Un *colgajo* es una sección del tejido de las encías que se ha liberado de su vínculo subyacente para obtener visión y acceso directo a las estructuras periodontales que están por debajo. Estas estructuras periodontales normalmente no son accesibles al paciente ni al dentista. El largo y la forma del colgajo están relacionados a la región particular de la cirugía y a la naturaleza del tratamiento requerido. Una analogía excelente es que el procedimiento es como levantar la solapa de un sobre para mirar al contenido y luego cerrarla cuando se ha terminado.

Indicaciones

Los procedimientos de colgajo están indicados en los casos de la enfermedad periodontal con bolsillos activos o que no responden fácilmente al tratamiento y que son demasiados profundos para ser tratados con éxito con el raspado, el alisado radicular o el curetaje. Se puede levantar el colgajo para tratar un diente, un sextante (seis dientes) o un cuadrante (ocho dientes). La ventaja del procedimiento de colgajo es el tiempo de tratamiento más corto necesario debido al acceso mejorado al área afectada. Las superficies de las raíces se pueden ver directamente para una limpieza mejor y más precisa. Los bolsillos se pueden reducir selectivamente o se puede intentar la regeneración de los tejidos perdidos. Muchas veces el procedimiento de colgajo se usa estrictamente para corregir los defectos en el tejido suave. Otras veces, cuando el daño es más severo, se usa el colgajo para ganar acceso a las estructuras duras de sostén periodontal para la cirugía ósea (de hueso).

Procedimientos

Las radiografías postoperatorias, la observación clínica y el registro de información en las gráficas periodontales ayudan a planear cuáles procedimientos se requieren durante el procedimiento de colgajo. Sin embargo, ninguno de estos procedimientos provee una vista directa del lugar de tratamiento. El procedimiento de colgajo frecuentemente es hecho por un especialista periodontal (un periodontista). Aunque el periodontista pudiera tener un plan específico para tratar las áreas enfermas, cuando se levanta el colgajo se puede modificar el método de tratar su problema particular. Puede envolver procedimientos regenerativos. Se puede hacer un injerto de hueso con hueso natural o sintético. Se puede intentar la regeneración guiada de tejido (RGT). Estos procedimientos se pueden hacer por separado y en conjunto uno con el otro. Otras opciones incluyen el raspado y alisado radicular directo del cálculo (sarro) que podrían existir y la reformación de un hueso en un área especialmente difícil.

El procedimiento envuelve el uso de un anestésico local para que no haya dolor durante el tratamiento. Después de hacer el procedimiento, normalmente hay un poco de incomodidad postoperatoria. Se puede proveer un medicamento recetado para manejar esto. Es raro que surjan problemas quirúrgicos después de cerrar el colgajo. Se usarán suturas y se puede colocar un vendaje periodontal (compresa) por una semana. Después de este tiempo, se puede eliminar la compresa o reaplicarla, dependiendo de su progreso individual de curación. Los colgajos normalmente sanan rápidamente y bien. El tejido parece normal en cuatro a ocho semanas después del procedimiento. Si es indicado, más odontología (empastaduras, coronas, etc.), se puede entonces completar.

Si usted tiene cualquier pregunta sobre los procedimientos de colgajo periodontales, favor de sentirse libre de preguntarnos.

Injertos Gingivales

Es más común asociar la cirugía periodontal (de las encías) con la eliminación del tejido suave. Sin embargo, hay veces cuando es necesario usar el tejido suave para cubrir un área donde hay muy poco tejido suave. La exposición de las raíces puede ser debido al cepillado inapropiado, la enfermedad periodontal o la estructura genética. El cepillado muy fuerte y/o con un cepillo duro puede causar que el tejido gingival desaparezca. El cambio del margen gingival (el borde de las encías), y uno o más milímetros de la estructura de la raíz puede quedar expuesta. La enfermedad periodontal activa también puede causar la pérdida de este tejido suave. En cualquier caso, esto puede resultar en dientes que son muy sensibles a los cambios de temperatura, en el deterioro de las raíces o en dientes bastante antiestéticos. La línea del tejido suave desfigurado puede crear una trampa para la placa, causando más enfermedad y más problemas.

Dos métodos de resolver estos problemas son los injertos libres y adheridos. Los dos son procedimientos quirúrgicos periodontales. En los dos casos se usa un anestésico local para adormecer el lugar de tratamiento. En el caso de un injerto adherido, el tejido gingival se toma de un lugar donante y se mueve al área donde se requiere una cobertura de raíz. El tejido de injerto se sutura en su lugar, y se coloca un vendaje sobre el área tratada. El vendaje permanece en el lugar por varias semanas y luego se elimina. Un injerto adherido no se remueve por completo del lugar donante. El lugar donante está adyacente al lugar que necesita la cobertura de la raíz. Se hace una incisión en el tejido de la encía y se mueve el tejido hacia los lados, hacia arriba o abajo y se sutura en su lugar. Nuevamente se coloca un vendaje protectivo para proteger el área mientras está sanando. Cualquier incomodidad postoperatoria anticipada se resuelve con medicamento. La mayor parte de la incomodidad vendrá de lugar donante del injerto libre.

Un periodontista (especialista de encías) normalmente hace estos procedimientos, y también otros tipos de injertos y tratamientos para cubrir raíces. Después de que el periodontista examina las áreas que necesitan tratamiento, usted tendrá una mejor idea de qué consistirá el tratamiento, cómo será la apariencia, el tiempo anticipado de curación, la incomodidad postoperatoria y el costo.

La mayoría de los pacientes han escuchado que deben cuidar mejor sus dientes—cepillar los dientes y usar el hilo dental. Algunos pacientes cepillan los dientes demasiado fuerte y con un movimiento hacia delante y hacia atrás; y algunas estructuras faciales y del hueso y las fuerzas de mordida son tales que ocurre la exposición de la raíz, resultando en dientes que se ven más largos. Los procedimientos de injerto que se mencionan aquí pueden restaurar la arquitectura marginal gingival correcta, prevenir el deterioro de la raíz, reducir o eliminar la sensibilidad termal y hacer que su sonrisa se vea magnífica otra vez.

Si usted tiene cualquier pregunta sobre los injertos gingivales, favor de sentirse libre de preguntarnos.

Procedimientos de Gingivectomía y Gingivoplastia

Hay dos razones para hacer los procedimientos de gingivectomía y gingivoplastia. Una es para corregir una patología o anormalidad periodontal y la otra es para reformar el tejido de la encía alrededor de un diente o unos dientes para que se pueda hacer una restauración, normalmente una corona.

Una *gingivectomía* es la eliminación de una porción del tejido periodontal (de las encías). La *gingivoplastia* es la reformación del tejido suave. Aunque las dos obviamente envuelven la eliminación de algún tejido suave, la gingivectomía envuelve más reducción de tejido. En ambos casos, no hay alteración del hueso de sostén subyacente a los dientes. Estos procedimientos pueden considerarse la forma más sencilla de la cirugía periodontal.

La razón más frecuente para una gingivectomía es que los tejidos de las encías sigan sangrando aún después que los dientes se han limpiado y pulido minuciosamente y el cuidado oral de sí mismo es excelente. Pueden haber áreas donde es imposible que el paciente las limpie efectivamente, debido a situaciones diferentes. Por lo tanto, el tejido nunca tiene la oportunidad de curarse y la inflamación y la infección permanecen. La eliminación de algún tejido suave ayuda a reposicionar las encías para que el área se pueda limpiar correctamente regularmente. Si el bolsillo es muy profundo, las bacterias no deseables colonizarán el área y causarán que la infección periodontal persista. El remover el tejido suave adicional le permite al paciente mejor acceso para el cuidado oral de sí mismo apropiado en ese lugar.

El tejido raramente crece de nuevo, a menos que estén presentes otros factores o si no se hace el cuidado oral de sí mismo. Estos procedimientos se pueden llevar a cabo con un láser o bisturí, dependiendo de la extensión de la terapia.

Aunque consumen tiempo para hacerse, los dos procedimientos son técnicamente sencillos de hacer. La visibilidad y el acceso a los lugares quirúrgicos normalmente son muy buenos, y se pueden predecir los resultados con mucha confianza.

En resumen, se administra un anestésico local, se elimina el tejido suave específico, se colocan las suturas (los puntos) o se puede usar un vendaje quirúrgico periodontal o un vendaje oral medicado para cubrir el área tratada. El vendaje se quitará después de alrededor de 7 días. A veces el vendaje puede ser reaplicado por otra semana. Esto depende de su progreso de curación. Mientras el vendaje esté puesto, es útil enjuagarse con un enjuague oral antibacteriano y no comer en el lado que se está tratando. Las comidas duras y crujientes o la goma de mascar pueden desplazar el vendaje periodontal, así que tenga cuidado.

Si usted va a tener este procedimiento para que haya más estructura de diente disponible para una corona, la impresión para la corona se demorará por este periodo de curación de 4 a 8 semanas.

Puede haber un poca de incomodidad postoperatoria. Se le puede recetar un medicamento anti-inflamatorio o para aliviar el dolor.

El tejido periodontal es una piel muy fina de color rosa. El tejido periodontal nuevo madurará y se pondrá más fuerte y alcanzará su posición final curada alrededor del diente durante las próximas 4 a 8 semanas.

Si usted tiene cualquier pregunta sobre los procedimientos de gingivectomía y gingivoplastia, favor de sentirse libre de preguntarnos.

Desbridamiento Completo

El desbridamiento completo define la eliminación a gran escala del cálculo (sarro) y de los restos que están alrededor de los dientes y las encías para permitir una evaluación clínica adecuada de los tejidos periodontales. Para que podamos hacer una evaluación y un examen correctos de los tejidos suaves de las encías, los tejidos tienen que verse y medirse fácilmente. Si los tejidos están inflamados (infectados), hinchados, sangran fácilmente o están cubiertos con cálculo, placa o restos de comida, esto no se puede hacer.

Normalmente un higienista dental registrado hace el desbridamiento completo. El higienista limpiará, en una o más citas, una gran cantidad de los restos visibles y fácilmente accesibles por encima del borde de la encía. Hay que permitirle al tejido algún tiempo para que se sane antes de proceder con el tratamiento. Frecuentemente, hay un sangrado cuantioso alrededor de los lugares que se están limpiando. Aun una cantidad menor de sangrado puede obscurecer la visibilidad. Este desbridamiento inicial siempre es seguido de un raspado y alisado radicular.

En algún momento un higienista o asistente dental pasará tiempo demostrando la manera correcta y más eficiente de usar un cepillo de dientes y el hilo dental y cualquier otro instrumento para ayudar a evitar los problemas periodontales futuros. Le pueden pedir que usted demuestre las técnicas del cepillado y del uso del hilo dental que le han mostrado. Repasaremos estas técnicas particulares con usted en las citas futuras para asegurar que usted las hace efectivamente.

Se le puede dar una receta para un enjuague oral antimicrobiano para que lo use por un período de tiempo después del desbridamiento completo. Frecuentemente es el gluconato de clorhexidina. Este enjuague (que no es un enjuague para el mal aliento) afectará las bacterias indeseables y ayudará a los tejidos de las encías a sanar más rápido. Usted sólo necesitará usar el enjuague de gluconato de clorhexidina por un tiempo limitado. Todavía debe cepillar sus dientes y usar el hilo dental diariamente, como le han enseñado.

Generalmente no hay necesidad de un anestésico local para el desbridamiento completo. La mayoría de los pacientes reportan que es sólo un poco incómodo. El sangrado que está presente se detendrá rápidamente. De hecho, la mayoría de las personas dicen que sus encías se sienten mejor inmediatamente después de que se hace—como una picor que se ha rascado. Raramente hay dolor postoperatorio de alguna importancia. La aspirina, Tylenol® y cualquier aliviador del dolor sin receta son todos suficientemente fuertes para aliviar cualquier dolor que pueda ocurrir. Los enjuagues de agua salada tibia pueden ayudar a los tejidos a sanar y a que se sientan mejor también.

Una vez que se haya completado el desbridamiento completo, el examen puede proceder correctamente y se puede sugerir otro tratamiento potencial. Mientras siga el cuidado oral de sí mismo que hemos recomendado y usted se adhiera a sus intervalos de cuidado dental rutinario, nunca habrá que repetir el desbridamiento completo.

Si usted tiene cualquier pregunta sobre el desbridamiento completo, favor de sentirse libre de preguntarnos.

Cirugía Ósea

Indicaciones

Cuando la enfermedad periodontal (de las encías) llega a una etapa avanzada, es común que el hueso subyacente se vea envuelto. Primero, se infecta y se inflama el tejido periodontal suave. Cuando aumenta la inflamación, el hueso reacciona a la infección. El hueso se destruye y no regresa. Usted generalmente no sentirá que las encías se están infectando ni que el hueso está desapareciendo. Desgraciadamente, no hay dolor. Generalmente, cuando el dolor aparece, la condición ya es bastante seria.

Como la enfermedad periodontal es específica al lugar, la pérdida de hueso no será uniforme. Algunos dientes mostrarán poca pérdida de hueso, algunos dientes mostrarán una pérdida más seria y algunos no exhibirán ninguna pérdida. La pérdida de hueso alrededor de un diente o dientes específicos puede ser de forma regular o irregular. La pérdida puede ser vertical, horizontal o ambas. Si es irregular, se necesitará cirugía para corregir la pérdida de hueso. En este momento no es posible regenerar todo el hueso perdido. Una vez que se va, se va. Investigaciones acerca de la posibilidad de regeneración del hueso periodontal se ha estad llevando a cabo por algún tiempo. Pero en este momento, hay pocas maneras de volver a crecer el hueso periodontal de sostén una vez se ha disuelto a causa de la enfermedad periodontal.

Tratamiento

Hasta hace poco tiempo, el único método de corregir el hueso irregular era alisar los puntos altos. La nueva altura de hueso entre los dientes se igualaría al nivel de la pérdida de hueso más severa. Aunque el problema ahora estaba corregido, los otros dientes podrían perder algún hueso saludable en el proceso de nivelación. Esto podría hacer, y hace, a los dientes menos estables, una consecuencia inevitable e indeseable. En algunos casos, la naturaleza del defecto del hueso todavía dicta que se haga este procedimiento.

Un mejor acercamiento sería aumentar o construir el hueso irregular en los lugares donde se ha perdido. Esto se hace con la colocación de hueso natural o sintético en un procedimiento conocido como injerto. Se ha usado el hueso natural por más de 3 décadas sin reportes de problemas con el sistema inmune. También existen injertos óseos autólogos que usan su propio hueso. Los aloinjertos son de hueso sintético o hueso secado por congelación.

Las radiografías preoperatorias, los exámenes clínicos y el registro de la gráfxica periodontal nos darán un entendimiento del tipo de cirugía ósea que es necesario. Sin embargo se podría no descubrir la extensión completa del problema hasta exponer el área durante la cirugía. Las radiografías son una representación en dos dimensiones y en blanco y negro de un área tridimensional, de color completo. Por esta razón, las metas del tratamiento quedarán igual, pero puede modificarse el método de la cirugía. Antes del tratamiento se le hablará del pronóstico para los dientes que necesitan la cirugía, de las opciones y del mejor estimado para el progreso del tratamiento.

Para llevar a cabo la cirugía ósea periodontal, hay que levantar un colgajo. (Favor de ver la página de los **Procedimientos de Colgajo Periodontal.**) Se usa un anestésico local y se maneja la incomodidad postoperatoria con medicamento. Después de este procedimiento quirúrgico, se colocan las suturas y un vendaje periodontal.

La cirugía ósea puede ser el único tratamiento que le ayudará con éxito a retener sus dientes después que la enfermedad periodontal severa ha estado presente por algún tiempo. Generalmente la retención de sus propios dientes naturales es mejor que tener una dentadura.

Si usted tiene cualquier pregunta sobre la cirugía ósea periodontal, favor de sentirse libre de preguntarnos.

Cirugía Periodontal

La cirugía periodontal es necesaria por una variedad de razones. Se iniciará cualquier cirugía sólo después de eliminar todas las señales de infección y cuando usted está envuelto en un cuidado oral de sí mismo de alta calidad. La cirugía periodontal envuelve la reformación de los tejidos suaves (de la encía) y duros (del hueso). El tipo de cirugía periodontal más sencillo envuelve la reformación y la reposición de los tejidos suaves solamente. La cirugía puede ser necesaria para eliminar o reducir las profundidades de los bolsillos problemáticos alrededor de uno, varios o todos los dientes. Las áreas problemáticas normalmente son lugares donde usted tiene alguna dificultad en mantenerlos sin infección, placa y cálculo.

También puede ser necesario reformar los tejidos suaves para mejorar su apariencia (cirugía periodontal cosmética) o para ganar acceso para la preparación y colocación correcta de cualquier tipo de restauración. Los diferentes procedimientos quirúrgicos periodontales que no envuelven el hueso subyacente pueden incluir la corrección de un frenillo (vínculo de músculo) que está mal posicionado y el injertar tejido en un área nueva donde hay una cantidad deficiente de tejido periodontal. Estos procedimientos pueden requerir alguna sutura del tejido de la encía.

Si usted ha experimentado una descomposición periodontal más severa, su hueso puede haber sido afectado por la enfermedad periodontal y puede requerir reformación. Esta cirugía es más extensiva que la cirugía del tejido suave. Si toda su boca ha sido afectada, se puede hacer la cirugía por secciones en citas separadas. Se colocan suturas y un vendaje periodontal (un vendaje intraoral) mientras ocurre la curación. Para estos procedimientos se usa un anestésico local. La incomodidad postoperatoria se aliviará con un medicamento con o sin receta.

Resultados

Una vez que la curación ha concluido, usted se dará cuenta de varias cosas. A menos que se haya colocado un injerto o se cortó un frenillo (músculo), se habrá eliminado algún tejido suave alrededor de los dientes. Normalmente esto significa que los dientes se verán más largos—porque más de los dientes estará expuesto. Desde el punto de vista cosmético, esto podría no ser de su agrado, pero puede ser inevitable. Si usted ha experimentado pérdida de hueso, podrá ser necesario reposicionar el tejido para conseguir la distancia correcta entre el hueso y la encía. El cambio en el tejido suave puede ser poco o significativo. Antes del procedimiento periodontal, le hablaremos acerca de la apariencia esperada de los dientes después de la cirugía. También hablaremos de que si hay o no otros métodos que se pueden usar para mejorar la apariencia de sus dientes después que los tejidos han sanado. Si se le envió a un especialista periodontal para estos procedimientos, también se le explicarán los resultados esperados.

Después de la cirugía, usted puede experimentar sensibilidad aumentada a la estimulación del frío y del calor—por ejemplo, el helado y las bebidas calientes o frías. La sensibilidad puede ser leve o severa; puede ser por un tiempo breve o durar por varios meses. No hay manera de predecir cómo usted va responder. Si la sensibilidad es severa y persistente, hay varios procedimientos que se pueden hacer para reducir o eliminar el problema.

Prevención de la Recurrencia

La pregunta más frecuentemente hecha por los pacientes que necesitan cirugía para corregir el daño causado por la enfermedad periodontal es si la enfermedad puede regresar después de terminar la cirugía. La contestación es, simplemente y claramente, sí. Si las mismas circunstancias que causaron la enfermedad periodontal vuelven a ocurrir después de la cirugía, usted puede desarrollar la enfermedad de nuevo. Usted ya ha demostrado una resistencia comprometida a la enfermedad periodontal. Sin embargo, si usted hace su parte con el cepillado y el uso del hilo dental según le hemos enseñado y mantiene su horario de visitas a la oficina para la higiene dental de cuidado repetido, las probabilidades a su favor aumentan. Usted reduce la probabilidad de que volverá a desarrollar la enfermedad periodontal. Su responsabilidad es entender la naturaleza de su problema periodontal y cepillar y usar el hilo dental y las ayudas periodontales recomendadas efectivamente.

Si usted tiene cualquier pregunta sobre la cirugía periodontal, favor de sentirse libre de preguntarnos.

Profilaxis

No hay nada más importante para su salud dental que mantener una boca limpia. La prevención o la ausencia de infección optimiza nuestra salud general. Una boca limpia estará sin enfermedad, infección y problemas. Una boca limpia no tiene la predisposición para desarrollar ni el deterioro ni la enfermedad periodontal (de las encías). Una de nuestras funciones muy importantes en la odontología es enseñarle cómo mantener sus dientes y encías correctamente y remover con regularidad cualquier cosa que usted no puede remover por sí mismo.

La teoría y práctica de la odontología preventiva ha pasado por unos cambios revolucionarios en los últimos años. Ahora sabemos que las necesidades preventivas son diferentes para cada individuo. El refrán de "visite su dentista regularmente, tenga una limpieza dos veces al año" también ha cambiado.

Su Plan Personal
El intervalo de examen y cuidado repetido que le hemos recomendado para usted está diseñado para su situación única. Y esto también puede cambiar. El intervalo entre las citas para la profilaxis (limpieza) regular que es establecido para usted es una función de muchas cosas.

Estas incluyen:
- la salud general
- la destreza y la coordinación de ojo/mano
- la edad
- la dieta
- los niveles de estrés
- los hábitos orales
- la posición y la alineación de los dientes
- la cantidad, los tipos, el tamaño y la localización de las restauraciones
- los materiales restaurativos usados
- la historia periodontal
- la localización de los tejidos periodontales y de hueso

Dicho en palabras sencillas, mientras más compleja sea su situación dental y más se desvíen de lo normal la posición y alineación de sus dientes, más difícil le será mantener sus dientes limpios y sus encías saludables.

Estudios recientes han identificado muchos de los microorganismos que causan la enfermedad y el deterioro de las encías. Estos se pueden controlar con su ayuda y con la nuestra. Estos estudios también demuestran que una "limpieza" cada 6 meses puede no ser adecuado para algunos pacientes. Para prevenir la enfermedad oral destructiva, pueden ser recomendables las citas de profilaxis en los intervalos de cualquier período entre 2 meses a un año. La enfermedad periodontal (de las encías) puede ocurrir donde sea en su boca y cuandoquiera.

¡Usted no tiene que permitir que le pase esto! Estamos aquí para ser su guía a la buena salud.

Si usted tiene cualquier pregunta sobre sus intervalos de mantenimiento de cuidado oral de sí mismos, favor de sentirse libre de preguntarnos.

Aumento de Reborde

Es una desgracia que a veces hay que extraer los dientes. Después de una extracción (con la excepción de las muelas cordales), la mayoría de las personas sabiamente escogen reemplazar los dientes que faltan. Cuando es posible, los pacientes quisieran tener un reemplazo que se acerque lo más posible a la apariencia del diente original. Normalmente esto indica un puente fijo, que consistirá en coronas en los dos lados del lugar de la extracción unidas por el pontic o diente de reemplazo.

Después de remover un diente, el tejido de la encía y el hueso en el lugar de la extracción comienzan a cambiar. Primero, el hoyo creado por el diente que falta comienza a llenarse con hueso nuevo. Los cambios en el lugar ocurren rápidamente durante los primeros pocos meses y luego los cambios son más lentos. El tejido se encoge en el lugar de la extracción. Si hubo una enfermedad periodontal significante, el encogimiento será bastante notable. Si hubo necesidad de una extracción quirúrgica, si se tuvo que remover o cortar el hueso o si hubo un trauma, habrá más encogimiento del tejido. Si usted fuera a pasara un dedo a lo largo de la encía de diente en diente, su dedo se hundiría en el lugar de la extracción. La arquitectura del hueso subyacente se ha alterado y como la encía sigue al hueso, la encía también cambiará.

Para construir un puente, se preparan (taladran) los dientes a ambos lados del espacio para permitir que se fabrique en metal y porcelana un diente de la forma y el ancho correcto. Estos se llaman los *dientes de anclaje*. Se reemplaza o "tiende un puente sobre" el diente que falta con un pontic. El pontic terminará en o se apoyará sobre el área del borde residual en el espacio de la extracción. Usted puede imaginarse que si hay mucho encogimiento de tejido, puede ser que el pontic necesite ser mucho más largo de lo que debe ser y muy diferente a su reflejo de espejo en el otro lado. Cuando ha ocurrido un encogimiento extensivo, frecuentemente es imposible conseguir un resultado estético agradable con un puente nuevo sin hacer un examen cuidadoso, un diagnóstico, un plan y un procedimiento de **aumento de reborde**.

El aumento de reborde envuelve la reconstrucción del tejido encogido hasta que llegue a su altura y ancho original. El procedimiento es quirúrgico y normalmente es hecho por un periodontista (especialista de las encías). El lugar defectuoso se reconstruye a través del uso de injertos de tejido suave libres o adheridos, relleno del hueso o bombeo del área deprimida. En la mayoría de los casos esto se hace en dos o tres citas de tratamiento. El lugar se construye en exceso con tejido y se deja sanar por varias semanas. Luego se hace un procedimiento de reformación para hacer el entallado fino necesario para que parezca que el pontic está saliendo de la encía, no meramente tocándola. Normalmente haremos este procedimiento de entallado fino para maximizar la apariencia y la función del futuro puente. Hecho correctamente, una nueva forma de pontic parecerá como si nunca se hubiera perdido el diente, sino que está creciendo en la encía (una forma de pontic ovoide). Los procedimientos se hacen en la oficina bajo un anestésico local y los pacientes los toleran bien. La incomodidad postoperatoria es mínima y se trata con un medicamento sencillo de aliviar el dolor.

Hecho correctamente, el aumento de reborde puede tomar algún tiempo para completarse. El lugar original de la extracción tiene que sanarse, hay que hacer el procedimiento de aumento y el procedimiento de reformar el tejido por separado y dejarlos sanar antes de que se puedan hacer las preparaciones finales y la impresión para el puente. Aunque puede tomar meses adicionales de trabajo, el resultado valdrá la pena.

Si usted tiene cualquier pregunta sobre el aumento de reborde, favor de sentirse libre de preguntarnos.

Hemisecciones y Amputaciones Radiculares

Indicaciones

A veces, una porción de un molar (o del hueso que rodea parte de él) está dañada y sin remedio, pero la otra porción todavía está sana. Dependiendo del problema individual, puede ser posible y deseable retener la parte buena del diente y remover la porción dañada. Los molares generalmente tienen dos o tres raíces. Una de las raíces puede estar severamente deteriorada, envuelta periodontalmente (con reducción de la encía y soporte del hueso) o partida. Comúnmente, si una raíz está partida, el diente ya ha tenido terapia endodóntica (un canal radicular). Si el problema es el deterioro, puede ser que no haya un canal radicular en ese diente y necesitará que se le haga un canal radicular en las raíces que se retendrán.

Procedimiento

Una *amputación radicular* es la eliminación de parte o de toda una raíz individual. Una *hemisección radicular* es la división del diente por el medio para hacer dos raíces separadas y dos dientes separados de lo que antes era un solo diente con dos raíces unidas. El procedimiento de hemisección se hace más frecuentemente en los molares inferiores.

El procedimiento para ambas es similar. Si el diente no tuvo un canal radicular, se hará esta terapia en la raíz o las raíces que permanecerán. Se levanta un colgajo periodontal (favor de ver la hoja **Procedimientos de Colgajo** para más información). Se mira directamente al área y se remueve la sección de raíz incurable o se divide el diente. Normalmente, remover la raíz no es un procedimiento difícil.

Luego se cierra el colgajo en la manera usual y el área sana en un mínimo de 6 a 8 semanas. Cuando está suficientemente sanado, el diente restante finalmente se restaura. En casi un 100% de los casos el diente necesitará una restauración de molde. Para una resección de la raíz, en la cual el diente molar se ha dividido en dos porciones de tamaño premolar, cada raíz recibirá un poste y base y luego se juntarán con coronas con férulas. Si es necesario, a otros dientes se le pueden colocar coronas y añadirlos al molar de la hemisección para apoyo adicional. Sus necesidades individuales dictarán qué es mejor para usted.

Los aspectos críticos para el éxito de estos procedimientos son el diagnóstico y la ejecución del tratamiento. Los postes y las bases podrían ser necesarios. Frecuentemente, hay que colocar una férula entre los dientes tratados y los dientes adyacentes. Hay que reformar las raíces y las coronas de molde para que se puedan limpiar fácil y minuciosamente con un cepillo de dientes y con el hilo dental u otras herramientas para el cuidado oral de sí mismo.

En algunos casos, los procedimientos de implante han reemplazado la hemisección y amputación radicular. Sin embargo, su situación particular puede indicar que uno de éstos es mejor para usted.

Si usted tiene cualquier pregunta sobre las hemisecciones o amputaciones radiculares, favor de sentirse libre de preguntarnos.

Raspado y Alisado Radicular

El Procedimiento

El *raspado* en un procedimiento dental periodontal en el cual se remueven la placa y el cálculo del diente tanto por encima (supragingival) como por debajo (subgingival) de la encía (gingiva). El *alisado radicular* es un procedimiento en el cual se remueven las porciones enfermas o alteradas de la superficie de la raíz, del cemento y de la dentina y la superficie nueva que resulta se hace lisa y limpia. Mientras más alterada y dañada la superficie de la raíz a causa del cálculo (sarro), mayor será la necesidad para el alisado radicular.

El propósito del raspado y alisado radicular es remover todos los restos de los dientes. Hay que eliminar cualquier cosa que puede causar inflamación del tejido de las encías. La superficie de la raíz tiene que hacerse lo más lisa como sea posible. Las irregularidades en la superficie de la raíz pueden contribuir a la inflamación de las encías. Las irregularidades son lugares donde se acumulan las bacterias y la placa. La bacteria y las toxinas que se producen en la placa son sostenidas contra los dientes por el cálculo. De esta manera, se ha asociado la ocurrencia de placa y cálculo en los dientes con la enfermedad de las encías.

Dependiendo de la severidad de su problema periodontal particular, el raspado y alisado radicular puede ser el tratamiento definitivo y no se requerirá ningún procedimiento adicional. En muchos casos el raspado y el alisado radicular son sólo una parte necesaria de la terapia total. Es un procedimiento exigente. Requiere mucho más tiempo que la conocida profilaxis adulta (limpieza). Normalmente se hace en citas múltiples y se trata un cuarto, la mitad o la boca completa en cada cita. En esta oficina encontramos que la mayoría de los pacientes están más cómodos si se adormece el área a tratarse durante el procedimiento del alisado radicular con un anestésico local.

Podría ser necesario repetir el raspado y alisado radicular en el futuro. Es habitual poner al paciente en un programa de higiene de cuidado repetido cada 3 a 4 meses. La evidencia científica demuestra claramente que un intervalo de 6 meses es muy largo para los individuos que han demostrado una predisposición a la enfermedad periodontal. Nosotros conocemos su situación periodontal particular y determinaremos el intervalo apropiado para usted. A medida que cambia su situación, también pueden haber cambios en el largo de estos intervalos.

Aparte de la leve sensibilidad de los dientes después del procedimiento de raspado y alisado radicular, hay poca incomodidad postoperatoria. La sensibilidad disminuirá con el tiempo. Si le han diagnosticado con una infección periodontal severa, la sensibilidad puede permanecer por bastante tiempo y procedimientos adicionales pueden ser necesarios para eliminarla. Aunque se puede considerar que muchos procedimientos en la odontología son electivos, nosotros consideramos que el raspado y alisado radicular es necesario para su salud dental.

Prevención de la Recurrencia

Una vez que se ha completado el raspado y alisado radicular, es más importante que usted practique las técnicas de cepillar los dientes y usar el hilo dental que le enseñarán. Si le hemos recomendado cualquier ayuda periodontal adicional, usted tiene que usarlas también. Su cooperación es vital para el éxito de los procedimientos. Para permanecer sin enfermedad, usted necesitará ser constante en su régimen de cuidado oral de sí mismo.

Si usted tiene cualquier pregunta sobre el raspado y alisado radicular, favor de sentirse libre de preguntarnos.

Raspado y Alisado Radicular: Instrucciones para después del Procedimiento

❏ La profilaxis dental recién completada ha sido de naturaleza preventiva debido a su cuidado oral de sí mismo completo. Esto significa que no había evidencia de enfermedad de las encías. La profilaxis fue completada rápidamente y con el trauma mínimo para sus dientes y sus tejidos suaves. En este caso, usted debe tener incomodidad postoperatoria insignificante en su boca. Felicitaciones por un trabajo bien hecho. Siga con el buen trabajo. Preferiríamos ayudarle a prevenir la enfermedad periodontal en vez de curar los problemas que la enfermedad periodontal puede causar.

❏ Se ha completado una profilaxis terapéutica. En este caso, el tejido gingival (de las encías) mostraba señales de infección e inflamación y usted puede haber tenido una acumulación significativa de cálculo (sarro). Usted podría haber notado que sus dientes se sienten diferentes donde se removió el cálculo. Los tejidos suaves podrían estar sensibles o adoloridos por aproximadamente un día mientras comienzan a sanarse. Usted puede encontrar que el tomar un aliviador de dolor sin receta (aspirina, ibuprofeno, etc.) le ayudará durante este período de 24 horas. También puede enjuagar la boca cada pocas horas con agua salada tibia. Asegúrese de cepillar los dientes y usar hilo dental durante este período de tiempo como le han enseñado. Hágalo suavemente porque las áreas cepilladas pueden estar adoloridas, ¡pero sea minucioso! Usted no quiere que la infección periodontal comience de nuevo.

❏ Cuando usted ha tenido un raspado y alisado radicular u otros procedimientos periodontales más complejos, puede esperar que sus tejidos gingivales (de las encías) estén bastantes adoloridos. Esto es normal cuando los tejidos de las encías han estado infectados e inflamados por algún tiempo. Mientras más severamente han sido afectados, más incomodidad usted puede esperar. Este dolor debe desaparecer muy rápidamente. Usted puede enjuagarse con agua salada tibia cada pocas horas hasta que desaparezca.

❏ Usted también podrá notar que después del raspado y alisado radicular, sus dientes están sensitivos a los cambios de temperatura. Esta sensación ocurre frecuentemente cuando se han limpiado las superficies de las raíces de los dientes. La eliminación de los restos que cubrían las raíces y estaban adheridos a ellas dejan las raíces descubiertas a los estímulos de temperatura. Si el problema persiste, favor de informarnos.

❏ Cuando usted examine sus encías de cerca en un espejo, observará también que el color, la textura y la posición de sus tejidos periodontales cambiarán durante la curación. El tejido hinchado y rojo de las encías se encogerá, se pondrá más firme y regresará a un color rosa saludable. Preste atención a estas señales de mejoría bienvenidas y anímese con el proceso de curación.

❏ Por favor no olvide de cepillar los dientes, usar el hilo dental y usar otras ayudas de limpieza periodontal como le han enseñado. Es importante que usted comience a establecer de inmediato los hábitos correctos de cuidado oral de sí mismo. Si usted encuentra que las áreas recién tratadas son sensibles al cepillado y al uso del hilo dental, hágalo suavemente—**¡pero sea minucioso!** Con las técnicas correctas usted no puede dañar ni los dientes ni los tejidos gingivales.

❏ Cepille los dientes después de todas las comidas con una pasta de dientes que contiene fluoruro. Enjuague una vez al día con un enjuague oral que contiene fluoruro.

❏ Use el irrigador oral con el accesorio periodontal como le han enseñado. Llene la reserva con
❏ agua ❏ gluconato de clorhexidina 0.12% ❏ otro_____

❏ Use las ayudas de limpieza periodontal como le han enseñado.

❏ Favor de regresar en _____ semanas para una cita de _____ minutos. Durante este tiempo, se evaluarán sus tejidos periodontales para la mejoría esperada y la efectividad de su cuidado oral de sí mismo y para determinar la posible necesidad de más tratamiento periodontal. Esta cita incluirá el sondeo de los tejidos periodontales.

❏ A causa de su condición periodontal, recomendamos enfáticamente que usted regrese para su próxima cita de examen y profilaxis en _____ meses.

Si usted tiene cualquier pregunta sobre estas instrucciones, favor de sentirse libre de preguntarnos.

Raspado y Alisado Radicular: Re-evaluación

La meta del raspado y alisado radicular es remover toda la placa, las toxinas y el cálculo tanto encima como debajo del borde de la encía. Después de sanarse, los tejidos se encogerán y una reevaluación de la condición de la encía y las estructuras de apoyo revelará cualquier área que puede necesitar re-tratamiento. Sus hábitos de cuidado oral de sí mismo serán reevaluados al mismo tiempo y se harán las revisiones necesarias a nuestras recomendaciones. Puliremos sus dientes en esta cita. Como usted recordará, no pulimos sus dientes durante las citas del alisado radicular y el raspado. Aunque teóricamente se puede hacer el pulido en este momento, creemos que permitirle a los tejidos el tiempo apropiado para que sanen nos permitirá hacer la mejor reevaluación de nuestro tratamiento y recomendaciones para el cuidado oral de sí mismo. Por eso hay un período de tiempo de varias semanas entre la cita del alisado radicular y raspado y esta profilaxis y evaluación. Una vez que todos los tejidos han respondido y se cumplen con las metas del raspado y alisado radicular, se establecerá un intervalo de cuidado repetido para usted.

En la cita de cuidado repetido, una vez más evaluaremos su cuidado oral de sí mismo para determinar si necesitamos recomendar procedimientos diferentes para mantener su salud oral lo mejor que sea posible. Reexaminaremos sus tejidos periodontales para evidencia de curación volviendo a medirlas por medio de sondear las profundidades alrededor de cada diente. Se observará y tratará cualquier área de sangrado; luego se pulirán sus dientes y se aplicará un tratamiento de fluoruro tópico.

El fluoruro tópico provee una acción bacteriostática para las bacterias orales durante el tratamiento y por varias horas después. Parece ser más difícil para las bacterias que causan enfermedad de las encías multiplicarse y causar problemas cuando se usa un fluoruro tópico.

Si no se han alcanzado las metas del raspado y alisado radicular, volveremos a tratar aquellas áreas que se han reinfectado o le enviaremos a un periodontista para cirugía periodontal específica. La cirugía periodontal corregirá algunos de los defectos en el tejido suave y duro (de hueso) causados por la infección periodontal.

En este momento también podemos considerar el uso de una o más de las nuevas terapias no quirúrgicas que están disponibles para los lugares localizados que no han sanado tanto como quisiéramos. La terapia específica al lugar puede ser recomendada por primera vez o como un retratamiento. Entonces, seguiremos los resultados de cerca para determinar si es apropiada una co-consulta con un periodontista.

Una nota final sobre cuán frecuentemente usted debe conseguir que le limpien los dientes: la odontología moderna considera que un paciente que ha tenido enfermedad de las encías siempre está en proceso de recuperación, y nunca está completamente "curado". Si usted no cuida sus dientes y encías, el problema puede regresar de nuevo. Está en el mejor interés de su salud oral que usted tenga sus dientes examinados y limpiados en un intervalo de 3 a 4 meses en la mayoría de los casos, y no cada 6 meses como le han dicho por años.

Si usted tiene cualquier pregunta sobre la cita de profilaxis y reevaluación, favor de sentirse libre de preguntarnos.

Manejo del Tejido Suave

Usted ha sido diagnosticado con enfermedad periodontal. Sus problemas periodontales específicos pueden ser leves y localizados, leves y generalizados, moderados o severos. Usted puede ser un paciente nuevo o un paciente que ha estado recibiendo tratamiento por parte nuestra por algún tiempo. El tratamiento puede ser simple o bastante complejo y arduo. Si usted ha estado recibiendo cuidado de higiene regular continuo por parte nuestra, puede haber ocurrido un cambio (un empeoro) en la condición de su periodonto (las encías y la estructura de hueso de apoyo) o usted puede haber tenido bolsillos existentes que no han respondido al tratamiento convencional. Si usted es un paciente nuevo, estamos comenzando el tratamiento necesario. La infección periodontal es específica al lugar y episódica: puede ocurrir alrededor de los dientes en cualquier momento.

La terapia inicial periodontal, también conocida como el *manejo del tejido suave*, es un método agresivo y a la vez el más conservador para tratar la enfermedad periodontal (de las encías). No es cirugía periodontal. Se hace para tratar de minimizar o eliminar la necesidad para la cirugía periodontal. La terapia periodontal inicial envuelve un alisado radicular minucioso de todas las áreas afectadas. El alisado radicular está diseñado para remover las toxinas producidas por las bacterias en la placa.

Cuando se une la terapia periodontal inicial con un régimen de cuidado oral de sí mismo de cepillado, uso del hilo dental y uso de las ayudas de limpieza periodontal como le han enseñado, ¡los resultados pueden ser dramáticos! Usted lleva mucha de la responsabilidad y puede afectar el resultado del tratamiento. Las instrucciones para el cuidado oral de sí mismo necesitarán ser seguidas cuidadosamente; de lo contrario, lo que hacemos por usted en nuestra oficina se puede deshacer en casa muy fácilmente.

Le han dado otra información escrita acerca de los procedimientos que se llevarán a cabo, tales como la irrigación subgingival. Se pueden requerir otros procedimientos, pero hablaremos con usted de éstos antes de hacerlos.

Lo que la odontología cree que es cierto acerca la enfermedad periodontal es muy diferente de lo que consideraba cierto hace varios años. Ahora sabemos que la enfermedad periodontal no es causada por un solo organismo. La causa muchos organismos que pueden estar activos e inactivos durante períodos diferentes del proceso de la enfermedad. Sabemos que usted no experimentará ningunos síntomas hasta que la destrucción del hueso esté avanzada. Esta enfermedad no duele hasta que llega a las etapas avanzadas. Mientras las investigaciones continúan y la odontología aprende hechos nuevos acerca del comienzo y el progreso de la enfermedad periodontal, el tratamiento recomendado y provisto por el dentista y/o el periodontista cambiará. Usted se dará cuenta de esto especialmente si le han tratado para esta enfermedad en el pasado, aquí o en otro lugar. Nuevos descubrimientos, nuevos tratamientos y nuevos medicamentos continuarán cambiando la manera en la que tratamos este proceso de enfermedad. Algunas personas podrían todavía pensar que el procedimiento correcto para mantener la salud periodontal es tener los dientes limpiados sólo dos veces al año. Esto no ha sido el caso por los últimos 20 años. Ahora sabemos que la enfermedad periodontal es una infección que afecta alrededor de 95 de cada 100 adultos. Puede ocurrir en arranques de actividad y puede causar una pérdida profunda de hueso.

Fomentamos la salud oral en todos nuestros pacientes. Sin embargo, cada paciente es diferente. El tratamiento que usted necesita será diferente al tratamiento de otro paciente. El hecho es que nuestras metas para usted son **prevenir** tanto el deterioro de los dientes como la enfermedad periodontal.

Si usted tiene cualquier pregunta sobre la terapia periodontal inicial (manejo del tejido suave), favor de sentirse libre de preguntarnos.

Colocar Férulas en los Dientes

En su estado normal, los dientes rodeados por las estructuras de sostén saludables exhiben muy poca movilidad. *Movilidad* en este caso se define como la movilidad de los dientes. Empujar los dientes con los instrumentos dentales puede causar que el diente se desvíe de la posición "de descanso", pero este movimiento será muy poco.

Por Qué los Dientes Pueden Necesitar Férulas

Cuando el hueso de sostén está comprometido y afectado por la enfermedad periodontal, los dientes exhibirán más movilidad. Si el diente o los dientes están sujetos a un trauma, pueden aflojarse en sus alvéolos. Los hábitos de bruxismo y rechinamiento también pueden aflojar los dientes.

Los dientes que no están dañados severamente por el trauma regresarán a su estabilidad anterior. Puede ser necesario colocar férulas temporales entre los dientes aflojados o entre ellos y otros dientes no dañados.

Si la movilidad es causada por el apretar o rechinar los dientes, se puede indicar un ajuste de la mordida (oclusión) y la fabricación de un aparato anti-rechinar/anti-bruxismo. En este caso, no se requería colocar férulas en los dientes.

La razón más común para colocar férulas en los dientes es la movilidad causada por la enfermedad periodontal. Los dientes exhiben más movimiento cuando su sostén de hueso disminuye. Los dientes de múltiples raíces (molares) normalmente exhiben menos movilidad que los dientes de una sola raíz con la misma cantidad de pérdida de hueso. Pero la necesidad de tratamiento es de igual importancia. Mientras más móviles sean los dientes, más daño ha ocurrido y más férulas se necesitarán.

El Procedimiento de Colocar Férulas

El primer paso en la eliminación de la movilidad de un diente es comenzar a corregir el problema periodontal. Si los dientes se mueven, el problema periodontal probablemente está avanzado y las medidas correctivas podrían ser complejas y consumir tiempo. Se pueden colocar férulas de inmediato. Esto envuelve el unir los dientes móviles, y quizás los no-móviles, con alambre, acrílico o combinación ambos. El unir los dientes les da más solidez. El uso de férulas puede considerarse temporal o final, dependiendo de su situación particular. Las férulas tienen una expectativa de vida limitada y tienen que arreglarse o reemplazarse periódicamente. Normalmente hay un honorario aparte asociado con estos procedimientos. Se le informará de lo que su condición particular requiere para la terapia a corto y largo plazo.

Una forma más extensiva envuelve el juntar los dientes con restauraciones de molde cementadas—las coronas, los puentes, los retenedores de metal fundido, etc. Este tipo de férula durará más tiempo y es más costosa. El propósito es idéntico al propósito de colocar férulas externas—juntar y atar los dientes móviles para que se fortalezcan y se muevan menos.

Los dientes que tienen férulas requerirán un cepillado y uso del hilo dental más complejos por su parte. Le demostremos estos procedimientos.

Honorarios

Los costos de los procedimientos de colocar férulas varían mucho. Esto dependerá de la cantidad de dientes que recibirán férulas, la severidad de la movilidad, el pronóstico de los dientes y el tipo de férula escogida.

Si usted tiene cualquier pregunta sobre el colocar férulas en los dientes, favor de sentirse libre de preguntarnos.

Ilustración en CD-ROM

Enjuague Oral de Gluconato de Clorhexidina 0.12%

El enjuague oral de gluconato de clorhexidina 0.12 % provee beneficios antimicrobianos a largo plazo. Es efectivo en reducir el enrojecimiento, la hinchazón y el sangrado de los tejidos de las encías, los cuales están presentes en la gingivitis y la periodontitis. No es una cura para la enfermedad periodontal y no se debe considerar como un tratamiento mayor para este tipo de infección. El uso de este enjuague por hasta 6 meses no parece causar ningunos cambios significativos en la resistencia bacterial o el crecimiento excesivo de las bacterias oportunistas ni otros organismos. No parece causar ningunos cambios adversos en el sistema microbiano normal que existe en la boca.

La dosis normal es $\frac{1}{2}$ onza fluida por uso. (Use la taza de medir provista o vea las marcas dentro de la tapa.)

Use durante la Terapia Periodontal
Si usted está actualmente recibiendo terapia periodontal, enjuague como le hemos enseñado. Enjuague dos veces al día, por 30 segundos cada vez, por la mañana y por la noche después de cepillar los dientes y usar el hilo dental. No coma, ni beba ni enjuague con agua por 30 minutos después de enjuagarse. Siga esta rutina hasta que se hayan completado todas las fases de su terapia periodontal. Si le instruyen a hacerlo, usted puede usar este enjuague en su irrigador oral (por ejemplo, WaterPik) también.

Use durante los Procedimientos de Corona y Puente
Si usted va a tener un procedimiento de corona, inlay, onlay o puente, favor de enjuagarse con el gluconato de clorhexidina 0.12% por dos (2) semanas antes de la cita de la preparación del diente hasta dos (2) semanas después de que se haya cementado o adherido la restauración en su lugar. Las investigaciones dentales han demostrado que el uso de este enjuague ayudará a que el tejido de las encías se ponga más ajustado y saludable. La cita de preparación e impresión será más fácil y más rápida y con menos sangrado. El tejido también se normaliza más rápido después de estos procedimientos. Para este uso, enjuáguese sólo una vez al día, antes de acostarse.

Precauciones
El uso de este enjuague puede causar manchas en los dientes, en la lengua y en algunos tipos de restauraciones. Las manchas se pueden remover con una limpieza profesional. Si usted cepilla sus dientes y usa el hilo dental minuciosamente, esto será menos problemático. Algunos pacientes pueden notar un leve cambio en la sensibilidad del gusto cuando usan el enjuague. Esta alteración del gusto se normalizará después de dejar de usar el enjuague.

No use este producto si están embarazada (o está intentando concebir). Este producto no se ha probado para el uso en niños menores de 18 años.

Si usted tiene cualquier pregunta sobre el uso de este enjuague, favor de preguntarnos.

Protocolo de Enjuague Oral

El estándar de cuidado recomendado para el tratamiento de la enfermedad periodontal moderada a severa es el uso selectivo de los procedimientos quirúrgicos periodontales. Estos procedimientos pueden envolver la eliminación de algunos tejidos de hueso y de las encías o el aumento de los tejidos de hueso y de las encías. Estas técnicas han demostrado un nivel previsible de éxito por muchos años. Usted ha sido diagnosticado con enfermedad periodontal y le han aconsejado tener uno de estos tratamientos periodontales estándares. Por cualquier variedad de razones(de edad, financiera, de salud, emocional, de tiempo, etc.), usted pudo haber rechazado esta recomendación. Sin embargo usted desea intentar retener sus dientes lo más tiempo posible. Lo siguiente describirá una técnica no quirúrgica basada en investigación respetada y de largo tiempo. Esto no es un sustituto para la cirugía periodontal. Es otra modalidad que podemos usar en el tratamiento de la enfermedad periodontal.

Si usted ha decidido que quiere rechazar la cirugía periodontal en este momento, sugerimos la siguiente rutina de mantenimiento en un esfuerzo para retener los dientes que tienen enfermedad periodontal. Los resultados pueden variar de paciente a paciente. Entienda también que usted puede tener algunos dientes con un pronóstico dudoso o incurable. Eventualmente estos dientes pueden necesitar removerse. Le dejaremos saber cuáles dientes pueden permanecer y cuáles se deben remover. Recuerde, si usted tiene una infección periodontal, hay una infección en su cuerpo por las 24 horas de cada día. Su sistema inmune tiene que combatirla por 24 horas al día, todos los días. Esto no es bueno para su salud general.

Protocolo
Inicial:
- ❏ Raspado/alisado radicular y irrigación subgingival donde sea indicado.
- ❏ Profilaxis de adulto.

Mantenimiento:
- ❏ Tratamiento profesional periódico: cada _____ meses.
- ❏ Profilaxis de adulto.
- ❏ Irrigación subgingival con cuatro enjuagues orales alternados.

Cuidado oral de sí mismo:
- ❏ Cepillar los dientes y usar el hilo dental diariamente como le han enseñado.
- ❏ Use los enjuagues recetados alternados una vez diaria.
- ❏ Cada ____ meses; después de la profilaxis de adulto en nuestra oficina dental, le aconsejaremos que cambie al próximo enjuague oral en el régimen (el mismo que se usa para la irrigación subgingival).
- ❏ Si usted tiene un irrigador intraoral (tal como un WaterPik) y los aditamentos apropiados, también puede usar la solución del enjuague oral para la irrigación subgingival diaria.

Los enjuagues orales recetados serán el gluconato de clorhexidina, los compuestos de fenol con aceites esenciales, el dióxido de cloro y el fluoruro estañoso. Le aconsejaremos cuándo debe cambiar a la próxima solución a base del progreso (o retroceso) de su enfermedad.

Si usted tiene cualquier pregunta sobre el protocolo de enjuague oral, favor de sentirse libre de preguntarnos.

Periostat: Dosis Submicrobiana Sistémica de Doxiciclina

Usted ha sido diagnosticado con enfermedad periodontal. Hasta ahora, el tratamiento para la periodontitis ha incluido la limpieza de los restos del área (la placa, el cálculo, etc.), las instrucciones para el cuidado oral de sí mismo apropiado, y donde sea necesario, la corrección de los defectos causados por la enfermedad.

En la década del 1980 se descubrió que el antibiótico de tetraciclina usado en dosis pequeñas diarias es útil para inhibir la destructividad de las enzimas que causan la descomposición del tejido que es resultado de las enfermedades periodontales.

PERIOSTAT es una doxiciclina (20 mg, dos veces diarias sistemáticamente) que se usa para reducir el número de enzimas destructivas. Los efectos secundarios son mínimos. No se puede dar a las personas que son alérgicas a la tetraciclina. Se ha demostrado que mejora la adhesión de las fibras a los dientes y reduce la profundidad de los bolsillos. No se debe considerar una cura para la enfermedad. Es un procedimiento adjunto al raspado y alisado radicular. Se administra al tomarla oralmente dos veces al día por un mínimo de 3 meses a 9 meses. Favor de tomar esta receta como le han enseñado: no salte ni un día. Investigaciones han demostrado que el uso de este medicamento junto con el tratamiento del raspado y alisado radicular tiene un efecto más positivo que cuando se hace sólo el alisado radicular y raspado.

Este medicamento trabaja más efectivamente en los dientes afectados con la enfermedad severa que en los lugares enfermos moderadamente. El uso de este medicamento como le han enseñado puede reducir o eliminar la necesidad de ciertos procedimientos quirúrgicos periodontales, o por lo menos "detener" el proceso destructivo por un tiempo limitado hasta que se puede hacer la cirugía correctiva y definitiva.

PERIOSTAT es una modalidad nueva, no quirúrgica o prequirúrgica, que ayuda en el manejo a largo plazo de la enfermedad periodontal adulta. Usted se puede beneficiar de esta receta si se usa en conjunto con el alisado radicular y raspado. No es "una bala mágica" que curará su enfermedad periodontal para siempre: no reemplaza su cepillado y uso del hilo dental diarios y usted tiene que tomarlo dos veces al día.

Si usted tiene cualquier pregunta sobre el Periostat, favor de sentirse libre de preguntarnos.

Terapia Antibiótica Específica al Lugar

Las bacterias orales son un factor principal en la enfermedad periodontal (de las encías). La enfermedad de las encías es una infección alrededor de uno o varios dientes y frecuentemente no hay síntomas. Usted puede enterarse que tiene enfermedad periodontal cuando le limpian sus dientes y registran información en la gráfica periodontal.

Por muchos años, los médicos han usado los antibióticos para tratar las infecciones en otras áreas de nuestros cuerpos. Ahora tenemos la habilidad de tratar las áreas infectadas individuales en nuestras bocas con un antibiótico específico al lugar. No hay que tomarlo oralmente y esperar que la corriente sanguínea lo lleve a través de todo el cuerpo. Hay varios tipos de medicamentos que se pueden colocar directamente en el lugar de la infección. Se puede colocar el material precisamente donde se necesite, por lo tanto sólo hay que administrar una cantidad pequeña del medicamento.

Generalmente se usa un antibiótico específico al lugar cuando un bolsillo tiene 5 mm o más de profundidad o donde se han hecho otros tratamientos que tuvieron éxito en mantener la infección bajo control. Es un tratamiento muy conservador y no es un procedimiento quirúrgico.

El Procedimiento

Generalmente el primer paso es una limpieza minuciosa.

Se coloca el material antibiótico escogido en el lugar afectado. Se pueden tratar múltiples lugares a la misma vez. Usted no debe cepillar los dientes ni usar el hilo dental en el área donde se ha colocado el material por algunos días como le han enseñado. Usted puede no darse cuenta de una mejoría inmediata en el área. El proceso de la curación puede tomar varios meses, durante los cuales podrá ser necesario repetir la colocación del medicamento. Esto no es raro. Durante cada cita de cuidado repetido de higiene dental, evaluaremos su condición periodontal total.

Éstas son varias de las terapias periodontales específicas al lugar que han evolucionado a través del tiempo. Aunque hace años que la industria de seguros dentales y la Asociación Dental Americana se pusieron de acuerdo en asignar un código de procedimiento para la terapia antibiótica específica al lugar, todavía podría no ser un beneficio pagable con su plan de seguro dental particular. No deje que la posible cobertura de seguros (o la falta de cobertura) dicte su tratamiento recomendado.

Seleccionaremos la forma de la terapia antibiótica específica al lugar que sea más apropiada para su condición periodontal.

❑ Atridox—Se coloca un gel de hiclato de doxiciclina directamente en el bolsillo enfermo, donde se disolverá en 7–10 días.
❑ Arestin—Se coloca un polvo de hiclato de minociclina directamente en el bolsillo enfermo, donde se disolverá en 7–10 días.
❑ Periochip—Se coloca un disco de gelatina de gluconato de clorhexidina en el bolsillo enfermo, donde se disolverá en 7–10 días.
❑ Otro_____.

Usted no debe cepillar los dientes ni usar hilo dental en esta área por _____ días. Evite masticar vigorosamente en el área tratada. Necesitará regresar a nuestra oficina en _____ días para una evaluación de este lugar.

Hasta que la terapia antibiótica específica al lugar se hizo disponible, una limpieza regular y minuciosa y el cuidado oral de sí mismo excelente eran las únicas opciones para algunas áreas difíciles en su boca. Ahora podemos ofrecerle una opción de tratamiento para las áreas que son difíciles de tratar.

Las otra opción que usted tiene es el no tratar el problema o una co-consulta con un periodontista para la posible corrección quirúrgica. El tratamiento específico al lugar es un método mucho más conservador que la cirugía. El tratamiento específico al lugar tiene el potencial de reducir o eliminar los procedimientos quirúrgicos correctivos.

Si usted tiene cualquier pregunta la terapia antibiótica específica al lugar, favor de sentirse libre de preguntarnos.

Irrigación Subgingival

La irrigación subgingival (enjuague) de los tejidos periodontales es un tratamiento adicional no quirúrgico para la enfermedad periodontal (de las encías).

En una boca saludable hay una grieta o espacio como una zanja alrededor de cada diente que se llama un *surco*. Tenemos un instrumento llamado una *sonda periodontal* para medir este espacio del surco cuidadosamente. El surco debe medir entre 1 y 3 milímetros, y no debe haber sangrado ni dolor mientras se hace el examen con la sonda. El tejido de las encías debe estar bien adherido al hueso que rodea de cada diente. Cuando el tejido de la encía está infectado y la enfermedad periodontal está presente, los tejidos se ponen rojos e hinchados. Cuando el surco mide más de 3 milímetros, es difícil, si no imposible, mantener los niveles de bacterias bajo control con el cuidado oral de sí mismo normal.

La irrigación subgingival puede ayudar a remover los restos, las bacterias y las toxinas que no se pueden remover rutinariamente con el cuidado oral de sí mismo normal. Un chorro de fluido bajo un poco de presión se dirige al lugar (o a los lugares) apropiado(s) debajo del tejido de la encía. El área se lava con el chorro. Normalmente se hace la irrigación en la oficina con un antimicrobiano que tiene un efecto positivo sustancial: las moléculas del antimicrobiano se afierran a sus dientes y sus tejidos y sigue trabajando por horas después de terminar la irrigación subgingival. También se puede usar agua u otros químicos. Si le dicen que la irrigación subgingival debe ser parte de su rutina diaria de cuidado oral de sí mismo, se le instruirá en cuanto a la solución correcta que debe usar.

Si se hace la irrigación subgingival correctamente, usted puede remover del surco un alto porcentaje de las bacterias y toxinas problemáticas que no se pueden alcanzar con los esfuerzos normales de cuidado. El área enjuagada y afectada debe mostrar un nivel reducido de bacterias. Puede tomar algún tiempo para que las bacterias y los restos se acumulen al nivel en que puedan causar problemas adicionales o continuados.

La irrigación subgingival no es un sustituto para el cuidado oral de sí mismo excelente ni para la cirugía periodontal, sino que es otra modalidad que podemos usar en el tratamiento o en la prevención de la enfermedad periodontal. Si usted está bajo la terapia periodontal inicial activa, la irrigación subgingival será parte de su tratamiento. Si está en mantenimiento, puede ser parte del tratamiento rutinario que se le hace cuando viene para su cita de cuidado repetido. Si le recomendamos que haga este procedimiento diariamente como parte de su cuidado oral de sí mismo normal, recibirá instrucciones adicionales.

Si usted tiene cualquier pregunta sobre la irrigación subgingival, favor de sentirse libre de preguntarnos.

Prostodoncia

Revisión del Contenido: Prostodoncia

Reemplazo de Dientes Que Faltan
Detalla los efectos adversos de no reemplazar los dientes que faltan lo antes posible.

Implantes, Coronas y Puentes versus Dientes Naturales
A la vez que sugiere fuertemente que los dientes naturales son la mejor selección, este documento describe las posibilidades de restauraciones con coronas, puentes y coronas de implante de apariencia natural.

Restauraciones Fijas
Coronas
Coronas: Una Visión General
Da una visión general de los procedimientos y el mantenimiento de los prostéticos fijos.

Diseño de Coronas
Explica el diseño y la construcción de las coronas y las posibilidades de cobertura por el seguro. Incluye una lista de verificación para las preferencias del paciente y los honorarios envueltos con cada una.

Coronas y Puentes: Una Visión General del Procedimientos
Provee al paciente una visión general de la técnica de coronas y puentes incluyendo las impresiones y los provisionales.

Honorarios por Coronas y Puentes
Elimina la confusión sobre los honorarios por las coronas y los puentes. Presenta una lista de verificación de lo que cubre el honorario por la corona o el puente y también de los procedimientos que, aunque necesarios, requerirán honorarios adicionales.

Instrucciones Preoperatorias para Coronas y Puentes
Examina los hábitos saludables que se deben seguir antes de las citas para las coronas y los puentes.

Opciones de Materiales
Opciones de Materiales: Una Visión General
Ventajas y desventajas de los materiales que se usan comúnmente en las restauraciones de coronas y puentes.

Restauraciones de Molde de Oro
Describe cuándo y por qué se usan estas restauraciones.

Restauraciones de Molde de Oro y Cerámica
Examina las ventajas y las restauraciones de molde de oro y de cerámica.

Restauraciones de Molde de Porcelana Unida a Metal
Examina las ventajas de las restauraciones de molde de porcelana unida a metal.

Restauraciones Completas de Porcelana/Cerámica
Examina las ventajas de las restauraciones de porcelana completa y cerámica completa.

Puentes
Puentes: Una Visión General
Explica los beneficios de reemplazar los dientes que faltan con puentes.

Puentes Completos de Cerámica y Porcelana
Describe las ventajas de los puentes completos de cerámica/ porcelana.

Puente de Maryland (Retenedor de Resina Adherida)
Una descripción de una alternativa al puente de dos anclajes.

Pontic Ovalado
Describe los beneficios en la estética del pontic ovalado.

Puentes Unidos de Cobertura Parcial
Explica la aplicación de puentes de cobertura parcial para conservar la estructura dental.

Revisión del Contenido: Prostodoncia—continuación

Implantes

Implantes: Opciones
Da una visión general de los implantes, el procedimiento, la información sobre el éxito y las alternativas.

Implantes: Una Visión General del Procedimiento
Una explicación detallada de las tres fases en el procedimiento de implantes dentales.

Procedimientos y Aplicaciones

Ancho Biológico
Define el ancho biológico y su importancia en las prostéticas.

Cementación: Instrucciones Postoperatorias
Una explicación de lo que puede esperar un paciente después de la cementación de su nueva restauración.

Procedimientos de Alargamiento de la Corona
Una explicación de por qué se necesita una estructura dental suficiente y del procedimiento.

Defecto en el Lugar de Extracción
Detalla por qué se debe resolver este problema antes de restaurar con un puente.

Estructura Coronaria Remanente (Abrazadera)
Describe una estructura coronaria remanente (abrazadera) y su importancia para la longevidad de la restauración.

Impresiones
Describe las impresiones, su uso y los procedimientos para tomar impresiones.

Postes
Da una descripción detallada de la composición, el uso y la ubicación de un poste.

Postes, Construcciones de Base-Corona y Alargamiento de la Corona
Informa al paciente sobre el uso de los postes y las construcciones de base-corona, con una información breve sobre la electrocirugía.

Coronas Provisionales
Explora las razones detrás del uso de las coronas provisionales.

Coronas Provisionales: Instrucciones Postoperatorias
Instrucciones para el paciente para prolongar la vida y la función de los provisionales.

Modelos de Estudio y Modelos de Cera
Explica el uso de los modelos diagnósticos de estudio y los modelos de cera en el desarrollo de los planes de tratamiento. Este mismo documento también aparece en la sección de "Odontología General".

Prostodoncia Removible

Dentaduras Completas
Explica cómo las dentaduras se hacen a la medida y se ajustan para los individuos. Motiva a los pacientes a retener sus dientes naturales donde sea posible, presentando las dentaduras completas como la última elección.

Dentaduras Inmediatas
Explica el rol de las dentaduras inmediatas en la extracción de los dientes y en los procedimientos de dentaduras.

Dentaduras Parciales
Describe la apariencia, la fabricación y la función de una dentadura parcial.

Reemplazo de Dientes Que Faltan

La mayoría de los adultos pueden esperar tener 32 dientes. Frecuentemente se extraen los cuatro terceros molares, o muelas cordales, porque no crecen bien en la boca o no hay suficiente espacio para que se queden en una alineación correcta. Es muy raro reemplazar las muelas cordales. Pero los otros 28 dientes son necesarios. Su boca, mandíbula y cuerpo se desarrollaron juntos a través de millones de años. Están diseñados para operar juntos con la máxima eficiencia. Cuando usted pierde un diente, la eficiencia disminuye y la función sufre. Cuando usted pierde un diente, pierde alguna habilidad de masticar la comida correctamente. Esto significa que usted pone más estrés sobre los otros dientes para masticar toda la comida que come o no mastica suficientemente bien y lo que traga no está totalmente listo para digerirse. Esto puede conducir a dificultades digestivas. O usted podría cambiar a una dieta que consiste de comidas más blandas que no hay que masticar tanto. Podría ser que usted tenga que eliminar ciertas comidas favoritas porque no las puede masticar bien. Por cada diente que falta, usted pierde aproximadamente el 10% de su capacidad restante de masticar la comida.

También ocurren otros problemas. Los dientes adyacentes al espacio dejado por el diente que falta eventualmente se moverán. Si, por ejemplo, se extrae un diente inferior, el diente contrario en la mandíbula superior se alargará lentamente (o a veces rápidamente) hacia abajo hacia el espacio del diente que falta. Esto se llama *extrusión* o *sobreerupción*. Los dientes a cada lado del diente que falta se moverán y se inclinarán fuera de su eje vertical correcto y se desplazarán hacia el espacio del diente que falta. Esto puede hacer a estos dientes más propensos al deterioro y a la enfermedad de las encías porque es mucho más difícil mantener limpios los dientes que no están bien alineados. Se puede exponer la estructura de la raíz que normalmente está cubierta por la encía y el hueso. Todo esto puede ocurrir si se pierde un diente. Otros problemas graves pueden ocurrir si se pierden múltiples dientes. Hay una pérdida del largo del arco, que es la distancia desde la parte de atrás del último diente en un lado de su boca hasta la parte de atrás del último diente en el otro lado de su boca. Con el colapso de la mordida y la pérdida de dimensión vertical, la distancia desde su mentón hasta la punta de su nariz disminuye, haciendo su cara más corta. La extrusión y el movimiento del hueso alveolar maxilar (superior) hasta que el tejido de la encía de la mandíbula superior puede tocar los dientes o el tejido de la encía de la otra mandíbula causa la pérdida del tono y forma facial. Los músculos faciales de los cachetes y la boca se hunden en el lugar desdentado (de extracción). También pueden haber problemas cosméticos severos cuando el espacio del diente extraído es -visible cuando usted habla o sonríe. Esto no es una visión atractiva para nadie. Hay una pérdida de imagen de sí mismo y de autoestima y un sentimiento que está envejeciendo. Una vez que usted comienza a perder los dientes, de veras puede comenzar a verse viejo. La pérdida de un diente es bastante seria. Cuanto más tiempo usted espera después de la extracción del diente, más difícil y más costoso podría ser para hacer el reemplazo que necesita. Con muy pocas excepciones, es mejor reemplazar los dientes que faltan lo antes posible. La evolución le diseñó para masticar su comida con 28 dientes.

Hablaremos con usted del tipo de reemplazo que sería mejor para usted. Usted puede escoger no hacer nada y quedarse con el espacio o los espacios, pero como usted se puede dar cuenta, normalmente no se recomienda esto. Usted puede conseguir que le hagan un reemplazo fijo que podría ser un implante, un puente convencional (coronas/caperuzas), un puente de resina adherida o una combinación de implantes y puentes. También podría conseguir que le hagan una dentadura parcial removible. Las ventajas de los reemplazos fijos son que no están diseñados para salir de su boca en ningún momento, es más fácil vivir con ellos, se sienten más como los dientes originales y quizás son más cosméticos que las dentaduras removibles. Una dentadura parcial removible se mantiene en su lugar con unas grapas que pueden ser visibles. Es más voluminosa y puede interferir con su manera de hablar por un período de tiempo. Sin embargo, las dentaduras generalmente cuestan menos que un reemplazo fijo.

Su aparato de masticar, las mandíbulas y los dientes evolucionaron para funcionar de un modo particular. La interacción es compleja y maravillosa. La pérdida de los dientes degrada esta función. Conserve su salud. Reemplace los dientes que faltan tan pronto que le sugieran que lo haga.

Si usted tiene cualquier pregunta sobre el reemplazo de los dientes que faltan, favor de sentirse libre de preguntarnos.

Implantes, Coronas y Puentes versus Dientes Naturales

Nada puede reemplazar los dientes naturales con los que usted nació para el masticar y el funcionamiento. Sin embargo, muy pocas personas pasan por la vida sin tener empastaduras en los dientes, coronas (caperuzas) o puentes e implantes para reemplazar los dientes que faltan. Las coronas, los puentes y los implantes son la mejor respuesta y lo más cercano a sus dientes naturales, pero no son iguales a los dientes naturales saludables.

Coronas

Se usan las coronas para reconstruir un solo diente descompuesto por el deterioro dental. Las coronas se hacen de materiales de cerámica, resina, porcelana, porcelana con metal o resina con metal. Éstas se adhieren o cementan al diente preparado y no se puede remover del diente fácilmente una vez que están puestas. Si el diente estaba bien alineado antes de preparar la corona, la corona estará bien alineada. Si el diente estaba mal alineado antes de la corona, a veces se puede formar la corona para obtener la forma y posición más ideal. Se limpia y se usa el hilo dental igual como si fuera un diente natural y se parece más a los dientes naturales.

Puentes

Los puentes consisten de las coronas ligadas, que suspenden la porción de la corona de un diente falso en o sobre el espacio dejado por el diente que falta. Se puede usar un puente para reemplazar uno o varios dientes. A veces se usa un puente como una férula para unir dientes flojos para hacerlos más estables. Normalmente se hacen los puentes de metal cubiertos con porcelana o resina. Algunos de los puentes nuevos están hechos totalmente de materiales de resina o totalmente de materiales de cerámica. Se cementan o se adhieren a los dientes existentes preparados y no se remueven fácilmente una vez que están puestos. Los dientes del puente se pueden cepillar igual a los dientes naturales, pero como están ligados, hay que usar el hilo dental de una manera diferente a través de un enhebrador u otro aparato.

Generalmente los dientes tienen la misma forma de los dientes naturales. Sin embargo, si los dientes existentes (los anclajes) que se usan para sujetar el puente se han movido de su posición original porque ha faltado un diente o unos dientes por varios años, el diente añadido (el pontic) puede ser más largo o más corto que el diente que está reemplazando. Con un puente, el diente falso normalmente colindará con el reborde de tejido suave donde estaba el diente extirpado.

La forma del lado lingual del diente falso varía. Normalmente el lado lingual es más pequeño y llena el espacio completamente. La comida tendrá una mayor tendencia de acumularse en esta área, por eso usted debe estar preparado para limpiarlo. Si el diente que falta ha faltado por mucho tiempo, el reborde puede haberse encogido bastante y el pontic será más largo que los dientes a cada lado. Si éste es el caso, hay varios procedimientos periodontales que se pueden hacer antes de la construcción del puente. Estos procedimientos reconstruirán el tejido hasta que alcance su altura anterior. Mientras más su boca haya cambiado de su estado normal, más difícil es conseguir que los dientes nuevos se vean y se sientan naturales.

Coronas de Implante

Las coronas de implante se usan para reemplazar uno o múltiples dientes que faltan. Éstas se cementen o se atornillan a un aparato de implante. Las coronas están hechas de porcelana o resina y metal. Sin embargo, tienen unas diferencias importantes de los dientes naturales que reemplazan. Los dientes están sostenidos por una raíz o por unas raíces que son de forma irregular. Los implantes son redondos. El corte transversal del implante nunca será igual al del diente que reemplaza. Un diente de múltiples raíces puede ser reemplazado por un solo implante, así que la manera en la cual una corona de implante sale del reborde del tejido suave se verá diferente a la de un diente natural. Habrá más espacio entre la raíz del implante y los dientes adyacentes. Frecuentemente se cementan las coronas de los implantes con un cemento provisional. Esto permite que el dentista pueda sacar la corona fácilmente y evaluar cómo está el implante. Normalmente se cementan las coronas en los dientes con un cemento final. Las coronas sostenidas por implantes son maravillosas, pero no son iguales a los dientes naturales con coronas. Prepárese para algunas diferencias. Esperé más mantenimiento por parte suya y en la oficina dental al tener coronas, puentes e implantes.

☞ *Fumadores tomen nota:* Hay un riesgo aumentado de fracaso de implante dental entre los fumadores—¡una razón de fracaso hasta 20% más alta!

Si usted tiene cualquier pregunta sobre los implantes, las coronas y los puentes versus los dientes naturales, favor de sentirse libre de preguntarnos.

Ilustración en CD-ROM

Coronas: Una Visión General

Normalmente hay tres razones para colocar las coronas (caperuzas) y los puentes.

La primera razón es que un diente está tan dañado por el deterioro o con tanta restauración de empastaduras que sólo se puede salvar con una restauración de molde.

La segunda razón es que se ha tratado un diente endodónticamente (tratamiento del canal radicular). Estos dientes casi siempre se restauran con una restauración de molde porque han perdido mucha estructura dental debido a la fractura, el deterioro o el proceso de taladrado. Estos dientes están propensos a fracturarse bajo las fuerzas de masticar normales y livianas.

La tercera razón por la cual se puede necesitar colocar una corona es que se necesita usar el diente como un pilar (anclaje) para un puente que reemplazará dientes que faltan.

El procedimiento envuelve:

❏ reparar (taladrar) el diente en el modo apropiado para el tipo de corona escogida.

❏ acer las impresiones del diente preparado, los dientes contrarios y las relaciones oclusales (de mordida).

❏ eleccionar un tono para las coronas del color del diente.

❏ abricar una restauración provisional que quedará en el lugar mientras se construye la corona.

❏ ementar o adherir la corona en su posición. Si el trabajo que se hará es extensivo, también podrán haber varias citas necesarias para el posicionamiento preliminar (prueba) de las coronas o de los moldes.

Las coronas se hacen de muchas clases de materiales. Hemos preparado una información escrita que describe las ventajas y desventajas de cada uno. Si usted no ha visto esta información, favor de pedirla. Si usted sabe que tiene alguna sensibilidad a los metales, favor de informarnos antes del tratamiento. Si prefiriese que no se use ningún metal en la construcción de las coronas, favor de informarnos. Discutiremos sus opciones antes de la preparación del diente (o de los dientes).

Para el éxito máximo de la(s) corona(s) es importante que usted entienda y pueda hacer la eliminación minuciosa de la placa. Usted debe comenzar a seguir de inmediato las instrucciones del cuidado oral de sí mismo que le han dado. Esto hará el procedimiento más cómodo y eficiente, y los resultados de la restauración se verán mejores. No se pueden tomar las impresiones finales hasta que el tejido de las encías esté saludable. Su cooperación es apreciada y necesaria.

Mantenimiento de Sus Prótesis Fijas

Al igual que con sus dientes naturales y especialmente con los dientes restaurados con cualquier material dental, usted debe evitar masticar comidas excesivamente duras o pegajosas después de que se cementen las coronas. Es especialmente importante no morder las comidas duras con fuerza con sólo un diente. Los materiales de porcelana se pueden fracturar de la subestructura de metal bajo fuerzas extremas. ¡Cualquier cosa que usted mastique que pueda fracturar un diente natural puede fracturar una corona!

Asegúrese de cepillar los dientes y usar el hilo dental diariamente como le han enseñado. También aconsejamos el uso de un enjuague bucal de fluoruro como parte de su rutina diaria. Favor de regresar para sus citas regulares de exámenes y de profilaxis (limpieza) en los intervalos de tiempo que sugerimos.

Después de observar estos tipos de procedimientos por muchos años, notamos que la gingiva (las encías) puede retirarse de los márgenes de las coronas y la estructura que rodea el diente puede hacerse visible. Este retiro normalmente ocurre durante un período de varios años y puede requerir el reemplazo de las restauraciones o un procedimiento de cirugía plástica periodontal para corregirse.

Esperamos que usted reciba muchos años de servicio de la restauración de molde.

Si usted tiene cualquier pregunta sobre las coronas y los puentes, avor de sentirse libre de preguntarnos.

Ilustración en CD-ROM

Diseño de Coronas

Hay muchos tipos de restauraciones de molde de cobertura completa (coronas) que se pueden usar para restaurar un diente o formar parte de un puente. También hay características imprescindibles en el diseño que no se pueden cambiar sin el riesgo de comprometer la restauración final. El diseño más común usa un metal noble para la subestructura y un material de porcelana adherido al metal que esconde la mayor parte del metal pero quizás no todo. Con el tiempo es posible que más metal quede expuesto si el tejido se retira del área. Este retiro puede ser el resultado del proceso normal de envejecimiento o el resultado de la patología dental. En la interfaz de la corona y el diente, hay un collar metálico de 0.4 mm de ancho que rodea al diente y marca los límites de la corona. Hay otros diseños que usan metales diferentes, tales como un contenido más alto de oro y cantidades diferentes de metal visible en la corona. Más metal puede ser deseable si el paciente tiene un hábito de bruxismo (rechinar) o si se hacen las coronas por razones de colocar una férula periodontal. Menos metal puede ser deseable si hay un compromiso cosmético.

Cuanto más complicada la construcción de las restauraciones de molde, más costará cada corona. Algunos de los costos son fijos, como la sustitución de un margen de metal por un margen de porcelana. Algunos costos cambian, como el precio del oro, del platino y de otros metales usados en la subestructura. La corona básica, menos costosa, tendrá algún metal visible. Contendrá un metal noble, un collar metálico circular y una cobertura de porcelana de 85% de la corona. Si usted tiene una alergia a cualquier tipo de material metálico o cerámico, tiene que informarnos antes de la fabricación de la corona. Una alergia al metal afectará la selección del metal.

La construcción de la corona también envuelve un laboratorio, el cual hará la fundición del metal y la aplicación de la porcelana. También hay una diferencia entre el nivel de pericia de los laboratorios. El componente estético de las coronas está relacionado directamente al nivel de habilidad del técnico del laboratorio y de la aptitud artística del dentista. Algunos laboratorios se especializan en las coronas estéticas. Las coronas que se ven bien y se ajustan correctamente cuestan más porque los mejores laboratorios cobran más por su trabajo. Nosotros usamos sólo los laboratorios que han demostrado que pueden producir coronas y puentes dentales excelentes consistentemente. En lo que concierne a su salud oral, no aceptamos nada que no sea de calidad.

La cobertura del seguro dental típicamente incluye sólo el tipo más básico de corona. No pagan por el componente estético de las coronas ni por ninguna mejoría sobre el tipo básico que usted ha escogido. Naturalmente esto reducirá su proporción de pago de ellos por el procedimiento. El reembolso a usted será aproximadamente 40% a 50% por cada corona. Quizás le han informado que es un 50% o más. Esto puede no ser necesariamente una declaración exacta; usted necesita saber precisamente qué clase de corona está cubierta por su seguro dental.

Favor de considerar las siguientes opciones para sus restauraciones de molde de cobertura completa. Ya se le han explicado las opciones verbalmente y/o en un documento por escrito. Mantenga esta información en mente al marcar las opciones que usted desea.

❑ Porcelana con metal semi-precioso, collar de metal completo de 360 grados, superficie
palatal y lingual de metal parcial (diseño normal de la corona) $
❑ Superficie facial (del lado del cachete) de porcelana en la juntura cabo a cabo $
❑ Metal precioso completo (no es metal semi-precioso) $
❑ Exposición mínima de metal en el lado lingual (palatal $
❑ Tipo CAPTEK® $
❑ Molde completo de porcelana o cerámica (sin usar metal, se puede adherir en su lugar) $
❑ Superficie oclusal (de masticar) completamente de metal; porcelana sólo en el lado facial $
❑ Otro:_____ $

                                                            Total $

**Si usted tiene cualquier pregunta sobre el diseño o los honorarios de las coronas, favor
de sentirse libre de preguntarnos.**

Coronas y Puentes: Una Visión General del Procedimiento

PREPARACIÓN DEL DIENTE, IMPRESIÓN Y RESTAURACIÓN PROVISIONAL

Expectativas de las Citas

La preparación del diente para una corona y un puente envuelve múltiples citas. La primera cita incluirá la preparación del diente (dientes), la toma de impresiones y el hacer una restauración provisional (temporal). Esta cita normalmente será la más larga y la más compleja. En su caso, usted puede esperar tener una cita de aproximadamente _____ hora(s). Cuantos más dientes preparemos para las coronas, más larga será la cita.

Preparación del Diente

La preparación de los dientes consiste de la reformación y eliminación de la estructura del diente. Esta reducción permite que se use el grueso ideal de metal, porcelana o metal con porcelana. La cantidad de reducción necesaria depende del material que hemos escogido; los diferentes tipos de coronas requieren diseños diferentes. Nos aseguraremos que usted esté cómodo durante todo el procedimiento adormeciendo el área como sea necesario.

A veces, a causa de la posición del tejido suave (las encías), puede ser necesario recortar o reformar el tejido suave alrededor de los dientes. Si encontramos que, debido a circunstancias imprevistas, la eliminación de tejido será complicada, le podemos enviar a un periodontista (especialista de encías) para este procedimiento. Si el tejido no necesita reformarse, normalmente usaremos una 'cuerda de retracción' que se ajusta y se coloca alrededor del diente. Esta cuerda temporalmente reposiciona el tejido de la encía más lejos de la porción preparada del diente y hace posible obtener una impresión mejor.

Toma de Impresiones

Una vez que los dientes se han preparados adecuadamente, se hace la impresión final. Durante este procedimiento de impresión, las porciones preparadas del diente tienen que estar claramente visibles. Mientras más limpios estén los dientes preparados, mejor será la impresión. Para asegurar la precisión frecuentemente tomamos una segunda impresión. Ésta es una tarea difícil y exigente, y algunos aspectos del obtener una impresión aceptable están fuera de nuestro control.

El material de impresión se mezcla y se coloca en una cubeta especial que se ajusta al tamaño de su boca. El material de impresión es bastante suave cuando se mezcla, similar a la melaza fría. Una vez que está puesto en su boca, el material de impresión se endurecerá en sólo unos pocos minutos. Dependiendo del tipo de la técnica de impresión usada, se puede hacer también otro modelo de los dientes contrarios.

Se usará una impresión de su mordida (registro de la mordida) para asegurar que su(s) corona(s) final(es) se asentará(n) bien con la mandíbula contraria, tal como lo hacía(n) anteriormente.

Restauraciones Temporales o Provisionales

Después de tomar la impresión, se construirá la(s) restauración(es) provisional(es) (temporales). La(s) corona(s) provisional(es) de plástico/resina reemplaza(n) la estructura dental preparada y protegerá(n) al diente mientras que se fabrica la corona final. Las restauraciones provisionales se mantienen en su lugar con un cemento provisional y normalmente permanecerán en su boca por un mínimo de 2 semanas—o más si el tratamiento requerido es complejo.

Su Nueva Apariencia

En la cita inicial haremos una determinación del tono de porcelana (o resina) que se usará para obtener los mejores resultados estéticos. Por supuesto, usted participará en este proceso. Muchas veces tomaremos fotos de sus dientes para igualar mejor el tono. La impresión, el registro de la mordida y la información del tono se envían a un laboratorio y se construye(n) la(s) corona(s) o puente(s) según nuestra orden de trabajo explícita. La restauración devuelta estará lista para la cementación (si es simple) o para la prueba de molde (si es más complicada).

Después de la Primera Cita

¿Cómo se sentirá usted después de concluir la cita? La mayoría de los pacientes notan que su tejido gingival (de la encía) les duele por uno o dos días. Cuanto menos modificación o manipulación de los tejidos gingivales, menos dolor usted sentirá. Algunos pacientes notan sensibilidad en los dientes, especialmente al frío, pero esto desaparece bastante rápido. Los analgésicos (medicamentos para aliviar el dolor) usualmente no son necesarios. Si creemos que usted estará más incómodo de lo normal, le informaremos al final de la cita.

Si usted tiene cualquier pregunta sobre la preparación del diente, impresión y restauración provisional para las coronas o puentes, favor de sentirse libre de preguntarnos.

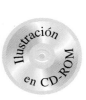

Honorarios por Coronas y Puentes

Aunque hacemos un gran esfuerzo para explicar el tratamiento específico y los honorarios relacionados, encontramos que para las restauraciones de molde (coronas, puentes, inlays, onlays de metal y/o porcelana; también conocidos como *caperuzas*) a veces queda alguna confusión. Favor de leer lo siguiente con cuidado de modo que entienda lo qué está incluido en los honorarios por cada procedimiento y dónde puede haber otros honorarios.

Restauraciones de Molde: Coronas y Puentes

El honorario por una restauración de molde incluye:
- ❏ Los impresiones y los modelos preliminares
- ❏ La anestesia local
- ❏ Preparación del diente (dientes)
- ❏ Una restauración provisional (temporal)
- ❏ Los registros de la mordida
- ❏ Los modelos
- ❏ Las impresiones finales y de retiro del diente preparado y sus dientes contrarios
- ❏ Los ajustes de prueba
- ❏ La selección del tono con fotografías donde sea indicado
- ❏ La cementación de experimental
- ❏ Los ajustes
- ❏ La cementación final
- ❏ Un año de seguimiento y ajustes

El honorario **no** cubre:
- ❏ La construcción de un poste y base necesario en un diente tratado anteriormente con un canal radicular
- ❏ Las construcciones para reemplazar la estructura dental donde faltan porciones significes del diente natural
- ❏ La cirugía periodontal (de la encía) para exponer una porción clínica adecuada para la retención de la corona
- ❏ Los procedimientos electroquirúrgicos para eliminar el tejido de la encía donde el deterioro del diente, la fractura del diente o la preparación previa del diente ha movido la estructura saludable del diente debajo de la encía hasta el punto que el diente no se puede preparar apropiadamente, no se puede ver o no se puede tomar una impresión

Desagraciadamente, la necesidad para una electrocirugía frecuentemente no se sabrá hasta que comience la preparación del diente. Normalmente podemos completar este procedimiento en nuestra oficina, pero para los casos más extensivos, le enviaremos a un especialista. Si hay un potencial para que usted necesite una construcción de poste y base para una corona o la eliminación de algún tejido suave, le informaremos del procedimiento y del honorario asociado antes de comenzar la preparación (cuando sea posible). Estos procedimientos tienen códigos de seguro dental individuales y se consideran como procedimientos separados y no están incluidos en el honorario por la corona o puente.

Si usted tiene cualquier pregunta sobre los honorarios por las coronas y los puentes, favor de sentirse libre de preguntarnos.

Instrucciones Preoperatorias para Coronas y Puentes

Como usted ha tomado la decisión de proceder con los procedimientos de las prótesis fijas (coronas, puentes, inlays u onlays) queremos enfatizar la importancia del cuidado oral de sí mismo. Cualquier infección del tejido suave, aun si parece ser menor, puede causar dificultad con la preparación o la impresión final y causar un atraso en el tratamiento. Si usted cepilla los dientes y usa el hilo dental tal como le hemos enseñado, no habrá ningún problema con las encías, y la preparación y la impresión serán más rápidas y fáciles para usted y para nosotros. El mantenimiento diario es necesario para asegurar la salud de las encías. Cuanto mejor cuidado usted tome de sus dientes y de las restauraciones procesadas en el laboratorio, más tiempo normalmente durarán y menos problemas tendrá usted en el futuro. Cualquier problema que se desarrolla normalmente será pequeño y se corregirá fácilmente. Recomendamos que usted continúe teniendo sus dientes examinados por nosotros en el intervalo de tiempo que hemos establecido para usted.

Cuando las encías están irritadas debido al cuidado oral de sí mismo inadecuado, el tejido se hinchará y se pondrá rojo y sangrará fácilmente. Cuando el tejido de la encía está hinchado, los márgenes de preparación del diente no son tan fáciles de aislar y secar para la impresión. El contorno verdadero del tejido puede desfigurarse, lo que hace virtualmente imposible tomar una impresión correcta de la preparación. Los materiales de impresión no trabajan bien en la humedad. Si la impresión no es correcta, la corona no se asentará correctamente. Cuando las condiciones del tejido se tornan muy difíciles para trabajar podemos decidir no hacer la preparación o la impresión y tendremos que fijar otra cita para después de que el tejido se mejore.

Es importante que usted practique la eliminación minuciosa de la placa, especialmente antes de que comencemos la preparación del diente. Usted necesitará continuar su cuidado excelente de sí mismo mientras la restauración provisional esté puesta, y durante el tiempo de la impresión y la cementación final de la restauración. ¡Por supuesto, esperamos que usted puede mantener estos hábitos buenos para siempre!

Como una medida adicional de protección le estamos recetando un enjuague antimicrobiano, que se ha demostrado que ayuda a mantener saludables los tejidos suaves y a reducir los problemas potenciales del sangrado. Favor de usar el enjuague _____ veces al día, comenzando 2 semanas antes de la cita de la preparación del diente y hasta 2 semanas después de la cementación final.

Otras Instrucciones:_____

_____

_____

Si usted tiene cualquier pregunta sobre estas instrucciones preoperatorias, favor de sentirse libre de preguntarnos.

Opciones de Materiales: Una Visión General

Cuando un diente natural ha sufrido daño extensivo no se puede restaurar con éxito a largo plazo con una "empastadura regular"—una que el dentista coloca en una sola cita en la oficina. Los materiales que se construyen y procesan en un laboratorio son más fuertes y durarán más tiempo. Todos los materiales para las restauraciones de molde tienen ventajas y desventajas. Lo siguiente es un resumen de los materiales que se pueden usar.

Restauraciones de Cobertura Parcial: Inlays y Onlays

Las restauraciones de cobertura parcial están indicadas cuando queda estructura dental saludable que no necesita incluirse en la preparación. Las ventajas de un inlay u onlay incluyen menos taladrado que para una corona de cobertura completa. Debido a la estética y preocupaciones sobre las posibles reacciones alérgicas al metal, la odontología se ha apartado de usar cualquier restauración que contiene metal.

❑ Aleación de Oro—El oro se ha usado con éxito en la restauración de los dientes por muchos años y tiene una historia larga de servicio. El color amarillo puede ser visible cuando usted habla o sonríe y por esta razón no se considera un material estético. Sin embargo, es útil para las restauraciones de tamaño pequeño a mediano y para las personas que bruxan o rechinan los dientes.
❑ Resina Procesada en el Laboratorio—Ésta es una selección cosmética excelente porque puede igualar muy de cerca el color natural del diente. Las resinas procesadas en el laboratorio son muy satisfactorias para las restauraciones de tamaño pequeño a mediano pero no son tan exitosas en los pacientes con hábito de rechinar los dientes. Las restauraciones tienen una tendencia a romperse bajo fuerzas compresivas extremas. Se puede recomendar un protector bucal para su protección.
❑ Porcelana/Cerámica—Excelentes para el uso en la odontología cosmética, las restauraciones de porcelana/cerámica se usan para restaurar las caries de tamaño pequeño a mediano. El material es más resistente al desgaste que la resina pero puede desgastar el esmalte contrario. No es tan exitoso para los pacientes que bruxan o rechinan los dientes y tiene la potencialidad de romperse bajo fuerzas de mordida extremas. Se puede recomendar un protector bucal para su protección.

Restauraciones de Cobertura Completa: Coronas y Puentes

Las restauraciones de cobertura completa están indicadas cuando toda la estructura remanente necesita protección o es vulnerable a la fractura. Una corona de cobertura completa requiere más preparación que un inlay u onlay.

❑ Oro (Noble Alto) de Molde Completo—Hecho de una aleación de oro, el oro de molde es el más duradero de todos los materiales procesados en el laboratorio—20 años o más. La aleación consiste de oro, plata, paladio, y a veces zinc, cobre y platino. Aunque es un material muy fuerte, el color amarillo lo hace no tan estéticamente agradable como las otras opciones.
❑ Metal Noble de Molde Completo—Tiene propiedades y calidades similares a las del oro de molde completo, este material contiene principalmente paladio más plata, oro y vestigios de otros metales. El material metal noble es más color plata que un metal noble de molde completo.
❑ Porcelana Fundida a Oro (Noble Alto o Aleación de Metal Noble)—Este material es muy estético y puede durar 10 a 20 años. La subestructura de oro está cubierta con porcelana, la cual puede desgastar los dientes contrarios o fracturarse con el rechinar o con el morder con fuerza. La porcelana se puede aplicar sólo en la superficie de la corona que enfrenta el cachete. El resultado no será tan estético pero durará más tiempo. Se puede recomendar un protector bucal para protegerla.
❑ De Cerámica o Porcelana Completa—Ésta es la tecnología más reciente en las restauraciones procesadas en el laboratorio y se considera muy estética. No se usa ningún metal en el proceso y por eso no habrá nunca ningún metal visible. Es excelente para restauraciones en los dientes de atrás; la vida de servicio esperada es 10 años o más. Este tipo de restauración puede ser cementada o adherida en su lugar. Las mismas precauciones existen como con cualquier material de porcelana o cerámica: puede desgastar el esmalte natural contrario y un protector bucal puede ser recomendable para protegerlo del bruxismo o del rechinar. Algunos procesos de la fabricación de la corona completa de cerámica o porcelana están controlados por una computadora.

Todas las restauraciones mencionadas arriba toman al menos dos citas para completarse. La preparación del diente, las impresiones y la corona, puente o inlay/onlay provisional se harán en la primera cita. La cementación permanente ocurrirá durante la segunda cita. A causa de la naturaleza altamente técnica del proceso y de nuestros estándares exigentes, podremos necesitar tomar más de una impresión. Si detectamos una irregularidad con la restauración devuelta por el laboratorio, tomaremos una impresión nueva y reharemos el onlay o la corona.

Recomendaremos el mejor material para cumplir con sus necesidades específicas y contestaremos cualquier pregunta que usted tenga. La longevidad de cualquier restauración depende de la calidad de los materiales (y usamos sólo los mejores), de las destrezas técnicas de la construcción y la colocación (y proveemos el mejor servicio posible) y de lo que usted hace con las restauraciones una vez estén en su boca. Los hábitos de apretar y rechinar abrevian significativamente la vida útil de cualquier restauración colocada. Lo que puede romper su diente natural puede romper cualquier restauración. Su cuidado oral de sí mismo afectará la duración del servicio de la restauración. Usted necesitará exámenes dentales regulares y el mantenimiento de higiene (limpieza) en los intervalos determinados por sus requisitos particulares de salud oral. Una regla general es mientras más restauraciones usted tiene en su boca, más cuidado usted (y ellas) necesitará(n). Cualquier problema que comience puede ser descubierto y corregido cuando es pequeño: con los exámenes dentales regulares, usted puede proteger su inversión.

Restauraciones de Molde de Oro

Una restauración de molde de oro le dará el servicio más duradero y menos problemático de todo tipo de material dental disponible hoy en día. Una corona completa en oro puede ser usada cuando un diente ha sufrido destrucción significativa. Cuando existe más esmalte y estructura del diente original se usa un tipo de restauración mucho más pequeña y conservadora llamado un *inlay*. Se ha conocido que las restauraciones de molde de oro duran por 25 a 40 años. Generalmente, una restauración de molde de oro no se rompe. El molde de oro se mantiene en su lugar con un cemento dental (pegamento). Hasta se puede fundir.

Estas restauraciones de oro se recomiendan especialmente para los pacientes que bruxan (rechinan) o aprietan sus dientes. Se indican para los pacientes que desean el tipo de restauración dental menos problemática y más duradera. Se recomiendan cuando hay destrucción del diente moderada a extensiva. Los moldes de oro se usan para cubrir las superficies de mordida y las áreas debilitadas y para prevenir la fractura durante el masticar normal. Sólo las restauraciones del molde pueden hacer esto. Las empastaduras de plata no pueden fortalecer los dientes. Las empastaduras adheridas de color del diente que no son fabricadas en el laboratorio no fortalecen los dientes como el de molde de oro. Un laboratorio está envuelto en la fabricación de la corona o inlay de oro. Por lo tanto se necesitarán dos visitas para completar la restauración. Un inlay o corona provisional de plástico permanecerá en el diente mientras se hace la restauración final. Las citas estarán separadas por alrededor de 2 semanas.

Inicialmente, las restauraciones de molde de oro son más costosas que las empastaduras de plata. Como no hay que rehacer las restauraciones de molde tan frecuentemente (si hay que rehacerlas) como las de plata, usted terminará economizando dinero a largo plazo. Cuanto más tiempo las restauraciones de oro están colocadas, menos usted gastará eventualmente en la restauración repetida del mismo diente. Otra desventaja potencial del molde de oro es el color. Tiene el color amarillo obvio de los "anillos de matrimonio". Si usted desea que las restauraciones sean del mismo color de sus dientes, el molde de oro no es para usted. Dependiendo del tipo de restauración que usted requiere, puede ser posible disfrazar o esconder el color del oro cuando usted sonríe, pero cuando abre la boca, el color puede ser visible. Si esto le es ofensivo, debe considerar un inlay u onlay del color del diente o una corona de porcelana unida a metal. Usted podría obtener la estética que desea: moldes de oro para los dientes de atrás que no se ven fácilmente y restauraciones del color de los dientes donde se podrían ver.

Para los pacientes que desean la restauración más duradera y menos problemática y que entienden la inversión inicial de tiempo y dinero y no encuentren ofensivo el despliegue de oro amarillo, ésta es la restauración preferida. Recomendamos favorablemente este tipo de restauración.

Si usted tiene cualquier pregunta sobre las restauraciones de molde de oro, favor de sentirse libre de preguntarnos

Restauraciones de Molde de Oro y Cerámica

Hoy en día hay varios tipos de materiales restaurativos disponibles para la cobertura parcial. Dos que parecen ser los más fuertes y tener la expectativa de vida más larga son los materiales de oro con cerámica/porcelana. Aunque hay algunas diferencias significativas entre ellos en su diseño y fabricación, en realidad son muy similares en su concepto.

Las ventajas principales del oro son su fiabilidad probada y su expectativa de vida larga. Las restauraciones de oro se han usado con éxito en la odontología por muchos años y pueden durar 40 años o más. El oro es el material restaurativo más duradero que los dentistas tienen para trabajar hoy en día. Dos desventajas del molde de oro son su alto costo inicial y un color amarillo que no se parece en nada a un diente verdadero. En comparación, una empastadura convencional cuesta menos inicialmente pero los costos del reemplazo repetido a través del curso de tiempo serán más que los de la restauración de molde de oro. A veces se puede enmascarar el color amarillo del oro de modo que no sea tan visible o tan ofensivo. Cuanto más pequeña la restauración y más hacia atrás en su boca, menos oro se verá. Como con los materiales de porcelana/cerámica, el oro puede usarse para reemplazar todo el diente (una corona completa) o parte del diente (cobertura parcial—inlay u onlay).

Dos ventajas de las restauraciones de porcelana/cerámica son una apariencia natural y un uso proyectado de largo plazo. Cuando son completadas, las restauraciones de porcelana/cerámica se adhieren al diente preparado (contraria a una restauración de molde de oro, que normalmente sólo se cementa) y como el oro, toman dos visitas para completarse. Las preparaciones para el oro y la porcelana/cerámica son similares. En la primera visita se hace una impresión de la preparación y se coloca una restauración provisional. La impresión se envía al laboratorio para la fabricación. Dos semanas más tarde, se coloca la restauración final. Las desventajas de las restauraciones de porcelana/cerámica incluyen el alto costo inicial y el alto grado de pericia técnica necesario por parte del dentista y el laboratorio.

Una restauración de oro se recomienda especialmente para los pacientes que bruxan (rechinan) o aprietan sus dientes. También se indica el oro para los pacientes que desean el tipo de restauración dental menos problemática y más duradera. Se recomienda cuando hay una destrucción moderada del diente. Los moldes de oro se usan para cubrir las superficies de mordida y las áreas debilitadas y para prevenir la fractura durante el masticar normal. Sólo las restauraciones de molde pueden hacer esto. Las empastaduras de plata no pueden fortalecer los dientes en esta manera. Las empastaduras adheridas del color del diente no se fabrican en el laboratorio y por eso no ofrecen fuerza adicional.

No se recomiendan las restauraciones de porcelana/cerámica para los pacientes que rechinan o bruxan sus dientes. Cuando se colocan en estos pacientes, el paciente debe esperar usar un aparato protectivo de anti-bruxismo para proteger las restauraciones. Estos materiales se recomiendan para los pacientes que exigen los materiales más fuertes, de la mejor apariencia y más estéticos que están disponibles hoy en día.

Si usted tiene cualquier pregunta sobre las restauraciones de molde de oro o de cerámica, favor de sentirse libre de preguntarnos.

Restauraciones de Molde de Porcelana Unida a Metal

Una restauración de porcelana unida a metal se puede usar en las mismas áreas que la restauración de molde de oro. Como el metal está cubierto con una capa de porcelana, tiene una apariencia mucho más natural que un molde de oro y asemeja más al diente natural. También tiene un largo de vida bastante largo de 8 a 10 años y puede durar más de 25 años. Este tipo más común de corona es la corona fabricada por los dentistas en los Estados Unidos. Cuando se hace con un metal noble o semi-precioso, normalmente tiene un contenido alto de oro, platino o paladio. Con las coronas de porcelana unida a metal, la porcelana normalmente cubre el metal o las superficies del lado de la mordida y del cachete y parte del lado de lengua. Frecuentemente hay una franja de metal no cubierta en el lado de la lengua. Algunas preparaciones necesitan tener un collar de metal en el lado del cachete, cerca de la encía. **Si usted cree que encontrará ofensivo cualquier despliegue de metal, déjenos saberlo antes de que se prepare el diente**. Hablaremos de sus preocupaciones y modificaremos la preparación para la corona de porcelana con metal o cambiaremos a una corona de cerámica completa, si es posible.

Un laboratorio externo está envuelto en la construcción de las coronas de porcelana con metal, lo que incrementa el costo y extiende el tiempo de tratamiento. Las coronas se mantienen en su lugar con un cemento dental que fija la corona permanentemente en el diente.

Algunas desventajas de las coronas de porcelana unida a metal son similares a las de la corona de molde de oro. Son costosas. Requieren por lo menos dos citas para completarse. Las coronas de porcelana unida a metal requieren más preparación del diente de lo que es necesario para las coronas de oro. Como es una restauración compuesta de varios materiales diferentes (metal, porcelana y opaco), potencialmente hay más problemas. La fractura cohesiva de la porcelana o una fractura de la porcelana del metal es posible. En estos casos, la corona podría todavía ser útil pero no estética. A veces se puede arreglar y a veces hay que reemplazarla. Como la porcelana es dura, puede desgastar el esmalte de los dientes contrarios a una razón de aproximadamente 100 microns (0.1 mm) por año. Esto puede no parecer como mucho desgaste, pero en el contexto de la boca, puede ser bastante significante. Las coronas de porcelana unida a metal normalmente no se consideran un tipo de restauración conservadora, pero en los casos donde ha ocurrido destrucción considerable de la estructura natural del diente, son la restauración más preferida. En la preparación (el taladrado) del diente natural, el nervio del diente se puede dañar y se puede requerir terapia endodóntica tratamiento del canal radicular). Aunque es desafortunado e impredecible, esto no es raro.

Si el retiro del tejido de la encía ocurre alrededor de la corona, una línea de metal oscuro puede aparecer o la raíz puede quedar expuesta. Esto no necesariamente significa que hay que reemplazar la corona. Puede todavía funcionar bien pero no tiene una apariencia estética tan agradable. La corrección por medio de la cirugía plástica periodontal es posible.

La restauración de molde de porcelana unida a metal produce una apariencia que se ve más natural que con una corona de oro, aunque alguna parte de la subestructura de metal puede ser visible. Esta restauración se puede usar con éxito para reemplazar mucho de la estructura que falta del diente. Pueden durar por mucho tiempo, con el cuidado apropiado.

Si usted tiene alguna alergia a los metales, favor de informarnos antes de que se comiencen las preparaciones.

Si usted tiene cualquier pregunta sobre las restauraciones de molde de porcelana unida a metal, favor de sentirse libre de preguntarnos.

Restauraciones Completas de Porcelana/Cerámica

Hoy en día una de las maneras más estéticas para restaurar los dientes es usar una corona de molde de cerámica o porcelana completa. La construcción de la corona es un poco diferente cuando se usa un material de cerámica o porcelana. La decisión de cuál de los materiales se usará se dejará a la discreción nuestra.

Este tipo de corona no contiene ningún metal y por eso aproxima más la apariencia total de un diente natural no dañado que cualquier otro tipo de corona completa de molde. Con la tecnología adhesiva de hoy, es más frecuente que estas restauraciones se adhieren en su lugar con un agente que adhiere el esmalte con la dentina. La corona fabricada de porcelana completa o cerámica completa es mucho más difícil de preparar y adherir en su lugar y técnicamente es más sensitiva y exigente. Normalmente tomará un poco más tiempo para terminarla. Los costos de laboratorio también son más altos. Por consiguiente, este tipo de corona es más costosa.

Como las superficies de la mordida o la incisión están cubiertas con porcelana, similares a las de una corona de porcelana con metal, el desgaste de los dientes contrarios será igual al de una corona de porcelana con metal. No hay otras diferencias significativas.

Aunque algunas de las coronas de cerámica parecen ser frágiles, al igual que los laminados de porcelana, están bien apoyadas y son muy fuertes una vez que se han adherido al diente. No se aconseja que usted mastique cubos de hielo, nueces o caramelos duros con estos tipos de restauraciones ni con sus dientes naturales. No se recomienda el uso de estas restauraciones en un paciente con un hábito de bruxismo o rechinar a menos que el paciente usará fielmente un protector bucal u otro aparato durante las horas de bruxismo.

Estas restauraciones son hermosas, posiblemente las restauraciones de cobertura completa más hermosas que hay disponibles. Estas restauraciones son más complicadas para llevar a cabo, pero las recompensas de verdad valen la pena. Usted puede esperar que duren mucho tiempo. Durarán tanto tiempo o casi tanto tiempo como las coronas de porcelana unida a metal. Si usted necesita una restauración de cobertura completa, y la estética le es de máxima importancia, debe considerar las coronas de porcelana y cerámica.

Si usted tiene cualquier pregunta sobre las coronas de porcelana completa y de cerámica completa, favor de sentirse libre de preguntarnos.

Puentes: Una Visión General

El reemplazo de los dientes frontales que faltan obviamente puede mejorar la apariencia de su sonrisa. Lo que la mayoría de las personas no piensan en qué pasa cuando no se reemplaza un diente de atrás que falta. El reemplazo de un diente de atrás le ayudará a recobrar su capacidad normal de masticar la comida y digerirla correctamente. Cada vez que usted pierde un diente, pierde alrededor de 10% de su capacidad de masticar. Cuando se pierde un diente, los otros dientes alrededor del espacio tienden a moverse hacia el espacio vacío. Esto contribuye a una oportunidad aumentada para el comienzo del deterioro y de la enfermedad de las encías, junto con los problemas de la mordida y la potencialidad de otros problemas dentales. Los dientes que faltan siempre se deben reemplazar—cuanto más temprano, mejor.

Los puentes fijos son una de las posibilidades que existen para el reemplazo de uno o más dientes que faltan. Otras alternativas son los implantes dentales, los puentes de Maryland (adheridos), puentes de cobertura parcial y las prótesis parciales removibles.

Las ventajas del puente fijo incluyen la fiabilidad y la longevidad probada. Las desventajas incluyen el costo, la dificultad aumentada para la limpieza correcta por parte del paciente, y ocasionalmente, la necesidad de preparar un diente para un anclaje (sostén de puente), que podía no haber sido empastado ni dañado anteriormente.

Se pueden remplazar uno o más dientes con un puente fijo. El diseño del puente es afectado por, entre otros factores, la cantidad, la fortaleza y la posición de los dientes restantes y por la habilidad del paciente de limpiar correctamente el puente terminado. Hablando en general, el sostén para el puente debe ser igual o mejor que el sostén de raíz que tenían los dientes que faltan.

Los dientes que serán los sostenes del puente se preparan similar a la preparación de una sola corona. El diente se empequeñece por 1 a 2 milímetros, dependiendo de la parte del diente taladrada. Se hace una impresión de los dientes preparados y se envía a un laboratorio. Mientras se hace el puente, se protegen los dientes preparados con un puente provisional bien diseñado. Una vez que se ha colocado el puente final con un cemento final, no es fácil sacarlo de nuevo sin dañar la porcelana y el metal permanentemente.

Su cuidado oral de sí mismo debe incluir la eliminación minuciosa de la placa, especialmente alrededor del puente. Le mostremos cómo limpiarlo correctamente. Es importante que usted siga nuestro horario de cuidado repetido de higiene dental. Los exámenes frecuentes son una manera de proteger su inversión y de mantener una salud oral óptima.

Si usted tiene cualquier pregunta sobre los puentes fijos, favor de sentirse libre de preguntarnos.

Puentes Completos de Cerámica y Porcelana

Por varios años la odontología ha provisto coronas muy fuertes de una sola unidad del color del diente. Los problemas de la sensibilidad al metal y de conseguir una igualación excelente de color con las coronas de porcelana unida a metal eran las fuerzas impulsoras en fomentar la investigación y el desarrollo de coronas sin metal.

Por varios años, los dentistas han sido capaces de colocar puentes de cerámica/porcelana completa para reemplazar un diente frontal que falta. La mordida en los dientes frontales no genera tanta fuerza como la mordida en los dientes de atrás. Recientemente, la investigación dental ha desarrollado un sustituto muy bueno para la subestructura de metal para reemplazar los dientes que faltan de atrás. Estos puentes de cerámica/porcelana completa se pueden usar para combinaciones de hasta cinco dientes que faltan y dientes de sostén. La subestructura cerámica no es tan fuerte como el metal, pero es clínicamente aceptable.

Las ventajas sobre los puentes de metal/porcelana incluyen una apariencia estética excelente, absolutamente ningún despliegue de metal y ningunas consideraciones de posible alergia al metal. Las desventajas incluyen un costo un poco más alto y más sensibilidad técnica. Al igual que los puentes sostenidos con metal, los hábitos orales del paciente, los tipos de comida que se comen y el cuidado oral de sí mismo diario tendrán un gran efecto en la longevidad del puente. Tenemos suficiente confianza en los puentes de cerámica y porcelana completa para ofrecerle este servicio.

El sistema LAVA es una nueva opción para las coronas y los puentes de cerámica/porcelana completa sin metal. Este sistema innovador usa una base de óxido de zirconio, que provee mayor fortaleza de la que era posible previamente en las coronas y los puentes de cerámica/porcelana completa. El sistema LAVA usa una impresión convencional tal como la que se usa con los otros procedimientos de coronas y puentes, pero la manufactura de la corona o el puente se lleva a cabo en una unidad fresadora controlada por computadora. Esta técnica requiere menos preparación del diente. Las coronas y los puentes producidos por este sistema son cuatro veces más fuertes que las coronas y los puentes de cerámica/porcelana completa, son altamente resistentes a la fractura y tienen propiedades estéticas excelentes.

Al igual que las coronas y los puentes de cerámica/porcelana completa, hay costos adicionales para producir estas restauraciones LAVA de alta calidad. Le proveeremos con información en cuanto a sus condiciones orales para ayudarle a escoger el material más fuerte y más duradero para su nueva restauración.

Si usted tiene cualquier pregunta sobre los puentes completos de cerámica y porcelana, favor de sentirse libre de preguntarnos.

Puente de Maryland (Retenedor de Resina Adherida)

El puente de Maryland, o retenedor de resina adherida, es una alternativa a los implantes y las coronas convencionales para reemplazar los dientes que faltan. Este tipo de procedimiento de reemplazo se puede considerar cuando el espacio a restaurarse está al lado de dientes que están bien alineados y que no están muy restaurados con materiales de empastadura. Como este tipo de puente se une adhesivamente al esmalte de los dientes de anclaje, es importante tener suficiente esmalte. Un puente de Maryland se fija en su lugar y no está hecho para ser removido durante la noche.

Una ventaja de este proceso sobre el puente convencional es que normalmente se puede reemplazar un diente que falta con una cantidad mínima de preparación (taladrado) de los dientes restantes. No es necesario preparar el diente al mismo grado extremo como con las restauraciones (coronas o caperuzas) que cubren el diente completo. Este método es un procedimiento extremamente conservador. También es menos costoso (aproximadamente un cuarto menos) que un puente convencional. Normalmente la salud del tejido alrededor de los dientes de anclaje es excelente porque se necesita poca o ninguna preparación de la estructura dental cerca del tejido gingival (la encía). Distinto a las restauraciones convencionales de cobertura completa, los dientes preparados para un retenedor de puente Maryland no necesitarán tratamiento endodóntico (terapia de canal radicular) en una fecha futura.

Si el paciente tiene hábitos abusivos de comer o bruxar (rechinar), este tipo de restauración está contraindicada. Aunque la consideramos más como una restauración para los dientes posteriores (de atrás) en vez de para los dientes anteriores (frontales), despliega metal más que un puente convencional. La mayor desventaja de un puente de Maryland es que su largo de vida puede no ser tan larga como la de un puente convencional de coronas de cobertura completa. Esta técnica se introdujo sólo en los primeros años de la década del 1980 y por eso no tiene la historia extensiva de éxito que tienen los puentes de cobertura completa. Aunque la fractura de un puente de Maryland no es probable, se puede despegar, lo cual requiere re-cementación. En algunos casos raros, podría ser necesario rehacerlo. En cualquier de los dos casos, se puede cobrar un honorario por el procedimiento. Un puente de Maryland es un reemplazo fijo por un diente que falta, pero es uno que tendrá que rehacerse en el futuro. La razón de éxito con 5 años de usar los puentes de Maryland en nuestra práctica es aproximadamente el 80%. Sin embargo, éste es un resultado mucho mejor que el promedio nacional que demuestra una razón de éxito de alrededor de 33% en 4 años. Los puentes de Maryland son más apropiados para el reemplazo de un solo diente.

Si los implantes dentales no son una opción para usted para reemplazar un diente y usted no desea que se preparen radicalmente sus dientes a cada lado del espacio (recortarlos o taladrarlos), entonces debe considerar la técnica del puente de Maryland. Para muchos pacientes, las ventajas de menos taladrado de los dientes y del costo reducido lo hace una alternativa deseable.

Si usted tiene cualquier pregunta sobre la técnica del puente de Maryland, favor de sentirse libre de preguntarnos.

Pontic Ovalado

Cuando se pierde un diente por medio del deterioro, trauma o enfermedad periodontal, la manera más común de reemplazarlo hoy en día es con un puente fijo. El puente más convencional usa porcelana unida a metal durante la fabricación. Avances recientes en la tecnología de resina y cerámica reforzada han resultado en puentes sin metal para reemplazar los dientes que faltan. Sin importar cuáles materiales se usan, un puente dental consiste de dientes de anclaje (dientes que sirven de pilar) a cada lado del espacio del diente que falta con un diente falso suspendido entre ellos. El diente falso (o pontic) está suspendido sobre el espacio del diente que falta. En muchos casos, este tipo de arreglo es suficiente para conseguir la restauración de la forma, función y estética requeridas, especialmente si es un diente posterior (de atrás). El lado del pontic que tiene contacto con el tejido de la encía se reforma para quede "sentado sobre" o "sobrepuesto a" el reborde del tejido suave, similar a una silla de montar puesta en el lomo de un caballo. Este tipo de forma del pontic se llama un *pontic sobrepuesto al reborde*. Una alteración posterior de este diseño se llama *pontic modificado sobrepuesto al reborde*. En este caso, se coloca la silla en el caballo, pero se sube un lado hasta la altura del lomo del caballo de modo que no pueda tocar el caballo. La ventaja de este diseño es que la comida tiene mucho menos tendencia de quedar atrapada debajo del pontic y el paciente puede limpiar debajo del diente falso más fácilmente. Hasta pocos años atrás se construyeron todos los pontics de esta manera.

Un diseño radicalmente diferente y más cosmético se ha usado recientemente con gran éxito. Se llama el *pontic ovalado* (*en forma de huevo*). Distinto al diseño *sobrepuesto al reborde* en donde el pontic toca el tejido suave, en el pontic ovalado, se crea una depresión en el reborde del tejido suave que imita la forma natural de la raíz y la corona. Entonces se hace que el diente falso parezca como si saliera del tejido de la encía y no sólo descansara en él. Cuando se hace bien, es difícil ver cuál diente es verdadero y cuál es un reemplazo. Entonces, ¿por qué no se hace esta forma de pontic siempre?

Este pontic ovalado toma más trabajo y más tiempo para llevar a cabo, así que costará más. Hay que preparar la forma ovalada del pontic en el reborde del tejido suave. Este procedimiento quirúrgico sencillo de invasividad mínima usa la electrocirugía o un láser para crear la depresión en forma de huevo en el reborde del tejido. Después de permitir que esta área se sane en la forma correcta, guiada por la forma del puente provisional (temporal), se toman las impresiones para la construcción de la prótesis final. Si un reborde está muy deformado por la extracción del diente o la contracción del reborde, un procedimiento quirúrgico adicional (aumento del reborde) puede ser necesario para reconstruir el reborde antes de reformarlo para el pontic ovalado. Esto también añadirá más costo y tiempo a la construcción del puente. Por eso, aunque se puede hacer la reformación en una cita, dos o aun tres procedimientos pueden ser necesarios.

El pontic ovalado le dará la máxima mejoría cosmética, se verá más natural y será más fácil de limpiar. Si usted tiene una línea del labio alta y muestra muchos de sus dientes cuando habla o sonríe o si usted exige la mejor estética disponible, entonces necesita considerar el pontic ovalado. Después de examinarle, evaluaremos el contorno de su tejido y su línea de sonrisa y determinaremos lo que estará envuelto en la creación del pontic ovalado. Éste es el diseño que más favorecemos, se ve mejor y es el más fácil de mantener limpio. Favor de entender que si el área ha estado sin el diente que falta por mucho tiempo o si el área se ha encogido de la posición normal de modo que la arquitectura normal está destruida, tomará un poco más esfuerzo para crear el pontic ovalado.

Si usted tiene cualquier pregunta sobre sus necesidades particulares, favor de sentirse libre de preguntarnos.

Ilustración en CD-ROM

Puentes Unidos de Cobertura Parcial

Usted puede conocer los tres métodos comunes para el reemplazo de los dientes que faltan—las coronas y los puentes (caperuzas), los implantes dentales y las dentaduras parciales removibles. Los primeros dos se cementan permanentemente en los dientes y por lo tanto permanecerán en la boca todo el tiempo. La tercera opción, una dentadura parcial removible, tiene que sacarse por las noches. Los puentes y los implantes trabajan muy bien como anclas para el reemplazo de los dientes que faltan. Una desventaja de los implantes es su costo y el tiempo necesario para completar la fabricación de la corona o el puente. Una desventaja del puente es la cantidad de diente que hay que preparar (reducir con el taladro) para permitir el uso del grueso suficiente de la aleación de oro y de porcelana. Aunque esto es aceptable en los dientes que tienen empastaduras grandes, no es aceptable taladrar cantidades significantes de la estructura dental en un diente que no ha sido restaurado anteriormente. Nuestra meta para el tratamiento es reemplazar un diente que falta sin eliminar la mayor parte de la estructura de un diente natural en los dientes adyacentes al diente que falta.

Recientemente, los puentes adheridos de cobertura parcial se han usado con gran éxito. Esta técnica nueva para los puentes de cobertura parcial requiere la eliminación de una cantidad mucho más pequeña de la estructura del diente. Si existe una restauración en el diente, se removerá la empastadura, y el puente de cobertura parcial se diseñara para que incluya esta área de preparación. Actualmente, éste es el diseño de puente más conservador que está disponible. Una ventaja adicional del puente adherido de cobertura parcial es que el costo puede ser menos que el costo de un puente convencional de metal/porcelana.

La cita para la preparación y las impresiones para el puente es similar a la cita para un puente convencional. El puente de cobertura parcial se hace de una resina procesada en un laboratorio y reforzada con una barra de titanio. La barra está totalmente escondida dentro del material de resina. El puente se adherirá (no se cementará) en su lugar. La igualación del color es normalmente excelente.

Estos tipos de puentes se han usado con éxito por años. El puente retenido de cobertura parcial es una opción altamente deseable para reemplazar un diente que falta, especialmente un diente posterior (de atrás) si hay pocas o ningunas empastaduras a cada lado del espacio del diente que falta.

Ilustración en CD-ROM

Implantes: Opciones

Hace veinticinco años, si alguien describiera cómo se podrían reemplazar los dientes que faltan con implantes, se le hubiera llamado un milagro. Hace diez años, el uso de los implantes dentales para reemplazar los dientes que faltan hubiera sido llamado asombroso. Hoy en día, los procedimientos de implante se llaman rutinarios. Quisiéramos que usted tuviera una comprensión básica de qué son los implantes, qué se puede esperar de ellos y qué limitaciones pueden tener en su área específica de necesidad.

Un implante dental es un sustituto metálico sintético de la raíz que se coloca o se implanta en el hueso de la mandíbula. Se puede usar para reemplazar un solo diente que falta, proveer un anclaje (ancla o retenedor), reemplazar varios dientes que faltan o proveer retención adicional para un aparato dental removible, tal como una dentadura completa. De hecho, si le faltan todos sus dientes naturales, es posible obtener reemplazos fijos maxilares (superiores) y mandibulares (inferiores). Los reemplazos no salen de la boca y usted no los puede remover por sí mismo.

Dos eventos separados son necesarios al reemplazar un diente que falta con un implante. Primero es la fase quirúrgica en la cual se coloca el implante. En la segunda fase, los dientes de reemplazo se construyen y se fijan en la posición correcta.

El procedimiento de colocar un implante envuelve el hacer una incisión pequeña en el área de la encía donde se colocará el implante, la preparación de un lugar en el hueso subyacente, la inserción del implante en el lugar preparado y el cierre del tejido sobre el implante con varias suturas. Esta área se deja sin tocar, por normalmente 4 a 6 meses. Más tiempo de curación puede variar debido a la densidad de su hueso. La mandíbula inferior está compuesta de hueso que es más denso que la mandíbula superior. Este tiempo de curación permite la integración lenta del implante dentro de su mandíbula. El hueso mantiene el implante en su lugar.

Después de la curación y la integración del implante, se reabre la encía para exponer el lugar de colocación. Luego se fija un poste al implante con cemento o con hilos internos. La corona, el puente u otro tipo de reemplazo estará unido a este poste. Algunos dentistas prefieren hacer todas las fases del procedimiento de implante por sí mismos, pero muchos escogen el hacer la parte quirúrgica o prostética (la verdadera construcción del aparato de reemplazo) solamente. Si éste es el caso, le enviaremos a un periodontista o un cirujano oral que hará la porción quirúrgica de la colocación del implante.

Los implantes son muy exitosos. Los implantes maxilares y mandibulares tienen más de un 90% de éxito. Los implantes inferiores tienen una razón de éxito un poco más alta que los implantes superiores. Ocasionalmente, los implantes fracasan, pero esto no es común. La probabilidad del fracaso de un implante, muchas veces, se puede determinar durante o después de la fase quirúrgica antes de construir el diente o los dientes de reemplazo.

☛ ***Fumadores tomen nota:*** *Hay un riesgo aumentado de fracaso de implante dental entre los fumadores—¡una razón de fracaso hasta 20% más alta!*

Hablaremos con usted sobre los requisitos y las opciones para su situación particular. Normalmente hay varias posibilidades para reemplazar efectivamente los dientes que faltan. Es importante tomar una decisión en cuanto al diseño del reemplazo retenido para el implante antes de hacer el verdadero procedimiento quirúrgico del implante. Hay que considerar la posición y la alineación de los dientes de reemplazo cuidadosamente antes de determinar el lugar del implante.

Si usted tiene cualquier pregunta sobre los implantes, favor de sentirse libre de preguntarnos.

Implantes: Una Visión General de los Procedimientos

En comparación con las empastaduras o coronas (caperuzas) dentales rutinarias, el reemplazo de un diente que falta con implantes es un proceso más complicado y más largo. Tomará varias fases. Un periodontista o un cirujano oral colocará el implante quirúrgicamente. Luego pondremos el diente o la porción visible.

Fase Uno
En la primera fase del tratamiento, el especialista evalúa la posición, la adaptabilidad y la fuerza del hueso que rodeará el implante. Esta información determinará el largo y el ancho de los implantes y cuántos implantes serán necesarios para reemplazar los dientes que faltan. Se tomarán impresiones de todos sus dientes para hacer modelos de estudio para diseñar la forma del diente o los dientes que se implantará(n). Se hará una guía quirúrgica para indicarle al cirujano dónde se deben colocar los implantes.

Fase Dos
La segunda fase consiste de los procedimientos quirúrgicos para colocar el implante en el hueso. Se da un anestésico local y se levanta el tejido de la encía para exponer el lugar del implante. El implante se coloca en el hueso y se cierra la encía sobre él. Usted no verá el implante durante su integración con el hueso. La integración toma 4 a 6 meses. Después de este tiempo, el lugar se abre de nuevo y se ensartará un collar curativo en el implante. Éste guiará al tejido a la forma que se necesita para la(s) corona(s) futura(s). El tiempo que el collar de curación necesita estar en el lugar variará de persona a persona pero será de por lo menos varias semanas.

Fase Tres
La tercera fase comenzará una vez la forma del tejido es suficiente. En esta fase, se colocan aditamentos y componentes específicos en el implante. Los componentes del implante son similares en función a las anclas de pared o de yeso que se usan para colgar retratos en las paredes de yeso. El collar de curación se remueve. Las cofias de transferencia del implante, los análogos y los otros aditamentos se usan para tomar una impresión del lugar. Luego se vuelve a colocar el collar de curación. Las impresiones y los componentes del implante se envían al laboratorio para fabricación de los postes del implante y las coronas acrílicas provisionales.

Cuando el puente o la corona provisional regresa del laboratorio, se remueve el collar de curación y se fijan los aditamentos del implante en el implante. Entonces se asientan y se ajustan las coronas provisionales. Éstas se mantendrán en su lugar con cemento provisional o con tornillos, dependiendo de su situación particular. Le explicaremos las desventajas y las ventajas de cada uno en su caso particular cuando usted decida tener el implante.

Las coronas provisionales se colocan porque el hueso que sostiene y rodea el implante tiene que tener la oportunidad de comenzar a funcionar gradualmente. Las técnicas de implante dictan que los implantes sean introducidos lentamente a la función de morder. Esto significa que usted regresará varias veces para que le añada más acrílico a la corona provisional. Después que el implante y la corona provisional hayan estado en función de morder por algunos meses, se fabricará(n) la(s) corona(s) finales y se cementará(n) o se atornillará(n) en su lugar.

Mantenimiento de Todos Sus Dientes
Para mantener sus implantes y sus dientes naturales saludables y funcionales por el tiempo más largo posible, limpie el implante y sus otros dientes diariamente como le han enseñado. También necesitará venir para las citas de higiene dental de cuidado repetido en un intervalo de 3 a 4 meses. Usted ha invertido tiempo y dinero en estos reemplazos de diente de última tecnología. El mantenerlos como le han enseñado le dará la mejor posibilidad de éxito.

Creemos que los beneficios de reemplazar los dientes con coronas y puentes sostenidos por implantes vale mucho más que la inconveniencia del largo tiempo entre el comienzo y la terminación. Esto es especialmente cierto cuando los dientes a cada lado del implante son dientes saludables sin empastaduras que en otras circunstancias no requerirían tratamiento dental. Los implantes le ayudan a preservar su estructura dental natural.

Si usted tiene cualquier pregunta sobre los implantes dentales, favor de sentirse libre de preguntarnos.

Ilustración en CD-ROM

Ancho Biológico

Cuando un diente está severamente dañado por el deterioro, trauma o fractura, su restauración se hace más difícil. La restauración preferida en estos casos es una corona procesada en el laboratorio o un onlay de cobertura parcial. Normalmente, es mucho mejor y menos costoso a largo plazo salvar el diente en vez de extraerlo y considerar un reemplazo artificial. Si el daño se extiende debajo del borde de la encía hasta cerca o más allá del borde del hueso, se requiere un tratamiento preliminar antes de poder colocar la restauración con éxito.

El *ancho biológico* es un término usado por los dentistas para describir una distancia de 2.5 mm que tiene que existir entre el borde del hueso (el más cercano a las superficies de la mordida del diente) y el extremo de cualquier restauración. Si no se mantiene esta distancia de 2.5 mm, el tejido suave (tejido de la encía) se inflamará crónicamente y la corona u onlay será un fracaso. La insuficiencia de ancho biológico tiene que corregirse.

Hay varias posibilidades para crear una ancho biológico suficiente. Lo que recomendamos dependerá de la severidad del daño, de cuál diente esté afectado y de la arquitectura del hueso y de la encía de los dientes adyacentes.

Para los dientes posteriores (de múltiples raíces), la terapia correctiva envuelve un procedimiento quirúrgico periodontal. Se hace una incisión en el tejido de la encía alrededor del diente. El material se vuelve hacia atrás y se observa el lugar de la fractura. Luego, se reforma la altura del hueso para que no esté cerca del lugar donde terminará la restauración. Sólo se remueve suficiente hueso para establecer el ancho biológico de 2.5 mm. Obviamente, habrá un límite de cuánto hueso se puede reformar. En la mayoría de los casos, esto se puede determinar antes de hacer la entrada quirúrgica. A veces esto no se conoce hasta que el lugar afectado está claramente visible. Las radiografías no siempre ofrecen la imagen completa. Después de la cirugía, habrá una espera de 3 a 4 meses para que el lugar se sane. Después de ese tiempo, se puede comenzar la restauración final.

Para los dientes de una sola raíz, se puede hacer la cirugía. Pero en vez de recortar la encía y el hueso, a veces es posible brotar ortodónticamente el diente de modo que el lugar de la fractura se aparta del borde del hueso. Esto se puede hacer en aproximadamente 4 meses. Si se mueve el diente de esta manera, el hueso vendrá lentamente con el diente. Después de que el diente haya alcanzado su posición final, el hueso necesitará recortarse para obtener la relación correcta con el diente adyacente. Para algunos dientes una erupción rápida puede ser posible. Cuando se hace en 3½ a 4 semanas, el hueso no se moverá con el diente que está brotando de modo que es posible que no hay que ajustarlo. Cuando se hace la ortodoncia, el diente tiene que estabilizarse en la nueva posición por alrededor de 6 meses antes que se pueda comenzar la restauración final. En algunas situaciones, se usará una combinación de los dos pasos.

Si usted necesita que le restauren el ancho biológico correcto antes de la restauración de un diente, éste se puede establecer ortodónticamente o quirúrgicamente o en una combinación de los dos. Si esto no se hace, la restauración final nunca será exitosa. Lo que le recomendaremos depende de la naturaleza de la fractura, de cuál diente está fracturado y de la posición de los dientes, tejidos gingivales (de la encía) y hueso adyacentes.

Si usted tiene cualquier pregunta sobre la necesidad de ancho biológico adecuado, favor de sentirse libre de preguntarnos.

Cementación: Instrucciones Postoperatorias

El laboratorio dental ha completado la fabricación de su siguiente trabajo dental:

❏ **corona(s)** ❏ **puente(s)** ❏ **inlay(s)** ❏ **onlay(s)**

Estas restauraciones se han cementado con:

❏ **ionómero de vidrio** ❏ **cemento de policarboxilato de fosfato de zinc** ❏ **pegado con un cemento adhesivo de resina**

Sensibilidad del Diente

Ocasionalmente, después de la cementación o el proceso de adhesión, puede haber alguna sensibilidad transitoria (que pasará) que puede durar desde varios días hasta varios meses. Esto no es raro y puede estar relacionado, en parte, al procedimiento de cementación/adhesión o a la cantidad de diente que fue removido durante la preparación para la restauración.

La sensibilidad también puede estar relacionada a la oclusión (mordida). Si se anestesiaron sus dientes para el procedimiento de cementación/adhesión, le puede ser difícil sentir si su mordida se siente normal después de la cementación/adhesión de una restauración nueva. Ocasionalmente esto resulta en una mordida que no es correcta. Cuando se disipa la anestesia, usted podría notar que la mordida no está bien. Sentirá que está alta y que la nueva restauración se encuentra muy pronto con los dientes contrarios. Esto puede causar que el nervio en el diente se ponga irritado y sensitivo al estímulo del calor o del frío. El ajuste de la oclusión normalmente rectificará este problema.

Ocasionalmente, esta sensibilidad no desaparece y de hecho puede empeorarse. Normalmente esto no está relacionado al procedimiento de la cementación/adhesión sino que es resultado de la cantidad de destrucción del diente original que usted experimentó a causa del deterioro. Aunque el diente puede parecer estar bien cuando la restauración provisional (temporal) está puesta, en realidad el nervio puede estar muriéndose lentamente. En esta situación, el diente restaurado puede experimentar la muerte eventual del nervio. Entonces el diente necesitará el tratamiento endodóntico.

Cuidado de Su Nueva Restauración

Después de la cementación o adhesión, es aconsejable **no** usar el diente para masticar comida hasta que regrese la sensación normal al área (si el área se anestesió). Los cementos se fijan sólo parcialmente mientras usted esté en la oficina y requieren por lo menos 24 horas para lograr mejores propiedades físicas. Por eso, no ponga estrés en los dientes cementados o adheridos por 24 horas (es decir—ningún masticar de goma de mascar, melcocha, nueces o roscas de pan, etc.)

Para su salud oral continua es muy importante cepillar los dientes y usar el hilo dental normalmente después de este procedimiento. Favor de regresar donde nosotros para sus citas normales de cuidado preventivo repetido en los intervalos de _____ meses. Entonces los problemas que pueden desarrollarse alrededor de las restauraciones (o de hecho, alrededor de cualquier otros dientes) puede encontrarse en una etapa temprana y repararse fácilmente. Le enviaremos una notificación cuando le toque la cita pero usted también debe marcar esta fecha en su propio calendario y llamar la oficina si no ha recibido la notificación.

También recomendamos el uso diario de un enjuague bucal que contenga fluoruro. Siga las instrucciones en la etiqueta. Se ha demostrado que la aplicación tópica regular del fluoruro reduce la incidencia de algunos tipos de problemas dentales.

Expectativas

Usted debe recibir muchos años de servicio de estas restauraciones. Hemos usado la mejor información y los mejores procedimientos y materiales disponibles hoy en día para su fabricación. Es posible que requieran un reemplazo si se fracturan debido a fuerza o trauma extrema—igual a los dientes naturales. No muerda los objetos extremadamente duros con los dientes que se han cementado o adherido. La gingiva (la encía) también puede retirarse de los márgenes de la restauración, y exponer el metal o la estructura dental original. Puede tomar varios años antes de que esto se note. Normalmente el retiro es un resultado del proceso normal de envejecer y no indica que la restauración es un fracaso. Sin embargo, si el retiro causa un problema cosmético, usted puede desear que se rehaga la restauración. El deterioro también puede comenzar cerca de la restauración. Si se atiende el deterioro en una etapa temprana, el arreglarlo no es un problema mayor.

Si usted tiene cualquier pregunta sobre estas instrucciones, favor de sentirse libre de preguntarnos.

Procedimiento de Alargamiento de la Corona

Un procedimiento para alargar la corona es necesario cuando clínicamente no hay suficiente estructura dental visible o accesible para la retención correcta de una restauración de molde (una corona o un onlay) o para una restauración rutinaria (una empastadura). También es necesario si el tejido de la encía tiene una mala posición o forma, o para mejorar la apariencia cosmética de los dientes. También se puede requerir para hacer una impresión exitosa para una restauración de molde. Los tejidos gingivales suaves se modificarán, se reposicionarán o se reformarán para que se pueda colocar una restauración. Si el diente se ha deteriorado severamente, una alargamiento de la corona puede ser necesario para exponer más completamente el área deteriorada y permitir una mejor preparación para la empastadura final.

Muchas veces, este alargamiento de la corona será mínimo y se puede hacer en nuestra oficina. Puede envolver la electrocirugía o un procedimiento de bisturí y suturas. Seleccionaremos el método basado en sus circunstancias individuales. Si la modificación es extensiva y envuelve muchos dientes o el hueso de apoyo, le podemos enviara a un periodontista (especialista de encías) para evaluación y tratamiento. A veces, después de completar el alargamiento de la corona y que el tejido se ha curado, el diente puede exhibir sensibilidad transitoria a los cambios termales. Con el tiempo, la sensibilidad disminuye. Tampoco queremos que el tejido que se ha eliminado crezca de nuevo. Si vuelve a crecer, lo cual puede pasar, podría necesitar que se remueva otra vez.

Las restauraciones colocadas en la estructura dental saludable durarán lo más posible. Un diente o varios dientes pueden estar envueltos en el procedimiento de alargamiento. En muchos casos, sería imposible obtener un resultado satisfactorio si no se hace el alargamiento de la corona. La incomodidad postoperatoria es normalmente mínima, a menos que el alargamiento ha sido extensivo, como cuando el hueso subyacente tiene que ser reformado. Los aliviadores de dolor sin receta normalmente son muy adecuados. El tiempo de curación varía dependiendo del grado del procedimiento. Algunas veces elegiremos terminar la restauración o hacer la impresión final en el momento del alargamiento de la corona; otras veces tendremos que esperar que el lugar se cure. El tiempo de curación puede ser de 4 a 6 semanas. Se le hablará de esto cuando se sugiera el procedimiento de alargamiento de la corona.

Si le recomiendan un alargamiento de la corona, usted debe conseguir que se haga, si no la restauración final puede tener problemas y la probabilidad de obtener una restauración clínicamente exitosa se reduciría seriamente.

Si usted tiene cualquier pregunta sobre el procedimiento de alargamiento de la corona, favor de sentirse libre de preguntarnos.

Defecto en el Lugar de Extracción

Los dientes se extraen por varias razones, incluyendo la enfermedad periodontal, el deterioro extremo y por razones ortodónticas. Una vez que se ha extraído un diente, la forma del reborde (es decir, el hueso de sostén y la encía donde el diente estaba situado y retenido) cambia. Si hubo una pérdida extensiva de hueso o si hubo que extraer el diente quirúrgicamente (se tuvo que recortar el hueso para ganar acceso al área), el cambio será más dramático. El reborde se encoge, colapsa hacia sí mismo y con el tiempo disminuye en su ancho y altura. Al pasar más tiempo después de la extracción, ocurren más cambios. Esto se llama un defecto en el lugar de extracción.

El defecto en el lugar de extracción presenta un problema cuando se va a restaurar el área con un puente o un implante. Cuando la arquitectura del reborde ha cambiado significativamente, el diente de reemplazo tendrá que desviarse de la forma ideal. Esto fácilmente podría hacer que el área sea más difícil de mantener limpia, difícil para que el dentista la restaure y bastante antiestética en su cosmética. Quizás la cosmética no le importe cuando se reemplaza en diente de atrás—uno que no es visible cuando usted habla o sonríe. Un defecto en el lugar de extracción en un área que es visible cuando usted habla o sonríe creará un problema estético severo. Cuanto más haya cambiado el reborde, más largo, ancho o grueso necesitará ser el pontic para llenar el lugar de extracción. Si usted tiene una línea de sonrisa que muestra el borde del diente o de la encía, el diente de reemplazo estará muy obviamente malformado. Nunca se verá bien y siempre será un fracaso cosmético.

Es claro que el lugar de la extracción tiene que reconstruirse para que el diente de reemplazo tenga una apariencia normal. Cuanto más cerca a lo ideal, mejor parecerá el diente de reemplazo. El lugar (o *reborde* como lo llama los dentistas) se restaurará a través de los procedimientos quirúrgicos periodontales menores en el tejido suave o en el tejido suave y duro. Si el reborde necesita sólo una pequeña cantidad de aumento, sólo se necesitarán los procedimientos de tejido suave. Si hay un defecto grande, también habrá que reemplazar el hueso subyacente de apoyo. Si el lugar es especialmente visible o necesita una cantidad extensiva de reconstrucción, puede ser necesario más de un procedimiento de aumento. Nuestra meta es hacer que el diente de reemplazo parezca crecer del lugar de extracción y no sólo descansar en el reborde del tejido suave.

Si se va a colocar un implante para que sirva de ancla para el diente de reemplazo, el lugar de extracción tiene que tener suficiente espesor y altura para rodear el implante correctamente. Estos procedimientos casi siempre envuelven la modificación del tejido duro (de hueso) y suave. Le informaremos lo que es más apropiado para usted.

Si usted tiene cualquier pregunta, favor de sentirse libre de preguntarnos.

Estructura Coronaria Remanente (Abrazadera)

Si un diente va a recibir una restauración de cobertura completa procesada en el laboratorio que será exitosa por mucho tiempo, hay varias variables que hay que atender. No puede haber ningún deterioro en el diente preparado. Su posición periodontal (de la encía y el hueso) tiene que estar saludable. La corona colocada en el diente tiene que tener un ajuste correcto, con la mordida ajustada bien y los márgenes de la interfaz de la corona/diente sellados y bien adaptados. Tiene que haber suficiente estructura dental para retener la corona y resistir las fuerzas externas que pueden desplazar la corona o fracturar el diente subyacente.

Aunque todas estas cosas son importantes, uno de los factores más importantes en una corona que será exitosa por mucho tiempo es que quede una estructura dental adecuada alrededor de la circunferencia del diente para que el diente pueda resistir las fuerzas laterales. Éstas son fuerzas que no se dirigen directamente hacia arriba y hacia abajo (paralelas) del eje largo del diente sino que son fuerzas vectoriales tangenciales aplicadas desde el lado (perpendicular al eje largo del diente).

Usted tiene un diente que ha sido dañado extensivamente debido al deterioro o fractura y queda muy poco del diente por encima del borde de la encía. En la odontología una abrazadera es un promedio de 2 mm de diente saludable no restaurado y no dañado que está disponible en los 360 grados alrededor del diente para que la corona lo "agarre". Aun si los postes (usados en los dientes tratados endodónticamente) o los pernos y las construcciones de base adherida se usan para restaurar la estructura dental debajo de una corona, a menos que esta abrazadera adecuada esté presente, el diente puede muy posiblemente ser demasiado débil para sostener una restauración y puede fracturarse bajo las fuerzas normales del masticar. La longevidad de la restauración está comprometida.

Si la abrazadera necesaria de 2 mm no está disponible alrededor de la circunferencia del diente, hay que crear una. Hay dos métodos para desarrollar una abrazadera. Si el diente se ha partido en o debajo del borde de la encía, se puede brotar ortodónticamente el diente (una extrusión forzada del diente remanente del hueso, se considera como una extracción sin dolor, lenta y muy controlada) hasta que haya suficiente diente disponible para que se pueda usar. Esto se puede hacer en aproximadamente un mes en la mayoría de los casos. El segundo método es eliminar tejido de la encía (y/o del hueso) para exponer los 2 mm necesarios del diente. Esto se puede hacer con un láser o con un procedimiento electroquirúrgico o con cirugía periodontal. El procedimiento seleccionado será una función de cuánto del diente hay que exponer, dónde está el diente, dónde está el borde de la encía con respecto a los dientes adyacentes y cuán lejos el área fracturada, a su distancia más profunda, del lugar del hueso subyacente. Tiene que haber por lo menos 2.5 mm de distancia entre el margen del diente preparado (y por ende, de la restauración final) y la parte superior del hueso. Este espacio se llama *ancho biológico*. Es crítico tener un ancho biológico suficiente. Si hay menos espacio disponible y no se crea más espacio, el tejido de la encía nunca se curará correctamente.

Después de usar las radiografías, la inspección clínica y una sonda periodontal para hacer medidas, determinaremos cuál curso de acción será mejor. Pueden haber tiempo y costo adicionales envueltos para establecer la abrazadera correcta, pero es vital hacer esto si se va a restaurar el diente con éxito por un tiempo largo.

Si usted tiene cualquier pregunta sobre el(los) procedimiento(s) necesario(s) para lograr una abrazadera clínicamente aceptable, favor de sentirse libre de preguntarnos.

Impresiones

Hay dos tipos de impresiones que tomamos rutinariamente en esta oficina. El primer tipo es para la fabricación de los modelos de estudio y los moldes diagnósticos. El segundo es para la construcción de las coronas, los puentes y las dentaduras parciales removibles procesadas en el laboratorio.

Impresiones Preliminares o para Modelos de Estudio

Las impresiones para los modelos de estudio son las impresiones más comunes que se hacen en una oficina dental. Se usa una cubeta de metal esterilizada o una cubeta plástica desechable para este procedimiento. La cubeta se ajusta aproximadamente a las dimensiones de su mandíbula superior o inferior y cubrirá sus dientes y su tejido de la encía. Una vez que esté ajustada, la cubeta se llena con un material suave y viscoso de impresión. Este material tiene la consistencia de una mezcla de masa de galletas dulces espesa. La cubeta de impresión se llena y se coloca sobre sus dientes y se presiona en su lugar. El material tomará desde 1 a 2 minutos para endurecerse. Las impresiones son absolutamente sin dolor y no requieren ninguna medicación ni preparación especial. El material tiene un sabor moderadamente agradable.

De esta impresión se harán modelos en piedra que son una replica muy semejante a sus dientes. Estos modelos nos permiten analizar sus dientes y diseñar su tratamiento dental correctamente. Investigamos las posibilidades de la ortodoncia (los frenillos), las cubetas hechas a la medida para blanquear/emblanquecer sus dientes y el reemplazo de dientes que faltan o están severamente dañados. Hacemos unas cubetas a la medida para impresiones finales, guías para las coronas provisionales, protectores bucales, férulas, etc.

Impresiones Finales

Este tipo de impresión es para la fabricación de coronas, puentes o dentaduras parciales. Las impresiones se hacen con un material diferente, uno que es mucho más preciso en demostrar las detalles más pequeños del área preparada. A causa del aumento en la necesidad de precisión, la impresión es diferente. Una cubeta fabricada a la medida muchas veces se hace del modelo hecho en la impresión preliminar. Este material se quedará en el lugar por 3 a 6 minutos. Frecuentemente, se ha usado un anestésico local para preparar el diente de modo que no debe haber ninguna incomodidad. No es raro que se tome una segunda o tercera impresión para asegurar que la restauración terminada tenga las proporciones precisas. Si la impresión no es correcta, la restauración final puede tener problemas.

Registro Oclusal

Con los dos tipos de impresiones, es una práctica estándar tomar un registro oclusal (de la mordida) durante la cita. Esto nos da la capacidad de relacionar los modelos de la mandíbula superior e inferior. La impresión se puede colocar en una cubeta o directamente en la superficie de mordida de sus dientes; entonces se le instruirá a morder y mantener esta mordedura hasta que el material se endurezca. La impresión para registrar la mordida se endurece muy rápidamente.

Si usted tiene cualquier pregunta sobre las impresiones, favor de sentirse libre de preguntarnos.

Postes

Después de sacar el tejido del nervio de un diente con la endodoncia (tratamiento del canal radicular), frecuentemente hay muy poca estructura dental remanente. Antes de poder colocar una corona (caperuza), una restauración de amalgama de plata o de resina adherida, se puede colocar un poste en el diente para ayudar a darle sostén y retención al diente remanente y a la restauración. El poste puede ser de molde hecho a la medida o un poste prefabricado.

Los postes prefabricados se pueden hacer de acero inoxidable, titanio o de cerámica o resina reforzada del color del diente. Se diseñan en varios diámetros y largos. Si usted cree que podría ser alérgico a cualquier metal, especialmente al níquel, déjenos saber antes de que seleccionemos cuál poste se va a usar. Se usa un taladro especial para eliminar parte del material de empastadura (guta percha) del canal radicular y para reformar el canal para el poste. El largo y el diámetro del poste corresponden a las dimensiones del espacio preparado en el canal. Una vez que se ha ajustado el poste, se cementa con un ionómero de vidrio u otro cemento o se adhiere en su lugar con una resina. La selección del medio de cementar es afectada por el largo y la posición del diente que recibirá el poste, el tipo de restauración que se pondrá sobre el poste y su historial pasado de deterioro dental.

Si se ha llenado un canal radicular con puntos de plata en vez de con guta percha, los puntos de plata probablemente necesitarán ser sacados y reemplazados, es decir que se rehará el canal radicular con el material de guta percha. El cemento que mantiene los puntos de plata en su lugar tiene la tendencia de disolverse y los puntos se aflojarán. Hay que colocar el nuevo poste y corona sobre una empastadura sólida del canal radicular para evitar problemas futuros que podrían requerir que se quite el poste y la corona que se acabó de colocar.

El poste ayudará a que la corona (o la empastadura) resista algunas de las tensiones que sufre un diente cuando usted mastica comidas duras o pegajosas. Reducirá la posibilidad de que el diente se parta en el borde de la encía. Servirá para retener cualquier empastadura, corona o construcción de base que se use para reconstruir el diente. Todavía es posible que el diente se parta en el borde de la encía, en la empastadura o en la corona o que se salga, aun con la corona en su lugar. Es más probable que se desplace si usted come comidas muy duras o pegajosas o las muerde de una manera incorrecta. Cuanto más estructura dental remanente sin dañar haya, menos probable será que esto ocurrirá. Se puede necesitar el alargamiento de la corona antes de colocar un poste y una corona para permitir el uso de más estructura dental.

Un poste de molde significa más trabajo por parte del dentista. Se necesitará al menos una visita adicional. De hecho, cuesta más que un poste prefabricado. No se usa tan rutinariamente como un poste prefabricado, sino en situaciones especiales. Se cementa o se adhiere en su lugar.

Si usted tiene cualquier pregunta sobre los postes, favor de sentirse libre de preguntarnos.

Ilustración en CD-ROM

Postes, Construcciones de Base-Corona y Alargamiento de la Corona

Postes

Después que la endodoncia ha extraído el tejido del nervio de un diente (tratamiento del canal radicular), frecuentemente queda muy poca estructura del diente que no está dañada. Antes de colocar una restauración, sea una corona (caperuza) o una empastadura adherida o de plata, se coloca un poste en el diente para ayudar a darle el sostén y la retención al diente remanente. El poste puede ser un poste hecho a la medida o uno prefabricado. El poste prefabricado se hace en varios diámetros, materiales y largos. Puede ser de metal o del color del diente. Se usa un taladro especial para eliminar parte del material de empastadura del canal radicular (guta percha) y para preparar y reformar el canal para el poste. Una vez que se ha ajustado el poste, se cementa en su lugar con un material de ionómero de vidrio o se adhiere con un cemento de resina. La selección del medio de cementar es afectada por el lago del poste, el lugar del diente donde se va a colocar el poste y la historia pasada de deterioro dental. Si el canal radicular existente se ha llenado con puntos de plata, hay que sacarlos antes de que se pueda construir la corona. Se ha demostrado que el cemento que mantiene los puntos de plata en los canales se disuelve rápidamente. La corona nueva tiene que colocarse sobre una empastadura de canal radicular sólida para evitar los problemas endodónticos futuros que pueden requerir que se saque la corona nueva.

El poste ayudará al diente a resistir algunas de las tensiones que sufre cuando usted mastica comidas duras o pegajosas. Reducirá la posibilidad que el diente se parta en el borde de la encía. También servirá para retener cualquier material de construcción de base, empastadura o corona que se haya usado en el diente. Todavía es posible que el diente se fracture, aun con el poste puesto. También es posible que el poste se desplace si usted come comidas especialmente duras o pegajosas y muerde de una manera incorrecta. Cuanto más diente original usted tenga, menos probable será que esto ocurra.

Construcción de Base-Corona

Una construcción de base o de corona se coloca cuando no resta suficiente estructura dental para retener la futura corona. Se puede hacer de amalgama de plata, de resina adherida o de ionómero de vidrio. La selección del material usado está relacionada a cuánto falta del diente y cuánto tiempo el diente tiene que estar en su lugar sin cementar la corona final. Normalmente, si se coloca un poste, también se requiere una construcción. Cuanto más estructura dental real o reconstruida haya disponible, mejor permanecerá en su lugar la corona final.

Alargamiento de la Corona

El alargamiento de la corona por medio de electrocirugía o cirugía convencional es un procedimiento hecho para corregir una de las siguientes condiciones:

- no queda suficiente estructura del diente para permitir la retención correcta de una corona
- estructura dental saludable/sólida que está debajo del tejido gingival (de la encía)
- tejido gingival que está en una posición o forma pobre

La electrocirugía permite la reposición, modificación o eliminación del tejido suave por medio de una corriente calibrada. La cirugía convencional se hace con un bisturí y envuelve la sutura. Cuando no hay suficiente estructura dental disponible para retener la corona, hay que exponer la estructura dental adecuada, y sacar el tejido de la encía necesario. Cuando el diente no se puede mantener aislado y seco durante los procedimientos dentales, es mucho más difícil, a veces imposible, obtener un resultado satisfactorio. La saliva, la sangre y el agua de su boca afectan el material dental en una manera adversa. Eliminar el tejido excesivo y no deseable permite que el diente se mantenga seco y así aumenta la posibilidad de un resultado bueno. Para decirlo más sencillamente, cuando el dentista no puede ver el área de trabajo, los resultados probablemente no serán satisfactorios.

Hay muy poco dolor postoperatorio asociado con el procedimiento electroquirúrgico. La mayoría de los pacientes dicen que lo sienten como una quemadura del queso caliente en una pizza. Un aliviador de dolor sin receta normalmente es adecuado. Ocasionalmente, el alargamiento de la corona no se puede terminar adecuadamente con la electrocirugía. El alargamiento de la corona con cirugía requerirá suturas y una demora en la impresión final para la corona mientras se cure el tejido. Cuatro a ocho semanas de tiempo de curación es normal. Cuando no se hace ninguno de los dos métodos de alargamiento de la corona, la posibilidad de éxito clínico se reduce seriamente.

Todos los postes y las construcciones de base-corona y el alargamiento de la corona están agrupados en esta página porque es muy común que estos problemas necesiten atenderse juntos. Si un diente necesita un tratamiento del canal radicular, normalmente está bastante descompuesto y difícil de restaurar. Cada procedimiento puede ser requerido individualmente o con uno o ambos procedimientos. Si hay que hacer cualquiera de estos procedimientos, se cobrará un honorario aparte del honorario para la corona.

Si usted tiene cualquier pregunta sobre los postes, las construcciones de base-corona y el alargamiento de la corona, favor de sentirse libre de preguntarnos.

Coronas Provisionales

Mientras se está fabricando una corona para usted, el diente o los dientes tratados tendrán una restauración provisional (temporal) que estará retenida por un cemento provisional. Esto es parte del tratamiento y no merece un honorario adicional. Sin embargo, hay varios casos cuando las coronas provisionales necesitan hacerse como un procedimiento separado e intermedio. A causa del tiempo y trabajo adicional envueltos, más allá de lo que se necesita para una corona o un puente, hay un honorario particular por el procedimiento.

Una situación donde la corona provisional merece un honorario particular envuelve un diente o unos dientes que están severamente deteriorados o fragmentados, en donde la vitalidad del nervio o la salud periodontal (de la encía) está en duda. Puede ser necesario reconstruir el diente lo antes posible de modo que la salud del nervio dentro del diente, y del tejido dental alrededor del diente, pueda ser evaluada a través del tiempo antes de proceder con la corona final. Cuando múltiples dientes necesitan este tratamiento, es habitual colocar coronas provisionales en cada uno a la vez. Si se completa cada diente individualmente antes de comenzar con el próximo diente, hay demasiada oportunidad para que los dientes restantes se deterioren más y así se complique el tratamiento y aumenten el costo total. Las coronas provisionales pueden estar colocadas por varios meses antes de comenzar el tratamiento adicional en el diente, después del cual el diente necesitará tener una preparación adicional y una corona provisional nueva.

Cuando el nervio en el diente dañado tiene la posibilidad de morirse, es más fácil salvar el diente con la terapia del canal radicular si no se ha colocado la corona final. Frecuentemente toma meses para determinar la salud del nervio. Y, de hecho, a pesar de usar una corona provisional de largo plazo, el nervio puede morirse años después de colocar la corona final. Cuando esto ocurre, el acceso para el tratamiento endodóntico se hace a través de la corona. En cuanto a los tejidos periodontales, si están infectados o en estado de salud pobre, tienen que curarse antes de tomar las impresiones finales. El tratamiento periodontal junto con una corona provisional bien ajustada fomentará la curación correcta. Después que el tejido periodontal esté saludable, su posición en cuanto a los márgenes de la corona cambiará y se preparará el diente de nuevo y se hará una segunda restauración provisional.

Otra razón para colocar las coronas provisionales de plazo es para estabilizar los dientes flojos y determinar el sostén necesario para las coronas de molde final. Cuando un diente que está envuelto en el sostén para un puente o una férula tiene un pronóstico dudoso, es buena idea hacer el puente provisional primero y dejar que funcione junto con el diente (o los dientes) por algún tiempo a ver cuán bien responden. Si el diente resulta no tener remedio, se puede extraer. Si los dientes son restaurados por cuadrantes (tres, cuatro, cinco o más dientes), puede ser necesario colocar coronas provisionales de largo tiempo en el arco contrario para establecer las relaciones oclusas (de mordida) entre los arcos.

Hay muchas y variadas razones porque se pueden necesitar puentes provisionales de largo plazo. Pueden permanecer en su lugar desde meses a años, especialmente en los casos muy complicados tales como cuando hay muchos dientes deteriorados y enfermedad de las encías moderada a severa que necesita corrección antes de finalmente colocar las coronas. En los casos más grandes, las limitaciones financieras pueden dictar que el tratamiento se introduzca paulatinamente durante un marco de tiempo más largo. En vez de dejar que los dientes se empeoren durante este tiempo, se hacen coronas provisionales de largo plazo para mantener las cosas en su lugar hasta que se pueda continuar el tratamiento.

Es importante que usted entienda por qué las coronas provisionales podrían ser necesarias para su salud dental.

Si usted tiene cualquier pregunta las coronas provisionales de largo plazo, favor de sentirse libre de preguntarnos.

Coronas Provisionales: Instrucciones Postoperatorias

Usted ha recibido una:

❑ restauración plástica provisional retenida con un cemento provisional
❑ restauración final que se ha cementado con un cemento provisional por un periodo de prueba

- El cemento provisional requiere más o menos 45 minutos para fijarse correctamente. Favor de evitar masticar comida durante este periodo de tiempo.
- Las restauraciones provisionales o finales ahora se mantienen en su lugar con un cemento provisional. Este cemento débil se usa para facilitar la remoción de la restauración para procedimientos adicionales. No mastique nada pegajoso mientras se está usando el cemento provisional. Estas restauraciones provisionales están diseñadas para estar colocadas sólo por un periodo de tiempo corto. El cemento final que se usará es mucho más fuerte.
- La restauración provisional puede no asemejarse a la restauración final en su tamaño, forma ni en ninguna otra manera.
- Ciertas comidas pueden adherirse al material de restauración provisional. Esto no pasará con las restauraciones finales de oro o porcelana.
- Las restauraciones provisionales **no** son fuertes. Pueden romperse o salirse. Si esto ocurre, llame a nuestra oficina y las atendremos. Si usted está en algún lugar donde no puede contactar a un dentista y la corona o puente provisional se sale, vaya a una farmacia y compre un tubo de adhesivo dental en crema. Limpie la restauración provisional y colóquela en su diente o dientes con un poco de adhesivo puesto en cada corona que se asienta sobre un diente preparado. Este adhesivo de dentadura mantendrá la restauración provisional colocada hasta que usted pueda regresar a nuestra oficina para una tratamiento adicional. **¡No deje la restauración provisional fuera de su boca por un periodo de tiempo extendido!** Los dientes que rodean los dientes preparados o los mismos dientes preparados pueden moverse y entonces la restauración final puede no encajar bien.
- Si usted tiene una **restauración final que está cementada por un tiempo corto con un cemento provisional,** favor de evitar las comidas pegajosas tales como la goma de mascar, etc. El masticar estos tipos de comidas puede causar que el cemento provisional falle; y el puente, corona, onlay o inlay final se afloje.
- Favor de cepillar sus dientes y usar el hilo dental diariamente tal como le han enseñado. Si usted tiene colocada una restauración provisional, cuando usa el hilo dental, comience como lo normal pero cuando es hora de sacar el hilo dental, suéltelo de una mano y sáquelo de entre los dientes con la otra mano. Esto reducirá la posibilidad que el hilo dental "se encaje" en el borde de la restauración provisional y la saque del diente.
- Es posible que los dientes preparados, ahora cubiertos con la restauración provisional, sean sensitivos al calor, frío o a los dulces. Esto no es raro. Las restauraciones provisionales pueden filtrar saliva u otros fluidos en el diente recién preparado (taladrado). Esto no ocurrirá con la restauración final.

Instrucciones Adicionales

❑ Enjuague con gluconato de chlorhexidina _____ veces al día por una semana después de la cementación final.
❑ Enjuague con agua salada tibia tal como le han enseñado.
❑ Enjuague con_____.
❑ Cepille los dientes y use el hilo dental como le han enseñado después de cada comida.

Modelos de Estudio y Modelos de Cera

Bastante frecuentemente un paciente tendrá problemas dentales que requieren un análisis más detallado para determinar las posibles soluciones. Se pueden examinar los dientes directamente, pero a causa de las limitaciones impuestas por la lengua, los labios, los cachetes y el pequeño ángulo visual desde el frente de la boca, la capacidad de proveer un plan de tratamiento apropiado puede estar comprometida. A medida que más dientes falten y más dientes se muevan de donde deben estar, especialmente en los casos donde el problema ha existido por muchos años, más opciones para el tratamiento son posibles. Esto puede ser el caso para el tratamiento dental extensivo o para sólo unos pocos dientes que necesitan restauración.

Necesitaremos hacer modelos de estudio (impresiones) de los dientes y también haremos un registro de cómo se encuentran para ayudar a planear el tratamiento. Podremos ver cosas en los modelos que no podemos ver clínicamente. También podemos trabajar con los modelos de sus dientes entre las citas. ¡Y esto definitivamente es una conveniencia para usted! Los modelos nos mostrarán muchos factores, especialmente en el movimiento de dientes, tales como, si los dientes se han movido, cuán lejos se han movido, cómo pueden afectar a los otros dientes y también otras consideraciones. Si usted está pensando en los puentes o coronas fijas o en los puentes removibles (parciales) para reemplazar los dientes que faltan, el diseño debe ser exacto desde el momento que comienza el tratamiento para obtener los mejores resultados.

Usamos un "modelo de cera" diagnóstico para ayudarnos (y a usted) a visualizar los cambios posibles en la forma y la alineación de sus dientes. El modelo de cera muestra los dientes y el tejido de la encía, normalmente en yeso blanco con la adición de cera blanca. Los modelos originales de estudio proveen una vista en tres dimensiones de la condición "anterior" de sus dientes y el modelo de cera dará un retrato de "después" en tres dimensiones de cómo se verán sus dientes, los reemplazos de los dientes, etc. cuando el tratamiento sea completado. El modelo de cera muchas veces se usa cuando hay que considerar los cambios cosméticos moderados a significantes. En conjunto con el modelo de cera, es posible tener el retrato anterior convertido a una imagen digital y luego modificarla en la computadora para mostrar una imagen de "después". El retrato digitalizado hará visibles sus labios, cachetes, tejido de la encía y cara y en el color apropiado.

El modelo de cera es valioso para usted también. Podrá juzgar los cambios propuestos y aprobarlos. Si no le gustan, es relativamente sencillo hacer que el modelo de cera se cambie para conseguir una apariencia diferente. Una vez que usted y nosotros hayamos aprobado el modelo de cera, se usará como la base para el tratamiento anticipado. Cuanto mejor se planee un tratamiento, mejor será la posibilidad de un resultado exitoso.

Hay un costo adicional por los modelos de estudio o por el modelo diagnóstico de cera. Los honorarios por los modelos de estudio son fijos. Los honorarios por el modelo diagnóstico de cera dependen de la cantidad de dientes que se están modificando. Para un cambio extensivo un honorario de varios cientos de dólares es posible.

Si usted tiene cualquier pregunta sobre la necesidad o el uso de los modelos diagnósticos de estudio o de cera, favor de sentirse libre de preguntarnos.

Dentaduras Completas

Las dentaduras completas reemplazan un arco completo de dientes que faltan para restaurar la apariencia facial y de mascar. Se puede construir una dentadura para reemplazar los dientes superiores que faltan, los dientes inferiores que faltan o los dos.

Una dentadura normalmente se construye de una base acrílica (plástica), teñida de color rosa para que parezca al tejido de la encía que cubre. Los dientes son plásticos o de porcelana. La selección de cuál tipo de material se usará para los dientes se basará en nuestro discernimiento y en cuáles son los dientes que están en el arco contrario. La porcelana va contra porcelana. El acrílico va contra acrílico o contra el diente natural.

Si usted ya tiene una dentadura o unas dentaduras, la construcción de una dentadura nueva es relativamente fácil. Su boca está familiarizada con la sensación de usar una dentadura. Las impresiones preliminares se hacen y se usan para diseñar y fabricar unas cubetas de impresión más exactas. Estas cubetas se usan para hacer una impresión maestra final de la cual se hará la dentadura. La alineación de los dientes y el grueso de la dentadura se establecen en cera y se verifican. Se escogen los dientes por su color, forma y material. Se colocan en la cera y se prueban en la boca. Cuando usted aprueba la forma, el diseño y la posición de los dientes, el laboratorio dental terminará el proceso en acrílico. Luego se regresan a la oficina y se entregan a usted. Se ajustarán en este momento. Usted debe esperar hacer varias visitas con nosotros mientras las dentaduras se establecen y se desarrollan áreas de dolor. No espere que las dentaduras nuevas le queden igual a las viejas. No se pueden duplicar dentaduras exactas. Siempre usted las sentirá diferentes. No peores, sólo diferentes.

Si le han extraído uno o algunos dientes recientemente o si le van a hacer una dentadura completa después de que usted ha usado una dentadura parcial removible, necesitará más tiempo para ajustarse a la nueva dentadura completa. Puede tomar 3 a 6 meses para que el tejido suave se cure y se reforme completamente después de una extracción. Cuanto más dientes se extraen, más cambio habrá y más tiempo tomará para curarse. Muchas veces, se hace una dentadura antes de pasar este periodo de tiempo. Debe esperar tener más áreas de dolor y más ajustes antes que la dentadura le quede cómoda. También puede esperar que le tengan que rebasar la dentadura después de algunos meses para compensar por ese cambio en el tejido. El rebasar llena el espacio que se desarrolla en el lugar de extracción debajo de la dentadura. Las dentaduras parciales tienen alguna retención mecánica de grapas en los dientes. Las dentaduras completas no tienen esta ayuda y son más difíciles de mantener en su lugar.

Si usted tiene una dentadura o unas dentaduras, asegúrese de sacarlas diariamente. No duerma con ellas puestas. Sus encías necesitan la oportunidad de recibir circulación de sangre fresca no impedida. Las dentaduras tienden a restringir el flujo de sangre. La placa puede acumularse en su dentadura y en su tejido de la encía. Use un cepillo de diente muy suave para cepillar sus encías suavemente. Asegúrese de mantener limpia sus dentaduras con el cepillado diario con un cepillo de dentadura y un producto para limpiar dentaduras—y asegúrese de guardarlas en agua cuando no la esté usando.

Si usted tiene cualquier pregunta las dentaduras completas, favor de sentirse libre de preguntarnos.

Dentaduras Inmediatas

Las dentaduras inmediatas completas o parciales se hacen cuando se extraen los dientes en el mismo día que se insertan las dentaduras terminadas. Las dentaduras inmediatas son diferentes de las dentaduras regulares porque las impresiones finales se hacen antes de que algunos o todos los dientes que serán eliminados sean extraídos. Las dentaduras fabricadas tradicionalmente se construyen para reemplazar una dentadura completa que ya existe. Ningún tiempo de curación es necesario y la dentadura se asentará mucho mejor porque las impresiones reflejarán precisamente los tejidos suaves en los cuales descansa la base de la dentadura.

Con la construcción de una dentadura inmediata, se aproxima el encaje correcto de la base de la dentadura. Como los dientes todavía están en su lugar cuando se construye y se prueba la dentadura, el ajuste no será tan exacto inicialmente. Es más difícil probar la dentadura inmediata para verificar su ajuste y apariencia cuando los dientes todavía están en su lugar. Esto es más cierto cuanto los dientes naturales que se extraerán se han desplazado lejos de su posición original. Se hacen las dentaduras inmediatas para que el paciente no se vea obligado a estar sin dientes mientras sanan los tejidos de la encía y los rebordes de tejido restantes alcanzan su forma final. Esta curación final puede tomar 3 a 6 meses después de extraer los dientes.

La dentadura inmediata se insertará en el mismo día que se extraen los dientes. Por esto, el paciente estará adormecido e hinchado por la anestesia local y no podrá decir mucho sobre la comodidad de la base de la dentadura y el encaje de los dientes de la dentadura con la mandíbula y los dientes contrarios. Debe esperar que haya varias citas con nosotros durante el periodo de curación mientras se baja la hinchazón y se establece la base de la dentadura. Su mordida cambiará y necesitará reajustarse. Cuanto más dientes se extraigan en el día que se entrega la dentadura inmediata, más tiempo tomará curarse y más áreas adoloridas usted tendrá.

A veces le aconsejaremos la extracción de algunos dientes mientras se hace la dentadura, dejando sólo algunos pocos dientes frontales en su lugar. Esto ayudará en conseguir un ajuste más preciso de la dentadura inmediata. Por supuesto, cada caso es único. Debe esperar que haya muchas áreas adoloridas y lugares donde el tejido se abra por la fricción. Cuando ocurra esto, quítese la dentadura y venga a vernos inmediatamente. Si usted sigue usando la dentadura sin ajustarla, el tejido de la encía se dañará mucho y tomará más tiempo para curarse. Aunque el proceso general de hacer una dentadura inmediata es similar al de hacer una dentadura completa tradicional, la construcción de la dentadura inmediata plantea unos problemas diferentes y más significantes.

Después que el tejido se cure por completo en el lugar de la extracción, la base de la dentadura necesitará que se le añada más plástico. Esto se llama *un rebase*. El plástico adicional llenará el espacio entre la base de la dentadura y la posición nueva del tejido suave. Originalmente, este espacio se estimó en los lugares donde los dientes todavía no se habían extraído. La contracción del tejido continuará por algún tiempo, pero después de aproximadamente 6 meses, es suficientemente lento para que sea práctico hacer el rebase. Con las dentaduras inmediatas, o después de usar dentaduras por algunos años, el cambio en el tejido puede ser suficiente para hacer necesario otros rebases. Cuando usted envejece y no tiene dientes, el hueso en las mandíbulas se vuelve más pequeño. La base plástica de la dentadura no cambia con los cambios en la mandíbula y por eso un rebase periódico es necesario.

Es posible que después de muchos años de tener dientes que faltan, el hueso en el cual se asienta la dentadura se ponga tan pequeño que es difícil, si no imposible, que una dentadura permanezca correctamente en su lugar. Los implantes dentales pueden ayudar a retener la dentadura. Algunos procedimientos quirúrgicos pueden ayudar.

Si usted tiene cualquier pregunta sobre las dentaduras inmediatas, favor de sentirse libre de preguntarnos.

Dentaduras Parciales

Una dentadura parcial está diseñada para reemplazar uno o varios dientes que faltan. Usted puede considerar una dentadura parcial removible para reemplazar los dientes que faltan si:

- usted tiene dientes que faltan
- los dientes restantes no pueden aceptar un puente fijo
- no hay suficiente hueso para implantes
- las finanzas son limitadas

Hace años que los dentistas han hecho y los pacientes han usado las dentaduras parciales removibles. Las dentaduras parciales están compuestas de tres materiales diferentes. Una base de molde de metal con brazos agarradores contiene un tejido de plástico de color rosa y dientes plásticos o de porcelana. Las grapas son de color plata y, dependiendo de las circunstancias individuales, pueden ser o no ser visibles cuando usted habla o sonríe. Estas grapas son absolutamente necesarias para mantener el parcial en su lugar. La forma y la posición de sus dientes restantes y cuáles dientes se reemplazarán dictan su ubicación y diseño. Le mostraremos dónde se ubicarán las grapas en su boca. En la mayoría de los casos, la cantidad de preparación (taladrado) que sus dientes necesitan es mínima para asegurar un diseño de grapa exitoso. Frecuentemente no hay necesidad de una inyección de un anestésico local. Esto no es como el puente fijo, que siempre requiere una reducción significativa del diente para obtener el diseño y ajuste correcto.

Si usted encuentra que la apariencia de las grapas es ofensiva, entonces podría considerar posibilidades diferentes. Es común colocar coronas en los dientes que son agarrados por los brazos metálicos y luego colocar las grapas **dentro** de las coronas. Esto le dará una apariencia más natural, pero aumentaría el costo final del tratamiento. Envuelve la preparación significativa del diente natural y usted podría desear repensar la posibilidad de los puentes fijos o los implantes.

La base de la dentadura parcial descansará levemente en el tejido de su encía. Se espera que usted necesitará ajustes a la base en algún momento en el futuro. Normalmente esto significa una adición de más material de color rosa a la base de la dentadura. Los brazos de la grapa se aflojarán y a veces necesitarán apretarse. La pérdida o el aumento de peso también afectará el ajuste de la base del parcial.

Aunque un parcial es menos costoso que un puente fijo, el cual consiste de metal y porcelana cementados en su lugar, hay varios posibles inconvenientes. Es mucho más voluminoso que un puente y es más difícil de usar inicialmente. Usted puede tener que ajustar la manera de hablar para acomodar el volumen adicional. Con el tiempo esto no será muy problemático. Y dependiendo de la posición de las grapas de retención, pueden ser visibles cuando usted habla o sonríe.

No duerma con las dentaduras parciales puestas. Definitivamente hay que sacarlas durante el tiempo de dormir para limpiarlas y dar a los dientes agarrados la oportunidad de descansar. El tejido de la encía debajo de la dentadura necesita la oportunidad de respirar y de restablecer la circulación sanguínea apropiada. La dentadura parcial puede comprimir el tejido y reducir el flujo de sangre en el área. La placa puede acumularse en su dentadura y en su tejido de la encía. Use un cepillo de dientes muy suave para cepillar sus encías suavemente. También cepille su dentadura parcial diariamente con un cepillo de dentadura y un producto para limpiar dentaduras. Siempre guarde su dentadura parcial en agua cuando no la esté usando.

Si usted tiene cualquier pregunta sobre las dentaduras parciales removibles, favor de sentirse libre de preguntarnos.

Odontología Restaurativa

Revisión del Contenido: Odontología Restaurativa

Restauraciones
Cada documento describe el uso, las ventajas y las desventajas de las siguientes restauraciones:

Restauraciones de Amalgama

Amalgamas y Resinas Adheridas:Instrucciones Postoperatorias

Restauraciones de Resina Adherida: Empastaduras del Color del Diente para los Dientes Posteriores

Microodontología: Restauración Preventiva de la Resina

Restauraciones de Cobertura Parcial

Inlays y Onlays de Porcelana

Inlays y Onlays de Resina

La Empastadura "Permanente"

Procedimientos Correctivos
Restauraciones Defectuosas
Explica que las restauraciones pueden degradar y/o fallar en cierto tiempo, y necesitan ser reparadas o reemplazadas. Describe los tipos de defectos y el servicio necesario.

Recontorno del Esmalte
Relata el uso del recontorno del esmalte, particularmente en relación con otros posibles tratamientos.

Restauraciones Sedativas
Las indicaciones y los procedimientos para el uso de restauraciones sedativas se discuten.

Seguridad y Garantía
Seguridad de la Amalgama de Plata y de los Metales Comunes
Asegura al paciente nuevamente que la amalgama de plata y los metales comunes no se utilizan en esta práctica. Incluye las razones.

Garantía de los Materiales Restaurativos
Documenta las condiciones de la política de la oficina para el reemplazo de restauraciones con énfasis en la adherencia de los intervalos cuidado repetido.

Garantía del Diente Severamente Comprometido
Este documento indica los límites de restaurar el diente severamente comprometido junto con los factores que pueden limitar la longevidad del tratamiento.

Restauraciones de Amalgama

Las restauraciones de amalgama de plata son los materiales de empastadura de plata tradicionales. Han sido utilizados con éxito por todos los dentistas por más de 150 años. Las empastaduras de amalgama de plata fueron creadas originalmente para ser un material de empastadura sustituto de bajo costo para aquellos pacientes que no tenían los recursos para pagar las restauraciones estándares de oro. Pueden ser utilizadas para sustituir cantidades pequeñas o grandes de la estructura del diente que es perdida por deterioro o fractura. No son sensibles a la técnica. Se componen de plata, estaño, mercurio, cobre y de otros metales. Algunos de los materiales más nuevos de amalgama de plata son libres de mercurio. No tenemos ningún estudio de largo plazo en cómo estas amalgamas sin mercurio servirán.

Las amalgamas de plata disponibles tienen una expectativa de vida de 14 años con una desviación de más o menos 14 años. Éstas pueden durar un tiempo largo o necesitan ser reemplazadas en menos de un año desde que se colocaron. Al igual que con las restauraciones de resina, mientras más pequeña la empastadura, más tiempo puede durar. Éste sigue siendo el material restaurativo predilecto para muchos dentistas pero este número está disminuyendo. La mayoría de las restauraciones para los dientes de atrás, sin importar el tamaño, son de amalgama de plata. Con la llegada de nuevos materiales de resina adherida, muchos dientes posteriores (de atrás) que previamente habrían sido restaurados con amalgama ahora se están restaurando con resinas del color del diente o materiales de porcelana que se conservan más y tienen una apariencia natural. Las empastaduras de amalgama de plata ahora pueden también ser unidas cuando queda poco del diente. Esto, claro, añadirá al honorario total cobrado por la restauración.

Las desventajas de las empastaduras de plata son estéticas. Es imposible hacer que parezcan naturales y la apariencia se deteriora mientras el tiempo pasa. Si el esmalte que le rodea es fino, el color gris/negro del metal se verá a través. Pueden hacer que el diente se vuelva oscuro. No añaden ninguna fuerza al diente (a menos que estén unidas). Debilitan el diente porque estas tienen una proporción expansión/contracción más grande que la del diente circundante. Estas fuerzas pueden, después de un tiempo, causar la fractura del diente. No se consideran una restauración conservadora porque requieren más preparación (taladrado) del diente que necesita ser removido debido al deterioro. Este taladrado adicional es estrictamente para permitir la retención de la restauración. En algunos casos, puede ser más costo efectivo y mejor para la salud gingival (de la encía) el colocar una restauración de molde (corona u onlay). Éste sería el caso cuando la empastadura de plata sería grande. Cuando hay cantidades extensas de la estructura del diente para ser reconstruidas/reemplazadas, frecuentemente es difícil el establecerle el contorno fisiológico apropiado al diente. La estructura restante del diente puede ser más propensa a fracturarse.

Las ventajas de las empastaduras de amalgama de plata son que son rápidas y fáciles colocar, relativamente baratas y tienen un historial de éxito probado.

Si las finanzas son una preocupación importante y la estética no es importante, entonces este material es conveniente para todos los tipos de restauraciones. Si la caries es pequeña o en una parte del diente no previamente dañada, una restauración de resina más conservadora será una mejor selección.

Si usted tiene cualquier pregunta sobre las restauraciones de amalgama de plata, favor de sentirse libre de preguntarnos.

Amalgamas y Resinas Adheridas: Instrucciones Postoperatorias

Usted acaba de tener uno o más dientes restaurados (empastados) con amalgama de plata o materiales de resina (color del diente/adherida), o preparado para un inlay/onlay o corona. Cuán rápido usted se ajusta a la nueva restauración depende del tamaño de la restauración y de la proximidad a la pulpa (nervio). Mientas más grande la restauración, usualmente, más tiempo le tomará el llegar a acostumbrarse.

Masticación

Si le han puesto un anestésico local, por favor no mastique en esa área hasta que vuelva la sensación completa. Cuando está "adormecido", no puede sentir si se está mordiendo su cachete o labio. Si le han colocado una empastadura de **plata/metal,** requerirá un mínimo de 2 horas después de que sale de la oficina antes de que pueda masticar en ella. Si usted come antes de que la empastadura de plata se fije adecuadamente, la empastadura se puede romper y requerir reemplazo. Si le han colocado una restauración de **resina,** la resina se fija inmediatamente, y puede comer cuando el efecto del anestésico se haya ido completamente.

Oclusión

La oclusión (mordida) de una restauración nueva ya se ha ajustado. Si le han anestesiado, puede que no pueda notar si la mordida se siente normal. Espere hasta que la anestesia se vaya y entonces, si la oclusión no es cómoda, llame a esta oficina para ajustarla. No creemos en una mordida "desgastándose", sin importar el material usado. Si le han colocado múltiples restauraciones, por favor deseé tiempo para ajustarse a ellas antes de que llame la oficina. Esto puede tomar uno o dos días. Sin embargo, si la mordida está fuera de lugar y no se corrige, usted podría romper la empastadura o el diente subyacente. Hemos verificado su oclusión antes de que saliera de nuestra oficina pero su diente todavía estaba anestesiado, y puede que no haya podido sentir la mordida bien. Es a menudo difícil hacer que los dientes se encuentren como normalmente se encuentran bajo estas circunstancias. No es infrecuente que una restauración nueva necesite un leve ajuste.

Tamaño

Las siguientes restauraciones eran: ❑ **normal en tamaño y forma**: diente #s _____

❑ **profunda y/o ancha**: diente #s _____

Cuando las restauraciones son muy grandes, es posible que en el futuro el diente se pueda fracturar y necesite una restauración de molde (corona u onlay) para ser restaurado correctamente. Si la restauración fue profunda, es posible que el nervio pueda morir y pueda necesitar terapia endodóntica (tratamiento del canal radicular). Esto puede llegar a ser evidente mañana o a 10 años de ahora. Si una amalgama de plata muy grande o una restauración adherida se rompe al poco tiempo de ser colocada, hay una gran probabilidad de que al material de empastadura se le está exigiendo que reemplace más estructura del diente de lo que fue diseñado para reemplazar. En esta situación el diente será mejor restaurado con una restauración de molde.

Exposición

La naturaleza del diseño de la preparación para la restauración o el grado del deterioro ha causado la **exposición** del nervio en el diente # _____ o una **exposición aproximada** en el diente # _____ . Cuando el nervio estuvo expuesto, se colocó un medicamento en el lugar de la exposición y puede haberse curado, pero es posible que sea necesario tratamiento endodóntico, (terapia del canal radicular) en algún momento en el futuro. Si había una exposición aproximada, también se colocó medicamento en el sitio, pero hay poca posibilidad de tratamiento endodóntico en el futuro. En cualquiera de los casos, espere que el diente sea muy sensible a los cambios de temperaturas, especialmente temperaturas frías, por varias semanas.

Sensibilidad

Cada vez que un diente es preparado (taladrado) para una empastadura, la estructura del diente es removida muy rápidamente. El proceso de desgaste natural que ocurre en los dientes de todos procede mucho más lentamente. La respuesta de un nervio vital, saludable a este desgaste es el retirarse y depositar una capa de aislamiento entre el nervio y la superficie del diente. Normalmente, el desgaste del diente prosigue más o menos el mismo paso mientras el nervio se retira y deposita aislamiento. Cuando se taladra un diente, la estructura del diente es removida mucho más rápido de lo que el nervio puede "defenderse". Una respuesta del nervio es llegar a ser sensible a los cambios de temperatura. Esto persistirá hasta que la recesión y el proceso de aislamiento puedan ponerse al día al retiro rápido de la estructura del diente causado por el taladro. Esta sensibilidad puede durar de varios días a varios meses. Generalmente, mientras más taladrado, más es la sensibilidad que experimenta y por más tiempo. Varios otros factores también contribuyen a la sensibilidad a la temperatura postoperativa, pero la selección del material de empastadura—la empastadura de amalgama de plata o la resina del color del diente adherida—**no** es una causa típica. Cuando están hechas correctamente, las empastaduras blancas no son más propensas a ser sensibles que las empastaduras de plata.

Cuidado Oral de Sí Mismo y Cuidado Repetido

Usted puede (¡y por favor hágalo!) cepillar y limpiar con hilo dental sus dientes después de que ha pasado el efecto del anestésico local. No hay necesidad de abstenerse de la rutina normal y diaria de cuidado oral de sí mismo normal, diaria. Continúe con sus citas de mantenimiento de la higiene oral en el intervalo que hemos recomendado previamente. Los problemas que pudieron desarrollarse alrededor de las restauraciones pueden ser encontrados en las etapas tempranas y ser reparados fácilmente. Si usted espera demasiado tiempo, la restauración entera puede tener que ser hecha de nuevo.

Si usted tiene cualesquiera preguntas sobre estas instrucciones, siéntase por favor libre preguntarnos.

Restauraciones de Resina Adherida: Empastaduras del Color del Diente para los Dientes Posteriores

Las restauraciones del color del diente se han utilizado en la odontología por mucho tiempo. Varias variaciones de estos materiales se han utilizado en los dientes delanteros por muchos años. La nueva generación de empastadura del color del diente (resinas) es también usada para restaurar caries en los dientes traseros. Esto es especialmente cierto cuando la restauración sería visible cuando usted habla o sonríe. El uso de los materiales de empastadura de amalgama de plata en restauraciones de tamaños de pequeñas a medianas está disminuyendo. Se puede esperar que estas resinas del color del diente posterior (de atrás) duren varios años. Una estimado razonable en este momento es aproximadamente de 10 a 12 años o más. La longevidad de las empastaduras de resina (y las empastaduras de plata) es una función de la posición y del tamaño de la empastadura, el cuidado que el paciente le da y los alimentos que el paciente come.

Las restauraciones de resina en los dientes de atrás requieren menos taladrado que para las empastaduras de plata. Debido al material de empastadura y los revestimientos de aislamiento y las bases usadas debajo de las resinas, puede haber una descarga de fluoruro y una inhibición subsiguiente de la formación de caries nueva. Son excelentes para las restauraciones pequeñas en una, dos y tres superficies en los premolares y molares. Las ventajas de las restauraciones de resina incluyen un aspecto natural similar al de su diente verdadero y la preparación más conservadora de su diente. Cuanto menos el dentista debe taladrar su diente, mejor es para usted y menos problemas dentales desarrollará en el futuro. También restauran un alto porcentaje de la fuerza original del diente. Cuando un diente se prepara (taladra), se vuelve más débil. El restaurarlo con un material de resina adherida ayudará a hacerlo fuerte otra vez. Requieren solamente una cita para la completarse.

Las desventajas incluyen la sensibilidad de la técnica, esto es, son más difíciles de colocar que las empastaduras de plata. También cuestan cerca de un 50% más que las empastaduras de plata. Pueden ser utilizadas solamente raramente en los pacientes que tienen hábitos de rechinar o bruxismo (apretar). No pueden ser utilizadas fácilmente en áreas donde no hay suficiente cantidad de la estructura original del diente. Requieren más tiempo para terminarlas.

Las restauraciones de resina están entre las restauraciones más conservadoras en la odontología de hoy. Requieren menos cantidad de taladrar. Cuanto más pequeña cualquier empastadura puede ser, más tiempo dura. Son las mejores para las empastaduras pequeñas a medianas. En áreas donde estaría fea la exhibición del metal de una empastadura de plata, son de gran importancia cosmética.

Si usted tiene cualquier pregunta sobre las restauraciones de resina adherida, favor de sentirse libre de preguntarnos.

Microodontología: Restauración Preventiva de la Resina

Con la llegada de la odontología adhesiva (adherida), el concepto de como un diente debe ser preparado para una empastadura ha cambiado. En los viejos tiempos, si usted iba a tener una empastadura de plata (la empastadura del material de amalgama de plata fue inventada al principio de los 1800s), el diente tendría que ser taladrado más allá de lo necesario para remover el deterioro. El taladrar adicional es necesario para tallar relieves para mantener la mecánica del material de plata. El diente adicional que fue quitado haría el diente más débil. Con la odontología adhesiva, y la capacidad del dentista de adherir (fijar) los materiales de resina compuestos al diente ha cambiado este concepto. Ahora, todo lo que el dentista necesita hacer es quitar el deterioro y después adherir la resina en la posición. Esto significa menos taladrar, y el diente se queda fuerte. La necesidad reducida para taladrar un diente permite que el dentista realice procedimientos de microodontología. La pericia técnica que necesita el dentista aumenta mientras que la remoción de la estructura del diente disminuye. Constantemente se están desarrollando maneras innovadoras de quitar deterioro. Con el uso de lupas magnificadoras, tintes que pueden manchar selectivamente el deterioro y nuevos materiales de unión, más del diente se preserva.

Una restauración preventiva de resina es una combinación de un procedimiento de la microodontología y un sellador de diente convencional. En los viejos tiempos, cuando un diente de atrás se deterioraba, los surcos no deteriorados cerca de la porción deteriorada eran removidos para prevenir que el deterioro futuro empezara. Con una resina preventiva, solamente se remueve el deterioro. La adhesión se coloca para restaurar el área y un sellador de resina se adhiere entonces sobre el resto del diente para prevenir deterioro adicional. De esta manera, menos taladrar es necesario y el resto de los dientes permanecen fuertes.

En la preparación de un diente para una resina preventiva, un taladro de una pieza de mano dental tradicional se puede utilizar para quitar el deterioro o la unidad recientemente reintroducida de la abrasión con aire puede ser utilizada. La unidad de abrasión con aire emite una corriente de óxido de aluminio u otro material de particulado, parecido a arena bajo alta presión. Esto es equivalente a limpiar con un chorro de arena—pero a una escala más pequeña. Las partículas que están bajo alta presión desgastan rápidamente el deterioro, frecuentemente sin la necesidad de una inyección anestésica local para adormecer el diente. Otra ventaja importante de la odontología de abrasión es que el "limpiar con un chorro de arena" no causa que se formen grietas en el frágil esmalte del diente. El taladro dental tradicional causa el que las grietas se irradien por la preparación. Con la odontología de la abrasión este problema puede ser eliminado. La abrasión con aire no se puede todavía utilizar para preparar coronas y puentes o ningún tipo de restauración de molde o fabricada en laboratorio.

Debido a que los procedimientos de microodontología requieren un nivel más alto de entrenamiento y pericia, los honorarios son levemente más altos que los de para una empastadura de plata. Las restauraciones de resina adherida tienen ventajas considerables sobre los materiales de empastaduras de plata. La naturaleza conservadora y el hecho de que protegen al diente, haciéndolo tan fuerte como puede ser, las hace dignas del costo adicional.

Si usted tiene cualquier pregunta sobre la microodontología y la restauración preventiva de resina, favor de sentirse libre de preguntarnos.

Ilustración en CD-ROM

Restauraciones de Cobertura Parcial

Una de nuestras metas fundamentales en proveerle el cuidado oral óptimo es preservar tanto de su dentición natural como sea posible. La prevención de la enfermedad oral es la mejor manera de lograr esta meta. Desgraciadamente, el deterioro dental es la enfermedad más común conocida al cuerpo humano. En las etapas tempranas el proceso de la caries se puede invertir con el uso del fluoruro. Sin embargo, si el deterioro progresa al punto cuando se requiere una empastadura, el deterioro puede ser quitado y el diente ser restaurado muy conservadoramente con una restauración directa adherida del color del diente. Una restauración directa significa que es comenzada y terminada en la oficina en una cita. Aunque la estructura del diente debe ser removida en este evento, la cantidad removida es pequeña y la solidez del diente no se daña. Ésta debe ser razón suficiente para ir al dentista y tener sus dientes examinados y limpiados en una base regular. Las necesidades pueden ser diferentes, pero la mayoría de los adultos deben ir de dos a cuatro veces cada año.

Si el diente tiene una cantidad moderada a grande de estructura dental a sustituir, una restauración directa no será tan exitosa. Para estos dientes, una restauración procesada en el laboratorio o externamente es más apropiada. Éstas no son iguales que una corona. Una corona implica el quitar una cantidad máxima de la estructura del diente. La restauración de molde es entonces hecha a la medida sobre el diente preparado, como un dedal se ajusta sobre la yema del dedo. Nada del diente natural puede ser visto. Mientras que las coronas de molde completo tienen un historial probado de éxito, se sacrifica una gran cantidad de la estructura del diente.

Las restauraciones de cobertura parcial pueden ser hechas de oro, resina, porcelana o materiales de cerámica. Las restauraciones de oro son las menos estéticas. El color es similar al de un anillo de matrimonio en oro. Los otros tres materiales son del color del diente y proveen una igualación maravillosa a la estructura natural del diente.

Hay varias ventajas que usted realizará con las restauraciones de cobertura parcial. Éstas requieren que se quite menos cantidad de la estructura del diente que para una corona, así que son pequeñas en tamaño. Esta preparación conservadora preserva mucho del diente adyacente al tejido de la encía, proveyendo una mejor oportunidad para una salud periodontal excelente. Con los bordes de la restauración por encima de la encía, la restauración se hace más fácil de verificar para el servicio continuado. El deterioro nuevo es visto más fácilmente y tratado en la etapa temprana. Al taladrar menos el diente, disminuye el riesgo potencial para el daño futuro del nervio y que resulta en un canal radicular.

En el lado negativo, las restauraciones de cobertura parcial son más difíciles para el dentista preparar y colocar. Son muy sensibles a la técnica y consumen mucho tiempo. Esto contribuye a un honorario más alto junto con los honorarios necesarios del laboratorio para procesar la restauración. Pero el resultado final es digno del esfuerzo y costo. La cantidad máxima del diente sano, natural se preserva. No hay nada que un dentista puede poner en su boca que sea tan bueno como un diente sin taladrar, sin daño. Cuanto menos el dentista debe taladrar, mejor para usted, a corto y largo plazo. Sugeriremos siempre el tratamiento y material más apropiado basado en sus necesidades orales individuales.

Si usted tiene cualquier pregunta sobre las restauraciones de cobertura parcial, favor de sentirse libre de preguntarnos.

Inlays y Onlays de Porcelana

Una manera innovadora de restaurar un diente que ha estado de moderadamente a extensivamente destruido por el deterioro, previamente taladrado o fracturado, es con inlay u onlay de porcelana. Un inlay es una restauración en la cual una parte de la superficie oclusal (mordida) es restaurada. Un onlay restaurará más de la superficie de mordida completa del diente. Puede ser que necesite un inlay solamente, un onlay solamente o una combinación de inlay/onlay. Esto se considera una restauración muy conservadora.

El material de porcelana produce un excelente resultado estético. El inlay u onlay de porcelana es adherido al diente, haciéndolo muy resistente. Puede ser usado con resultados excelentes en restauraciones pequeñas, medianas o aún grandes durante más de 12 años, relativamente libre de problemas.

Un laboratorio del exterior está implicado en la construcción de este tipo de restauración. Durante el tiempo de transformación de 2 o 3 semanas mientras el inlay u onlay se está haciendo, el diente será protegido con una restauración temporal. Los inlays y onlays de porcelana tienen algunas desventajas. Son más costosos de hacer y colocar y toman dos citas para completarse. Deben ser ajustados y pulidos bien o pueden causar el desgaste del esmalte de oposición, exactamente como una porcelana fundida a una corona de metal.

Las ventajas incluyen una estética excelente, mucha solidez, longevidad predicha y preparación conservadora. Si la porcelana se astilla, puede ser reparada. Sin embargo, usted no debe masticar cubos de hielo, "trituradores de la mandíbula" u otros dulces duros con ésta o cualquier otro tipo de restauración. Cualquier cosa que usted pone en su boca que puede fracturar un diente real puede fracturar este tipo de material restaurativo.

Para los pacientes que desean una restauración resistente, duradera, conservadora que iguale muy de cerca un diente, la porcelana es posiblemente la mejor selección. Todas las cosas consideradas, no es tan costosa como puede ser que parezca. Una vez que se acabe, el diente, si es cuidado correctamente, no debe tener que ser taladrado otra vez por años. Permite la conservación de la mayoría del diente natural. Recuerde, nuestra meta es preservar tanto de su estructura natural del diente como sea posible.

Si usted tiene cualquier pregunta sobre los inlays y onlays de porcelana, favor de sentirse libre de preguntarnos.

Inlays y Onlays de Resina

Los inlays y onlays de resina son de apariencia muy natural y se adhieren en el lugar. Son restauraciones extremadamente conservadoras. Requieren dos citas para completarse y, como con el inlay u onlay de porcelana, la ayuda del laboratorio es necesaria. El diente será protegido con un inlay u onlay de plástico temporal mientras el laboratorio procesa la restauración final.

La fabricación en el laboratorio dental toma cerca de 2 semanas. El desgaste de las resinas es similar a la del esmalte. Distinto a la porcelana, no desgastará la estructura natural de oposición del diente.

El material de resina puede ser levemente "más débil" que la porcelana. Sin embargo, porque la porcelana es más frágil y más difícil de reparar, la diferencia en solidez no es significativa. La resina perdona más y se acaba o repara más fácilmente y la resina es más fácil de trabajar. Las restauraciones de resina, sin embargo, no se aconsejan para los pacientes que tienen el hábito de bruxismo (rechinar) o apretar a menos que se construya un protector bucal.

Nosotros seleccionaremos y recomendaremos el material restaurativo apropiado basado en sus necesidades dentales. Ambos tipos son opciones excelentes y se consideran altamente conservadoras en la cantidad de taladrado necesitado.

Una manera excelente de restaurar un diente con un deterioro moderado a extenso es con un inlay u onlay.

Si usted tiene cualquier pregunta sobre los inlays y onlays de resina, favor de sentirse libre de preguntarnos.

Ilustración en CD-ROM

La Empastadura "Permanente"

Una de las preguntas más frecuentes que los pacientes hacen es, "¿Es esto una empastadura permanente?" Sin envolverse mucho en los aspectos técnicos de los materiales restaurativos modernos, la contestación generalmente es no. Todos los materiales de empastaduras tienen un largo de vida de varios a muchos años, dependiendo del material restaurativo usado. Como regla general para restauraciones moderadas a grandes, mientras más cuesta, más tiempo durara.

Los materiales restaurativos dentales construidos y procesados en un laboratorio dental serán más resistentes y duros y durarán más tiempo que las empastaduras de amalgama de plata (metal) y los materiales de empastadura compuestos colocados en la oficin (del color del diente/adheridos). Estos materiales construidos en el laboratorio incluyen restauraciones indirectas tales como coronas de molde completo, inlays y onlays de porcelana, oro y aleaciones de oro, cerámicas y resinas. Aunque el dentista tendrá ciertas preferencias, usted tiene la decisión final sobre de que material debe ser utilizado. Para hacer el proceso de decisión más fácil, aquí hay un breve resumen de las ventajas y desventajas de los materiales usados comúnmente en restauraciones de cobertura parcial. La porcelana fundida a coronas de aleación de oro no están incluidas aquí ya que éstas son una categoría diferente.

Moldes de Oro: El color del molde de oro es amarillo, igual que un anillo de matrimonio. Puede durar de 25 a 40 años o más—el más largo de cualquier material dental. El oro tiene una historia larga de éxito. La estética es de pobre a regular. El costo es alto. Sin embargo, el uso de moldes de oro resulta en menos problemas postoperatorios. Es excelente para restauraciones dentales medianas a grandes. Dos citas son necesarias para terminar la restauración.

Requisitos de la Técnica: Alto

Porcelanas, Cerámicas y Resinas Adheridas Procesadas en el Laboratorio: Estos materiales producen una estética excelente: igualan el color del diente casi perfectamente. El costo es moderado a alto. En cuanto a longevidad, probablemente no es tan larga como el molde de oro, pero debe durar por 12 años o más. Generalmente requiere menos preparación del diente (taladrado) que al utilizar oro. Éstos son procedimientos dentales relativamente nuevos. No tienen el historial de éxito a largo plazo que tiene el oro. Estos materiales pueden romperse si se fuerzan demasiado. La resina es más fácil de reparar que la porcelana, y es menos costosa que la porcelana y la cerámica, y una selección excelente para restauraciones medianas a grandes. Dos citas son necesarias completar estas restauraciones.

Requisitos de la Técnica: Alto

Resinas Directas: Las resinas directas también proporcionan una estética excelente. La preparación del diente implicada es mínima. Éstos son los mejores materiales para las restauraciones dentales pequeñas a medianas. Las resinas directas implican menos costo que el oro o porcelanas. Éstas son adheridas al diente. La expectativa de vida del material es 12 años o más, y esta tecnología nueva le da solidez al diente. Las resinas directas se pueden completar en una visita.

Requisitos de la Técnica: Alto

Metal de Amalgama de Plata: La amalgama de plata primero fue utilizada como material de empastadura en 1816. Longevidad probada de 14 años, más o menos 14 años. La amalgama de plata no le da solidez al diente. No es una preparación del diente conservadora. La estética es pobre. Se ennegrece, corroe y expande con el pasar del tiempo. Es el de costo más bajo de todos los materiales restaurativos.

Requisitos de la Técnica: Bajo

Nosotros seleccionaremos y recomendaremos los materiales restaurativos más apropiados para satisfacer sus necesidades dentales. La cobertura del seguro (o la falta de) **nunca** dictará qué tratamiento dental sentimos usted necesita y se merece. Nuestra meta es poder proporcionar las mejores y más duraderas restauraciones posibles. Estaremos contentos de discutir estas opciones con usted.

Si usted tiene cualquier pregunta sobre la empastadura "permanente", favor de sentirse libre de preguntarnos.

Restauraciones Defectuosas

Nada dura para siempre. En la odontología, esto es un verdadero problema. **Cada** material restaurativo—ya sea empastadura, corona, puente, cemento, etc.— tiene una vida limitada. Ahora estamos viviendo vidas mucho más largas. La mayoría de los materiales dentales no fueron diseñados para servir el tiempo que ahora podemos esperar vivir. Algunos materiales pueden durar muchos años, y otros, considerablemente menos. No hay realmente tal cosa como una empastadura permanente. Como regla general, cuanto más costosa la restauración o material dental, más tiempo dura. Si usted desea una restauración que dure más tiempo, probablemente necesitará un inlay, un onlay o una corona procesada en un laboratorio. Los materiales de empastaduras directos (colocados en una visita de oficina) no se esperan que duren tanto tiempo. La longevidad de estas restauraciones dependerá del tipo de material, la localización del diente y el tamaño de la preparación en el diente. Hay también consideraciones exteriores tales como las habilidades y el conocimiento del dentista en ese entonces, las clases de alimento que usted come, sus hábitos de cuidado oral de sí mismo y del abuso estructural que usted pone sobre sus dientes. Hábitos tales como el apretar y rechinar sus dientes, masticar dulces duros o hielo, etc. tienden a degradar rápidamente el material de empastadura, así como sus dientes, mucho más rápido.

Aun las empastaduras mejor colocadas se ponen viejas. El cemento de la corona se disuelve, la porcelana se rompe, los metales se fatigan, las resinas se degradan, y así sucesivamente. Eventualmente, pedazos del material de empastadura o diente se pueden fracturar o astillar. Una caries nueva puede comenzar en una superficie sin empastar del mismo diente. La restauración necesita ser reemplazada. Las empastaduras de amalgama de plata (las empastaduras negras o grises que la mayoría tenemos) pueden absorber la humedad de la saliva, expandirse y causar la rotura del diente. La expansión de la empastadura puede causar que la empastadura y el borde entre el diente y la empastadura lleguen a ser ásperos. Esto puede promover la retención de la placa y el comienzo del nuevo deterioro. Cuando esto sucede, es mejor sustituir la restauración cuanto antes por una resina adherida, que requerirá menos taladrado. Cuanto mejor sea el material, menos drástico serán los ciclos termales (café caliente/helado frío y cualquier variación de temperatura) y menos abusivos sean sus hábitos personales, más tiempo la restauración durará. Si usted tiene cualquiera de estos problemas restaurativos, usted debe hacerlos corregir cuanto antes. El esperar puede causar que aumente la severidad, y un tratamiento más extenso y costoso puede ser requerido, o el problema puede llegar a ser imposible de reparar.

Definiciones

Fractura: Se llama al material de empastadura que se ha roto en dos o más pedazos. Los pedazos pueden o no moverse y el paciente a menudo no lo siente. La restauración debe ser substituida.

Filtración: Los líquidos penetran entre la empastadura y el diente, causando deterioro. Un paciente nota generalmente esta condición cuando el diente llega a ser sensible a los líquidos, dulces o al caliente o al frío. La restauración debe ser substituida.

Corona Floja: El medio de la cementación de la corona pudo haber fallado, en el caso del tratamiento endodóntico, el poste que sostiene la corona pudo haberse roto o su medio de cementación ha fallado. Puede ser causado por una relación incorrecta de mordida, comer los alimentos incorrectos o los hábitos parafuncionales de la boca. La restauración se puede reparar y reutilizar a veces, sino debe ser hecha totalmente nueva.

Contacto Abierto: Cuando dos dientes que deben tocarse, no lo hacen se refiere a un *contacto abierto*. Puede ser debido al movimiento indeseado del diente después de una extracción, pero generalmente es el resultado una empastadura de contorno insuficiente. Puede atrapar el alimento y causar la infección severa de la encía, sangrado y la pérdida del hueso alrededor de los dientes afectados. La empastadura (o empastaduras) puede necesitar ser reemplazada.

Margenes Abiertos: Cuando una empastadura no se encuentra con la preparación del diente, el resultado es un margen abierto. Básicamente, existe una grieta entre la empastadura y el diente. La placa se atrapa fácilmente, predisponiendo el diente al deterioro adicional. Esto puede ser especialmente serio en coronas. Un margen abierto se puede reparar infrecuentemente, pero debe ser reemplazado generalmente.

Sobrecontorno: Cuando una empastadura o una corona se forma incorrectamente, especialmente cuando es demasiada ancha, puede causar la infección y sangrado de las encías. La restauración debe ser reformada o reemplazada.

Sobresalir: El tipo de defecto más común de la restauración es el sobresalir. Cuando el material restaurativo se extiende más allá del contorno normal del diente debajo de la encía, causa una trampa de placa. Una indicación común es la rasgadura o trituración del hilo dental. El sobresalir causa infección de la encía (encías rojas que sangran fácilmente). El exceso de material debe ser quitado puliendo o reemplazando la restauración.

Deterioro Recurrente: El deterioro nuevo es visto alrededor del diente/borde de la empastadura o debajo de la empastadura. Usted puede o no notar esta condición. Lo notamos generalmente en un examen clínico o en una radiografía dental. El deterioro recurrente requiere el reemplazo inmediato.

Resinas Manchadas: Una resina compuesta manchada es a menudo una muestra de la degradación de la resina. Las resinas viejas son más propensas a mostrar manchas. La mancha indica que la matriz de la resina que retiene los componentes inorgánicos juntos es vieja, se ha forzado demasiado y ya no está resistiendo la humedad. En este caso podemos determinar la urgencia de reemplazo. Cuando es un problema cosmético, recomendamos que la reemplace más pronto.

De Contorno Insuficiente: Cuando una empastadura o corona es de una forma incorrecta, especialmente deficiente en ancho, está con contorno insuficiente. Esta condición causa impacción de los alimentos y infección de la encía.

Si usted tiene cualquier pregunta sobre las restauraciones defectuosas, favor de sentirse libre de preguntarnos.

Recontorno del Esmalte

La mayoría de las personas desean dientes derechos, maravillosamente alineados, blancos. Desgraciadamente, la mayoría de las personas no nacen naturalmente de esa manera. Cuando los dientes están pobremente alineados, rotados, inclinados y/o apiñados, una manera obvia de corregir el problema es con la ortodoncia (frenillos). Sin embargo, hay situaciones donde puede no ser posible o deseable utilizar frenillos para enderezar los dientes. Puede ser que usted sienta que es demasiado viejo, (aunque esto es raramente el caso), el costo de la ortodoncia puede imposibilitar su uso, puede que usted no quiera usar frenillos o quizás hay solamente algunas áreas que necesitan atención y la ortodoncia completa no sería apropiada.

En ciertos casos, la apariencia de los dientes superiores e inferiores puede mejorar levemente o dramáticamente con el recontorno del esmalte. Los incisivos y caninos superiores e inferiores pueden ser alterados rutinariamente. A veces los dientes que están más atrás en su boca también se pueden mejorar cosméticamente. El recontorno es útil cuando hay superposición leve a moderada de los dientes frontales, un desgaste no igual o unos dientes que no tienen sus bordes de la mordida e incisión en armonía, lo que crea una apariencia no igual de "cerca de estacas puntiagudas". El recontorno del esmalte generalmente es un procedimiento sin dolor y no se necesita anestesia local. El esmalte que está superpuesto o mal formado se remueve, se recontorna y se pule. Dependiendo de sus necesidades individuales, uno o varios dientes pueden requerir alguna reformación. Se pueden remover cantidades diferentes de esmalte de diversos dientes. Los dientes reformados no son más propensos al deterioro, no se ponen más sensibles a los cambios de temperatura y no son significativamente más débiles o dañados por el procedimiento.

Muchas veces, el recontorno es todo lo que se necesita para mejorar su apariencia significativamente. Otras veces, cuando la pobre alineación es más pronunciada, se puede hacer en conjunto con la adhesión de resina o porcelana a los dientes. Su tratamiento dependerá de sus condiciones actuales y de lo que le gustaría ver cambiado.

El procedimiento no es difícil para el paciente y muchas veces se puede hacer en sólo una cita. El cambio es inmediato y permanente. Requiere cierto don artístico por parte del dentista para ver cuáles son las posibilidades de cambio. Necesitamos determinar qué cantidad de esmalte necesita removerse, dónde debemos añadir material y dónde la ortodoncia es el mejor tratamiento. Los honorarios son razonables y dependen del grado del tratamiento.

Si usted tiene cualquier pregunta sobre el recontorno del esmalte, favor de sentirse libre de preguntarnos.

Restauraciones Sedativas

Las restauraciones sedativas se colocan por diversas razones. La razón más común es dolor del diente. El dolor puede ser constante, intermitente o una reacción a dulces o a un estímulo frío o caliente. Si la sensibilidad es debido al deterioro y es muy profundo y cerca del nervio, hay la posibilidad de la exposición de la pulpa (nervio) una vez que se quite todo el deterioro. Si la caries es especialmente profunda, tanto del deterioro como sea posible será quitado, y una empastadura medicada, sedativa será colocada en el diente. Esto servirá para calmar el nervio y para darle la oportunidad de curar. La restauración sedativa, si es hecha por esta razón, debe permanecer en su boca por _____ semanas. Entonces la restauración sedativa será quitada y el diente será examinado para determinar la necesidad de tratamiento adicional. Puede ser restaurado con una empastadura o una restauración de molde. Sin embargo, si el deterioro era demasiado profundo y el nervio no cura, tratamiento endodóntico (terapia del canal radicular) será requerido para aliviar el dolor y para salvar el diente.

Si usted tiene caries múltiples grandes y/u otros problemas dentales serios, podemos elegir restaurar primero todos los dientes con restauraciones sedativas. Esto estabilizará rápidamente todos los dientes de modo que no continúen deteriorándose. Entonces los otros, quizás más serios, problemas dentales pueden ser atendidos y tratados. Una vez que esté fuera de la situación de emergencia, tendremos tiempo de planear a fondo los mejores métodos para restaurar sus dientes.

Un tercer uso para una restauración sedativa es como ayuda en diagnosticar dientes sensibles. Usted puede tener un problema con un solo diente, o quizás no puede establecer claramente el diente exacto. Si el diente (dientes) ya tiene una restauración, podemos necesitar quitar la restauración y ver directamente las partes preparadas del diente. Si no sentimos que es apropiado colocar una restauración final en ese momento, pondremos una restauración sedativa para permitir que el diente se normalice para recibir la empastadura final. En su caso, esperamos que la restauración sedativa esté en el lugar por aproximadamente _____ semanas. De vez en cuando, el diente se siente mejor tan pronto como se coloca la restauración sedativa. Sin embargo, todavía será necesario observar el diente por algunas semanas antes de colocar una restauración final.

Infrecuentemente, la colocación de la restauración sedativa no ofrece ningún alivio evidente. En este caso otras posibilidades deben ser exploradas. La mayoría de las veces el diente requerirá tratamiento endodóntico. Otras veces, solo toma varios días para obtener un resultado positivo. Si es posible, dele tiempo a la restauración sedativa para trabajar. Pero bajo ninguna circunstancia usted debe vivir en constante dolor. No tenga miedo de llamar y pedir ser visto si la restauración sedativa no parece ser eficaz.

Si usted tiene cualquier pregunta sobre las restauraciones sedativas, favor de sentirse libre de preguntarnos.

Seguridad de la Amalgama de Plata y de los Metales Comunes

La práctica del arte y de la ciencia de la odontología ha cambiado enormemente durante los últimos 15 a 20 años. En ninguna parte es esto más evidente que en la variedad de materiales dentales disponibles para la restauración del diente. Las resinas compuestas (plásticos adheridos del color del diente) nos permite restaurar el diente con menos remoción (taladrado) de la estructura sana del diente. Los compuestos se ven como la estructura natural del diente, están adheridos al diente para un sellado apretado, una larga duración y añadir solidez al diente preparado. Las amalgamas de material de plata (empastaduras de metal) no se ven como diente natural, filtran fluidos en la superficie de contacto del diente con el metal; pueden agrietar el diente por la expansión volumétrica y termal; requieren más remoción de la estructura del diente de la que es requerida para eliminar el deterioro; hacen al diente más débil; pueden durar por mucho tiempo pero a menudo dañan seriamente el diente mientras está colocada. Las empastaduras de plata fueron inventadas alrededor del año 1814 por los franceses como un material de empastadura temporal, no muy costoso para usarse hasta que el paciente pudiera pagar una restauración de oro de mejor calidad. En aquel entonces, los dentistas en los Estados Unidos estaban horrorizados por el uso del material de plata/mercurio que no era permitido a ser importado en los Estados Unidos, o aun ser enseñado en las escuelas dentales, por muchos años.

Los metales comunes han sido usados en la odontología como una alternativa económica a los metales noble y noble alto. Los metales noble y noble alto contienen metales preciosos como el oro, paladio y platino, en varios porcentajes. Los metales comunes están compuestos de metales que pueden tener altas propiedades alérgicas, tóxicas o aun carcinogénicas. Desde el 1976, nunca hemos especificado que se usen metales comunes en ninguna restauración procesada en el laboratorio. Hemos estado usando metales de moldes de alta calidad probada. Porque somos considerados de su salud médica en general, no ofrecemos los metales comunes como opción para cualquier corona, puente o implante de molde.

Hemos tomado una decisión en nuestra práctica de proveerle los mejores y más apropiados procedimientos y materiales que la odontología tiene para ofrecer. Esto no significa necesariamente el tratamiento más costoso. Quisiéramos que se vieran bien, sean funcionales y cómodos, también. Sentimos que los materiales de amalgama de plata no le ayudarán a satisfacer esta meta. Sentimos que la rutina de utilizar nuevas empastaduras de plata y de metal común no tiene ningún lugar en la odontología de hoy. Hemos elegido el eliminar este material y procedimiento de nuestra práctica.

Si Usted Tiene Seguro Dental
Los portadores de seguro proporcionan rutinariamente beneficios para restauraciones compuestas adheridas del color del diente para los dientes de atrás que reflejan el honorario por empastaduras de metal de plata. Los contratos con el portador indican casi siempre que el beneficio es por el servicio menos costoso posible (cláusula alternativa del beneficio). El portador de seguro no le está diciendo a usted o al dentista qué tratamiento usted debe tener, solamente cuál es su responsabilidad de pago. Cuanto más alta es la prima de seguro, más es pagado en beneficios. Cuanto más baja la prima de seguro, más bajos son los beneficios. Como un ejemplo tonto, un seguro dental de costo muy bajo puede pagar el 100% del honorario de una dentadura de madera. Pero eso no significa que cualquier dentista le tallará un juego. Si mejores materiales son usados basados en la discreción del dentista, usted es responsable por la diferencia.

En Conclusión
Por su salud en general, no pondremos moldes de metal común en su boca. Por la salud y longevidad de sus dientes, no colocaremos empastaduras de plata nuevas en dientes con nuevo deterioro o como reemplazo para una restauración existente.

Si usted tiene cualquier pregunta sobre la amalgama de plata y los metales comunes, favor de sentirse libre de preguntarnos.

Garantía de los Materiales Restaurativos

Usted acaba de tener un tratamiento restaurativo ('empastaduras') o le han colocado un prostético fijo (coronas, puentes, inlays u onlays procesados en el laboratorio). En todos los casos usamos los materiales y técnicas mejores disponibles y más apropiados. El tratamiento completado debe servirle bien por varios años. Como cualquier otra cosa, los materiales dentales tienen un largo de vida eficaz y requieren un mantenimiento rutinario y continuo. No hay nada disponible en la odontología hoy en día que sea tan bueno o mejor que su diente natural. Como cualquier pieza de una maquinaria fina o un automóvil, mientras mejor cuidado le dé, y a menos abuso esté sometida, más tiempo durará.

Sujeto a algunas condiciones, lo que sigue es la garantía para los materiales y el tratamiento que usted ha recibido. Cuatro posibilidades podrían invalidar esta garantía. (1) Si le han diagnosticado como un apretador o bruxista y/o si le han aconsejado tener un protector bucal y usted no lo usa o no lo mandado a hacer. **(2) Si usted no se adhiere al intervalo continuo profesional de la higiene dental (limpiezas por el higienista dental) que se ha determinado en base a sus necesidades orales actuales. Recomendamos que usted tenga sus dientes examinados y que se realice una profilaxis dental cada _____ meses.** (3) Nuevo deterioro que requiere que la restauración sea hecha de nuevo. (4) Trauma, accidente, negligencia o tratamiento al diente tratado o al diente adyacente que envuelve el diente restaurado.

Los dentistas no tienen ningún control sobre lo que un paciente coloca en su boca—alimento u otras cosas. La masticación de cubos de hielo o bombones congelados o duros, rechinar o apretar puede envejecer sus dientes naturales o cualquier material restaurativo **mucho** más rápido que su velocidad normal. Por favor no chupe bombones o mentas—esto puede causar un deterioro rápido alrededor de las restauraciones recién colocadas.

GARANTÍA

Para las restauraciones de colocación directa (completada en una sola cita en la oficina): Si la restauración necesita ser hecha de nuevo en el plazo de **dos (2) años** de la colocación inicial, la restauración será substituida sin ningún honorario adicional para usted.

Para las restauraciones procesadas en el laboratorio: Si la restauración procesada en el laboratorio necesita ser hecha de nuevo en el plazo de **dos (2) años** de la colocación inicial, la corona, puente, inlay u onlay será sustituido sin ningún honorario adicional para usted. **De 2–3 años,** el paciente es responsable por el 40% del costo de volver a dar tratamiento. **De 3–4 años,** el paciente es responsable por el 60% del costo de volver a dar tratamiento. **De 4–5 años,** el paciente es responsable por el 80% del costo de volver a dar tratamiento. **A los 5 años de la colocación inicial,** se termina la garantía.

Si usted tiene cualquier pregunta sobre la garantía, por favor pregúntenos. Con el cuidado apropiado, usted debe conseguir años de servicio de sus nuevas restauraciones. Haga el cepillado oral y la limpieza con hilo dental diariamente y tenga un examen de sus dientes y limpiezas en el intervalo sugerido. Nada (usualmente) dura para siempre, pero si usted toma cuidado de su boca según lo dirigido, las restauraciones estarán sirviendo satisfactoriamente por cierto tiempo.

Esta garantía cubre lo siguiente:

Diente#_____   **Tipo de Restauración**_____   **Fecha**_____

Garantía del Diente Severamente Comprometido

La naturaleza creó los dientes suficientemente fuertes para soportar años de servicio diario en la boca. Sin embargo, los dientes pueden cambiar y debilitarse por un número de razones, algunas de las cuales son:

- Deterioro
- Taladrado del diente para remover el deterioro
- Empastaduras de metal que se expanden y rompen el diente
- Dientes rotos (fracturados) que solamente pueden ser restaurados con coronas (caperuzas)
- Enfermedad de las encías resultando en pérdida del hueso que rodea el diente
- Tratamiento endodóntico (tratamiento del canal radicular)
- Apretar y rechinar
- Movimiento del diente después de la extracción de diente adyacente u opuesto

Un diente que ha experimentado una o más de estas condiciones puede terminar en tal mala condición que se vuelve difícil para restaurar y proporcionar un buen pronóstico a largo plazo.

Aunque un dentista puede restaurar casi cualquier diente gravemente dañado, hay riesgos. La pregunta verdadera no es si la restauración se puede hacer pero, más bien, ¿si el diente que estará bajo este procedimiento será lo suficientemente fuerte para durar por un largo considerado de tiempo?

Nos gusta dar una garantía para las restauraciones que colocamos. Usted tiene un diente que esta severamente comprometido. Aunque sentimos que el diente puede ser restaurado a la función clínica, no podemos dar nuestra garantía acostumbrada para longevidad. Todo depende de la fuerza del diente, y cuando un diente está roto, esto a menudo es difícil de determinar.
La restauración puede ser excelente pero su diente natural podría romperse. Esto puede ocurrir pronto después que el diente se restaura o después de varios años. Dependiendo de la naturaleza de la rotura, el diente podría ser reparado otra vez o podría estar roto tan gravemente que ningún otro tratamiento trabajaría y el diente debe ser sacado.

Pensamos que salvar los dientes es muy importante. Reconocemos, además, que en un cierto punto, salvar un diente llega a ser impráctico debido al costo: $2,500 para salvar un diente por 5 años hace sentido económico, pero $2,500 para salvar un diente 6 meses no es una buena inversión. Basado en sus necesidades orales y nuestro juicio clínico, recomendamos que usted tenga el diente en cuestión restaurado, conforme a las limitaciones descritas. Entienda por favor que hay muchos factores fuera de nuestro control que se relacionan con el éxito a largo plazo de este diente y restauración. El diente puede que no sea lo suficientemente fuerte para durar por mucho tiempo.

Si usted se propone salvar el diente en cuestión, por favor firme abajo, demostrando que usted ha leído y entiende la información en este documento, y aunque los mejores esfuerzos y materiales serán utilizados, el diente mismo puede demostrar ser inadecuado para apoyar correctamente una restauración a largo plazo.

Diente(s) # que está(n) severamente comprometido(s): _____

Firmado: _____   Fecha: _____

Paquetes para la Educación del Paciente

Construcción de los Paquetes Educativos

El material en esta sección le ayudará a montar paquetes educativos útiles para sus pacientes. Estos paquetes pueden ser montados en un sin número de temas dentales utilizando documentos de este paquete de comunicación dental. Utilice las portadas de las páginas de esta sección y las añada páginas de la lista de los temas sugeridos. Podrá encontrar beneficioso el recopilar y preparar a su gusto sus propios paquetes.

Revisión del Contenido: Paquetes para la Educación del Paciente

Bienvenido a Nuestra Práctica: *Teniendo la Sonrisa Que Usted Desea*

Recopilar un sin número de temas en un paquete atractivo para un paciente nuevo dice mucho acerca de su práctica y de cómo los pacientes pueden esperar ser tratados. Este paquete cubre temas desde una bienvenida general hasta las políticas de la oficina para animar a los pacientes a tener el cuidado dental que ellos se merecen.

Paquete Educativo de Odontología Pedriática: *Odontología para Niños*

Los documentos sugeridos para este paquete cubren prevención y las preguntas frecuentemente preguntadas con respecto al paciente niño. Los documentos adicionales pueden ser igualmente apropiados para incluir y se pueden incluir fácilmente.

Paquete Educativo de Periodoncia: *Diagnóstico y Tratamiento de la Enfermedad de las Encías desde Temprana hasta Moderada*

Este paquete educativo ayuda a los pacientes que buscan la terapia periodontal a tener un entendimiento claro de la naturaleza de su enfermedad y de los procedimientos de tratamiento recomendados. Los documentos adicionales pueden ser igualmente apropiados para incluir y se pueden incluir fácilmente.

Paquete Educativo de Periodoncia: *Diagnóstico y Tratamiento de la Enfermedad de las Encías Avanzada*

Este paquete está diseñado para el paciente que no está en la fase avanzada de la enfermedad periodontal y que necesita entender el papel del cuidado oral profesional regular y los hábitos apropiados del cuidado oral de sí mismo.

Paquete Educativo de Prostodoncia: *Consideraciones en el Reemplazo de Dientes*

Este paquete educativo ayuda al paciente que está reemplazando dientes que faltan a entender la necesidad de la odontología prostética y las muchas opciones de tratamiento disponibles hoy en día. Los documentos adicionales pueden ser igualmente apropiados para incluir y se pueden incluir fácilmente.

Paquete Educativo de Prostodoncia: *Consideraciones en el Reemplazo de Dientes Avanzado*

Los documentos sugeridos para este paquete ayudan a informar al paciente que está contemplando el procedimiento de una corona a entender más completamente el proceso y la selección del material apropiado. Los documentos adicionales pueden ser igualmente apropiados para incluir y se pueden incluir fácilmente.

Paquete Educativo de Odontología Restaurativa: *Restaurando Sus Dientes*

Este paquete ayudará al paciente buscando la odontología restaurativa a entender la razón fundamental para la selección del material, el cuidado postoperatorio de las nuevas restauraciones y los puntos acerca de la garantía. Los documentos adicionales pueden ser igualmente apropiados para incluir y se pueden incluir fácilmente.

Cómo Montar Sus Propios Paquetes Educativos

Instrucciones para asistirle con la creación de paquetes individualizados según las necesidades de su práctica.

Bienvenido a Nuestra Práctica

TENIENDO LA SONRISA QUE USTED DESEA

Ahora que comenzamos esta relación en el cuidado de salud, hay algunos asuntos que nos gustaría que usted conociera acerca de nuestra filosofía de tratamiento y las políticas de nuestra oficina. Este paquete está diseñado para que conozca algunos de esos puntos y esperamos que le conteste una o dos de las preguntas que usted pueda tener.

Por favor siéntase libre de llamarnos en cualquier momento para hacer preguntas o discutir las opciones de tratamiento. Sentimos que mientras más educación usted tenga acerca de la odontología, mejor será su resultado del tratamiento.

Estamos esperando ansiosos para proveerle con una magnífica salud oral y una sonrisa ganadora.

Paquete Educativo de Odontología Pedriática

ODONTOLOGÍA PARA NIÑOS

Su salud oral, y ciertamente, la salud oral de sus niños es una parte importante del bienestar total. Hemos preparado los siguientes materiales para proveerle información acerca de la prevención de enfermedades y una guía de referencia practica de cuándo su niño perderá los dientes de leche.

Por favor lea la siguiente información cuidadosamente. Si usted tiene preguntas relacionadas a este material o tiene otras preguntas relacionadas a la odontología, por favor siéntase libre de llamar a esta oficina en cualquier momento.

Paquete Educativo de Periodoncia

DIAGNÓSTICO Y TRATAMIENTO DE LA ENFERMEDAD DE LAS ENCÍAS DESDE TEMPRANA HASTA MODERADA

Por favor lea la información incluida cuidadosamente.

Usted ha sido diagnosticado con la etapa más temprana de la enfermedad periodontal activa—gingivitis. Las siguientes páginas le ayudarán a entender nuestras recomendaciones de tratamiento, por qué estos procedimientos necesitan ser realizados, sus opciones y las consecuencias y riesgos de la acción o de no tomar acción por su parte.

Este paquete contiene información que le ayudará a entender:
- Un método efectivo para cepillar y limpiar con hilo dental sus dientes. Le demostraremos estas destrezas a usted.
- El proceso de la enfermedad periodontal. Usted será capaz de entender completamente el tipo exacto de enfermedad que usted tiene.
- La teoría del tratamiento no quirúrgico propuesto, qué es logrado y cómo usted se beneficiará de esta terapia.
- Los procedimientos exactos que son necesarios para tratar esta enfermedad.
- Los procedimientos para el cuidado oral de sí mismo adjuntos o adicionales que puedan ser necesarios para tratar la enfermedad y mantener la salud periodontal.

Por favor note que toda la información es respecto al tratamiento no quirúrgico. En este momento su salud periodontal está en una etapa critica. Si se deja sin tratar, la condición actual, qué es reversible, puede conducir a la próxima etapa de la enfermedad, la cual es irreversible. Cualquiera de las opciones de tratamiento que sentimos es apropiada para su tratamiento será discutida antes de comenzar el tratamiento.

Ocasionalmente, los pacientes con seguro dental preguntan si estos procedimientos son beneficios cubiertos o si son de naturaleza cosmética y no estarían cubiertos. El tratamiento recomendado para la enfermedad periodontal no es cosmético y la mayoría de los planes lo incluyen como un beneficio pagable. Una excepción puede ocurrir para los procedimientos como la irrigación subgingival o la colocación de una terapia en un lugar especifico. Si usted quiere, podemos someter un pre-estimado a su portador de seguro para determinar qué beneficios serán cubiertos y hasta que grado. Sin embargo, debido a que los procedimientos deben ser realizados en la secuencia correcta, esto puede causar un retraso en el tratamiento. Más daños pueden ocurrir a sus estructuras de soporte mientras esperamos la respuesta de su portador de seguro. Adicionalmente, ya sea éste un beneficio cubierto o no, es parte de nuestra recomendación de la terapia periodontal el tratar su enfermedad.

Por favor lea la siguiente información cuidadosamente. Ha sido escrita para explicar claramente qué usted necesita saber acerca del proceso de la enfermedad y los pasos necesarios para tratarla.

Ilustración en CD-ROM

Paquete Educativo de Periodoncia

DIAGNÓSTICO Y TRATAMIENTO DE LA ENFERMEDAD DE LAS ENCÍAS AVANZADA

Por favor lea la información incluida cuidadosamente.

Usted ha sido diagnosticado con enfermedad periodontal activa y las siguientes páginas le ayudarán a entender nuestras recomendaciones de tratamiento, por qué estos procedimientos necesitan ser realizados, sus opciones y las consecuencias y riesgos de la acción o de no tomar acción por su parte.

Este paquete contiene información que le ayudará a entender:
- Un método efectivo para cepillar y limpiar con hilo dental sus dientes. Le demostraremos estas destrezas a usted.
- El proceso de la enfermedad periodontal. Usted será capaz de entender completamente el tipo exacto de enfermedad que usted tiene.
- La teoría del tratamiento no quirúrgico propuesto, qué es logrado y cómo usted se beneficiará de esta terapia.
- Los procedimientos exactos que son necesarios para tratar esta enfermedad.
- Los procedimientos para el cuidado oral de sí mismo adjuntos o adicionales que puedan ser necesarios para tratar la enfermedad y mantener la salud periodontal.

Por favor note que toda la información es respecto al tratamiento no quirúrgico. Es posible que usted pueda necesitar tratamiento quirúrgico para corregir los problemas causados por la enfermedad periodontal después de completar el tratamiento no quirúrgico. Mientras mejor usted se cepille, limpie con hilo dental y use otras ayudas de limpieza como le hemos enseñado y mejor usted sanará, y menos cirugía será indicada. Así que haga el mejor trabajo que usted pueda—¡diariamente! Si usted necesita cirugía como parte de su terapia, le proveeremos información adicional. A menudo, referimos los procedimientos periodontales quirúrgicos a un especialista (periodontista). Usted también está bienvenido a tener la porción no quirúrgica de este tratamiento completada con un periodontista y no en esta oficina. Si esto es algo que le gustaría discutir, por favor déjenos saber.

Ocasionalmente, los pacientes con seguro dental preguntan si estos procedimientos son beneficios cubiertos o si son de naturaleza cosmética y no estarían cubiertos. El tratamiento recomendado para la enfermedad periodontal no es cosmético y la mayoría de los planes lo incluyen como un beneficio pagable. Una excepción puede ocurrir para los procedimientos como la irrigación subgingival o la colocación de una terapia en un lugar especifico. Si usted quiere, podemos someter un pre-estimado a su portador de seguro para determinar qué beneficios serán cubiertos y hasta que grado. Sin embargo, debido a que los procedimientos deben ser realizados en la secuencia correcta, esto puede causar un retraso en el tratamiento. Más daños pueden ocurrir a sus estructuras de soporte mientras esperamos la respuesta de su portador de seguro. Adicionalmente, ya sea éste un beneficio cubierto o no, es parte de nuestra recomendación de la terapia periodontal el tratar su enfermedad.

Por favor lea la siguiente información cuidadosamente. Ha sido escrita para explicar claramente qué usted necesita saber acerca del proceso de la enfermedad y los pasos necesarios para tratarla.

Paquete Educativo de Prostodoncia

CONSIDERACIONES EN EL REEMPLAZO DE DIENTES

Por favor lea la información incluida cuidadosamente.

En consideración de tener dientes que faltan reemplazados, encontramos provechoso el proveerle con información de trasfondo importante. Las siguientes páginas le ayudarán a entender nuestras recomendaciones de tratamiento, por qué estos procedimientos necesitan ser realizados, sus opciones y las consecuencias y riesgos de la acción o de no tomar acción por su parte.

Este paquete contiene información que le ayudará a entender:
- Por qué los dientes que faltan deberían ser reemplazados.
- La variedad de las opciones de tratamiento disponibles hoy en día.
- Los procedimientos exactos que son necesarios para tratar esta condición.
- Los muchos materiales dentales contemporáneos disponibles.

Ocasionalmente, los pacientes con seguro dental preguntan si estos procedimientos son beneficios cubiertos o si son de naturaleza cosmética y no estarían cubiertos. El tratamiento recomendado para el reemplazo de un diente que falta no es cosmético y la mayoría de los planes lo incluyen como un beneficio pagable. Una excepción, sin embargo, puede ocurrir. Si usted quiere, podemos someter un pre-estimado a su portador de seguro para determinar qué beneficios serán cubiertos y hasta que grado. Sin embargo, debido a que los procedimientos deben ser realizados en la secuencia correcta, esto puede causar un retraso en el tratamiento. Más daños pueden ocurrir a sus estructuras de soporte mientras esperamos la respuesta de su portador de seguro. Adicionalmente, ya sea éste un beneficio cubierto o no, es parte de nuestra recomendación de la terapia periodontal para tratar su enfermedad.

Por favor lea la siguiente información cuidadosamente. Si usted tiene preguntas relacionadas a este material o tiene otras preguntas relacionadas a la odontología, por favor siéntase libre de llamar a esta oficina en cualquier momento.

Ilustración en CD-ROM

Paquete Educativo de Prostodoncia

CONSIDERACIONES EN EL REEMPLAZO DE DIENTES AVANZADO

Por favor lea la información incluida cuidadosamente.

En consideración de un procedimiento restaurativo avanzado, como una corona, encontramos provechoso el proveerle con información de trasfondo importante. Las siguientes páginas le ayudarán a entender nuestras recomendaciones de tratamiento, por qué estos procedimientos necesitan ser realizados, sus opciones y las consecuencias y riesgos de la acción o de no tomar acción por su parte.

Este paquete contiene información que le ayudará a entender:
- Por qué una corona es el mejor procedimiento restaurativo para su condición.
- La variedad de las opciones de tratamiento disponibles hoy en día.
- Los procedimientos exactos que son necesarios para tratar esta condición.
- Los muchos materiales dentales contemporáneos disponibles.

Ocasionalmente, los pacientes con seguro dental preguntan si estos procedimientos son beneficios cubiertos o si son de naturaleza cosmética y no estarían cubiertos. El tratamiento recomendado para el reemplazo de un diente que falta no es cosmético y la mayoría de los planes lo incluyen como un beneficio pagable. Una excepción, sin embargo, puede ocurrir. Si usted quiere, podemos someter un pre-estimado a su portador de seguro para determinar qué beneficios serán cubiertos y hasta que grado. Sin embargo, debido a que los procedimientos deben ser realizados en la secuencia correcta, esto puede causar un retraso en el tratamiento. Más daños pueden ocurrir a sus estructuras de soporte mientras esperamos la respuesta de su portador de seguro. Adicionalmente, ya sea éste un beneficio cubierto o no, es parte de nuestra recomendación de la terapia periodontal el tratar su enfermedad.

Por favor lea la siguiente información cuidadosamente. Si usted tiene preguntas relacionadas a este material o tiene otras preguntas relacionadas a la odontología, por favor siéntase libre de llamar a esta oficina en cualquier momento.

Ilustración en CD-ROM

Paquete Educativo de Odontología Restaurativa

RESTAURANDO SUS DIENTES

Por favor lea la información incluida cuidadosamente.

En consideración de cualquier tratamiento dental restaurativo, encontramos provechoso el proveerle con información de trasfondo importante. Las siguientes páginas le ayudarán a entender nuestras recomendaciones de tratamiento, por qué estos procedimientos necesitan ser realizados, sus opciones y las consecuencias y riesgos de la acción o de no tomar acción por su parte.

Este paquete contiene información que le ayudará a entender:
- Por qué una restauración defectuosa debe ser reemplazada.
- La variedad de las opciones de tratamiento disponibles hoy en día, incluyendo asuntos de seguridad.
- Asuntos del desgaste y la longevidad de las restauraciones dentales.

Ocasionalmente, los pacientes con seguro dental preguntan si estos procedimientos son beneficios cubiertos o si son de naturaleza cosmética y no estarían cubiertos. El tratamiento recomendado para el reemplazo de un diente que falta no es cosmético y la mayoría de los planes lo incluyen como un beneficio pagable. Una excepción, sin embargo, puede ocurrir. Si usted quiere, podemos someter un pre-estimado a su portador de seguro para determinar qué beneficios serán cubiertos y hasta que grado. Sin embargo, debido a que los procedimientos deben ser realizados en la secuencia correcta, esto puede causar un retraso en el tratamiento. Más daños pueden ocurrir a sus estructuras de soporte mientras esperamos la respuesta de su portador de seguro. Adicionalmente, ya sea éste un beneficio cubierto o no, es parte de nuestra recomendación de la terapia periodontal el tratar su enfermedad.

Por favor lea la siguiente información cuidadosamente. Si usted tiene preguntas relacionadas a este material o tiene otras preguntas relacionadas a la odontología, por favor siéntase libre de llamar a esta oficina en cualquier momento.

Ilustración en CD-ROM

Cómo Montar Sus Propios Paquetes Educativos

Usted puede montar fácilmente sus propios paquetes acerca de cualquier tema que usted normalmente discute con sus pacientes Le recomendamos que comience casi todos los paquetes con el documento p. 485, *Antes de Comenzar el Tratamiento*. Usted puede entonces encontrar el documento que trata específicamente los problemas que usted está discutiendo, luego las soluciones, seguido por una descripción de los procedimientos específicos. Puede añadir información financiera, la cual está disponible para muchos temas como un documento final. Asegúrese de usar las portadas atractivas para los paquetes provistas en el CD-ROM.

Mientras más revise los documentos en este paquete de comunicación, más usos usted encontrará durante cada fase de las interacciones con el paciente.

Ilustraciones

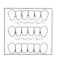
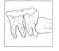

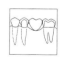

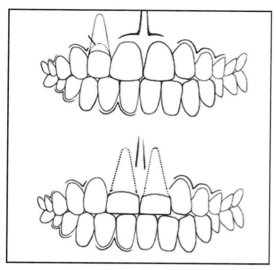

Erupción pasiva alterada

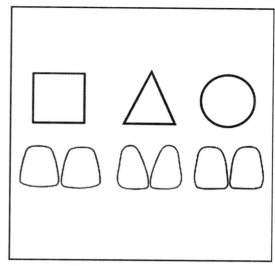

Forma de diente—anterior

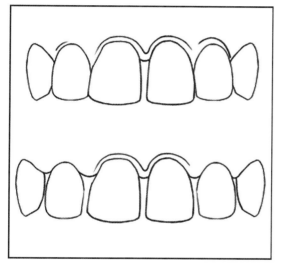

Diastemas

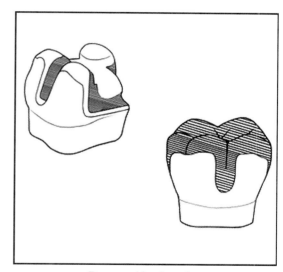

Preparación de onlay

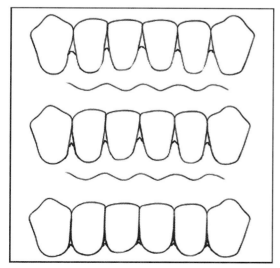

Contactos interproximales

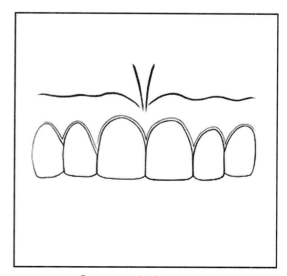

Contorno gingival normal

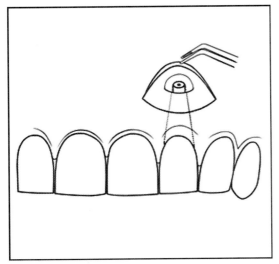

Apicectomía

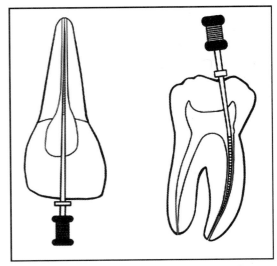

Terapia endodóntica—anterior y posterior

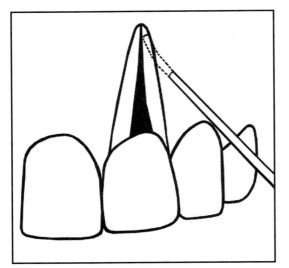

Trecho de fístulas

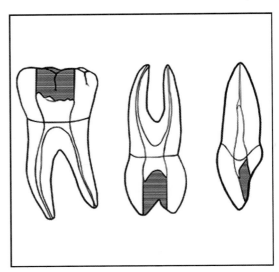

Acceso endodóntico

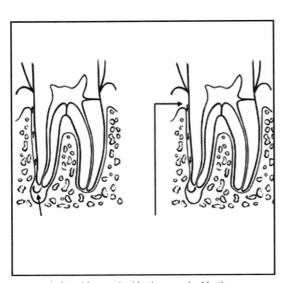

Infección endodóntica-periodóntica

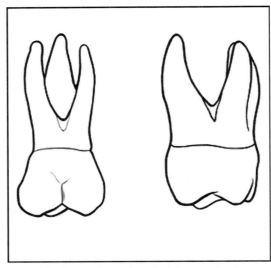

Maxilar molar—vista facial y proximal

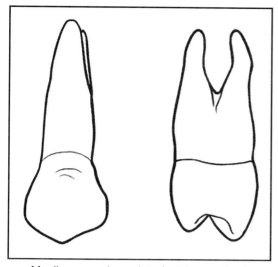

Maxilar premolar—vista facial y proximal

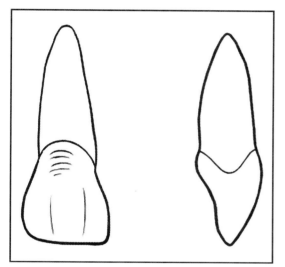

Maxilar central—vista facial y proximal

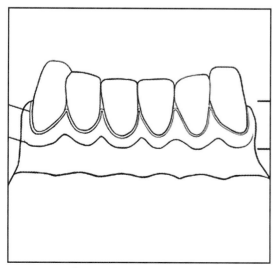

Anatomía gingival normal

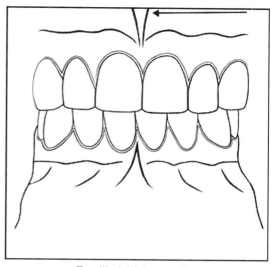

Frenillo labial—maxilar

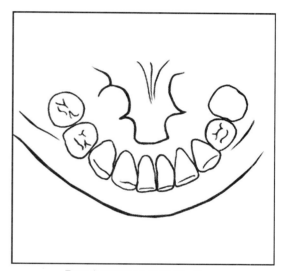

Protuberancias mandibulares

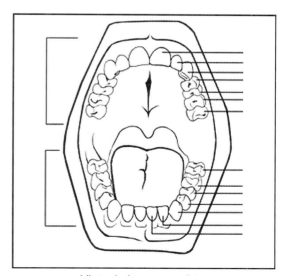

Vista de boca completa

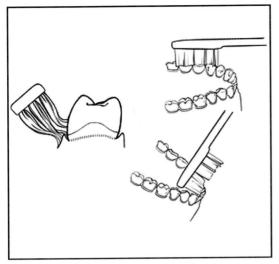

Posicionar el cepillo de dientes

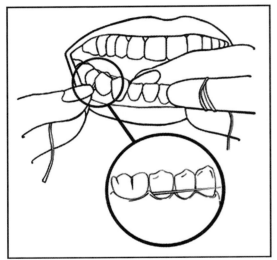

Colocación de hilo dental

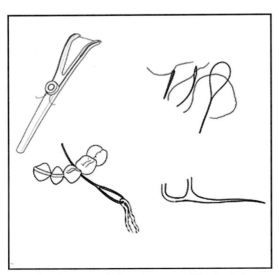

Ayudas para la limpieza con hilo dental

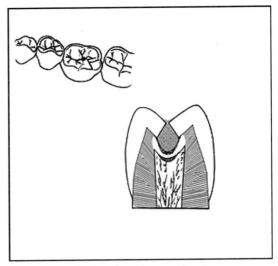

Caries dentales—oclusal

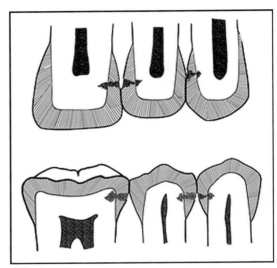

Caries dentales—proximal

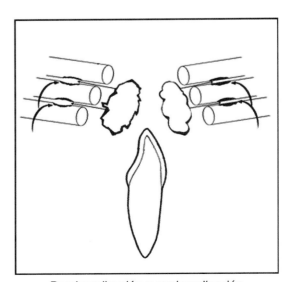

Demineralización y remineralización

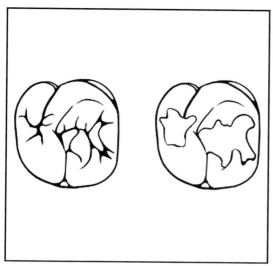

Sellador dental en un molar

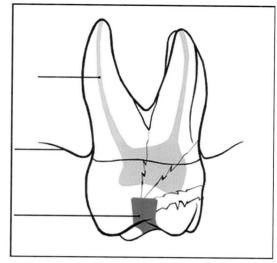

Fractura del diente

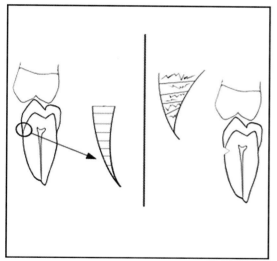

Abfracción

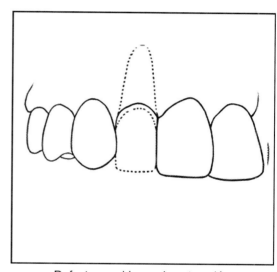

Defecto en el lugar de extracción

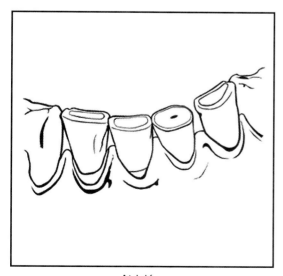

Atrición

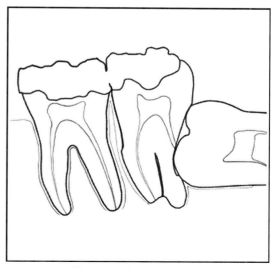

Tercer molar impactado

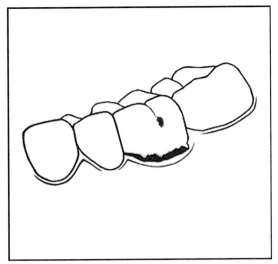

Caries dentales—margen gingival y facial

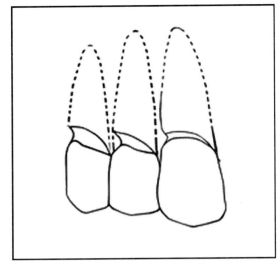

Abrasión por el cepillo de dientes

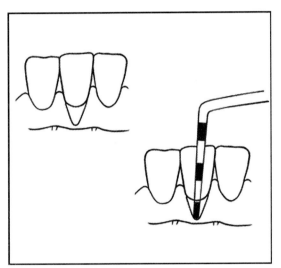

Recesión

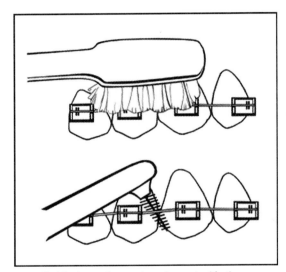

Cuidado oral para bandas ortodónticas

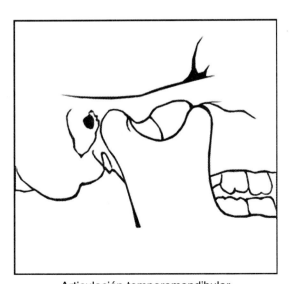

Articulación temporomandibular

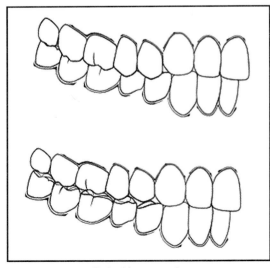

Oclusión cruzada

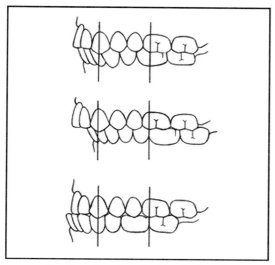

Clasificación de oclusión de ángulo

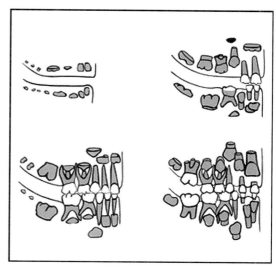

Patrón normal de erupción de dientes

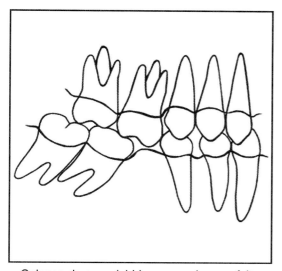

Colapso de arco debido a un molar que falta

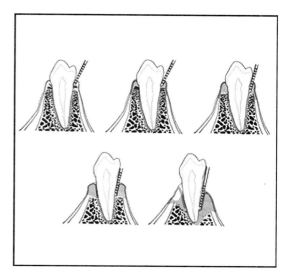

Progreso de la enfermedad periodontal

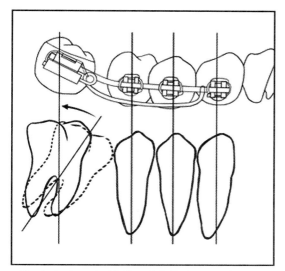

Movimiento ortodóntico del diente—enderezar
un molar inclinado

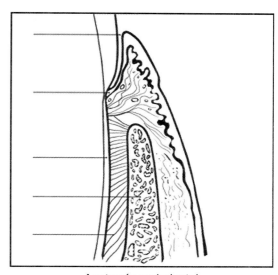

Anatomía periodontal

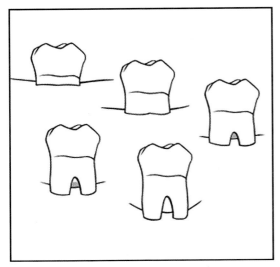

Involucración de la furcación

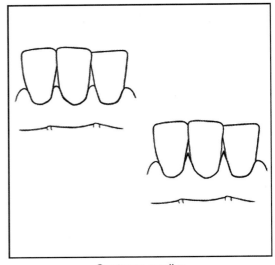

Contorno papilar

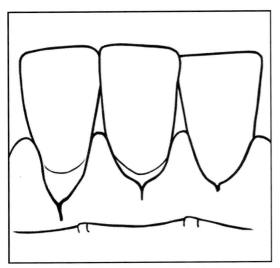

Recesión y hendidura gingival

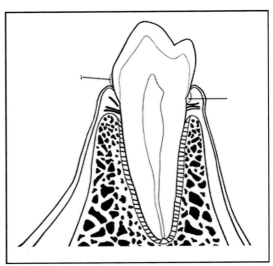

Cálculo—super y subgingival

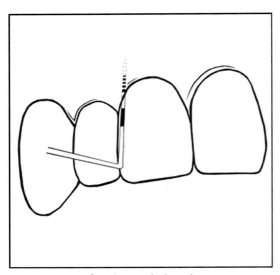

Sondeo periodontal

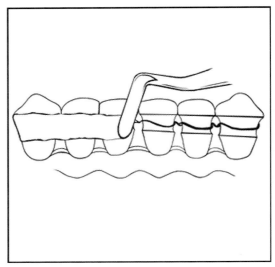

Procedimiento de colocar férulas

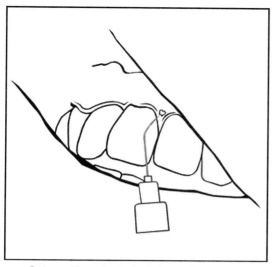

Colocación subgingival de medicamento

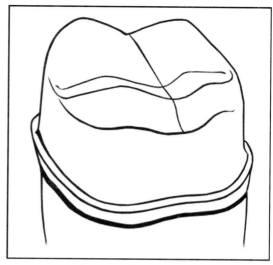

Preparación de corona

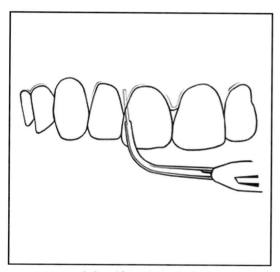

Irrigación subgingival

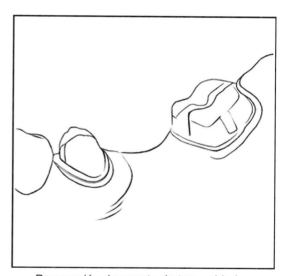

Preparación de puente de tres unidades

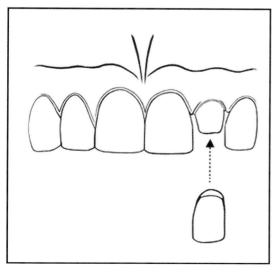

Corona sencilla

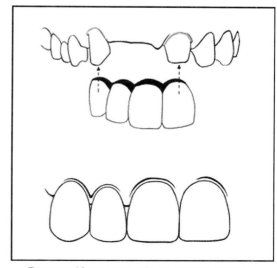

Preparación y acomodo de puente anterior

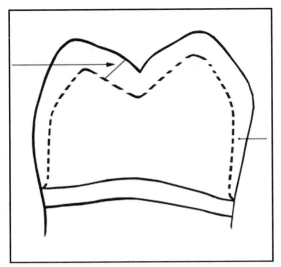

Corona completa en metal

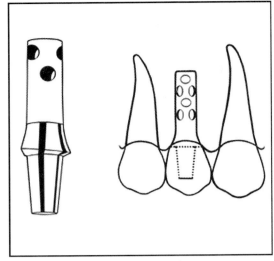

Implante dental

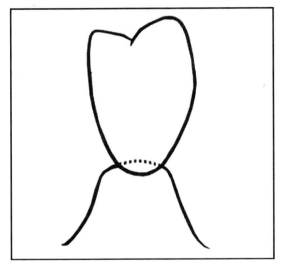

Pontic ovalado

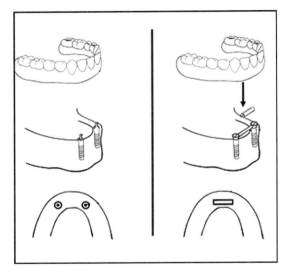

Implante dental sobredentadura

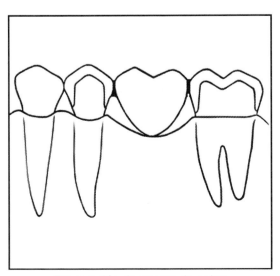

Preparación de puente de onlay

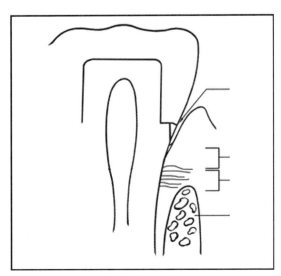

Ancho biológico

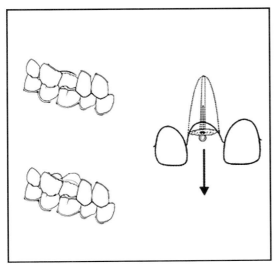

Opción de alargamiento de la corona

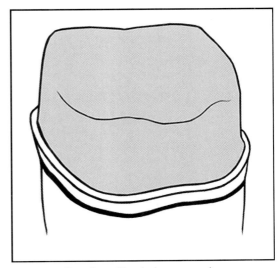

Construcción de base—molar

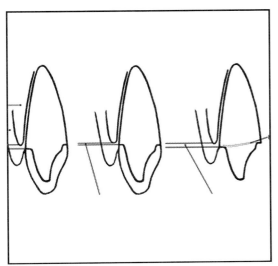

Ancho biológico y abrazadera

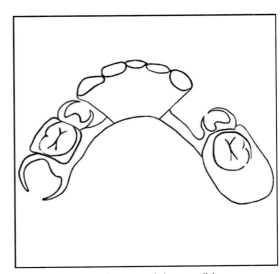

Dentadura parcial removible

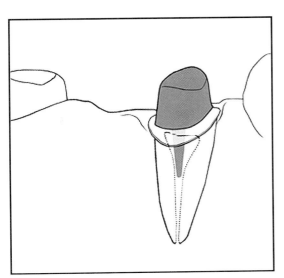

Poste y base—premolar

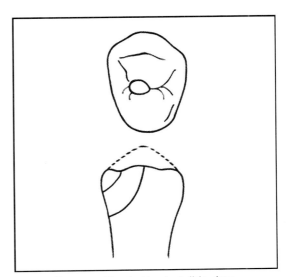

Preparación de túnel—tejido duro

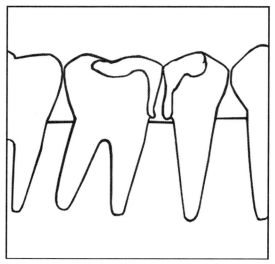

Restauración de amalgama de contorno pobre

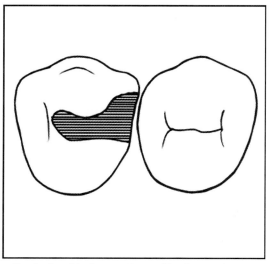

Contacto abierto—restauración de amalgama

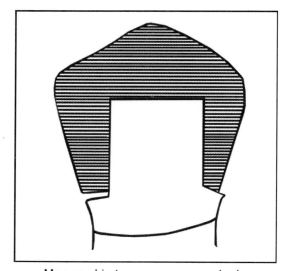

Margen abierto y margen no acabado

Arte para la Portada del Paquete Educativo

Esta sección contiene siete piezas de arte que pueden ser usadas como atractivas portadas para cualquier paquete educativo que usted quiera preparar a su gusto para un paciente. Los tópicos para los cuales usted puede proporcionar paquetes educativos incluyen lo siguiente:

Teniendo la Sonrisa Que Usted Desea
Odontología para Niños
Diagnóstico y Tratamiento de la Enfermedad de las Encías desde Temprana hasta Moderada
Diagnóstico y Tratamiento de la Enfermedad de las Encías Avanzada
Consideraciones en el Reemplazo de Dientes
Consideraciones en el Reemplazo de Dientes Avanzado
Restaurando sus Dientes
El texto que es incluido en la portada con arte puede ser cambiado a su gusto para reflejar sus preferencias personales.

Teniendo la Sonrisa Que Usted Desea

Como paciente nuevo a nuestra práctica, quisiéramos que usted supiera que usted puede contar con el mejor cuidado oral. Nuestra meta es determinar el tratamiento dental que usted necesita y quiere, ayudarle a explorar opciones financieras, y proporcionarle su cuidado dental en una manera eficiente y atenta. Repase por favor la información en este paquete antes de su primera cita. Estaremos alegres de discutir cualquier pregunta o preocupación que usted pueda tener concerniente a su salud oral antes que el tratamiento comience.

Este paquete incluye los siguientes materiales:

Bienvenido al Vecindario
Bienvenido a Nuestra Práctica
Política de Cancelación y de No Presentarse a una Cita
Emergencias Dentales
Cobertura del Seguro Dental
Seguro Dental – Puntos a Considerar
Examen Oral Inicial
Obtenga la Odontología Que Usted Necesita, Quiere y Se Merece
Para una Vida con una Magnífica Salud Oral

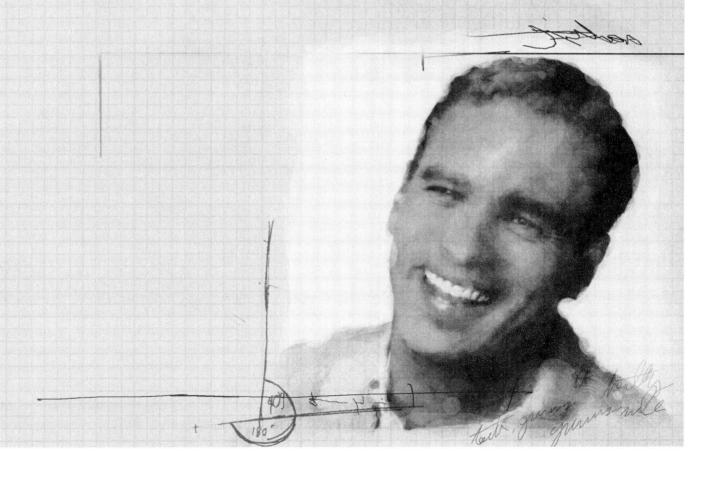

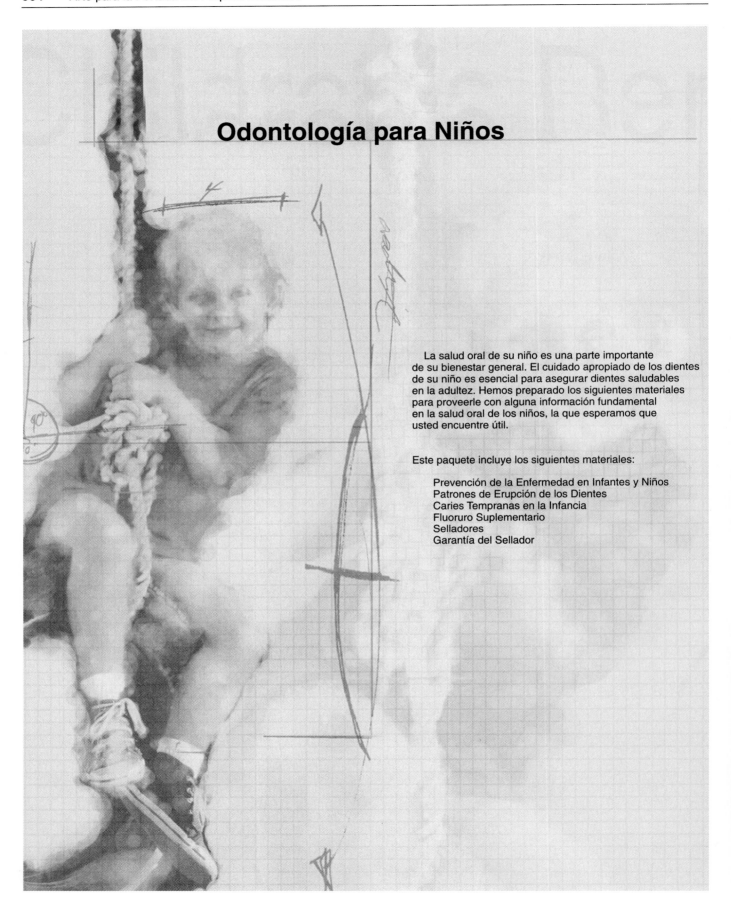

Odontología para Niños

La salud oral de su niño es una parte importante
de su bienestar general. El cuidado apropiado de los dientes
de su niño es esencial para asegurar dientes saludables
en la adultez. Hemos preparado los siguientes materiales
para proveerle con alguna información fundamental
en la salud oral de los niños, la que esperamos que
usted encuentre útil.

Este paquete incluye los siguientes materiales:

Prevención de la Enfermedad en Infantes y Niños
Patrones de Erupción de los Dientes
Caries Tempranas en la Infancia
Fluoruro Suplementario
Selladores
Garantía del Sellador

Diagnóstico y Tratamiento de la Enfermedad de las Encías desde Temprana hasta Moderada

La enfermedad periodontal es una infección que afecta los tejidos de las encías y el hueso alrededor de sus dientes. Usted ha sido diagnosticado con enfermedad periodontal activa que debe ser tratada. La información en este paquete le ayudará a entender nuestras recomendaciones de tratamiento y la parte que usted tomará en asegurar el éxito del tratamiento.

Repase por favor estas hojas de información antes de su cita. Estaremos alegres de discutir cualquier pregunta o preocupación que usted pueda tener antes que el tratamiento comience.

Este paquete incluye los siguientes materiales:

Antes de Comenzar el Tratamiento
Gingivitis
Se ñales Tempranas de la Enfermedad Periodontal
¡Cómo Cepillarse! ¡Cómo Limpiarse con Hilo Dental!
Profilaxis
Para una Vida con una Magnífica Salud Oral

Diagnóstico y Tratamiento de la Enfermedad de las Encías Avanzada

La enfermedad periodontal es una infección que afecta los tejidos de las encías y el hueso alrededor de sus dientes. Usted ha sido diagnosticado con enfermedad periodontal activa que debe ser tratada. La información en este paquete le ayudará a entender nuestras recomendaciones de tratamiento y la parte que usted tomará en asegurar el éxito del tratamiento.

Repase por favor estas hojas de información antes de su cita. Estaremos alegres de discutir cualquier pregunta o preocupación que usted pueda tener antes que el tratamiento comience.

Este paquete incluye los siguientes materiales:

Antes de Comenzar el Tratamiento
Enfermedad Periodontal
Clasificación de la Enfermedad Periodontal
Medida de la Profundidad de los Bolsillos
Manejo del Tejido Suave
Raspado y Alisado Radicular
Reevaluación del Raspado y Alisado Radicular
Irrigación Subgingival
Periostat
Enjuague Oral de Gluconato de Clorohexidina 0.12%
Terapia Antibiótica Específica al Lugar

Consideraciones en el Reemplazo de Dientes

Hay muchas opciones disponibles para restaurar los dientes a su función completa. La decisión de rellenar un diente, colocar una corona, o reemplazar un diente que falta con un puente o implante será basada en las condiciones que son únicas para su boca. Este paquete le proveerá información para ayudarle a entender nuestras recomendaciones de tratamiento y discute las diferentes opciones disponibles.

Repase por favor la información en este paquete antes de su cita. Estaremos alegres de discutir cualquier pregunta o preocupación que usted pueda tener antes que el tratamiento comience.

Este paquete incluye los siguientes materiales:

    Antes de Comenzar el Tratamiento
    Reemplazo de Dientes Que Faltan
    Coronas y Puentes: Una Visión General del Procedimiento
    Honorarios por Corona y Puente
    Opciones de Materiales: Una Visión General
    Moldes de Porcelana Fundidos a Restauraciones de Metal
    Puentes: Una Visión General
    Puentes Completos de Cerámica y Porcelana

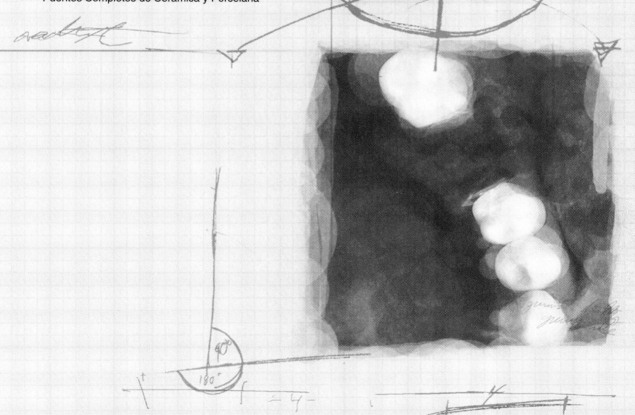

Consideraciones en el Reemplazo de Dientes Avanzado

Hay muchas opciones disponibles para restaurar los dientes a su función completa. La decisión de rellenar un diente, colocar una corona, o reemplazar un diente que falta con un puente o implante será basada en las condiciones que son únicas para su boca. Este paquete le proveerá información para ayudarle a entender nuestras recomendaciones de tratamiento y discute las diferentes opciones disponibles.

Repase por favor la información en este paquete antes de su cita. Estaremos alegres de discutir cualquier pregunta o preocupación que usted pueda tener antes que el tratamiento comience.

Este paquete incluye los siguientes materiales:

Antes de Comenzar el Tratamiento
Implantes, Coronas y Puentes versus Dientes Naturales
Coronas: Una Visión General
Honorarios por Corona y Puente
Coronas y Puentes: Una Visión General del Procedimiento
Opciones de Materiales: Una Visión General
Restauraciones con Moldes de Oro
Restauraciones con Molde de Oro y Cerámica
Moldes de Porcelana Fundidos a Restauraciones de Metal
Restauraciones Completas de Porcelana/Cerámica

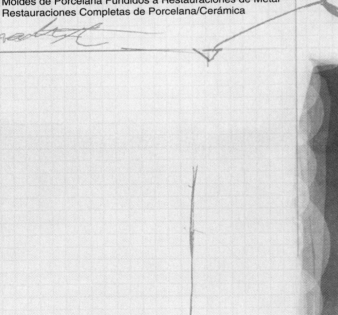
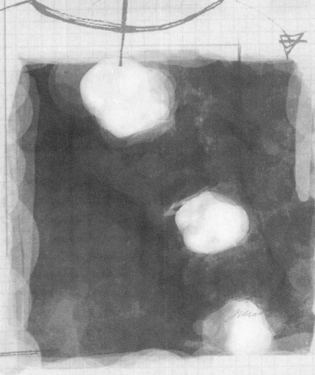

Restaurando sus Dientes

Hay muchas opciones disponibles para restaurar los dientes a su función completa. La decisión de rellenar un diente, colocar una corona, o reemplazar un diente que falta con un puente o implante será basada en las condiciones que son únicas para su boca. Este paquete le proveerá información para ayudarle a entender nuestras recomendaciones de tratamiento y discute las diferentes opciones disponibles.

Repase por favor la información en este paquete antes de su cita. Estaremos alegres de discutir cualquier pregunta o preocupación que usted pueda tener antes que el tratamiento comience.

Este paquete incluye los siguientes materiales:

Antes de Comenzar el Tratamiento
Restauraciones de Amalgama
Restauraciones de Resina Adherida
Restauraciones Defectuosas
Seguridad de la Amalgama de Plata y de los Metales Comunes
Garantía de los Materiales Restaurativos

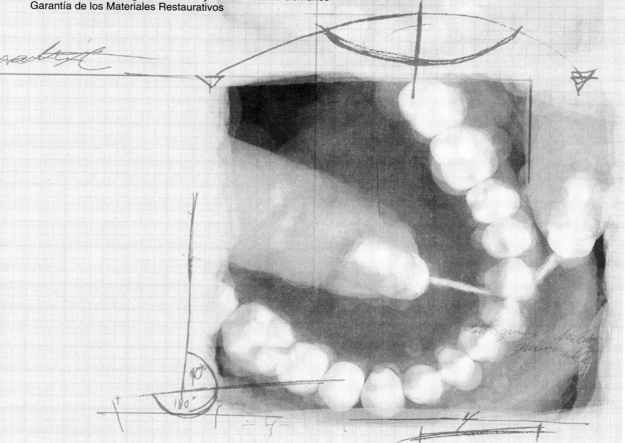

Índice